Instructional Course Lectures

Volume XXXVIII 1989

American Academy
of Orthopaedic Surgeons

Instructional Course Lectures

Volume XXXVIII 1989

Edited by
Joseph S. Barr, Jr., MD
Assistant Clinical Professor
Department of Orthopaedic Surgery
Harvard Medical School
Boston, Massachusetts

With 528 illustrations

American Academy
of Orthopaedic Surgeons

American Academy of Orthopaedic Surgeons

Instructional Course Lectures
Volume XXXVIII

Assistant Director, Publications: Marilyn L. Fox, PhD
Director of Communications and Publications: Mark W. Wieting
Senior Editor: Wendy O. Schmidt
Editorial Assistant: Alice Michaels Levine

Design: James Buddenbaum Design, Wilmette, Illinois
Typesetting: Impressions, Inc., Madison, Wisconsin
Printing: Mack Printing Company, Easton, Pennsylvania
Stock: Acid-free Warrenflo

The material presented in this volume has been made available by the American Academy of Orthopaedic Surgeons for educational purposes only. This material is not intended to represent the only, or necessarily best, methods or procedures for the medical situations discussed, but rather is intended to present an approach, view, statement, or opinion of the author(s) or producer(s), which may be helpful to others who face similar situations.

International Standard Book Number 0-89203-028-3

Library of Congress Catalog Card Number 43-17054

Contributors

Erwin A. Aguilar, PharmD, Director, Section of Medical Informatics and Graphics, Department of Orthopaedic Surgery, School of Medicine, Louisiana State University Medical Center, New Orleans, Louisiana

David W. Altchek, MD, Sports Medicine and Shoulder Service, The Hospital for Special Surgery, New York, New York

Thomas E. Anderson, MD, Section of Sports Medicine, Department of Orthopaedic Surgery, Cleveland Clinic Foundation, Cleveland, Ohio

James H. Beaty, MD, Clinical Assistant Professor of Orthopaedic Surgery, University of Tennessee, Memphis, Chief, Tennessee Crippled Children's Service, Staff, The Campbell Clinic, Inc., Memphis, Tennessee

Ralph M. Belle, MD, Research Resident, Division of Orthopaedic Surgery, University of Western Ontario, London, Ontario, Canada

Wanda K. Bernreuter, MD, Assistant Professor of Radiology, University of Alabama at Birmingham, Birmingham, Alabama

Louis U. Bigliani, MD, Assistant Professor of Orthopaedic Surgery, College of Physicians and Surgeons, Attending Orthopaedic Surgeon, New York Orthopaedic Hospital, Columbia-Presbyterian Medical Center, New York, New York

Sidney J. Blair, MD, Dr. William M. Scholl Professor and Chairman, Department of Orthopaedics and Rehabilitation, Stritch School of Medicine, Loyola University Medical Center, Maywood, Illinois

Henry H. Bohlman, MD, Professor of Orthopaedic Surgery, Case Western Reserve University School of Medicine, Chief, Acute Spinal Cord Injury Service, Cleveland Veterans Administration Medical Center, Cleveland, Ohio

Michael J. Bolesta, MD, Senior Instructor, Orthopaedic Surgery, Case Western Reserve University School of Medicine, Associate Chief, Acute Spinal Cord Injury Service, Cleveland Veterans Administration Medical Center, Cleveland, Ohio

Stephen W. Burke, MD, Associate Attending Surgeon, The Hospital for Special Surgery, Associate Professor of Clinical Surgery (Orthopaedics) and Pediatrics,

Cornell University Medical College, New York, New York

S. Terry Canale, MD, Clinical Associate Professor of Orthopaedic Surgery, University of Tennessee, Memphis, Chief of Pediatric Orthopaedics, Le Bonheur Children's Medical Center, Staff, The Campbell Clinic, Inc., Memphis, Tennessee

Robert P. Castleberry, MD, Professor of Pediatrics, Director, Division of Pediatric Hematology/Oncology, University of Alabama at Birmingham, Birmingham, Alabama

Anthony Catterall, M Chir, FRCS, Children's Orthopaedic Unit, Royal National Orthopaedic Hospital, Stanmore, London, Great Britain

Jeffrey Ciolek, PT, ATC, Section of Sports Medicine, Department of Orthopaedic Surgery, Cleveland Clinic Foundation, Cleveland, Ohio

William G. Clancy, Jr., MD, Professor of Orthopedic Surgery, Head, Section of Sports Medicine, University of Wisconsin, Madison, Wisconsin

Sherman S. Coleman, MD, Chief Surgeon, Shriners Hospital for Crippled Children, Salt Lake City, Utah

Alvin H. Crawford, MD, Director of Orthopaedic Surgery, Professor of Pediatrics and Orthopaedic Surgery, Children's Hospital Medical Center, Cincinnati, Ohio

James E. Culver, Jr., MD, Head, Section of Hand Surgery, Department of Orthopaedic Surgery, Cleveland Clinic Foundation, Cleveland, Ohio

Eugene J. Dabezies, MD, Professor, Department of Orthopaedic Surgery, School of Medicine, Louisiana State University Medical Center, New Orleans, Louisiana

Robert D. D'Ambrosia, MD, Professor and Chairman, Department of Orthopaedic Surgery, School of Medicine, Louisiana State University Medical Center, New Orleans, Louisiana

Lisa T. DeGnore, MD, Resident, Division of Orthopaedics, University of North Carolina School of Medicine, Chapel Hill, North Carolina

William K. Dunham, MD, Professor of Surgery, University of Alabama at Birmingham, Birmingham, Alabama

Gordon L. Engler, MD, Clinical Professor of Orthopaedic

Surgery, Director, Scoliosis and Spinal Deformities, New York University Medical Center, New York, New York

Harvard Ellman, MD, Associate Clinical Professor, Division of Orthopedic Surgery, University of California, Los Angeles, Center for the Health Sciences, Los Angeles, California

Bruce L. Evatt, MD, Director, Division of Host Factors, Centers for Disease Control, Department of Health and Human Services, Atlanta, Georgia

Carl D. Fackler, MD, Clinical Assistant Professor of Orthopaedics, Emory University School of Medicine, Associate, Peachtree Orthopaedic Clinic, Atlanta, Georgia

Paul D. Fadale, MD, Assistant Professor, Department of Orthopaedic Surgery, University of Pittsburgh School of Medicine, Pittsburgh, Pennsylvania

James Floyd, MD, Chief Resident, Department of Orthopaedics, University of Florida, Gainesville, Florida

Walter B. Greene, MD, Associate Professor of Orthopaedic Surgery and Pediatrics, University of North Carolina School of Medicine, Division of Orthopaedics, The University of North Carolina School of Medicine, Chapel Hill, North Carolina

Richard J. Hawkins, MD, FRCS(C), Clinical Professor of Orthopaedic Surgery, St. Joseph's Health Centre, Division of Orthopaedic Surgery, University of Western Ontario, London, Ontario, Canada

John A. Herring, MD, Chief of Staff, Texas Scottish Rite Hospital, Dallas, Texas

Frank W. Jobe, MD, Kerlan-Jobe Orthopaedic Clinic, Centinela Hospital Medical Center, Inglewood, California

Robert B. Keller, MD, Associate Professor of Orthopaedic Surgery, University of Massachusetts Medical School, Worcester, Massachusetts

Thomas A. Lange, MD, Department of Orthopedics, St. Paul-Ramsey Medical Center, St. Paul, Minnesota

Dale N. Lawrence, MD, Medical Epidemiologist, Division of Host Factors, Centers for Disease Control, Department of Health and Human Services, Atlanta, Georgia

Robert D. Leffert, MD, Associate Professor of Orthopaedic Surgery, Harvard Medical School, Chief, Surgical Upper Extremity Rehabilitation Unit and the Department of Rehabilitation Medicine, Massachusetts General Hospital, Boston, Massachusetts

Terry R. Light, MD, Professor, Department of

Orthopaedics and Rehabilitation, Loyola University School of Medicine, Attending Surgeon, Shriners Hospital for Crippled Children, Chicago Unit, Maywood, Illinois

John E. Lonstein, MD, Minnesota Spine Center, Clinical Associate Professor, Department of Orthopedics, University of Minnesota, Minneapolis, Minnesota

John T. Makley, MD, Professor of Orthopaedic Surgery, Case Western Reserve University, Director of the Musculoskeletal Tumor Center, University Hospitals, Department of Orthopaedics, Case Western Reserve University, Cleveland, Ohio

Paul R. Manske, MD, Chairman and Fred C. Reynolds Professor of Orthopedic Surgery, Washington University Medical School, St. Louis, Missouri

Frederick A. Matsen III, MD, Department of Orthopaedics, University of Washington, School of Medicine, Seattle, Washington

Leslie S. Matthews, MD, Assistant Professor of Orthopaedic Surgery, Johns Hopkins Hospital, Department of Orthopaedic Surgery, Union Memorial Hospital, Baltimore, Maryland

Campbell W. McMillan, MD, Professor of Pediatrics, University of North Carolina School of Medicine, Chapel Hill, North Carolina

Raymond T. Morrissy, MD, Medical Director and Chief of Orthopaedics, Scottish Rite Children's Hospital, Clinical Professor of Orthopaedics, Emory University, Atlanta, Georgia

Colin F. Moseley, MD, CM, University of California, Los Angeles, Shriners Hospital for Crippled Children, Los Angeles, California

Jeffrey L. Myers, MD, Assistant Professor of Pathology, University of Alabama at Birmingham, School of Medicine, Birmingham, Alabama

Thomas J. Neviaser, MD, Associate Clinical Professor of Orthopaedic Surgery, George Washington University, Fairfax, Virginia

Robert P. Nirschl, MS, MD, Orthopaedic Consultant and Medical Director, Virginia Sportsmedicine Institute, Senior Attending Orthopaedic Surgeon, Arlington Hospital, Arlington, Virginia, Assistant Clinical Professor of Orthopaedic Surgery, Georgetown University Medical School, Washington, D.C.

Clayton A. Peimer, MD, Associate Professor of Orthopaedic Surgery, Clinical Assistant Professor of Anatomical Sciences and of Rehabilitation Medicine, School of Medicine, State University of New York at Buffalo, Chief of Hand Surgery, Department of Orthopaedic Surgery, Millard Fillmore Hospital and Erie County Medical Center, Buffalo, New York

Charles T. Price, MD, Director of Pediatric Orthopaedics, Orlando Regional Medical Center, Orlando, Florida

Cecil H. Rorabeck, MD, FRCS(C), Professor of Surgery, Division of Orthopaedic Surgery, University of Western Ontario, Chief, Department of Orthopaedic Surgery, University Hospital, London, Ontario, Canada

Carter R. Rowe, MD, Associate Clinical Professor of Orthopaedic Surgery (Emeritus), Harvard Medical School, Senior Orthopaedic Surgeon, Massachusetts General Hospital, Boston, Massachusetts

Merle M. Salter, MD, Professor and Chairman of Radiation Oncology, University of Alabama at Birmingham, Birmingham, Alabama

Michael J. Skyhar, MD, Sports Medicine and Shoulder Service, The Hospital for Special Surgery, New York, New York

Robert J. Sollaccio, MD, Department of Radiation Oncology, University of Alabama at Birmingham, Birmingham, Alabama

Suzanne S. Spanier, MD, Associate Professor, Department of Orthopaedics and Pathology, University of Florida, Gainesville, Florida

Jeanette K. Stehr-Green, MD, Medical Epidemiologist, Division of Host Factors, Centers for Disease Control, Department of Health and Human Services, Atlanta, Georgia

James W. Stone, MD, Clinical and Research Fellow in Sports Medicine, Massachusetts General Hospital, Boston, Massachusetts

Alfred B. Swanson, MD, Professor of Surgery, Michigan State University, Lansing, Michigan, Director of Orthopaedic and Hand Surgery Training Program of the Grand Rapids Hospitals, Director of Hand Fellowship and Orthopaedic Research, Blodgett Memorial Medical Center, Grand Rapids, Michigan

Genevieve de Groot Swanson, MD, Assistant Clinical Professor of Surgery, Michigan State University, Lansing, Michigan, Coordinator of Orthopaedic Research Department, Blodgett Memorial Medical Center, Grand Rapids, Michigan

Timony F. Swoop, MBA, Director, Computer and Management Advisory Services, Touche Ross & Company, New Orleans, Louisiana

James S. Thompson, MD, Assistant Professor of Orthopaedic Surgery, Johns Hopkins University School of Medicine, Baltimore, Maryland

Vernon T. Tolo, MD, Professor of Orthopaedic Surgery, University of Southern California School of Medicine, Head, Division of Orthopaedics, Children's Hospital, Los Angeles, California

John J. Ward, MD, Assistant Professor of Orthopaedic Surgery, Louisiana State University School of Medicine, Shreveport, Louisiana

Russell F. Warren, MD, Director, Sports Medicine and Shoulder Service, The Hospital for Special Surgery, New York, New York

Dennis S. Weiner, MD, Chairman, Department of Pediatric Orthopaedic Surgery, Children's Hospital Medical Center of Akron, Professor of Orthopaedic Surgery, Northeastern Ohio Universities College of Medicine, Department of Pediatric Orthopaedic Surgery, Children's Hospital Medical Center of Akron, Akron, Ohio

Stuart L. Weinstein, MD, Ignacio V. Ponseti Professor of Orthopaedic Surgery, Department of Orthopaedic Surgery, The University of Iowa Hospitals and Clinics, Iowa City, Iowa

Dennis R. Wenger, MD, Department of Orthopaedic Surgery, Children's Hospital, Associate Clinical Professor, Orthopaedic Surgery, University of California, San Diego, California

Frank C. Wilson, MD, Professor and Chief, Division of Orthopaedics, University of North Carolina School of Medicine, Chapel Hill, North Carolina

Bertram Zarins, MD, Assistant Clinical Professor of Orthopaedic Surgery, Harvard Medical School, Chief, Sports Medicine Unit, Massachusetts General Hospital, Boston, Massachusetts

Preface

The Instructional Course Lectures are widely recognized as one of the most important educational offerings at the Annual Meeting of the Academy. Timely publication of selected lectures further enhances their value to Academy fellows and others. This is the third volume that has been produced entirely "in-house" by the Academy staff. Authors were asked to have their manuscripts ready by the Annual Meeting in Atlanta in February of 1988. Their cooperation with this request was crucial to the completion of Volume 38 in time for the 1989 Annual Meeting.

We have attempted to make available in this volume timely dissertations on the practice of orthopaedics. Lectures selected for publication are a mix of those offered for the first time in Atlanta as well as others that have been tested and refined over one or more Annual Meetings. We feel that the material in Volume 38, along with that in other recent volumes in the series, represents an excellent cross section of contemporary orthopaedic practice and an important resource for practitioners.

Volume 38 contains chapters on a variety of topics, with sections on the hand, the spine, and the shoulder, as well as on pediatric disorders of the lower extremity, soft-tissue sarcomas, and sports medicine.

Thanks are due to committee members Frank H. Bassett, III, MD, Walter B. Greene, MD, Paul P. Griffin, MD, and Hugh S. Tullos, MD, who helped formulate the 1988 Instructional Courses, and particularly to Kathie Niesen of the Academy staff who worked tirelessly to organize the courses and ensure their success.

As editor of Volume 38, it has been my pleasure to work with the following Academy staff members: Marilyn L. Fox, PhD, directed the development, editing, and production efforts of Volume 38. She was ably assisted in these areas by Wendy O. Schmidt, who not only supervised the editorial process, but did the layout and indexing for the volume. Alice Michaels Levine edited manuscripts, communicated with authors and did the permissions work, as well as assisting Dr. Fox in the day-to-day management of the project. Finally, Mark W. Wieting provided valuable consultation and general oversight. Their tireless efforts brought Volume 38 to fruition.

Joseph S. Barr, Jr., MD
Boston, Massachusetts
Chairman, Committee on Instructional Courses

Frank H. Bassett III, MD
Durham, North Carolina

Walter B. Greene, MD
Chapel Hill, North Carolina

Paul P. Griffin, MD
Baltimore, Maryland

Hugh S. Tullos, MD
Houston, Texas

Contents

The Hand

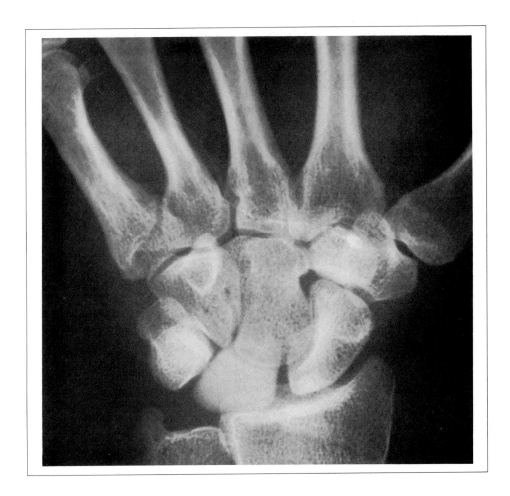

Complications and Salvage of Trapeziometacarpal Arthroplasties

James S. Thompson, MD

Introduction

Posttraumatic or degenerative painful arthrosis of the trapeziometacarpal joint (thumb basal joint) is the most common cause of dysfunction of the critical thumb ray (Fig. 1–1). Women who are more than 50 years of age account for 80% to 90% of patients treated surgically[1-3] after nonoperative modalities have failed. Solid arthrodesis remains the procedure of choice for young, vigorous patients who work as manual laborers and for those with connective-tissue disorders contributing to painful trapeziometacarpal joint hypermobility. However, the orthopaedic surgeon has many surgical options when trapeziometacarpal joint arthroplasty is considered:

Partial or complete trapeziectomy;
silicone trapezium replacement implants;
silicone or other synthetic interposition materials;
total joint arthroplasties;
trapeziectomy and ligament reconstruction, with or without autogenous interposition; and
other tissue interposition (allogenic fascia lata, tendo Achillis, patellar tendon, etc.).

Various complications leading to painful failure of trapeziometacarpal joint arthroplasty are occurring more frequently as the number and variety of trapeziometacarpal joint arthroplasties increase. This chapter presents the most common complications of trapeziometacarpal joint arthroplasty and a surgical method for salvage of this difficult clinical situation.

Complications

Scaphometacarpal Impingement

Painful scaphometacarpal impingement (Fig. 1–2) may occur after any trapeziometacarpal joint arthroplasty that involves trapeziectomy. The competence of the intermetacarpal ligament (Fig. 1–3) determines whether the first metacarpal will subside after the trapezium is removed. If the ligament is competent, the metacarpal settles proximally to the limit of ligamentous restraint. If the ligament is destroyed, either by attrition through osteophyte formation (Fig. 1–4) or by the surgical act of trapeziectomy, painful scaphometacarpal impingement occurs. The importance of the intermetacarpal ligament is gradually being recognized.[4-8] Scaphometacarpal impingement is disabling to the patient, re-

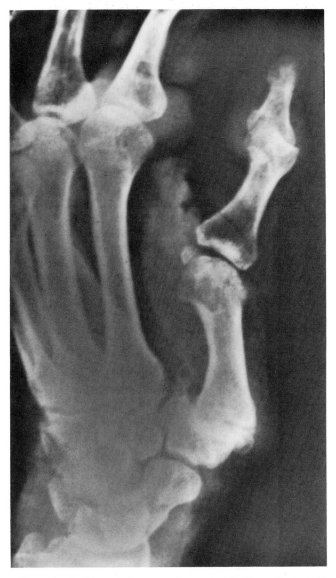

Fig. 1-1 Radiograph demonstrating typical findings of advanced trapeziometacarpal arthrosis: (1) radial subluxation of the first metacarpal base; (2) flexion adduction deformity of first metacarpal; (3) compensatory hyperextension of the metacarpophalangeal joint. (Reproduced with permission from Thompson JS: Surgical treatment of trapeziometacarpal arthrosis. *Adv Orthop Surg* 1986;10:105–120.)

sulting in a short, adducted, weak, unstable, and painful thumb.

There are cases of painful scaphometacarpal impingement following trapeziectomy without intermetacarpal ligament reconstruction or with the removal of

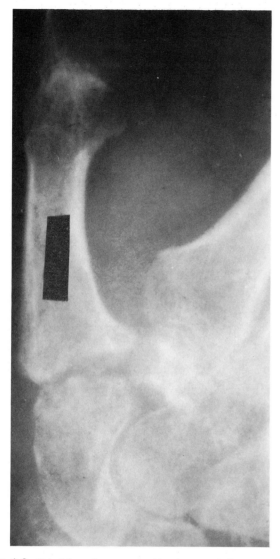

Fig. 1–2 Painful scaphometacarpal impingement after removal of silicone trapezium implant and capsular imbrication. Note marked subsidence of first metacarpal secondary to either pathologic or iatrogenic destruction of the intermetacarpal ligament. (Reproduced with permission from Thompson JS: Surgical treatment of trapeziometacarpal arthrosis. *Adv Orthop Surg* 1986;10:105–120.)

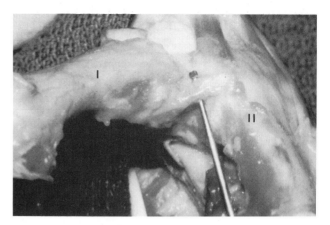

Fig. 1–3 Anatomic specimen showing the intermetacarpal ligament (beneath probe). I, first metacarpal; II, second metacarpal. (Reproduced with permission from Thompson JS: Surgical treatment of trapeziometacarpal arthrosis. *Adv Orthop Surg* 1986;10:105–120.)

silicone trapezium replacements (Fig. 1–2). This problem stimulated the development of the "suspensionplasty"[9–11] procedure described later in this chapter.

Silicone Trapezium Dislocation

All silicone rubber trapezium replacements serve as spacers between the scaphoid and first metacarpal. If the implant has a stem that extends into the medullary canal of the first metacarpal (Fig. 1–5), the metacarpal is lengthened by the implant, and this increased length (metacarpal plus implant) yields an increased lever arm on the base of the implant. Complex schemes have been

devised in an attempt to stabilize these implants.[12] If the implant is firmly fixed by soft-tissue repair, dislocation (Fig. 1–6) may not occur, but motion will take place around the stem of the implant and contribute to fracture of the implant (Fig. 1–7) and endosteal erosion by the implant stem (Fig. 1–8).

Silicone Trapezium Fracture

In addition to dislocation, silicone implant fractures occur, although actual rates of implant fracture are unknown. Figure 1–7 demonstrates a combination of implant dislocation and fracture.

Silicone Deformation and Wear

Deformation and wear of silicone trapezium replacements are common. Pellegrini and Burton[13] observed a 50% deformation rate at the four-year follow-up visit. Deformed implants also tend to fracture (Fig. 1–8).

Silicone Synovitis

Although stable implants tend to compress and deform, implants with true gliding at a bone-cartilage or bone-silicone interface are subjected to compression and shear forces. As a result of these forces, silicone particles may shed, producing a synovitis that is driven by the presence of these particles. This synovitis is being seen more frequently (Fig. 1–9) and necessitates the removal of many silicone carpal replacements.[13–16] Hofammann and associates,[17] in a review of silicone trapezium replacements in 33 hands followed for an average of 7.8 years, reported a 50% incidence of destructive changes in the host bone. Peimer and associates[15] have shown that elemental silicone is highly concentrated within the erosive cysts formed by the locally invasive synovitis. The statement: "between 30% and 90% of these implants would be expected to fail

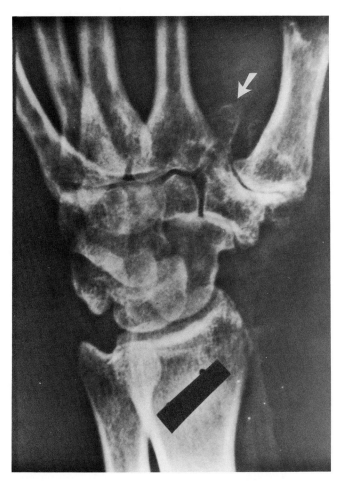

Fig. 1–4 Pantrapezial arthrosis. The large osteophyte that develops between the base of the first and second metacarpals (arrow) probably results from instability and abnormal motion of the first metacarpal base. It may result in or contribute to further attrition and attenuation of the intermetacarpal ligament. (Reproduced with permission from Thompson JS: Surgical treatment of trapeziometacarpal arthrosis. *Adv Orthop Surg* 1986;10:105–120.)

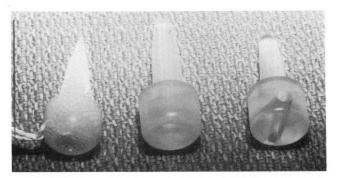

Fig. 1–5 Silicone trapezium replacement implants. **Left:** Niebauer "tie-in" prosthesis. **Center:** Swanson prosthesis. **Right:** Eaton prosthesis with round stem and hole for tenodesis. (Reproduced with permission from Thompson JS: Surgical treatment of trapeziometacarpal arthrosis. *Adv Orthop Surg* 1986;10:105–120.)

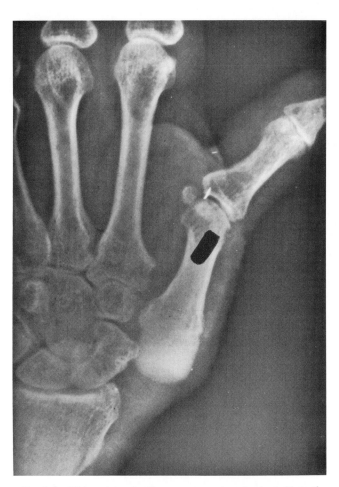

Fig. 1–6 Dislocation of a Swanson trapezium implant. Note the subsidence of the first metacarpal secondary to the incompetent intermetacarpal ligament. (Reproduced with permission from Thompson JS: Surgical treatment of trapeziometacarpal arthrosis. *Adv Orthop Surg* 1986;10:105–120.)

because of wear-induced synovitis . . ."[15] may be conservative. In my opinion, silicone is not indicated for replacement of carpal bones.

Problems With Constrained Implants

All "total joint" arthroplasties that have been attempted in the hand have had a high incidence of failure, and those used at the trapeziometacarpal joint are no exception. The Caffiniere prosthesis[18,19] has been used (Fig. 1–10), and there has been a recent report on the early results after Steffee total joint replacement of the trapeziometacarpal joint.[20] The long-term problems of loosening, implant failure, or dislocation associated with all constrained, articulated, and cemented prostheses in the hand are likely to develop in most of these patients. Fibrosis about these implants also limits

range of motion, as demonstrated by the patient in Figure 1–10.

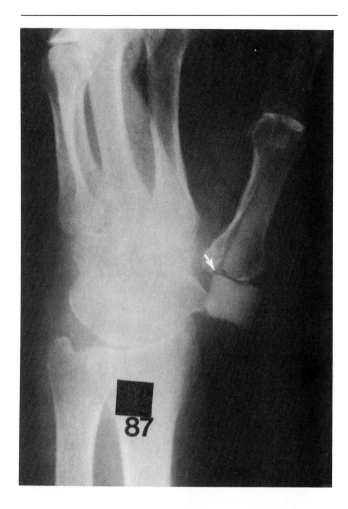

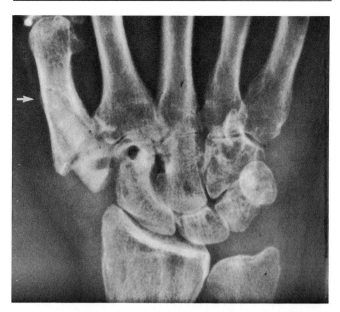

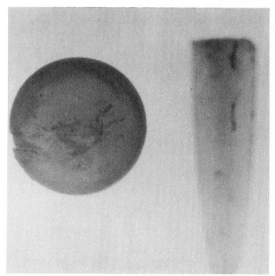

Fig. 1–7 **Top:** Radiograph of a patient who had silicone trapezium implant dislocation followed by fracture at the stem-body junction of the implant (arrow). **Bottom:** Photograph of the implant after removal.

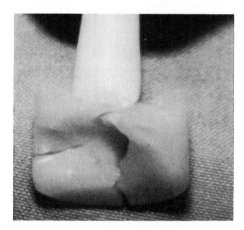

Fig. 1–8 Three-year follow-up on Eaton trapezium implant. **Top:** The implant is subluxated and deformed, and the implant stem is eroding through the cortex of the first metacarpal (arrow). (Reproduced with permission from Thompson JS: Surgical treatment of trapeziometacarpal arthrosis. *Adv Orthop Surg* 1986; 10:105–120.) **Bottom:** Eroded, fractured Eaton trapezium implant removed at the time of suspensionplasty.

Table 1–1
Failed trapezium implant arthroplasty* (1977 to 1988)

Causes	No. of Patients
Painful dislocation	8
Silicone synovitis	8
Implant fracture	6
Combinations†	4
Infection	0

*All stemmed silicone implants in situ at least three years.
†All permutations of dislocation, deformation, fracture, and synovitis.

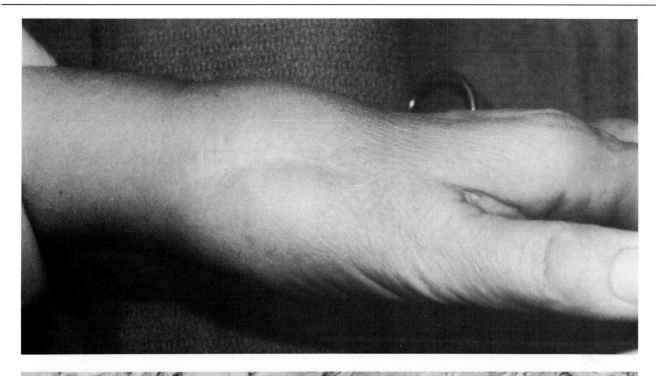

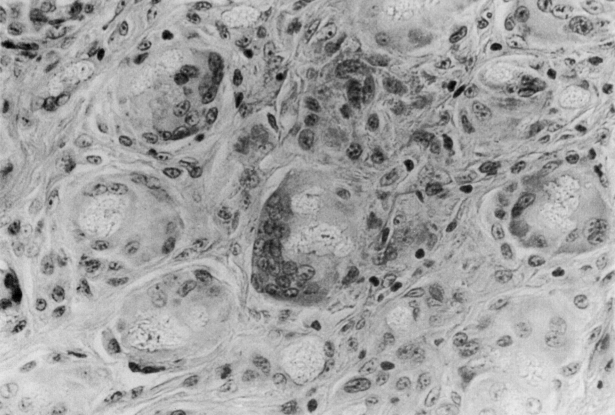

Fig. 1–9   Top: Clinical findings of silicone synovitis 12 years after trapezium implant arthroplasty. Progressive swelling and tenderness are usual; the inflammation is not acute. **Bottom:** Histologic specimen of silicone synovitis. Clumps of intracellular silicone particles are clearly visible within giant cells of a typical foreign-body reaction.

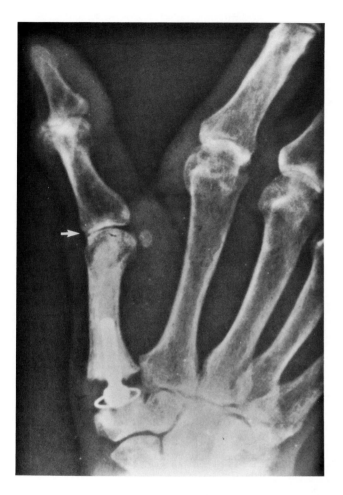

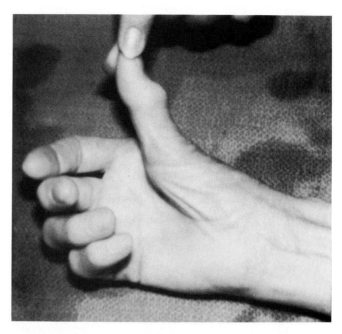

Fig. 1–10 Caffiniere total joint replacement. **Top left:** The first metacarpal is adducted and abduction is limited. Secondary hyperextension at the metacarpophalangeal joint resulted in progressive metacarpophalangeal arthrosis, especially at the dorsal joint margins (arrow). **Top right:** Limited abduction at the site of the trapeziometacarpal joint replacement has resulted in compensatory metacarpophalangeal hyperextension and arthrosis. **Bottom:** Operative photograph demonstrating complete loss of articular cartilage over the dorsal 40% of the metacarpophalangeal joint. Arthrodesis of the metacarpophalangeal joint was performed. (Reproduced with permission from Thompson JS: Surgical treatment of trapeziometacarpal arthrosis. *Adv Orthop Surg* 1986;10:105–120.)

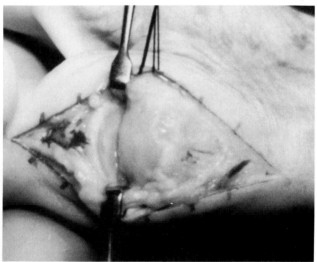

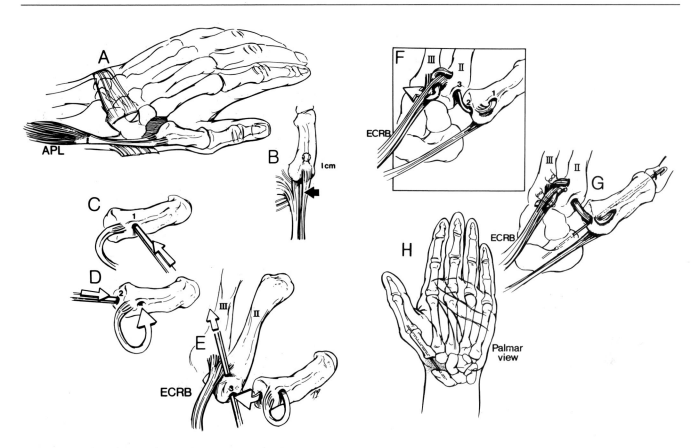

Fig. 1-11 Surgical technique of suspensionplasty. **A:** After complete trapeziectomy (lined area), the most dorsal slip of abductor pollicis longus (APL) is divided at the muscle-tendon junction. **B:** The relationship between the insertion point of the dorsal slip of the APL on the dorsoradial base of the first metacarpal and the cortical hole in the first metacarpal. **C:** The cortical hole in the first metacarpal is made 1 cm proximal to and directly in line with the APL insertion. **D:** The second hole is made directly in the center of the base of the first metacarpal. **E:** The hole in the base of the second metacarpal is made from volar-radial to dorso-ulnar. This hole establishes the "suspension point" of the suspensory ligament; it can be placed more distal at the surgeon's discretion. **F:** Demonstration of the route of the APL transfer as it is turned 180 degrees distal from its insertion, brought through the cortical hole in the first metacarpal, the basilar hole in the first metacarpal, and the "suspension point" hole in the second metacarpal to be secured with an interweave-type tendon juncture to the extensor carpi radialis brevis (ECRB). **G:** Completed transfer and K-wire placement. **H:** Palmar view of completed procedure demonstrating scaphometacarpal distraction, interposition material (dotted area), and K-wire placement. (Reproduced with permission from Thompson JS: Surgical treatment of trapeziometacarpal arthrosis. *Adv Orthop Surg* 1986;10:105–120.)

Table 1-2
Revision of trapezium implant arthroplasties

Type of Procedure	No. of Procedures
Implant replacement, soft-tissue reconstruction	3*
Implant removal, capsular imbrication	2†
Suspensionplasty	24

*Two of the three patients had unrecognized silicone synovitis when their implants were replaced in 1977 to 1978. Ultimately, they required implant removal and underwent suspensionplasty.
†One of these two patients developed painful scaphometacarpal impingement and the arthroplasty was salvaged by suspensionplasty.

Table 1-3
Grading criteria for trapeziometacarpal joint salvage

Grade	Criteria
Excellent	Near-full range of motion, no pain, functional pinch*
Satisfactory	Mild limitation of range of motion, occasional pain, functional pinch
Failure	Rest pain, nonfunctional pinch

*Pinch strengths were measured and were below the 12 to 15 lb (5 to 7 kg) that many consider normal. However, all patients in the excellent and satisfactory categories had an increase in pinch strength to measurable levels that allowed completion of normal daily functional tasks that were impossible preoperatively.

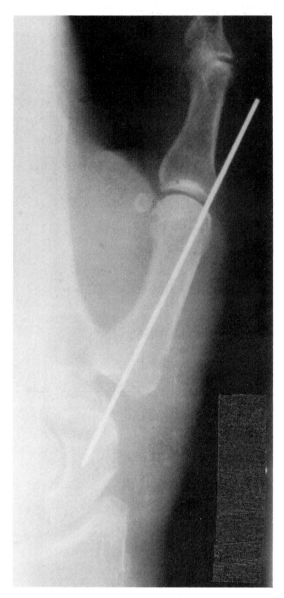

Fig. 1-12 Postoperative radiograph demonstrating K-wire placement.

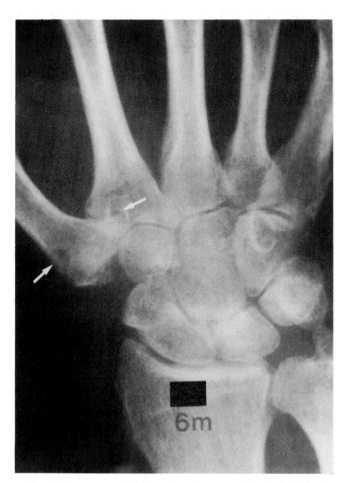

Fig. 1-13 Radiograph six months after suspensionplasty. Note the maintenance of a wide scaphometacarpal interval. Cortical holes for passage of the abductor pollicis longus in the first and second metacarpals are marked by white arrows.

Suspensionplasty

The suspensionplasty procedure is a simple method in which the base of the first metacarpal is suspended at approximately its normal level and then stabilized by reconstruction of a strong intermetacarpal ligament. Suspensionplasty evolved as a salvage procedure[21] for revisions of failed silicone trapezium replacements associated with painful dislocation, fracture, stem erosion of the metacarpal, silicone synovitis, and scaphometacarpal impingement after implant removal (Fig. 1-2).

Technique

Careful placement of incisions, prevention of damage to the dorsal sensory branch of the radial nerve and deep branch of the radial artery, and attention to other details of the surgical technique[11] are critical to success. The suspensionplasty procedure uses the most dorsal slip of the abductor pollicis longus, which is divided at or just proximal to the muscle-tendon junction (Fig. 1-11, *A*), as the donor tendon. This particular slip of the abductor pollicis longus is used because it has an anatomically constant and reliably strong bony insertion at the radial base of the first metacarpal (Fig. 1-11, *B*). This insertion is left intact. Use of this portion of the abductor pollicis longus reduces the deforming forces on the base of the first metacarpal and maintains the potential for full range of motion through the other insertions of the abductor pollicis longus.

After complete or partial removal of the trapezium (hemitrapeziectomy may be done if it is clear that the scaphotrapezial and scaphotrapezoidal joints are normal, but preservation of the proximal portion of the trapezium increases the difficulty of the procedure and has not been shown to improve results), openings are

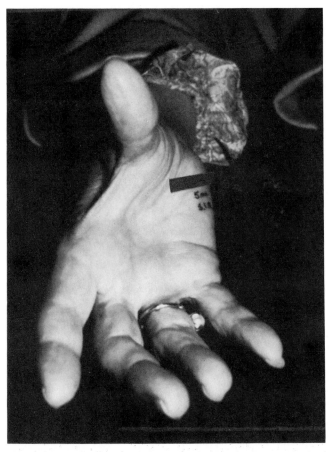

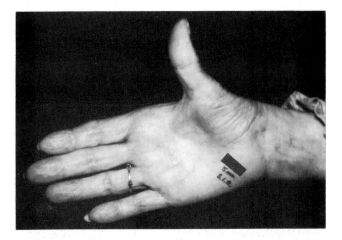

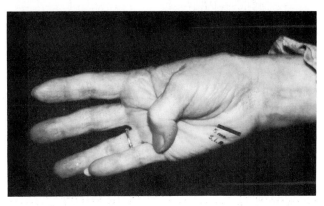

Fig. 1–14 Range of motion five months after suspensionplasty. **Top left:** Palmar abduction-opposition. **Top right:** Extension-abduction. **Bottom right:** Flexion-adduction. (Reproduced with permission from Thompson JS: Surgical treatment of trapeziometacarpal arthrosis. *Adv Orthop Surg* 1986;10:105–120.)

made (1) in the dorsoradial cortex of the first metacarpal 1 cm distal to and directly in line with the abductor pollicis longus insertion (Fig. 1–11, *C*); (2) in the center of the base of the first metacarpal (Fig. 1–11, *D*); and (3) through the base of the second metacarpal from volar-radial to dorso-ulnar (usually this hole is made through the trapezial facet at the base of the second metacarpal) (Fig. 1–11, *E*). This hole establishes the "suspension point" of the abductor pollicis longus sling, and it can be moved more distal at the surgeon's discretion.

The abductor pollicis longus is (1) dissected distally free of the joint capsule to its undisturbed insertion, and (2) turned 180 degrees and brought through the holes (described in the previous paragraph) from the first opening to the second and then the third (Fig. 1–11, *F*). At this point, tension on the abductor pollicis longus slip distracts the first metacarpal base away from the scaphoid and suspends the base of the first metacarpal from the "suspension point" on the second metacarpal (Fig. 1–11, *F*). The space between the bases of the first and second metacarpals must be debrided completely and all joint debris and osteophytes removed.

Also, all protruding osteophytes at the base of the first metacarpal should be removed to provide smooth contact between the metacarpal base and the abductor pollicis longus transfer.

A longitudinal Kirschner wire is passed through the first metacarpal medullary canal (Figs. 1–11, *G* and *H*, and 1–12), maintaining the metacarpophalangeal joint in slight flexion and penetrating the scaphoid to its mid or proximal third.

After K-wire placement, the free end of the abductor pollicis longus is sutured under tension to the extensor carpi radialis brevis tendon using an interweave-type juncture (Fig. 1–11, *G*).

Autogenous interposition material (for example, palmaris longus, fascia lata, extensor pollicis brevis) may be placed in the trapeziectomy defect, if desired. The interposition may be sutured to the tendon of the flexor carpi radialis or it may be secured to the K-wire itself. The capsule is then imbricated and closed over the defect. It is uncertain whether or not interposition is necessary, but it remains a routine part of the suspensionplasty procedure.

The bulky, postoperative splint-dressing and sutures

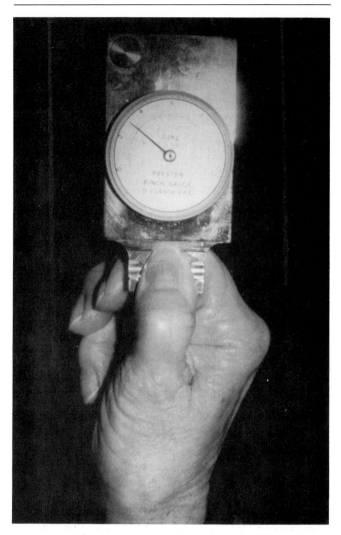

Fig. 1–15 Key-pinch power of 3 kg (7 lb) five months after suspensionplasty.

Table 1–4
Advantages of suspensionplasty utilizing the abductor pollicis longus (APL)

Advantage	Achieved by
Pain relief	Diseased joint resected
Biologic	No foreign material
Biomechanical	Maintains thumb-ray length
Stability	Intermetacarpal ligament
Mobility	Near-normal range
Strength	Comparable to implant, less than arthrodesis
Reduced deforming stress	Use of APL reduces proximally directed forces on metacarpal base*
Proper direction of ligament	IML reconstruction suspends first metacarpal†
Preserves FCR	Laceration, weakening, or adherence of important wrist flexor avoided

*The procedures using the flexor carpi radialis (FCR) potentially weaken wrist flexor power and have no effect on deforming forces of the APL.
†The intermetacarpal ligament (IML) direction of pull is 20 to 30 degrees more distal than procedures using FCR, and the suspension point is several millimeters more distal than the insertion of the FCR (the limit of the suspension point in those procedures).

are removed at ten to 14 days. A comfortable thumb spica cast is applied for three additional weeks and the K-wire is removed five to six weeks after surgery. Range-of-motion exercises are started and intermittent static splinting is used for comfort. Power grip and pinch activities are not instituted until 12 weeks after surgery.

Trapeziometacarpal Joint Arthroplasty Salvage Series

Since 1977, 26 patients with failed trapezium implant arthroplasties (Table 1–1) have had 29 surgical procedures (Table 1–2). All patients have been followed up and the results graded as excellent, satisfactory, or failure on the basis of the simple criteria listed in Table 1–3. Of the 24 suspensionplasties performed, 22 were graded as excellent and two as satisfactory. Follow-up is now six months to six years and, to date, suspensionplasty has proved to be a promising procedure. Postoperative radiographs, taken at six months (Fig. 1–13) and every two years thereafter, confirm main-

tenance of first metacarpal suspension. Range of motion in the group graded as excellent is impressive (Fig. 1–14) and pinch is markedly improved (Fig. 1–15).

Conclusion

The requirements for the ideal trapeziometacarpal reconstruction are that it be simple to perform, of autogenous material, biomechanical (to maintain thumb-ray length and motion at the metacarpal base), stable (to allow functional pinch and grip), mobile, and able to provide pain relief (long-term satisfactory results in more than 90% of patients). As follow-up lengthens, all types of implants are exhibiting clear disadvantages.[9] The category of procedure that offers the most promise of reaching the ideal in trapeziometacarpal joint arthroplasty is a combination of ligament reconstruction and autogenous tissue interposition.[9,17,22,23]

Many investigators[21,23,24] have reported excellent results following procedures that combined stabilization of the first metacarpal base and interposition of biologic tissue at the trapeziometacarpal joint. Hofammann and associates[17] also recommended interposition-type arthroplasty "in all but the most sedentary patients." Most of the procedures described use the flexor carpi radialis for the ligament reconstruction and tendon interposition.[22-24] In my practice, nonbiologic, nonautogenous methods of trapeziometacarpal joint arthroplasty have not been used since 1982.

Thus far, suspensionplasty has proved satisfactory and I prefer it for several reasons (Table 1–4). Continued observation of these patients is necessary to ascertain whether or not late rupture of the reconstructed intermetacarpal ligament occurs (a potential disadvantage of the procedure). It is hoped that patients suffering disabling pain and weakness of the thumb caused by failed trapeziometacarpal joint arthroplasty may benefit from suspensionplasty.

Acknowledgment

Robert L. Merkow, MD, performed the dissection shown in Figure 1–3 and provided the original photograph.

References

1. Amor B: Rhizarthrose du pouce: Clinique et traitement médical. *Ann Chir* 1976;30:877–881.
2. Dell PC, Brushart TM, Smith RJ: Treatment of trapeziometacarpal arthritis: Results of resection arthroplasty. *J Hand Surg* 1978;3:243–249.
3. Graber-Duvernay J, Graber-Duvernay B, Graber-Duvernay JL: Remarques sur la rhizarthrose du pouce (d'après 500 observations). *Rev Lyon Med* 1970;19:209–224.
4. Biddulph SL: The extensor sling procedure for an unstable carpometacarpal joint. *J Hand Surg* 1985;10A:641–645.
5. Epping W, Noack G: Die operative Behandlung der Sattelgelenksarthrose. *Handchirurgie* 1983;15:168–176.
6. Kuczynski K: Carpometacarpal joint of the human thumb. *J Anat* 1974;118:119–126.
7. Pagalidis T, Kuczynski K, Lamb DW: Ligamentous stability of the base of the thumb. *Hand* 1981;13:29–36.
8. Pieron AP: The mechanism of the first carpometacarpal (CMC) joint: An anatomical and mechanical analysis. *Acta Orthop Scand* 1973;1(suppl):1–104.
9. Thompson JS: Surgical treatment of trapeziometacarpal arthrosis. *Adv Orthop Surg* 1986;10:105–120.
10. Thompson JS: Suspensionplasty: A method of trapeziometacarpal arthroplasty, in Saffar P (ed): *Degenerative Arthritis of the Thumb Column*. Paris, Groupe D'Etude de la Main, in press.
11. Thompson JS: Suspensionplasty. *J Orthop Surg Tech*, in press.
12. Swanson AB: Disabling arthritis at the base of the thumb: Treatment by resection of the trapezium and flexible (silicone) implant arthroplasty. *J Bone Joint Surg* 1972;54A:456–471.
13. Pellegrini VD Jr, Burton RI: Surgical management of basal joint arthritis of the thumb: Part I. Long-term results of silicone implant arthroplasty. *J Hand Surg* 1986;11A:309–324.
14. Carter PR, Benton LJ, Dysert PA: Silicone rubber carpal implants: A study of the incidence of late osseous complications. *J Hand Surg* 1986;11A:639–644.
15. Peimer CA, Medige J, Eckert BS, et al: Reactive synovitis after silicone arthroplasty. *J Hand Surg* 1986;11A:624–638.
16. Smith RJ, Atkinson RE, Jupiter JB: Silicone synovitis of the wrist. *J Hand Surg* 1985;10A:47–60.
17. Hofammann DY, Ferlic DC, Clayton ML: Arthroplasty of the basal joint of the thumb using a silicone prosthesis: Long-term follow-up *J Bone Joint Surg* 1987;69A:993–997.
18. de la Caffiniere JY, Aucouturier P: Trapezio-metacarpal arthroplasty by total prosthesis. *Hand* 1979;11:41–46.
19. Braun RM: Total joint replacement at the base of the thumb: Preliminary report. *J Hand Surg* 1982;7:245–251.
20. Ferrari B, Steffee AD: Trapeziometacarpal total joint replacement using the Steffee prosthesis. *J Bone Joint Surg* 1986;68A:1177–1184.
21. Thompson JS: The failed trapezium implant arthroplasty, salvage with suspension interposition arthroplasty. Presented at the meeting of the Eastern Orthopaedic Association, Palm Beach, Florida, October 1983.
22. Burton RI, Pellegrini VD Jr: Surgical management of basal joint arthritis of the thumb: Part II. Ligament reconstruction with tendon interposition arthroplasty. *J Hand Surg* 1986;11A:324–332.
23. Eaton RG, Glickel SZ, Littler JW: Tendon interposition arthroplasty for degenerative arthritis of the trapeziometacarpal joint of the thumb. *J Hand Surg* 1985;10A:645–654.
24. Burton RI: The arthritic hand, in Evarts CM (ed): *Surgery of the Musculoskeletal System*. New York, Churchill Livingstone, 1983, vol 1, pp 621–692.

Arthroplasty of the Hand and Wrist: Complications and Failures

Clayton A. Peimer, MD

The interphalangeal, metacarpophalangeal, thumb carpometacarpal or basilar joints, and the wrist are often sites of symptomatic arthritic dysfunction secondary to both inflammatory systemic and oligoarticular or poly-articular osteoarthritis. Nonsurgical treatments frequently do not produce adequate long-term relief of symptoms and, therefore, arthroplasties are necessary. I have become increasingly aware of complications that arise long after joint replacement or reconstructive surgery has been performed. The nature of these complications strongly suggests that host tolerance of implants and prosthetic wear may be more of a problem than was originally believed.

Degeneration of the surfaces of bone and cartilage, loss of alignment, and incompetence of ligaments occur in the later stages of all forms of arthritis. The recommended techniques for arthroplasty aim to preserve or improve joint and ligament stability in the reconstructed site. Swanson pioneered silicone implant interposition arthroplasty in the 1960s and has been responsible for its success and widespread acceptance. Although the majority of arthroplasties in the hand and wrist employ silicone elastomer implants,[1-23] surgical options may include ligament reconstruction or joint fusion, bone excisions, and interposition of fascia or biologic materials.[16,24-42] Short-term complications and failures usually result from inadequate or incorrect surgical techniques, residual bone abutment, and unstable or dislocated prostheses. Long-term problems reflect the individual patient's disease and the way in which physical demands on the joint affect implant durability and host tolerance. Unfortunately, the ability to evaluate surgical results is frequently impaired because serious failures may not become evident until many years have elapsed, when patients are no longer being actively followed.

Frequency of Complications

In the last several years, reports have increased of destructive synovitis and osteolysis in the presence of both silicone implants and cemented metal-plastic prostheses.[43-71] Joint mobility and the forces exerted on a joint may challenge even the most sturdy prosthetic materials.[72] If the prosthesis is unstable or the ligament support inadequate, subluxation or dislocation may occur. If a prosthetic joint is constrained, the prosthesis is subjected to increased cyclic (loading) forces.

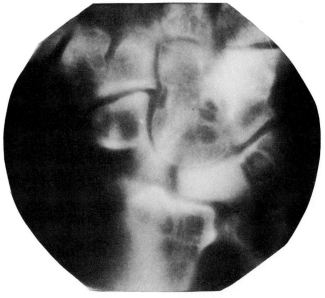

Fig. 2-1 Wrist tomography (30 months after silicone lunate arthroplasty) demonstrates osteolytic lesions of scaphoid, capitate, hamate, triquetrum, ulnar head, and radius; also note flattening of implant contours and loss of volume.

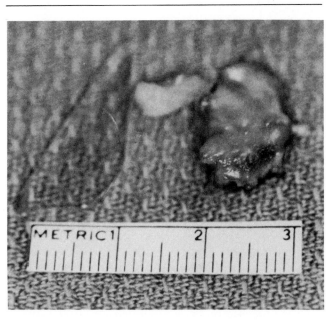

Fig. 2-2 Foreign-body reaction (fibrous encapsulation) of a storm-door glass fragment after 14 weeks.

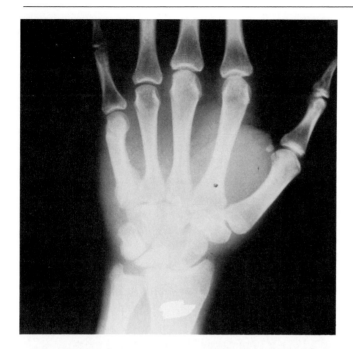

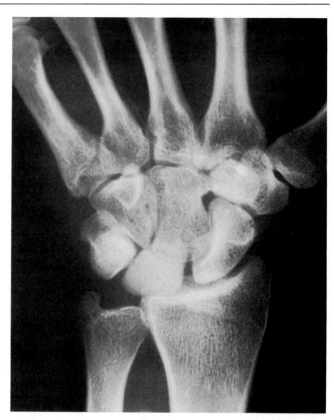

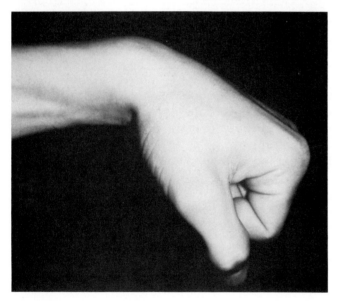

Fig. 2-3 Symptomatic Kienböck's disease in a 16-year-old adolescent who had ulnar minus variance. Radiographs were taken before (**top left**) and eight months after (**top right**) silicone lunate arthroplasty. Prosthetic stabilization stem can be seen in the triquetrum (**top right**). **Bottom:** Active palmar flexion eight months after surgery. The patient was then "lost" to further follow up.

The most frequent early complication of silicone arthroplasty is postoperative instability. Reports of the incidence of this complication at the basilar joint of the thumb range from 10% to 35%.[34,36,37,73–77] Postoperative instability occurred in 25% of Swanson and de Groot Swanson's[78] cases. Attempts to remedy the instability have included reinforcing or reconstructing surrounding ligaments and modifying implants to incorporate a ligament.[40,71,74,75,79] The potential hazard of stabilizing the prosthetic joint is that significant physiologic loads are then focused on the synthetic materials and on the interface of bone and prosthesis.

Published reports of the incidence of fractures of silicone implants at the metacarpophalangeal joint range from 2% to 30%.[22,44,45,47–49,52,53,59,80–88] However, I believe that the most serious hazard is not implant fracture with gross fragmentation. Rather, it is the insidious development of microparticulate (wear-induced) debris that incites the most destructive change (Fig. 2–1).[58,62,73,89,90] The physiologic and biomechanical factors that cause implants to fail deserve serious attention and review.

Causes of Failure

Implantable silicone polymers have been produced in a variety of forms. The solids are all similar to rubber

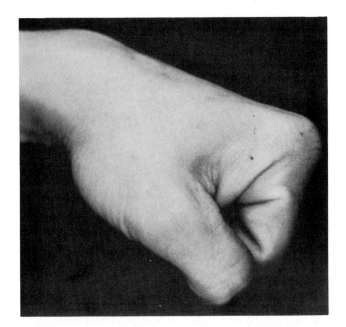

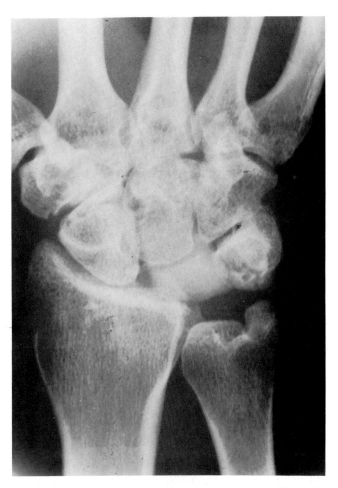

Fig. 2–5 Radiograph of a 28-year-old patient taken 31 months after silicone lunate arthroplasty shows circumscribed osteolysis in each of the carpals and the base of the fifth metacarpal.

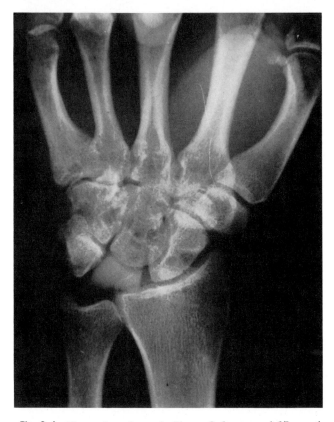

Fig. 2–4 The patient shown in Figure 2–3 returned 37 months after arthroplasty complaining of increasing wrist pain and swelling. Photograph (**top**) demonstrates loss of postoperative palmar flexion. Radiograph (**bottom**) reveals diminished implant volume and wear and discrete lytic lesions in the scaphoid, capitate, and hamate. Synovectomy and proximal row carpectomy were required.

in their physical properties and are referred to as silicone elastomers. Several high-molecular-weight polymers are available commercially. Tissue culture and subcutaneous animal implantation studies have shown that silicones are not cytotoxic.[91-98]

Implantation of silicones in various mammalian species has demonstrated repeatedly that the typical biologic interface is characterized by a surrounding fibrous capsule containing a histiocytic or mesothelial inner layer. This biologic phenomenon of fibrosis is the host response to foreign material that is generated to maintain an equilibrium of destructive and isolating cellular mechanisms and is found uniformly in vertebrate and invertebrate species.[52,53,92,99-109] Similarly, fibrous reactions to parasites, inorganic substances, and manufactured prostheses have been noted.[81,99,107-110] As a necessary final stage of the chronic inflammatory process, the host forms a fibrous capsule to isolate the foreign "irritant" that is too resistant or too large to be eliminated by cellular phagocytosis (Fig. 2–2).[77,99,107,109] Sil-

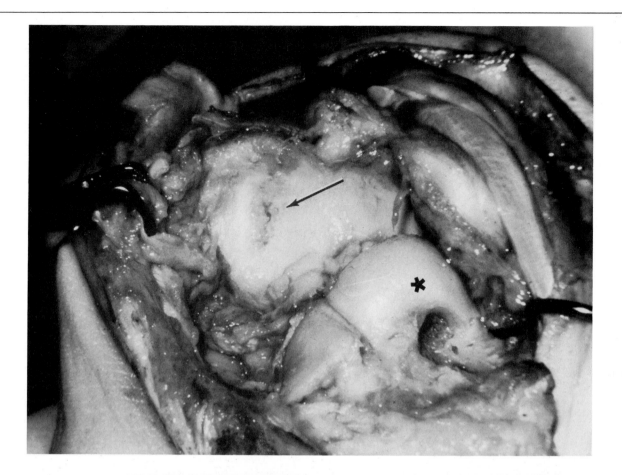

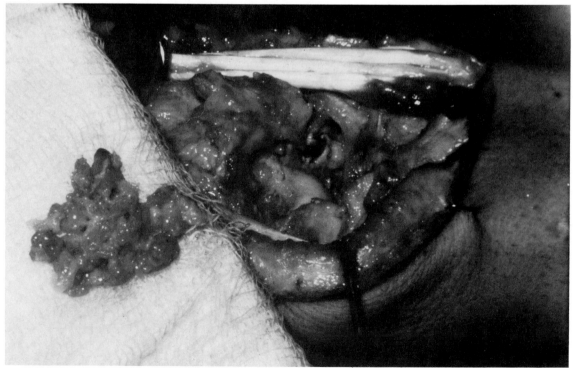

Fig. 2-6 Same patient shown in Figure 2–5. **Top:** At surgery, with wrist flexed, cartilage destruction was found in the previously normal lunate fossa of the radius (arrow). A curetted lytic lesion (synovial tumor) of the dorsum of the body of the capitate is also shown (asterisk). Salvage by proximal row carpectomy was successful, because he had surgery before advanced destruction. **Bottom:** Photograph of the portion of synovium removed from the intraosseous and cartilaginous surfaces in this wrist.

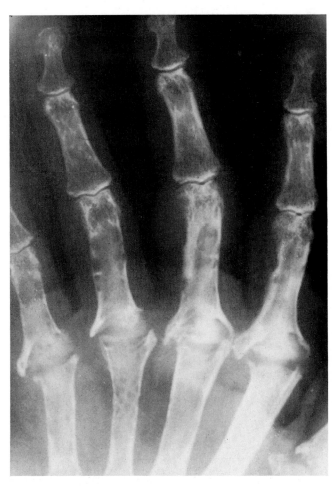

Fig. 2-7 Radiograph shows endosteal scalloping, erosion, and phalangeal cortical perforations 35 months after multiple metacarpophalangeal arthroplasties in a 49-year-old woman. Note prosthetic erosion and dissolution in addition to the prefracture bone changes.

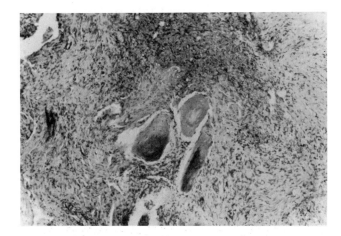

Fig. 2-8 Inflammatory synovium from microparticulate (silicone) synovitis includes widespread presence of foreign bodies and fibrosis, and partially viable and nonviable bone fragments secondary to invasion reaction (hematoxylin and eosin, × 43).

icone implants have no inherent stability; therefore, the effectiveness of these implants depends on the foreign-body reaction to produce the desired "pseudojoint" capsule. Implantation of a cytotoxic substance or potentially degradable material, however, produces a prolonged inflammatory phase.[110]

Although cytotoxicity implies that the implant material causes tissue destruction and cellular death, one cannot conclude that noncytotoxic prostheses are biocompatible or even safe. Biocompatibility signifies that the host cannot damage or degrade the implant *and* that the implant induces no host response. The only conclusion that can be drawn from all available literature is that implants currently available are neither cytotoxic *nor* biocompatible.

Tests of Implant Materials

Manufacturers of so-called "higher performance" materials often cite the physical durability of their implants in tests standardized by the American Society for Testing and Materials (ASTM). Tests have included elongation prevention (No. D412–83), tear resistance (No. D624–81), and crack growth (No. D813–59 [1976]). However, the ASTM tests are all performed on standardized slabs of material, using carefully designed machines, in air at a temperature of 25 C.[111-113] The flexion test (No. D813–59 [1976]) was designed for the stiff rubbers used in shoe soles and automobile tires. The ASTM itself cautions that specific test results do not reflect potential service value of the material in vivo and that the biocompatibility of the class of silicone materials has never been established (ASTM No. F604–78, section 1.4).[111]

My associates and I[62] have not found an applicable, standardized test for abrasion wear of silicone elastomers. I am not aware of any published scientific data to support or refute claims by commercial manufacturers of silicone elastomers about the efficacy of titanium grommets or other elastomers in resisting abrasion.

The ASTM tests of silicones do not measure the effects of shear, compression, or bearing stress, either singly or in combination.[107,110,114,115] Thumb carpometacarpal and intercarpal loading primarily reflects compression from ligament and musculotendinous forces, and secondarily reflects compression from shear as a consequence of the motions of the implant and adjoining bones. These normal physiologic forces may be of great significance if there is a potential for axially loading an implant spacer. Lack of exact congruity at the bone-implant interface can result in the generation of moments within the prosthesis; if the curvature radius of a concave implant surface is larger than that of the opposing convex bone surface onto which it is loaded, bearing stress occurs. Conversely, if the cur-

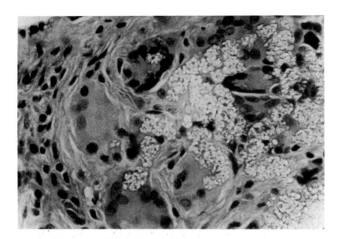

Fig. 2-9 Synovitis showing multinucleated giant cells engulfing microparticulate silicone (hematoxylin and eosin, × 150).

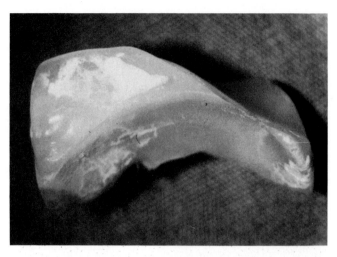

Fig. 2-11 Worn, eroded, and fragmented lunate implant removed 53 months after arthroplasty; note multiple powdery areas (white) in zones of wear.

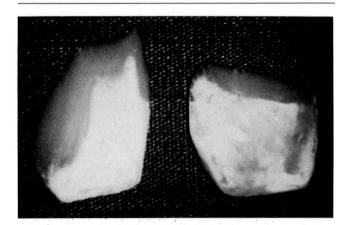

Fig. 2-10 Broken and worn scaphoid implant shows no resemblance to original prosthetic shape. The broken surfaces are incongruous, worn, and polished. Note the extensive powdery surface deposits (white).

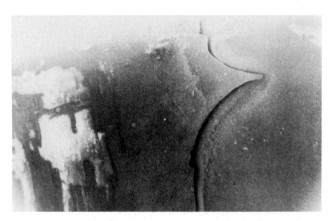

Fig. 2-12 Scanning electron micrograph of bearing surface of a carpal implant reveals large, irregular fatigue crack and multiple zones of wear deformation (× 26).

vature radius of a convex implant surface is smaller than the opposing concave bone surface, bending occurs. There is no dispute that these physiologic forces occur in combination, repetitively, and cyclically (Figs. 2–3 and 2–4). Repetitive loading causes an implant to wear or deteriorate; secondary surface irregularity may produce increased friction and abrasion, speeding the generation of free microparticles.[57,60,61,107,110,116–119] The uptake of lipids in the host environment by prostheses has negative effects on the physical properties of many implanted materials, including silicones.[54,57,107,110,114,120] Hagert[121] demonstrated frequent and significant fractures, fragmentation, and surface deformation and wear in the majority of Niebauer and Swanson finger prostheses[4,19] implanted in rabbit knees that were subjected to physiologic forces not evaluated by ASTM tests.

The choice of metal implants and the effects of secondary physiologic loading at metal-bone and bone-cement interfaces have been a concern in orthopaedics for more than half a century.[122–126] Nonetheless, manufacturers often continue to focus on bond strength of coating and resistance to traction (pull-out) at bone-cement interfaces, whereas the more important (and untested) question may be how much angular and shear support is required by fixation or ingrowth to maintain stability at an interface.[69,127–132]

Deterioration of the Implant

Formation of microparticulate debris is now recognized as a predictable and direct consequence of the

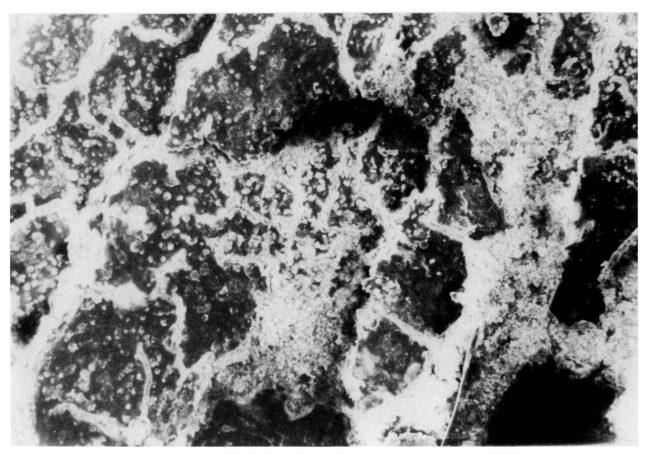

Fig. 2-13 Higher magnification of micrograph shown in Figure 2–12 demonstrates material deterioration and multiple fissures to a depth of nearly 200 μ below the implant surface (× 72).

normal use of silicone and polyethylene implant materials.[43,45,48,55,58,60,61,63,78,81,82,132–134] The underlying microparticulate pathophysiology and its relationship to secondary synovitis, joint destruction, and bone resorption have been described only recently.[55,58,60–62,90,133] Wear-induced deformation of the implant surface incites an inflammatory and cell proliferation response in the host that may affect potentially 75% or more of carpal implants.[62,73] One recent experimental study suggested that there may also be a humeral (IgG) immune response.[135] Particle size is crucial to the host response to noncytotoxic implant materials in experimental and human models.[58,62,73,90,107,109,110]

Clinical Findings

The published literature, confirmed by evidence from my own patients with silicone implants in the hand and wrist, reveals a pattern of predictable, progressive deterioration following implant surgery that, in the initial postoperative period, had shown good to excellent clinical and radiographic results.[36,39,61,62,73–75,89,136] The outcome for many patients was so good that they frequently failed to appear for re-examination at regular intervals, or physicians ceased requiring them to return, and they were "lost to follow up." An average of one to three years after surgery, increasing swelling and pain at the surgically treated joint caused the patient to return to the surgeon (Figs. 2–5 and 2–6). At examination, moderate to significant swelling was observed at the joint operated on previously. Although none of the patients complained of severe pain, all noted chronic discomfort often associated with, and proportionate to, routine activities or palpation of the inflamed zone. Few took pain medication regularly, and none could describe a specific event or injury associated with the onset of their recent problem; symptoms increased gradually in all patients.

Radiographic Findings

Radiographic examination of these patients who had silicone implants revealed focal zones of osteolysis and erosions in bone adjacent to implants, and in both con-

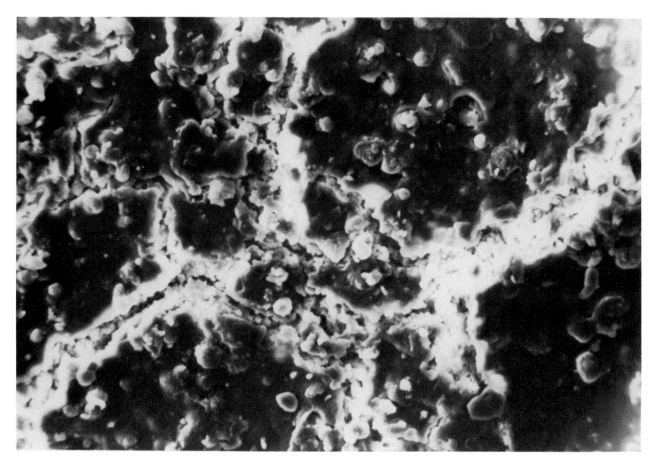

Fig. 2–14   Further increased magnification of micrograph shown in Figures 2–12 and 2–13 demonstrates fatigue zone detail with numerous surface microparticles in this same specimen (× 360).

tiguous and noncontiguous bones if carpal spacers were used. I observed a deteriorating radiographic pattern that showed additional bone destruction and an increasing number and size of areas of circumscribed osteolysis in patients who were followed over time.[62] The volume and contour of the implants of all patients had been lost progressively. In the wrist, intercarpal relationships were not maintained and carpal height diminished in implants that included carpal spacers. Many prostheses were stabilized with a Kirschner wire or nonabsorbable suture when they were implanted, as recommended in the manufacturer's protocol, and in most instances these "pin tracts" were zones of osteolysis.

Destruction seen radiographically was never confined to the areas of pin or suture placement, nor to articular structures immediately adjacent to failing implants (Figs. 2–1; 2–3, *top right*; 2–4, *bottom*; and 2–5). If an intramedullary implant was used, such as for metacarpophalangeal and wrist joints, radiographs often revealed extensive endosteal widening and scalloping rather than site-specific areas of circumscribed osteolysis. Retrospectively, I recognized that the radio-

graphic "internal rim" of cortical bone usually anticipated to be beneath a successful, symptom-free intramedullary implant[137] was either not seen or had been lost in these patients. Indeed, destruction observed on radiographs may be so advanced as to compromise the cortical integrity and strength of the bone in which the prosthesis was implanted, resulting in secondary, pathologic fractures (Fig. 2–7).[138]

Treatment

Nonsurgical

Conservative measures, such as rest, splinting, avoidance of activity, and oral or local medications may give transient relief of symptoms. All patients eventually require surgery to relieve their complaints and prevent additional destruction. Because osteolysis in the presence of swelling and pain is nonspecific and may be compatible with infection, tissue specimens should be taken routinely at surgery for culture of aerobic and anaerobic organisms, tuberculosis, atypical microbacteria, and fungi. All such studies of my cases have been negative.

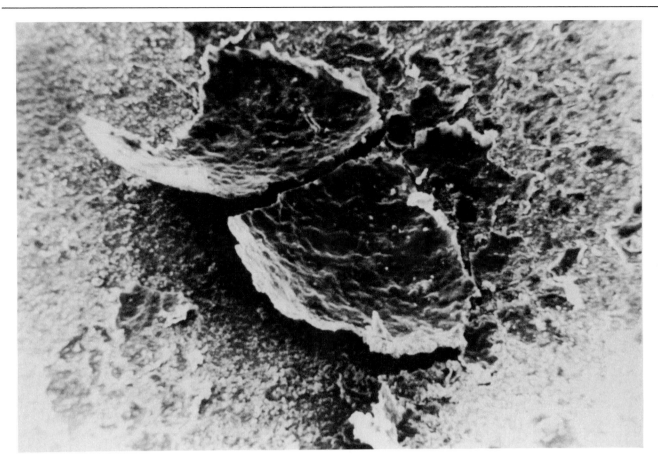

Fig. 2-15 High magnification of the same area shown in Figures 2–12 through 2–14 delineates shedding and flaking silicon microparticles in area of material destruction (× 1000).

Surgical

The surgeon should perform a fusion or an alternative arthroplasty to salvage function. The pathophysiology of the problem and my experience lead me to recommend that a degenerated silicone prosthesis not be removed and replaced with another even larger prosthesis of the same material. The surgical procedure that is consistently required is synovectomy. Osseous lesions exceeding 5 mm in diameter should be thoroughly curetted. Large areas of osteolysis associated with bone destruction and loss of articular cartilage require the addition of bone graft following synovectomy and curettage. The smaller lytic lesions can often be treated with curettage alone. Inaccessible lesions or truly small lesions, as seen radiographically, need not be curetted. In my experience, the radiographs of such lesions have remained unchanged for more than four years after synovectomy and implant removal.

Surgical Findings

Findings at surgery correspond to the duration of the patient's symptoms and the specific joints involved.

A rather dry, proliferative synovitis is always present in relative proportion to the severity of symptoms and radiographic changes. The synovium is typically a whitish yellow, and fluid is not usually present in the pseudojoints. If the prostheses originally were placed to articulate with normal hyaline cartilage, there is destruction and loss of underlying cartilage and bone (Fig. 2–6). The synovium on the surface of cartilage, capsule, and ligaments is indistinguishable from that found in discrete intraosseous lesions and within endosteal canals. A surface pannus may be the only indication that a large zone of synovial destruction lies within the bone. The preoperative radiographs and tomograms should be inspected frequently to avoid missing potentially large intraosseous lesions. These are not empty or fluid-filled cysts nor are they arthritic cysts. Rather, they are sites of microparticulate-induced synovial osteolysis and osteonecrosis. The lytic lesions are far more like synovial tumors than degenerative cysts (Figs. 2–8 and 2–9).

Appearance of Implants

Often, the most striking changes are found in the implants that have advanced and marked destruction,

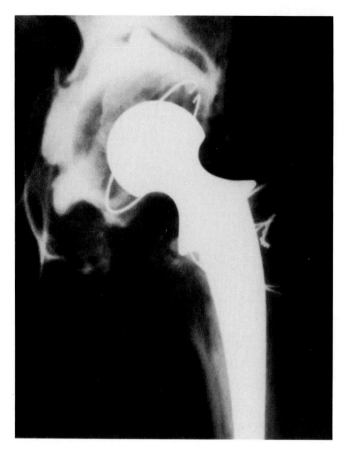

Fig. 2-16 Osteolysis is seen adjacent to acetabular component and bone cement following total hip arthroplasty.

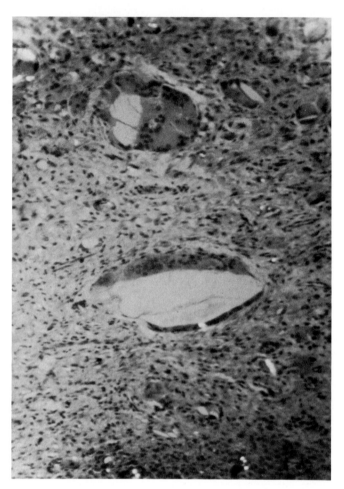

Fig. 2-17 Acetabular tissue curetted at revision arthroplasty reveals multinucleated giant cells, fibrosis, and refringent microparticles when viewed under polarized light (hematoxylin and eosin, × 43).

erosion, grooving, multiple infractions, and surface defects. Prostheses may be yellowed and, in certain zones, have worn so thin that there is only a translucent remnant of silicone remaining. Broken surfaces often have the smooth and polished appearance of a stone at the ocean's edge that has been repeatedly subjected to the pounding of waves and sand (Fig. 2–10).

Implant deterioration generally correlates with the duration and symptom level of the clinical problem and the radiographic appearance.

Once removed and dried, the implants have ubiquitous zones of powdery surface deposits in areas of wear, and these deposits flake and shed particulate matter readily to the touch. I have examined numerous implants under light microscopy and scanning electron microscopy, confirming the surface erosions and wear, material disintegration and fragmentation, and the presence of numerous free microparticles, the average size of which is 15 μ or less (Figs. 2–11 through 2–15). Implants that I have cut at the bearing surface show deterioration, often more than 100 to 200 μ below the eroded face. These worn areas confirm that there is a continuous process of implant deterioration occurring in a moving front at and below the bearing surface of the implant. The accompanying shedding and extrusion of microparticles induce the destructive inflammatory synovitis.

Histopathology

Intra-articular inflammation is a serious consequence of constant microparticulate production from implant destruction and produces significant secondary joint and bone damage. The uniform histologic lesion is proliferative synovitis (Figs. 2–8 and 2–9). The synovial and capsular tissues surrounding implants contain microfragments of particulate silicone. In some instances, these fragments appear to be aggregates of microscopic pieces of similar size, never more than 60 to 80 μ. Transmission electron microscopy of selected synovial tissue specimens discloses numerous amorphous foreign particles, ranging in size from 0.2 to 1.0 μ, distributed among collagen fibers and within cells. Osteoclastic osteolysis is mediated by the proliferating synovium, and the lytic lesions and endosteal destruction, apparent on radiographs, result from this intraos-

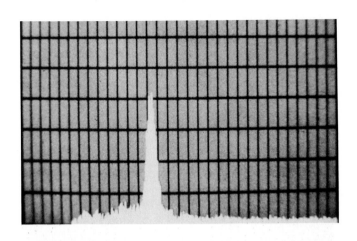

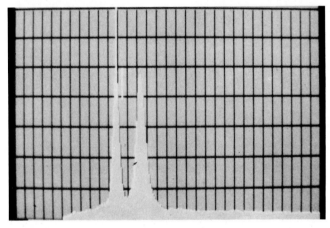

Fig. 2-18 Energy-dispersive X-ray spectrographic analysis on a control specimen of animal tendon (**top**) shows only a gold (Au) elemental spectrum peak, whereas analysis of a specimen from a patient with silicone synovitis (**bottom**) reveals a nearly 4+ silicon (Si) peak to the left of (and noted by the thin vertical marker line) the standard quantity gold (Au) peak used to coat all specimens.

seous synovial invasion. The histologic process is reminiscent of invasive pigmented villonodular synovitis and may be from a similar initial pathophysiologic mechanism of bone invasion via the vascular foramina.[61,62] This process is markedly different from the synovitis associated with benign small and large degenerative cystic lesions and intraosseous ganglia, often noted as a consequence of an arthritic process. Microparticulate synovitis is a dose-related phenomenon typified by multinucleated giant cells with many intracellular foreign bodies, fibrosis, and frequent macrophages. The synovitis is arrested by removal of the implant, aggressive synovectomy, and curettage of lesions (Figs. 2–16 and 2–17).

Electron Imaging and X-ray Spectrographic Analysis

I have used backscattered electron imaging and energy-dispersive X-ray spectrographic analysis[62] to ascertain the presence of certain elements in extracted surgical specimens. A spectrographic system is pro-

grammed so that emission peaks of selected elements can be identified in the output. All tissue samples are coated with a uniform quantity of gold, allowing the use of a gold emission peak as a quantitative reference (arbitrarily equal to 2+). This method permits estimation of the relative amounts (0 to 4+) of any other elements present. Since atomic silicon is not found in normal tissues and is absent from control specimens and the testing equipment, it can be concluded that any silicon peaks found in surgical specimens have come from silicone that was contained within the excised tissue (Fig. 2–18). My studies of tissues from cases of "silicone synovitis" have uniformly revealed positive peaks. In addition, backscattered electron imaging can locate visually specific elements in given tissue samples. Backscattered imaging is the electron microscopy equivalent of viewing foreign material on light microscopy. Imaging, however, not only locates the material but identifies it elementally.

Discussion

Retrospective studies of silicone implants for carpal bones,[61,62,78] wrist joint replacements,[90,132,136] and the thumb carpometacarpal joint[24,28,36,37,39,63] do not demonstrate that silicones offer any long-term advantages in comparison to bone resection and ligament reconstruction for the thumb carpometacarpal joint or to resection or alternate arthroplasty in the wrist. The short-term incidence of subluxation is greater for silicone implants; in the long run, the silicones show progressive deterioration functionally and radiographically. Although destructive synovitis is a well-established entity, it is rarely seen in older patients, even in those whose implants fracture, such as in (rheumatoid) metacarpophalangeal joints. The explanation is that they probably do not place as much stress on their flexible hinge implants as younger people do. Reactive changes and problems subjacent to cemented acetabular and femoral components, which have been noted clinically and radiographically, have also been identified in experimental studies[64,90,116] (Figs. 2–16 and 2–17).

These observations suggest to some that results from using silicone carpal spacer implants might be more predictable if they are "stress shielded" or "off loaded" by surrounding them with zones of intercarpal arthrodesis to prevent cyclic loading and destruction.[139] The conceptual basis for this approach is not necessarily well founded. If the implant is effectively shielded, not loaded, why put it in? If shielding is not complete, deterioration is likely to occur and progress, albeit with the potential for a later onset. Studies of limited intercarpal arthrodeses in patients with Kienböck's disease indicate that intercarpal fusion alone, with or without lunate excision,[140] produces satisfactory comfort,

Fig. 2-19 Silicone hinge implant wear and deterioration caused by titanium grommet in ten-week experimental implantation in a rabbit knee (**top**). **Bottom left and right**: Cracking and tearing at implant shoulder (on grommet edge) and abrasive erasure (beneath grommet surface).

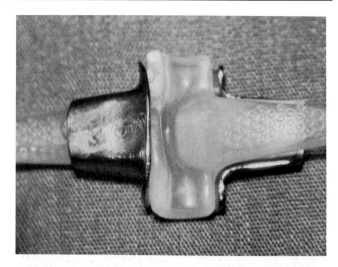

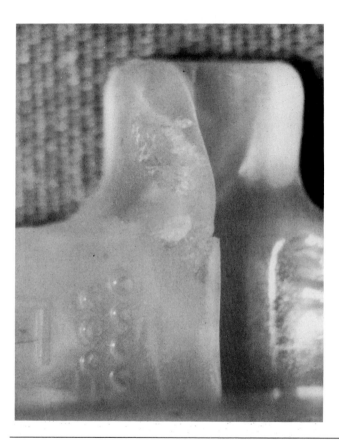

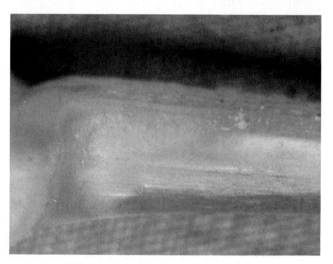

strength, and motion; motion achieved from limited intercarpal arthrodeses is equivalent to that predicted in experimentally simulated arthrodeses.[141]

Similarly, there is a theoretical problem with advocating the use of titanium grommets. Swanson and associates[137] presented data that demonstrated bone remodeling subjacent to flexible silicone implants in the hand; unfortunately, to my knowledge the details of these studies have never been published. Nonetheless, if weight transfer really occurs (and both success and failure data support this notion), then force transmission at a metal-bone interface will result, predictably, in subjacent bone resorption rather than silicone deterioration. No data have been published reporting long-term results using grommets in any series of such patients, although the problem of bone reaction beneath metal implants has been the subject of study and reports for more than 50 years.[122,123,125,142] The notion that metal collars will actually protect silicone implants from abrasive wear may be of little importance because the greatest forces are generated in bearing, shear, and compression; interestingly, the best reported clinical results with these devices are in the hinge locations, which, historically, have been unshielded. The experience in my laboratory (C.A. Peimer and Y. Minamikawa, unpublished data) reveals that implants in rabbit knees actually wear on the grommet edge as badly as on bone (Fig. 2-19).

The data and experience relating to a metal-bone prosthetic interface in the carpus and forearm lead to serious questions regarding the wisdom of recommending titanium (or other metal) thumb carpometacarpal and carpal implants without experimental or retrospective human data to support their efficacy.[143-146] As first employed more than 40 years ago,[143] metallic carpal "bones" were associated with a high incidence of dislocation, erosion, and even infraction of the spheres (H.C. Fett, Jr., December 1987; K.G. Jones, March 1988; and D.G. Murray, March 1988; personal communications). What successful experience exists with

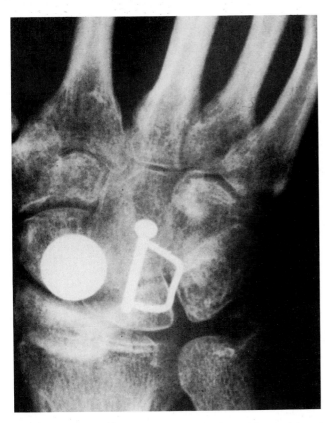

Fig. 2-20 Hollow vitallium sphere prosthesis used for partial proximal scaphoid replacement in conjunction with capitate-lunate arthrodesis.

spheres and other metal carpal implants[147] probably constitutes less than 18 published cases, many of which are anecdotal; but one investigator is convinced that if used for partial carpal bone replacements, spherical implants represent the best results he has ever achieved (K.G. Jones, personal communication, March 1988) (Fig. 2-20).

Recommendations

I recommend the following guidelines for the use of prosthetic implants:

(1) Patients with prosthetic implants must be followed indefinitely, at regular intervals of 12 to 24 months, by both clinical and radiographic examinations.

(2) Silicone implants should not be used if they will be subjected to prolonged, repetitive, and cyclic bearing, shear, and compression forces either singly or in combination. These conditions occur in the carpals, and to some degree at the thumb basilar joint. There are no published data to support the assumption that silicone carpal bone spacers are any safer or more efficacious when used in association with intercarpal fusions or metal collars.

(3) The severity of destructive changes revealed on radiographs, by clinical complaints, and by surgical pathologic findings are directly related to the length of time since prosthetic implantation, typically three years or more. Therefore, reports of any series of patients observed for a shorter period of time should be viewed with suspicion.

(4) All patients who are planning to have implants should be advised preoperatively that wear, deformation, or destruction may be consequent to normal physiologic use and that such complications may necessitate additional surgery and salvage.

(5) Even if asymptomatic, patients who show radiographic evidence of bone destruction and osteolytic lesions must be advised of the findings and informed that implant removal will arrest progression of the process and permit surgical salvage by arthroplasty or arthrodesis. Those individuals who decline treatment should be followed with semiannual to annual examinations and radiographs and advised of progressive changes. Further destruction will eventually lead to symptoms, and potentially to fewer salvage options.

References

1. Beckenbaugh RD, Dobyns JH, Linscheid RL, et al: Review and analysis of silicone-rubber metacarpophalangeal implants. *J Bone Joint Surg* 1976;58A:483–487.
2. Björnsson HA, Gestsson J, Ekelund L, et al: Silastic scaphoid implants in osteoarthritis of the radioscaphoid joint. *J Hand Surg* 1984;9B:177–180.
3. Cracchiolo A III, Swanson A, Swanson GD: The arthritic great toe metatarsophalangeal joint: A review of flexible silicone implant arthroplasty from two medical centers. *Clin Orthop* 1981;157:64–69.
4. Goldner JL, Gould JS, Urbaniak JR, et al: Metacarpophalangeal joint arthroplasty with silicone-Dacron prostheses (Niebauer type): Six and a half years' experience. *J Hand Surg* 1977;2:200–211.
5. Goldner JE, Urbaniak JR: The clinical experience with silicone-Dacron metacarpophalangeal and interphalangeal joint prostheses. *J Biomed Mater Res* 1973;7:137–163.
6. Lichtman DM, Alexander AH, Mack GR, et al: Kienböck's disease: Update on silicone replacement arthroplasty. *J Hand Surg* 1982;7:343–347.
7. Lichtman DM, Mack GR, MacDonald RI, et al: Kienböck's disease: The role of silicone replacement arthroplasty. *J Bone Joint Surg* 1977;59A:899–908.
8. Mannerfelt L, Andersson K: Silastic arthroplasty of the metacarpophalangeal joints in rheumatoid arthritis. *J Bone Joint Surg* 1975;57A:484–489.
9. Nalebuff EA: The rheumatoid hand: Reflections on metacarpophalangeal arthroplasty. *Clin Orthop* 1984;182:150–159.
10. Nalebuff EA: Metacarpophalangeal surgery in rheumatoid arthritis. *Surg Clin North Am* 1969;49:823–832.
11. Roca J, Beltran JE, Fairen MF, et al: Treatment of Kienböck's disease using a silicone rubber implant. *J Bone Joint Surg* 1976;58A:373–376.
12. Stark HH, Zemel NP, Ashworth CR: Use of a hand-carved silicone-rubber spacer for advanced Kienböck's disease. *J Bone Joint Surg* 1981;63A:1359–1370.
13. Summers B, Hubbard MJ: Wrist joint arthroplasty in rheumatoid arthritis: A comparison between the Meuli and Swanson prostheses. *J Hand Surg* 1984;9B:171–176.

14. Swanson AB: Silicone rubber implants for replacement of arthritic or destroyed joints in the hand. *Surg Clin North Am* 1968;48:1113–1127.

15. Swanson AB: Silicone rubber implants for the replacement of the carpal scaphoid and lunate bones. *Orthop Clin North Am* 1970;1:299–309.

16. Swanson AB: Flexible implant arthroplasty for arthritic finger joints: Rationale, technique, and results of treatment. *J Bone Joint Surg* 1972;54A:435–455.

17. Swanson AB: Flexible implant arthroplasty for arthritic disabilities of the radiocarpal joint: A silicone rubber intramedullary stemmed flexible hinge implant for the wrist joint. *Orthop Clin North Am* 1973;4:383–394.

18. Swanson AB: Flexible implant arthroplasty in the hand. *Clin Plast Surg* 1976;3:141–157.

19. Swanson AB: Implant arthroplasty in the hand and upper extremity and its future. *Surg Clin North Am* 1981;61:369–382.

20. Swanson AB, Swanson GG: Pathogenesis and pathomechanics of rheumatoid deformities in the hand and wrist. *Orthop Clin North Am* 1973;4:1039–1056.

21. Swanson AB, de Groot Swanson G, Maupin BK: Flexible implant arthroplasty of the radiocarpal joint: Surgical technique and long-term study. *Clin Orthop* 1984;187:94–106.

22. Swanson AB, deGroot Swanson G, Frisch EE: Flexible (silicone) implant arthroplasty in the small joints of extremities: Concepts, physical and biological considerations, experimental and clinical results, in Rubin LR (ed): *Biomaterials in Reconstructive Surgery*. St. Louis, CV Mosby, 1983, pp 595–623.

23. Zemel NP, Stark HH, Ashworth CR, et al: Treatment of selected patients with an ununited fracture of the proximal part of the scaphoid by excision of the fragment and insertion of a carved silicone-rubber spacer. *J Bone Joint Surg* 1984;66A:510–517.

24. Amadio PC, Millender LH, Smith RJ: Silicone spacer or tendon spacer for trapezium resection arthroplasty: Comparison of results. *J Hand Surg* 1982;7:237–244.

25. Ashworth CR, Blatt G, Chuinard RG, et al: Silicone-rubber interposition arthroplasty of the carpometacarpal joint of the thumb. *J Hand Surg* 1977;2:345–357.

26. Braun RM: Total joint replacement at the base of the thumb: Preliminary report. *J Hand Surg* 1982;7:245–251.

27. Carroll RE, Hill NA: Arthrodesis of the carpo-metacarpal joint of the thumb. *J Bone Joint Surg* 1973;55B:292–294.

28. Dell PC, Brushart TM, Smith RJ: Treatment of trapeziometacarpal arthritis: Results of resection arthroplasty. *J Hand Surg* 1978;3:243–249.

29. Engel J, Ganel A, Patish H, et al: Osteoarthritis of the trapeziometacarpal joint: Results of treatment with a silicone cap implant. *Acta Orthop Scand* 1982;53:219–223.

30. Ferlic DC, Busbee GA, Clayton ML: Degenerative arthritis of the carpometacarpal joint of the thumb: A clinical follow-up of eleven Niebauer prostheses. *J Hand Surg* 1977;2:212–215.

31. Froimson AI: Tendon arthroplasty of the trapeziometacarpal joint. *Clin Orthop* 1970;70:191–199.

32. Gervis WH: Excision of the trapezium for osteoarthritis of the trapezio-metacarpal joint. *J Bone Joint Surg* 1949;31B:537–539.

33. Gervis WH, Wells T: A review of excision of the trapezium for osteoarthritis of the trapezio-metacarpal joint after twenty-five years. *J Bone Joint Surg* 1973;55B:56–57.

34. Haffajee D: Endoprosthetic replacement of the trapezium for arthrosis in the carpometacarpal joint of the thumb. *J Hand Surg* 1977;2:141–148.

35. Lucht U, Vang PS, Munck J: Soft tissue interposition arthroplasty for osteoarthritis of the carpometacarpal joint of the thumb. *Acta Orthop Scand* 1980;51:767–771.

36. Pellegrini VD Jr, Burton RI: Surgical management of basal joint arthritis of the thumb: Part I. Long-term results of silicone implant arthroplasty. *J Hand Surg* 1986;11A:309–324.

37. Burton RI, Pellegrini VD Jr: Surgical management of basal joint arthritis of the thumb: Part II. Ligament reconstruction with tendon interposition arthroplasty. *J Hand Surg* 1986;11A:324–332.

38. Slocum DB: Stabilization of the articulation of the greater multangular and the first metacarpal. *J Bone Joint Surg* 1943;25:626–630.

39. Smith RJ, Amadio PC: Controversies in hand surgery: Resection arthroplasty versus silicone replacement arthroplasty for trapeziometacarpal osteoarthritis, in Strickland JW, Steichen JB (eds): *Difficult Problems in Hand Surgery*. St. Louis, CV Mosby, 1982, pp 183–188.

40. Swanson AB, deGroot Swanson G, Watermeier JJ: Trapezium implant arthroplasty: Long-term evaluation of 150 cases. *J Hand Surg* 1981;6:125–141.

41. Weilby A: Surgical treatment of osteoarthritis of the carpo-metacarpal joint of the thumb: Indications for arthrodesis, excision of the trapezium, and alloplasty. *Scand J Plast Reconstr Surg* 1971;5:136–141.

42. Wilson JN, Bossley CJ: Osteotomy in the treatment of osteoarthritis of the first carpometacarpal joint. *J Bone Joint Surg* 1983;65B:179–181.

43. Aptekar RG, Davie JM, Cattell HS: Foreign body reaction to silicone rubber: Complication of a finger joint implant. *Clin Orthop* 1974;98:231–232.

44. Barker DE, Retsky MI, Schultz S: 'Bleeding of silicone' from bag-gel breast implants, and its clinical relation to fibrous capsule reaction. *Plast Reconstr Surg* 1978;61:836–841.

45. Christie AJ, Weinberger KA, Dietrich M: Silicone lymphadenopathy and synovitis: Complications of silicone elastomer finger joint prostheses. *JAMA* 1977;237:1463–1464.

46. Donahue WC, Nosanchuk JS, Kaufer H: Effect and fate of intra-articular silicone fluid. *Clin Orthop* 1971;77:305–310.

47. Ellenbogen R, Rubin L: Injectable fluid silicone therapy: Human morbidity and mortality. *JAMA* 1975;234:308–309.

48. Ferlic DC, Clayton ML, Holloway M: Complications of silicone implant surgery in the metacarpophalangeal joint. *J Bone Joint Surg* 1975;57A:991–994.

49. Foster WC, Springfield DS, Brown KL: Pseudotumor of the arm associated with rupture of silicone-gel breast prostheses: Report of two cases. *J Bone Joint Surg* 1983;65A:548–551.

50. Gayou R, Rudolph R: Capsular contraction around silicone mammary prostheses. *Ann Plast Surg* 1979;2:62–71.

51. Hastings H III, Thornberry RL, Kleinman WB, et al: Carpal collapse deformity following lunate resection for Kienböck's disease. *Orthop Trans* 1983;7:34.

52. Hausner RJ, Schoen FJ, Pierson KK: Foreign-body reaction to silicone gel in axillary lymph nodes after an augmentation mammoplasty. *Plast Reconstr Surg* 1978;62:381–384.

53. Pearl RM, Laub DR, Kaplan EN: Complications following silicone injections for augmentation of the contours of the face. *Plast Reconstr Surg* 1978;61:888–891.

54. Rose RM, Paul IL, Weightman B, et al: The role of stress-enhanced reactivity in failure of orthopaedic implants. *J Biomed Mater Res* 1973;7:401–418.

55. Rosenthal DI, Rosenberg AE, Schiller AL, et al: Destructive arthritis due to silicone: A foreign-body reaction. *Radiology* 1983;149:69–72.

56. Smahel J: Foreign material in the capsules around breast prostheses and the cellular reaction to it. *Br J Plast Surg* 1979;32:35–42.

57. Weightman B, Simon S, Rose R, et al: Environmental fatigue testing of Silastic finger joint prostheses. *J Biomed Mater Res* 1972;6:15–24.

58. Worsing RA Jr, Engber WD, Lange TA: Reactive synovitis from particulate Silastic. *J Bone Joint Surg* 1982;64A:581–585.

59. Mayhall WS, Tiley FT, Paluska DJ: Fracture of Silastic radial-head prosthesis: Case report. *J Bone Joint Surg* 1981;63A:459–460.

60. Sollitto RJ, Shonkweiler W: Silicone shard formation: A product of implant arthroplasty. *J Foot Surg* 1984;23:362–365.

61. Smith RJ, Atkinson RE, Jupiter JB: Silicone synovitis of the wrist. *J Hand Surg* 1985;10A:47–60.
62. Peimer CA, Medige J, Eckert BS, et al: Reactive synovitis after silicone arthroplasty. *J Hand Surg* 1986;11A:624–638.
63. Peimer CA: Long-term complications of trapeziometacarpal silicone arthroplasty. *Clin Orthop* 1987;220:86–98.
64. Harris WH, Schiller AL, Scholler JM, et al: Extensive localized bone resorption in the femur following total hip replacement. *J Bone Joint Surg* 1976;58A:612–618.
65. Moreland JR, Gruen TA, Mai L, et al: Aseptic loosening in total hip replacement: Incidence and significance, in *The Hip: Proceedings of the Eighth Open Scientific Meeting of the Hip Society.* St. Louis, CV Mosby, 1980, pp 281–291.
66. Amstutz HC, Markolf KL, McNeice GM, et al: Loosening of total hip components: Cause and prevention, in Evarts CM (ed): *The Hip: Proceedings of the Fourth Open Scientific Meeting of the Hip Society.* St. Louis, CV Mosby, 1972, pp 102–116.
67. Beckenbaugh RD, Ilstrup DM: Total hip arthroplasty: A review of three hundred and thirty-three cases with long follow-up. *J Bone Joint Surg* 1978;60A:306–313.
68. Stauffer RN: Ten-year follow-up study of total hip replacement: With particular reference to roentgenographic loosening of the components. *J Bone Joint Surg* 1982;64A:983–990.
69. Buchert PK, Vaughn BK, Mallory TH, et al: Excessive metal release due to loosening and fretting of sintered particles on porous-coated hip prostheses: Report of two cases. *J Bone Joint Surg* 1986;68A:606–609.
70. Amstutz HC: Arthroplasty of the hip: The search for durable component fixation. *Clin Orthop* 1985;200:343–361.
71. Carter PR, Benton LJ, Dysert PA: Silicone rubber carpal implants: A study of the incidence of late osseous complications. *J Hand Surg* 1986;11A:639–644.
72. Cooney WP III, Chao EY: Biomechanical analysis of static forces in the thumb during hand function. *J Bone Joint Surg* 1977;59A:27–36.
73. Braunohler W, Waddell R: Thumb metacarpal-trapezium implant-scaphoid instability. *Orthop Trans* 1982;6:77.
74. Eaton RG: Replacement of the trapezium for arthritis of the basal articulations: A new technique with stabilization by tenodesis. *J Bone Joint Surg* 1979;61A:76–82.
75. Eaton RG, Littler JW: Ligament reconstruction for the painful thumb carpometacarpal joint. *J Bone Joint Surg* 1973;55A:1655–1666.
76. Kessler I: Silicone arthroplasty of the trapezio-metacarpal joint. *J Bone Joint Surg* 1973;55B:285–291.
77. Weilby A, Søndorf J: Results following removal of silicone trapezium metacarpal implants. *J Hand Surg* 1978;3:154–156.
78. Swanson AB, de Groot Swanson G: Flexible implant resection arthroplasty: A method for reconstruction of small joints in the extremities, in American Academy of Orthopaedic Surgeons *Instructional Course Lectures, XXVII.* St. Louis, CV Mosby, 1978, pp 27–60.
79. Braun RM: Stabilization of Silastic implant arthroplasty at the trapezometacarpal joint. *Clin Orthop* 1976;121:263–270.
80. Ben-Hur N, Ballantyne DL Jr, Rees TD, et al: Local and systemic effects of dimethylpolysiloxane fluid in mice. *Plast Reconstr Surg* 1967;35:423–426.
81. Bullough PG: Letter to the editor (reply). *J Bone Joint Surg* 1983;65A:281.
82. Engber WD: Letter to the editor (reply). *J Bone Joint Surg* 1983;65A:281.
83. Nalbandian RM: Letter to the editor. *JAMA* 1977;238:939.
84. Nalbandian RM: Letter to the editor. *J Bone Joint Surg* 1983;65A:280–281.
85. Nalbandian RM, Swanson AB, Maupin BK: Long-term silicone implant arthroplasty: Implications of animal and human autopsy findings. *JAMA* 1983;250:1195–1198.
86. Swanson AB: Letter to the editor. *JAMA* 1977;238:939.
87. Weeks PM, Vannier MW, Stevens WG, et al: Three-dimensional imaging of the wrist. *J Hand Surg* 1985;10A:32–39.
88. Wintsch W, Smahel J, Clodius L: Local and regional lymph node response to ruptured gel-filled mammary prostheses. *Br J Plast Surg* 1978;31:349–352.
89. Fatti JF, Palmer AK, Mosher JF: The long-term results of Swanson silicone rubber interpositional wrist arthroplasty. *J Hand Surg* 1986;11A:166–175.
90. Howie DW, Vernon-Roberts B, Oakeshott R, et al: A rat model of resorption of bone at the cement-bone interface in the presence of polyethylene wear particles. *J Bone Joint Surg* 1988;70A:257–263.
91. Imber G, Schwager RG, Guthrie RH Jr, et al: Fibrous capsule formation after subcutaneous implantation of synthetic materials in experimental animals. *Plast Reconstr Surg* 1974;54:183–186.
92. Irving IM, Castilla P, Hall EG, et al: Tissue reaction to pure and impregnated Silastic. *J Pediatr Surg* 1971;6:724–729.
93. Hernández-Jáuregui P, Esperanza-García C, González-Angulo A: Morphology of the connective tissue grown in response to implanted silicone rubber: A light and electron microscopic study. *Surgery* 1974;75:631–637.
94. Marzoni FA, Upchurch SE, Lambert CJ: An experimental study of silicone as a soft tissue substitute. *Plast Reconstr Surg* 1959;24:600–608.
95. Rees TD, Ballantyne DL Jr, Seidman I, et al: Visceral response to subcutaneous and intraperitoneal injections of silicone in mice. *Plast Reconstr Surg* 1967;39:402–410.
96. Rigdon RH, Dricks A: Reaction associated with a silicone rubber gel: An experimental study. *J Biomed Mater Res* 1975;9:645–659.
97. Robertson G, Braley S: Toxicologic studies, quality control, and efficacy of the Silastic mammary prosthesis. *Med Instrum* 1973;7:100–103.
98. Roggendorf E: The biostability of silicone rubbers, a polyamide, and a polyester. *J Biomed Mater Res* 1976;10:123–143.
99. Coleman DL, King RN, Andrade JD: The foreign body reaction: A chronic inflammatory response. *J Biomed Mater Res* 1974;8:199–211.
100. Eskeland G, Eskeland T, Hovig T, et al: The ultrastructure of normal digital flexor tendon sheath and of the tissue formed around silicone and polyethylene implants in man. *J Bone Joint Surg* 1977;59B:206–212.
101. Neuman Z, Ben-Hur N, Tritsch IE: Induction of tendon sheath formation by the implantation of silicone tubes in rabbits. *Br J Plast Surg* 1966;19:313–316.
102. Rayner CR: The origin and nature of pseudo-synovium appearing around implanted Silastic rods: An experimental study. *Hand* 1976;8:101–108.
103. Smahel J: Histology of the capsules causing constrictive fibrosis around breast implants. *Br J Plast Surg* 1977;30:324–329.
104. Smahel J, Meyer V: Structure of capsules around silicone implants in hand surgery. *Hand* 1983;15:47–52.
105. Swanson JW, Lebeau JE: The effect of implantation on the physical properties of silicone rubber. *J Biomed Mater Res* 1974;8:357–367.
106. Urbaniak JR, Bright DS, Gill LH, et al: Vascularization and the gliding mechanism of free flexor-tendon grafts inserted by the silicone-rod method. *J Bone Joint Surg* 1974;56A:473–482.
107. van Noort R, Black MM: Silicone rubbers for medical applications, in Williams DF (ed): *Biocompatibility of Clinical Implant Materials II.* Boca Raton, CRC Press, 1981, p 79.
108. Vistnes LM, Bentley JW, Fogarty DC: Experimental study of tissue response to ruptured gel-filled mammary prostheses. *Plast Reconstr Surg* 1977;59:31–34.
109. Vistnes LM, Ksander GA, Kosek J: Study of encapsulation of silicone rubber implants in animals: A foreign-body reaction. *Plast Reconstr Surg* 1978;62:580–588.
110. Willert HG, Semlitsch M: Tissue reactions to plastic and metallic wear products of joint endoprostheses, in Gschwend N, De-

brunner HU (eds): *Total Hip Prosthesis.* Baltimore, Williams & Wilkins, 1976, pp 205–239.

111. American Society for Testing and Materials: *Annual Book of ASTM Standards, V9.01–.02. Rubber Material and Synthetic-General Test Methods: Carbon Black.* Philadelphia, American Society for Testing and Materials, 1986.

112. Frisch EE: Technology of silicones in biomedical applications, in Rubin LR (ed): *Biomaterials in Reconstructive Surgery.* St. Louis, CV Mosby, 1983, p 73.

113. Frisch EE: Biomaterials in foot surgery. *Clin Podiatry* 1984;1:11–27.

114. Leyshon RL, Channon GM, Jenkins DH, et al: Flexible carbon fibre in late ligamentous reconstruction for instability of the knee. *J Bone Joint Surg* 1984;66B:196–200.

115. Watson HK, Ryu J, DiBella A: An approach to Kienböck's disease: Triscaphe arthrodesis. *J Hand Surg* 1985;10A:179–187.

116. Jasty MJ, Floyd WE III, Schiller AL, et al: Localized osteolysis in stable, non-septic total hip replacement. *J Bone Joint Surg* 1986;68A:912–919.

117. Kahn AJ, Stewart CC, Teitelbaum SL: Contact-mediated bone resorption by human monocytes in vitro. *Science* 1978;199:988–990.

118. Vernon-Roberts B, Freeman MAR: The tissue response to total joint replacement prostheses, in Swanson SAV, Freeman MAR (eds): *The Scientific Basis of Joint Replacement.* Tunbridge Wells, Pitman Medical, 1977, pp 86–129.

119. Willert HG, Ludwig J, Semlitsch M: Reaction of bone to methacrylate after hip arthroplasty: A long-term gross, light microscopic, and scanning electron microscopic study. *J Bone Joint Surg* 1974;56A:1368–1382.

120. Pazzaglia U, Byers PD: Fractured femoral shaft through an osteolytic lesion resulting from the reaction to a prosthesis: A case report. *J Bone Joint Surg* 1984;66B:337–339.

121. Hagert CG: Implants designed for finger joints: A roentgenographic study and a study of implant wear and tear. *Scand J Plast Reconstr Surg* 1975;9:53–63.

122. Venable CS, Stuck WG: Electrolysis controlling factor in the use of metals in treating fractures. *JAMA* 1938;111:1349–1352.

123. Venable CS, Stuck WG: Results of recent studies and experiments concerning metals used in the internal fixation of fractures. *J Bone Joint Surg* 1948;30A:247–250.

124. Fink CG, Smatko JS: Bone fixation and the corrosion resistance of stainless steels to the fluids of the human body. *Trans Electrochem Soc* 1948;94:271.

125. Bowden FP, Williamson JBP, Laing PG: The significance of metallic transfer in orthopaedic surgery. *J Bone Joint Surg* 1955;37B:676–690.

126. Cave EF, Mayfield FH, McLaughlin HL, et al: Report of the joint committee for the study of surgical materials. *J Bone Joint Surg* 1954;36A:411–424.

127. Halawa M, Lee AJ, Ling RS, et al: The shear strength of trabecular bone from the femur, and some factors affecting the shear strength of the cement-bone interface. *Arch Orthop Trauma Surg* 1978;92:19–30.

128. Huiskes R: Properties of the stem-cement interface and artificial hip joint failure, in Lewis JL, Galante JO (eds): *The Bone-Implant Interface: Workshop Report.* Park Ridge, American Academy of Orthopaedic Surgeons, 1985, pp 86–101.

129. Engh CA, Bobyn JD: The influence of stem size and extent of porous coating on femoral bone resorption after primary cementless hip replacement. *Clin Orthop,* in press.

130. Geesink RGT, deGroot K, Klein CPAT: Chemical implant fixation using hydroxyl-apatite coatings, in *Proceedings of the 15th Open Scientific Meeting of the Hip Society.* St. Louis, CV Mosby, 1987.

131. Georgette FS, Davidson JA: The effect of HIPing on the fatigue and tensile strength of a case, porous-coated Co-Cr-Mo alloy. *J Biomed Mater Res* 1986;20:1229–1248.

132. Comstock CP, Louis DS, Eckenrode JF: Silicone wrist implant: Long-term follow-up study. *J Hand Surg* 1988;13A:201–205.

133. Gordon M, Bullough PG: Synovial and osseous inflammation in failed silicone-rubber prostheses. *J Bone Joint Surg* 1982;64A:574–580.

134. leNobel J, Patterson FP: Guepar total knee prosthesis: Experience at the Vancouver General Hospital. *J Bone Joint Surg* 1981;63B:257–260.

135. Smith DJ, Sazy JA, Crissman JD, et al: Immunogenic potential of carpal implants. Presented at the meeting of the American Society for Surgery of the Hand, San Antonio, Tex, Sept 10, 1987.

136. Brase DW, Millender LH: Failure of silicone rubber wrist arthroplasty in rheumatoid arthritis. *J Hand Surg* 1986;11A:175–183.

137. Swanson AB, Poitevin LA, deGroot Swanson G: Bone remodeling phenomena in flexible hand implants: Kappa Delta Awards. *Orthop Rev* 1982;11:129–130.

138. Peimer CA, Taleisnik J: Pathologic fractures from Silastic synovitis. *J Hand Surg,* in press.

139. Watson HK, Ballet FL: The SLAC wrist: Scapholunate advanced collapse pattern of degenerative arthritis. *J Hand Surg* 1984;9A:358–365.

140. Pisano S, Peimer CA: Scaphocapitate intercarpal arthrodesis: Results and functional analysis. *Orthop Trans,* in press.

141. Douglas DP, Peimer CA, Koniuch MP: Motion of the wrist after simulated limited intercarpal arthrodeses: An experimental study. *J Bone Joint Surg* 1987;69A:1413–1418.

142. Weinstein A, Amstutz H, Pavon G, et al: Orthopedic implants: A clinical and metallurgical analysis. *J Biomed Mater Res* 1973;7:297–325.

143. Fett HC: The treatment of carpal fractures, including Kienböck's disease, Preiser's disease, etc. *Comps Med* 1953;4:15–20.

144. Metcalfe JW: The vitallium sphere prosthesis for nonunion of the navicular bone. *J Int College Surg* 1954;22:459–461.

145. Speed K: Ferrule caps for the head of the radius. *Surg Gynecol Obstet* 1941;73:845–850.

146. Waugh RL, Reuling L: Ununited fractures of the carpal scaphoid: Preliminary report on the use of vitallium replicas as replacements after excision. *Am J Surg* 1945;67:184–200.

147. Jones KG: Replacement of the proximal portion of the scaphoid with spherical implant for post-traumatic carporadial arthritis. *J Hand Surg* 1985;10B:217–226.

Congenital Malformations and Deformities of the Hand

P A R T   A

General Concepts

Terry R. Light, MD

Introduction

An estimated 11.4 of every 10,000 live births result in one or more congenital deformities or malformations of the hand. Five percent of the patients who have these abnormalities also have other syndromes.[1] Each child with a congenital hand malformation should be examined carefully for other malformations that may exist.[2] Conditions that have hereditary implications should be identified and parents of patients who have these conditions should be referred to a geneticist for counseling.[3]

Malformations are primary structural defects that result from a localized developmental failure, for example, syndactyly. Deformities result from secondary changes of form or structure that occur after normal development has begun, for example, congenital constriction band amputation.[4]

Surgical reconstruction often begins during the first year of life. Complex conditions may require multiple-stage procedures. Surgical reconstruction of the congenitally anomalous hand can be completed before the child is 4 or 5 years old—the age at which children begin to face the difficulty of school socialization. Children should be reexamined periodically until they reach skeletal maturity to identify progressive growth abnormalities or recurrence of a surgically corrected deformity.

The goals and techniques of surgical reconstruction must be individualized to balance function and appearance. Without reconstruction, most children are resourceful enough to effectively accomplish a wide range of tasks. Surgical reconstruction may allow them to do these tasks with greater ease, speed, and dexterity. Aesthetic considerations are vital. Skin incisions should be planned carefully. Parts that are without function and have a grossly abnormal appearance are often best removed rather than reconstructed by elaborate multistage procedures. It may be preferable to reconstruct a four-digit hand that functions well rather than trying to preserve or reconstruct a less functional five-digit hand.

Classification

A number of classification systems have been proposed for categorizing congenital limb malformations and deformities. The classification system proposed by Swanson[5] has been adopted by the American Society for Surgery of the Hand and the International Federation of Societies for Surgery of the Hand. This system is straightforward and emphasizes the morphologic appearance of the hand. The seven categories of hand malformations and deformities in this classification system are (1) failure of formation of parts, (2) failure of differentiation (separation) of parts, (3) duplication, (4) congenital constriction band syndrome, (5) overgrowth, (6) hypoplasia, and (7) generalized skeletal abnormalities.

International acceptance of this schema has allowed centers in various parts of the world to define the relative incidence of different anomalies in their centers and to compare their figures to those of other centers.[1] Monitoring such as this will enable investigators to detect an increase in the rate of malformations in their region, and thus may alert them to the presence of new exogenous factors that are responsible for the increased incidence of malformations such as maternal thalidomide ingestion.

Limb Bud Development

The upper limb bud appears during the fourth week of gestation as a mesenchymal condensation covered by ectoderm. The mesodermal tissue gives rise to muscle, tendon, nerve, and bone and the ectoderm gives rise to skin, hair, and nails. The limb bud elongates and definition of elements proceeds in a proximal to distal sequence. The development of the upper limb generally precedes that of the lower limb by a few days. At 33 days of gestation, the hand is recognizable as a paddle without individually defined digits. By 41 days, mesenchymal elements coalesce and congregate to define each of the five rays of metacarpals and proximal phalanges. A process of programmed cell death controlled by the apical ectodermal ridge leads to resorption of interdigital web space cells through lysosomal destruction. This process separates each of the five rays by creating four web spaces while the middle and distal phalanges gain definition. Digital separation begins at 47 days and is complete by 54 days.[6,7]

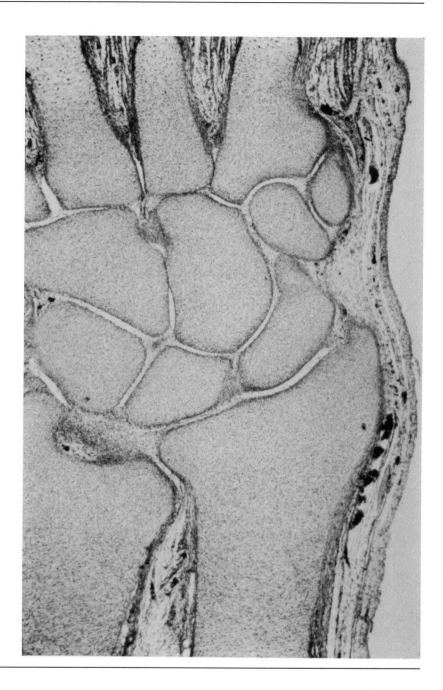

Fig. 3A-1 At 10 weeks (crown-rump length = 60 mm) embryologic development has concluded. A cartilage model has formed for each future bone of the forearm, carpus, and hand. (Reproduced with permission from the Patten Embryology Research Collection, Department of Anatomy and Cell Biology, the University of Michigan Medical School.)

A critical interactive relationship exists between the mesenchymal tissue and the overlying apical ectodermal ridge. The mesenchymal cells induce the development and maintenance of the apical ectodermal ridge by elaborating a factor called apical ectodermal ridge maintenance factor. The apical ectodermal ridge itself directs the differentiation of the underlying mesenchymal tissue.

The skeleton of the upper limb begins to form in the proximal mesenchymal tissues. The mesenchymal elements form cellular concentrations identifiable as the future bones by six weeks of gestation. By seven weeks, the condensations that will give rise to each of the bones

of the hand are evident. By the eighth week, each of the major bones of the appendicular skeleton has been defined. At the end of the embryonic period, all future bones are cartilaginous models of their adult form (Fig. 3A–1), and the tufts of the distal phalanges have begun ossification.

The embryonic period ends as ossification begins in the clavicle and in the humerus. The embryonic period is characterized by the definition of new organs. The fetal period is concerned primarily with the increase in size of established organs. Primary ossification centers appear in the humerus, radius, ulna, metacarpals, and phalanges during fetal development. As the primary

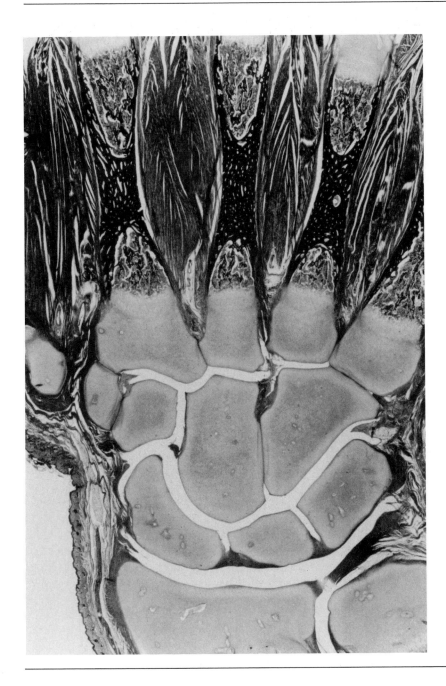

Fig. 3A–2 At 21 weeks (crown-rump length = 195 mm) extensive fetal development is evident. Cartilage canals are visible within the carpal bones. Primary ossification centers have formed and expanded in each tubular bone, defining physes that will shape postnatal growth. (Reproduced with permission from the Patten Embryology Research Collection, Department of Anatomy and Cell Biology, the University of Michigan Medical School.)

ossification centers expand in size, the physes become defined at the ends of each of the long bones (Fig. 3A–2). The carpals remain cartilaginous.

During postnatal growth, secondary ossification centers appear at the ends of each of the tubular bones while each of the cartilaginous carpals ossifies sequentially. By the time of skeletal maturity, each of the physes has closed.

In many anomalous upper limbs this orderly pattern of ossification is modified. Elements that normally ossify during fetal growth may persist as entirely cartilaginous tissue at the time of birth. These elements may begin to ossify during postnatal development or may persist into adulthood as cartilage or fibrocartilage.[6,7]

Mechanisms of Malformation

The exact mechanism of most hand malformations is poorly understood. Many malformations may be either single- or multiple-gene disorders. Generally, bilateral disorders are hereditary, particularly when both the hands and feet demonstrate similar malformations. The absence of a family history of a malformation does not exclude the possibility of a hereditary disorder because the condition may be the result of a recessive trait or a new inheritable mutation. Because the face, eye, and ear develop at the same time as the upper limb, many hand malformation syndromes involve abnormalities of the face, eye, ear, and upper extremity.

The thalidomide tragedy demonstrated that exogenous factors, such as drugs, may have a profound effect on limb development. The resulting malformations vary with the timing of the insult.[4] In general, the earlier the exposure to the drug or other exogenous factor, the more severe the resultant deformity. Many of the early exposures may be so severe that they are lethal, resulting in spontaneous first-trimester abortion.

An example of a failure of separation of parts is syndactyly, a persistence of the embryonic paddle shape of the hand that results from a failure of the normally programmed cell death between digital rays. Some forms of duplication, particularly preaxial polydactyly, may be an overly aggressive splitting or segmentation of the most radial ray anlage. When the anlage is inappropriately split, cell death occurs within a digital ray and leads to its partial or complete division into separate rays.[8,9]

References

1. Lamb DW, Wynne-Davies R, Soto L: An estimate of the population frequency of congenital malformations of the upper limb. *J Hand Surg* 1982;7:557–562.
2. Poznanski AK: *The Hand in Radiologic Diagnosis: With Gamuts and Pattern Profiles*, ed 2. Philadelphia, WB Saunders, 1984.
3. Temtamy S, McKusick V: *The Genetics of Hand Malformations.* New York, Alan R Liss, 1978.
4. Buck-Gramcko D: Congenital malformation, in Nigst N, Buck-Gramcko D, Millesi H, et al (eds): *Hand Surgery*. New York, Thieme Medical Publishers, 1988, vol 1, chap 12.
5. Swanson AB: A classification for congenital limb malformations. *J Hand Surg* 1976;1:8–22.
6. Christ B, Jacob HJ, Jacob M, et al: Principles of hand ontogenesis in man. *Acta Morphol Neerl Scand* 1986;24:249–268.
7. Light TR: Growth and development of the hand and carpus, in Carter P, Toledo K (eds): *Reconstructive Surgery of the Child's Hand*. Philadelphia, Lea & Febiger, in press.
8. Kitayama Y, Tsukada S: Patterns of arterial distribution in the duplicated thumb. *Plast Reconstr Surg* 1983;72:535–542.
9. Nogami H, Oohira A: Experimental study on pathogenesis of polydactyly of the thumb. *J Hand Surg* 1980;5:443–450.

P A R T B

Duplication, Failure of Differentiation, Congenital Constriction Band Syndrome

Terry R. Light, MD

Duplication

Duplication and syndactyly are the two most common congenital hand malformations. Duplication is manifest in a variety of forms. The most common forms are postaxial polydactyly in black children and preaxial or radial polydactyly (duplicate or bifid thumb) in white children.

Postaxial Polydactyly

Among blacks, postaxial polydactyly is a common autosomal dominant condition. Postaxial polydactyly is distinctly uncommon in white children in whom its presence may signal a syndrome such as trisomy 13, or Ellis-van Creveld, or Laurence-Moon-Bardet-Biedl syndromes. Most often, the most ulnar digit lacks a well-developed base and may be simply excised. However, when two proximal phalanges each articulate with a single fifth metacarpal head, reconstruction is more complex than simply removing the most ulnar digit. The reconstruction is approached through a dorsal zig-zag incision. The ulnar collateral ligament and ulnar intrinsic insertions should be peeled off of the most ulnar phalanx. The metacarpal head is narrowed by longitudinal osteotomy to accommodate the remaining phalanx, and the ulnar collateral ligament and intrinsic insertions are reconstructed on the ulnar surface of the retained little finger.

Central Polydactyly

Central polydactyly[1] is an uncommon, often hereditary, form of preaxial polydactyly. Many instances of central polydactyly are associated with a concealed polydactylous digit embedded in a syndactylized web between the middle and ring or the ring and little fingers. Surgical excision usually involves syndactyly release. Proximal interphalangeal joint contractures are common and often resistant to surgical release. In some instances, it is better to delete more than one digit and create a well-aligned four-digit hand than to attempt to preserve five inadequate, angled, syndactylized digits.[1]

Preaxial Polydactyly

Preaxial polydactyly may vary from a broad-thumb distal phalanx with a central hole to a hand with two separate and independent thumbs. Wassel's system classifies patients based on the skeletal level of duplication.[2] Type I thumbs have a broad distal phalanx that bifurcates distally, and type II thumbs have two separate distal phalanges articulating with a single proximal phalanx. Type III thumbs have a bifurcating proximal phalanx, with each half of the bifurcation supporting a distal phalanx. Type IV thumbs, the most common pattern, have two thumbs each with a proximal phalanx that articulates with a broad shared metacarpal (Fig. 3B–1). Type V thumbs have a Y-shaped bifurcating metacarpal and each limb supports proximal and distal phalanges. Type VI duplicated thumbs each have a metacarpal and proximal and distal phalanges. Type VII thumbs are duplicated thumbs with triphalangeal components.

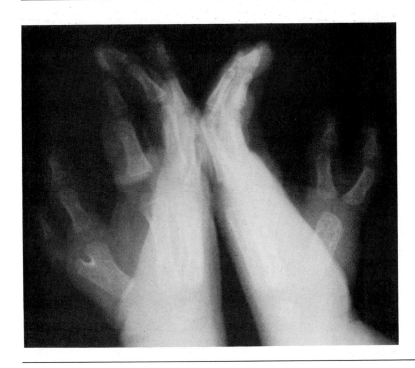

Fig. 3B–1 When preaxial polydactyly is bilateral, the type of thumb duplication is often asymmetric. This radiograph shows a child who has a Wassel type V thumb on the left and a Wassel type IV thumb on the right.

An important consideration in the surgical management of the bifid or bifurcated thumb is that, in most cases, neither component thumb has bulk equivalent to the contralateral normal thumb. The goal of surgical reconstruction is to create a single aesthetically acceptable, well-aligned, stable, and mobile digit.[3–7] Usually the bony skeleton is managed by excising the skeletal elements of one of the component digits. In most instances, the more completely developed ulnar thumb is retained and the skeletal elements of the more radial thumb are excised. When the level of duplication involves either the interphalangeal or metacarpophalangeal joints, as in Wassel types II and IV duplications, the proximal articular surface is broader than normal. Longitudinal osteotomy narrows the phalangeal or metacarpal articular surface to a width appropriate to the retained digit.[8] The alignment of the metacarpophalangeal and interphalangeal joints should be assessed. Osteotomies should be located proximal to the articular surface to ensure parallel alignment of the joints perpendicular to the long axis of the retained digit. The bone graft necessary for an opening wedge osteotomy can be harvested from the deleted skeletal elements.

Soft-tissue components of both digits should be combined to create a single optimal digit. Central skin incisions, originally advocated by Bilhaut,[9] are useful in providing exposure and optimal soft-tissue closure contour (Fig. 3B–2). In Wassel types II and IV, collateral ligament reconstruction is important to achieve joint stability. The collateral ligament is lengthened by a periosteal strip taken from the outer border of the excised skeletal element. Digital flexor and extensor tendons should be carefully defined and centralized on the retained digit. Intrinsic muscle insertions should be detached from the deleted digit and reattached to the skeleton of the retained digit.

In some proximal duplications, the basilar joint of one digit may be combined with the more distal joints of the other digit. This can be accomplished through a modified pollicization called an on-top-plasty procedure.[3]

Mirror Hand

The extremely rare mirror hand deformity is the most profound form of duplication. Two ulnae, two ulnar carpal components, and two sets of ulnar digits combine to form a seven- (or, less commonly, eight-) digit thumbless hand.[10] Forearm rotation is always limited and elbow and wrist motion is usually restricted. Surgical treatment consists of pollicization of one of the digits along the preaxial surface, deletion of the redundant preaxial digits, and consolidation of musculotendinous elements.[11]

Failure of Differentiation

Failure of differentiation is an abnormality in the separation or segmentation of either skeletal or soft-tissue elements, or both.

Syndactyly

Syndactyly results from a failure of the embryologic separation of adjacent digital rays. Syndactyly is clas-

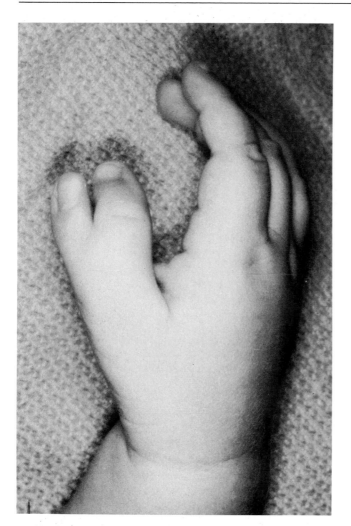 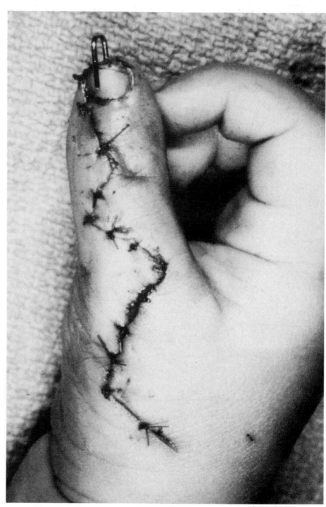

Fig. 3B-2   **Left:** Preoperative photograph of a Wassel type IV thumb duplication shows two small component thumbs. **Right:** Central zig-zag exposure permits osteotomy, collateral and intrinsic insertion reconstruction, and the combination of soft tissue from both components.

sified as simple when only soft tissue is joined and complex when there is union of bony or nail elements. Complete syndactyly refers to syndactyly in which the entire lengths of adjacent digits are joined, and incomplete syndactyly refers to the joining of only a portion of adjacent digits. The term complicated syndactyly has been suggested to describe cases in which abnormally shaped phalanges, often delta-shaped or triangular, result in angular deformity of one or more of the syndactylized digits.[3]

When syndactyly involves adjacent digits of distinctly unequal lengths, such as the thumb and index finger or the ring and little fingers, joint development is frequently distorted. This is particularly true in complex syndactyly. These syndactylies should be released surgically first because the longer that unequal adjacent digits remain joined, the more fixed the underlying joint deformity will become. When a central digit has syndactyly along both its radial and ulnar borders, it is

generally unwise to risk devascularizing the digit by releasing both sides in a single surgical procedure.

A variety of surgical techniques have been advocated for the release of syndactyly.[3,8,12–19] The creation of a properly situated web space floor that has true anatomic dimensions of width and breadth is common to all effective techniques. This floor can be created with tissue flaps based either volarly or dorsally. Alternative techniques use a volarly based rectangular flap, a combination of interdigitated volarly and dorsally based triangular flaps, or a dorsally based rectangular flap. I prefer the technique that uses a dorsally based rectangular flap advocated by Bauer and associates[16] because it provides the best color match and is technically straightforward (Fig. 3B–3).

The base of the dorsal flap is just distal to the corresponding metacarpophalangeal joints. Its length may be determined by measuring the cross-sectional distance to the intended volar edge of the web space. This

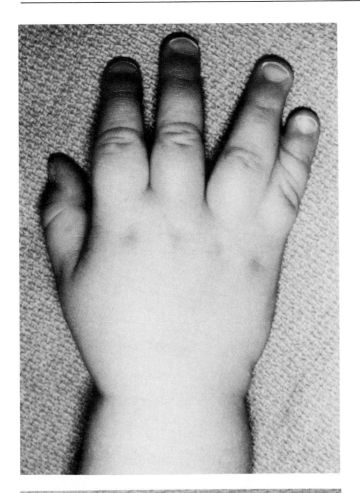

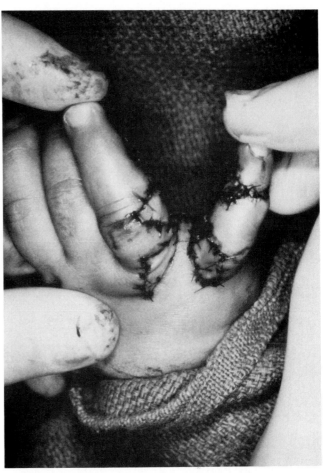

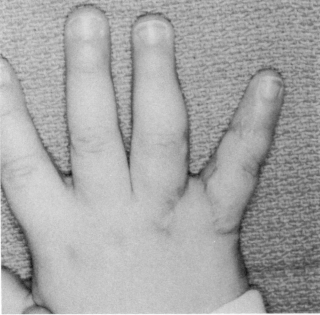

Fig. 3B-3 **Top left:** Photograph of incomplete simple syndactyly of ring and little fingers. **Top right:** Photograph of a dorsally based flap set into a newly deepened web space. The full-thickness groin skin graft has been sutured to areas not covered by volar and dorsal zig-zag flaps. **Bottom:** Photograph shows a well-maintained web space six months after release.

is measured most directly with an eye muscle caliper. The most proximal volar flap is based upon the digit that will require a second contralateral release, if pres-

ent. Flaps are developed from zig-zag incisions on both the volar and dorsal aspect of the digits. The flaps provide partial coverage of the exposed surfaces of the

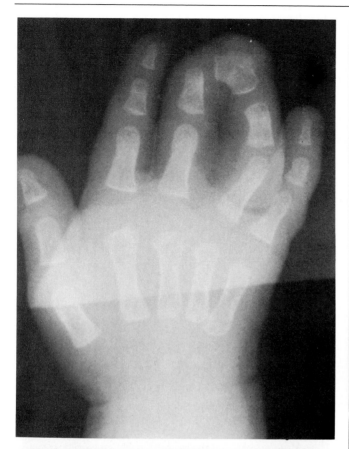

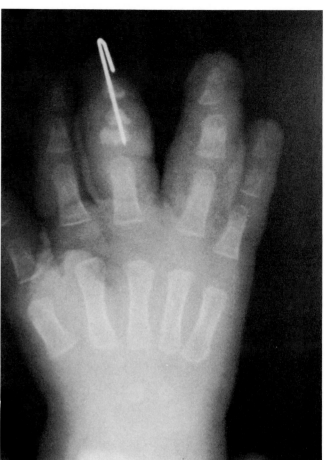

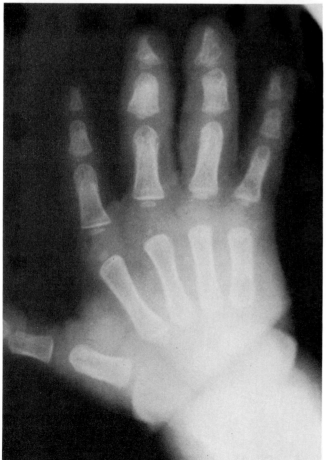

Fig. 3B–4   Top left: Complex complete syndactyly of middle and ring fingers is associated with markedly distorted distal interphalangeal joint of middle finger. **Top right:** For complex syndactyly, osteotomy through combined distal phalanges allows digital separation, and osteotomy through the middle phalanx of the middle finger allows realignment of the distal interphalangeal joint. **Bottom:** One year after surgery for complex syndactyly, osteotomy has healed and correction is well maintained.

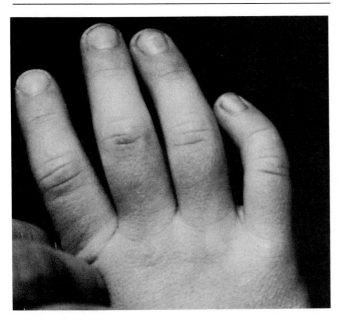

Fig. 3B–5 Clinodactyly of the little finger is due to a trapezoid-shaped middle phalanx.

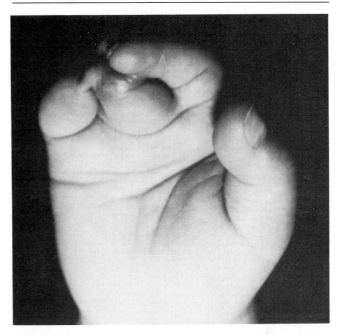

Fig. 3B–6 Congenital constriction band syndrome has resulted in partial amputation and distal syndactyly of index, middle, ring, and little fingers. The thumb has been spared.

released digits. A full-thickness skin graft is required in all but the most proximal syndactyly to cover one or both digits after surgical release. A skin graft is usually harvested from the groin crease.

Neurovascular structures should be preserved carefully when syndactylized digits are separated. When the common digital nerve bifurcates distally, it is teased apart, beginning distally and continuing proximally until the bifurcation of the digital nerve components has been shifted proximal to the planned web space floor. Occasionally, a common digital artery bifurcates distal to the planned web space. Establishing this web space floor level requires ligation of one of the two proper digital arteries. The proper digital artery should be preserved to the digit along the side opposite the planned syndactyly release. If the vascularity to the digit deprived of the digital artery is questionable, the perfusion of the two digits may be assessed by applying microvascular clamps to both digital arteries and deflating the tourniquet.

Complex syndactyly requires osteotomy of shared bony elements and attention to nail contour (Fig. 3B–4). Local pulp flaps may provide tissue for reconstruction of lateral paronychial nail borders.[19]

Poland's syndrome is a condition in which there is simple syndactyly and brachydactyly principally of the index, middle, and ring fingers and absence of the sternocostal portion of the pectoralis major.[20,21] Syndactyly release is performed as described above. Although the functional deficit in the chest is slight, the cosmetic defect may be significant. In females, hypoplasia of the ipsilateral breast and chest may be improved by plastic

reconstructive procedures done at about the time of skeletal maturity.

Apert's syndrome is a form of acrocephalosyndactyly in which premature closure of cranial sutures is associated with complex syndactyly of both the hands and feet.[22,23] The interphalangeal joints are stiff, the middle phalanx is frequently suppressed, and angular deformity of the thumb is common. Surgical reconstruction improves complex syndactyly involving all fingers (spoon hand), or all the fingers but the thumb (mitten hand). At least two stages are usually required. The first stage should release the thumb from the index finger and the little finger from the ring finger. Then, it is often helpful to delete the skeletal elements of the middle finger to create a hand with three fingers and a thumb. Resection or opening wedge osteotomy of the commonly encountered triangular or delta-shaped phalanx corrects the radial angular deformity of the thumb.

Trigger Thumb and Trigger Finger

Trigger thumb or trigger finger often occurs in young children. Although they are commonly referred to as congenital, only a few of these abnormalities are evident at birth. Many other abnormalities are first seen during the first few years of life.[3,12,24,25] Some trigger digits may be present at birth with a minimal, not easily detected degree of fixed flexion. With growth, the flexion contracture increases to a more detectable extent.[3] Trigger thumb is more common than trigger fingers and may be present bilaterally. Multiple digits may be involved within one hand.[25] Spontaneous resolution oc-

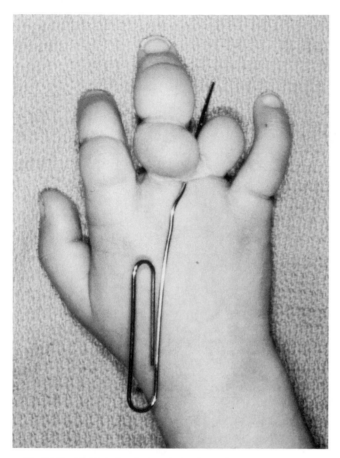

Fig. 3B-7 Multiple-level constriction bands have resulted in partial ring finger amputation and multiple areas of residual constriction. A paper clip has been passed through a palmar-dorsal sinus proximal to the syndactyly.

curs in one third of the digits diagnosed at the time of birth and in only 10% of the digits diagnosed after birth.[3,24]

Typically, children do not experience clicking, locking, and localized pain as adults who have a trigger digit do. The interphalangeal joint is locked in flexion with an apparently fixed flexion contracture of the interphalangeal joint. Thickening of the flexor pollicis longus tendon is palpable over the metacarpal head just proximal to the first anular pulley. This mass is often referred to as Notta's node.[26] Splinting, although a logical measure, has never permanently cured a trigger thumb or trigger finger.

When flexion posture persists after 18 months of age, surgical release is usually recommended. A transverse skin incision allows digital nerve retraction and exposure of the first anular pulley. Because the radial digital nerve crosses over the flexor sheath obliquely to assume its ultimate position radial to the sheath, dissection of the subcutaneous tissue overlying the first anular pulley must be done carefully. The proximal pulley is incised longitudinally. The finger or thumb may be extended

passively without difficulty. The tendon thickening resolves gradually after the constricting pulley has been opened. It is not necessary to resect or trim areas of tendon redundancy. Postoperative splinting is not necessary. Although some digits may rest in their former flexed position initially, this tendency disappears spontaneously as normal activity is resumed.

Camptodactyly

Camptodactyly is a nontraumatic flexion deformity of the proximal interphalangeal joint. This condition may be seen at birth in any finger or may first become evident in adolescence, usually in the little finger. This latter form is more common in girls and is often familial.

The cause of camptodactyly remains uncertain. Each of the proposed explanations for camptodactyly suggests an imbalance of forces across the proximal interphalangeal joint. Some plausible explanations are (1) hypoplasia of the extensor mechanism, (2) lumbrical insertion abnormalities, and (3) flexor superficialis overpull.[27-30]

Camptodactyly that has been present for some time is associated with secondary proximal interphalangeal joint changes. With time, the proximal phalanx articulates with the dorsal half of the middle phalanx articular surface, molding the growing articular contours into a position that favors continued flexion by creating an eccentric center of joint motion. Fixed joint contracture involves tightening of soft-tissue structures, including the checkrein ligaments that tether the volar plate.[31] The metacarpophalangeal joint usually hyperextends to accommodate the flexed finger and allow the hand to lie flat.

Splinting is an integral part of the management of camptodactyly. Hori and associates[32] suggested that fulltime splinting with an extension assist coil splint will gradually stretch out a fixed contracture. Once passive mobility of the proximal interphalangeal joint is achieved, splinting can be limited to only eight hours per day but must be continued until skeletal maturity.

Surgical treatment of camptodactyly may be unrewarding, particularly when fixed flexion contracture of the proximal interphalangeal joint is present.[33] When there is a fixed contracture, splinting should eliminate or diminish the fixed contracture. Surgical reconstruction aims either to diminish flexion forces or augment extension forces across the proximal interphalangeal joint, or both. An abnormal lumbrical insertion is resected or reinserted. Sublimis tenotomy may be helpful, particularly when the contracture diminishes with wrist flexion. A chevron or zig-zag palmar exposure permits delineation of the lumbrical insertion and sublimis tenotomy proximal to the first anular pulley. A postoperative splinting program similar to that used preoperatively may be necessary to retain correction. Other surgical techniques include the transfer of either the

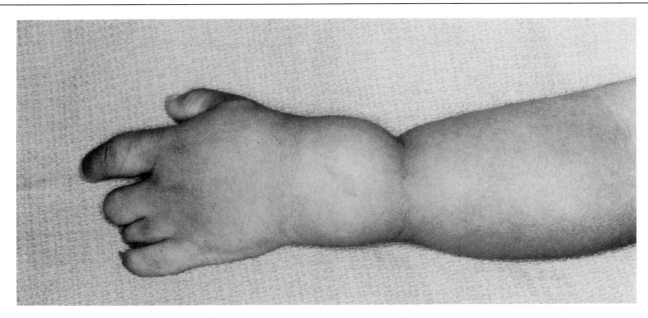

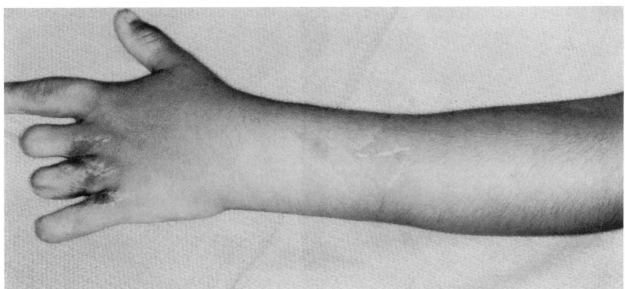

Fig. 3B–8 **Top:** Mid-forearm congenital constriction band associated with middle, ring, and little finger syndactyly and distal amputation of digits. **Bottom:** Forearm contour has been improved by band excision and Z-plasty and effective digital length has been increased by web space deepening.

sublimis or the adjacent fourth dorsal interosseous tendon into the dorsal hood aponeurosis to augment proximal interphalangeal joint extensor forces. When the deformity is profound in skeletally mature individuals, a dorsal closing wedge proximal phalangeal osteotomy or proximal interphalangeal joint arthrodesis may be used as a salvage procedure.

Clinodactyly

In clinodactyly a finger is angled, usually the little finger, as the result of a trapezoid-shaped middle phalanx. This condition is often an autosomal dominant trait. Clinodactyly of the little finger is associated with

numerous syndromes, many of which are characterized by mental retardation.[3,19,34,35]

In the common form of clinodactyly involving the little finger, the digit angles radially (Fig. 3B–5). When the index finger is involved, the digit angles ulnarly. When the proximal phalanx of a biphalangeal thumb is affected, the thumb angles in a radial direction. The eccentric intermediate phalanx of a triphalangeal thumb causes the thumb to angle in an ulnar direction.[19]

When the angulation is small, surgical treatment is usually not necessary. When angulation is severe, the finger may underlap an adjacent finger when the digits are flexed. Closing wedge osteotomy through a midlateral exposure corrects angulation but shortens further an already short digit. Opening wedge osteotomy with radial bone graft is preferred for length preservation and augmentation. Z-plasty skin transposition may be required to relieve skin tension.[3] Temporary Kirschner wire fixation of the osteotomy is required with both opening and closing wedge osteotomies.

Congenital Constriction Band Syndrome

Congenital constriction band syndrome, also known as anular grooves or amniotic bands, occurs sporadically and may be associated with abnormalities of the extremities or the face.[36-40] Theories concerning amniotic bands involve either endogenous cell degeneration, a theory made popular by Streeter,[41] or an exogenous amniotic band, a theory made popular by Torpin.[40,42] Manifestations of congenital constriction band syndrome may include total digital loss, severe indentation with neurovascular compromise, massive distal lymphedema, mild indentation, and syndactyly[40-44] (Fig. 3B–6).

Syndactyly secondary to amniotic bands can be distinguished from other forms of syndactyly by the presence of a small sinus (cleft, skin tunnel, or fenestration) proximal to the skin bridge of the distal digit syndactyly (Fig. 3B–7). Often one finger may be pushed palmar or dorsal to the other joined digits. Adjacent digits often become so entwined in a grape-like cluster that it is difficult to determine the corresponding proximal digit for each of the distal elements.

When the area of syndactyly is narrow, distal, and involves many digits, simultaneous release of multiple digits may be done. Because the residual web space is usually situated distally, proximal relocation of the floor of the web space is necessary. The techniques described by Flatt[12] may allow slight proximal shifting of the web space without the need for skin grafting.

At birth, if edema is profound distal to a tight constriction band, the viability of the extremity may be threatened. In these children, Z-plasty release should be done in the neonatal period. Traditionally, release of only half of the circumference of a constricted digit or limb was advised for the initial surgical procedure. A number of recent reports have challenged this concept and suggested that a one-stage procedure may be satisfactory.[3,45,46] The skin band itself should be excised (Fig. 3B–8). The underlying soft tissue should be dissected sufficiently to ensure that an underlying subcutaneous or fibrous band does not remain beneath the skin. Residual unreleased indentation of the soft tissue beneath the skin level may cause a recurrent deformity or persistent neurologic deficit. In patients who have a neurologic deficit, the peripheral nerve should be directly exposed and explored. Neurolysis or nerve

grafting may be necessary.[47] Z-plasty flaps are transposed to ensure that the skin is closed without tension.

W-plasty is a particularly effective alternate technique when there is extensive soft-tissue redundancy. After the band is excised, a "W" configuration is created by excising additional tissue both proximally and distally to the band. With either Z-plasty or W-plasty it is important to have flaps large enough to ensure that the circumferential band is truly broken up.

Digital amputations are most common in the index, middle, and ring fingers, presumably because these digits are longer and thus most likely to become ensnared by amniotic tissue. A pointed, tapered tip with inadequate soft-tissue coverage may occur when amputation is through a phalanx. Correction may require diaphyseal shortening, soft-tissue recontouring of the tip, or amputation by phalangeal excision or ray resection.

If the thumb has been amputated through the proximal phalanx, or more proximally, microvascular free toe transfer may be considered. Because the deformity is principally distal, appropriate neurovascular and musculoskeletal elements will be found in the hand to attach to the transferred toe. The second toe is most often selected for this transfer.[36-40]

References

1. Wood VE: Treatment of central polydactyly. *Clin Orthop* 1971;74:196–205.
2. Wassel HD: The results of surgery for polydactyly of the thumb: A review. *Clin Orthop* 1969;64:175–193.
3. Dobyns JH, Wood VE, Bayne LG: Congenital hand deformities, in Green DP (ed): *Operative Hand Surgery*, ed 2. New York, Churchill Livingstone, 1988, vol 1, pp 255–536.
4. Cheng JC, Chan KM, Ma GF, et al: Polydactyly of the thumb: A surgical plan based on ninety-five cases. *J Hand Surg* 1984;9A:l55–164.
5. Miura T: Duplicated thumb. *Plast Reconstr Surg* 1982;69:470–481.
6. Marks TW, Bayne LG: Polydactyly of the thumb: Abnormal anatomy and treatment. *J Hand Surg* 1978;3:107–116.
7. Tada K, Yonenobu K, Tsuyuguchi Y, et al: Duplication of the thumb: A retrospective review of two hundred and thirty-seven cases. *J Bone Joint Surg* 1983;65A:584–598.
8. Blauth W, Schneider-Sickert F: *Congenital Deformities of the Hand: An Atlas of Their Surgical Treatment*, Weil UH (trans). Berlin, Springer-Verlag, 1981.
9. Bilhaut M: Guérison d'un pouce bifide par un nouveau procédé opératoire. *Ann Orthop Chir Prat* 1890;3:33–37.
10. Barton NJ, Buck-Gramcko D, Evans DM: Soft-tissue anatomy of mirror hand. *J Hand Surg* 1986;11B:307–319.
11. Barton NJ, Buck-Gramcko D, Evans DM, et al: Mirror hand treated by true pollicization. *J Hand Surg* 1986;11B:320–336.
12. Flatt AE: *The Care of Congenital Hand Anomalies*. St. Louis, CV Mosby, 1977.
13. Barsky AJ: *Congenital Anomalies of the Hand and Their Surgical Treatment*. Springfield, Charles C Thomas, 1958.
14. Kelikian H: *Congenital Deformities of the Hand and Forearm*. Philadelphia, WB Saunders, 1974.
15. Lewis RC, Nordyke MD, Duncan KH: Web space reconstruction with an M-V flap. *J Hand Surg* 1988;13A:40–43.
16. Bauer TB, Tondra JM, Trusler HM: Technical modification in repair of syndactylism. *Plast Reconstr Surg* 1956;17:385–392.

17. Toledo LC, Ger E: Evaluation of the operative treatment of syndactyly. *J Hand Surg* 1979;4:556–564.

18. Cronin TD: Syndactylism: Results of zig-zag incision to prevent postoperative contracture. *Plast Reconstr Surg* 1956;18:460–468.

19. Buck-Gramcko D: Congenital malformation, in Nigst N, Buck-Gramcko D, Millesi H, et al (eds): *Hand Surgery*. New York, Thieme Medical Publishers, 1988, vol 1, chap 12.

20. Poland A: Deficiency of the pectoralis muscle. *Guys Hosp Rep* 1841;6:191.

21. Ireland DC, Takayama N, Flatt AE: Poland's syndrome. *J Bone Joint Surg* 1976;58A:52–58.

22. Hoover GH, Flatt AE, Weiss MW: The hand and Apert's syndrome. *J Bone Joint Surg* 1970;52A:878–895.

23. Apert ME: De l'acrocéphalosyndactylie. *Bull Mem Soc Med Hosp* 1906; 23:1310–1330.

24. Dinham JM, Meggitt BF: Trigger thumbs in children: A review of the natural history and indications for treatment in 105 patients. *J Bone Joint Surg* 1974;56B:153–155.

25. Sprecher EE: Trigger thumb in infants. *Clin Orthop* 1953;1:124–128.

26. Notta A, cited by Dobyns JH, Wood VE, Bayne LG: Congenital hand deformities, in Green DP (ed): *Operative Hand Surgery*, ed 2. New York, Churchill Livingstone, 1988, vol 1, pp 255–536.

27. McFarlane RM, Curry GI, Evans HB: Anomalies of the intrinsic muscles in camptodactyly. *J Hand Surg* 1983;8:531–544.

28. Miura T: Non-traumatic flexion deformity of the proximal interphalangeal joint: Its pathogenesis and treatment. *Hand* 1983;15:25–34.

29. Smith RJ, Kaplan EB: Camptodactyly and similar atraumatic flexion deformities of the proximal interphalangeal joints of the fingers: A study of thirty-one cases. *J Bone Joint Surg* 1968;50A:1187–1203.

30. Maeda M, Matsui T: Camptodactyly caused by an abnormal lumbrical muscle. *J Hand Surg* 1985;10B:95–96.

31. Watson HK, Light TR, Johnson TR: Checkrein resection for flexion contracture of the middle joint. *J Hand Surg* 1979;4:67–71.

32. Hori M, Nakamura R, Inoue G, et al: Nonoperative treatment of camptodactyly. *J Hand Surg* 1981;6:1061–1065.

33. Engber WD, Flatt AE: Camptodactyly: An analysis of sixty-six patients and twenty-four operations. *J Hand Surg* 1977;2:216–224.

34. Burke F, Flatt A: Clinodactyly: A review of a series of cases. *Hand* 1979;11:269–280.

35. Poznanski AK, Pratt GB, Manson G, et al: Clinodactyly, camptodactyly, Kirner's deformity, and other crooked fingers. *Radiology* 1969;93:573–582.

36. Miura T: Congenital constriction band syndrome. *J Hand Surg* 1984;9A:82–88.

37. Moses JM, Flatt AE, Cooper RR: Annular constricting bands. *J Bone Joint Surg* 1979;61A:562–565.

38. Kurata T, Tsuge K: A study of congenital constriction band syndrome of the upper extremities. *Hiroshima J Med Sci* 1972;21:23–34.

39. Walsh RJ: Acrosyndactyly: A study of twenty-seven patients. *Clin Orthop* 1970;71:99–111.

40. Torpin R: *Fetal Malformations Caused by Amnion Rupture During Gestation*. Springfield, Charles C Thomas, 1968.

41. Streeter GL: Focal deficiencies in fetal tissues and their relation to intrauterine amputations. *Carnegie Inst Contrib Embryol* 1930;22:1–44.

42. Torpin R: Amniochorionic mesoblastic fibrous strings and amnionic bands: Associated constricting fetal malformations or fetal death. *Am J Obstet Gynecol* 1965;91:65–75.

43. Kino Y: Clinical and experimental studies of congenital constriction band syndrome, with an emphasis on its etiology. *J Bone Joint Surg* 1975;57A:636–643.

44. Opgrande JD: Constriction ring syndrome: Unusual case report. *J Hand Surg* 1982;7:11–12.

45. Hall EJ, Johnson-Giebink R, Vasconez LO: Management of the ring constriction syndrome: A reappraisal. *Plast Reconstr Surg* 1982;69:532–536.

46. Di Meo L, Mercer DH: Single-stage correction of constriction ring syndrome. *Ann Plast Surg* 1987;19:469–474.

47. Weeks PM: Radial, median, and ulnar nerve dysfunction associated with a congenital constricting band of the arm. *Plast Reconstr Surg* 1982;69:333–336.

P A R T C

Radial Deficiency

Paul R. Manske, MD

Longitudinal Failure of Formation

The failure of formation of the structures of the upper extremity is related to longitudinal or transverse deficiencies of the embryonic limb bud. The deficiencies that develop along longitudinal axes include preaxial (radial) deficiencies, postaxial (ulnar) deficiencies, and central ray deficiencies. It is tempting to speculate that these axially oriented failures of formation result from teratogenic or genetic influences at specific locations on the apical ectodermal ridge or the supporting mesodermal cells of the limb bud.[1] This axial alignment is particularly true for radial deficiency presentations, which characteristically affect only the structures on the radial border of the forearm and hand. However, the relationship between the origin and specific presentation of ulnar and central deficiencies is not as clearly defined. Ulnar deficiency frequently includes dysplasia of the thumb and radial rays in addition to the ulnar structures. Central deficiency (cleft hand) has a frequent association with polydactyly (duplication) and syndactyly (failure of differentiation) of the central digits. These more complex presentations of postaxial and central deficiencies suggest that the concept of upper extremity deficiencies related to focal failures of formation of limb bud cells is too simplistic. Nevertheless, it provides a basis for categorizing and discussing the clinical presentations.

Radial deficiency describes a spectrum of osseous, musculotendinous, and neuromuscular congenital dysplasias of the radial border of the upper limb.[2] There are associated skeletal, hematologic, cardiac, renal, and gastrointestinal defects[3–9] that may be overlooked initially because of the more obvious manifestations of radial dysplasia. It is important to identify hematologic and cardiac abnormalities, particularly when a corrective surgical procedure is anticipated.

The dysplastic manifestations differ in each patient, ranging from the minimal findings noted in congenital hypoplasia of the thenar muscles to the more severe anatomic and functional abnormalities of an absent thumb or radial club hand. This section discusses the individual characteristics and potential treatment op-

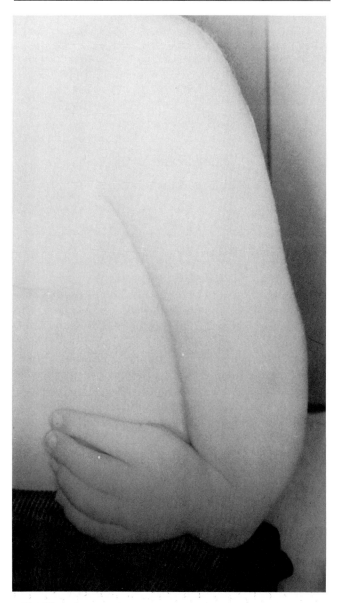

Fig. 3C-1 Patient who has radial club hand shows clubbed appearance of the left upper extremity.

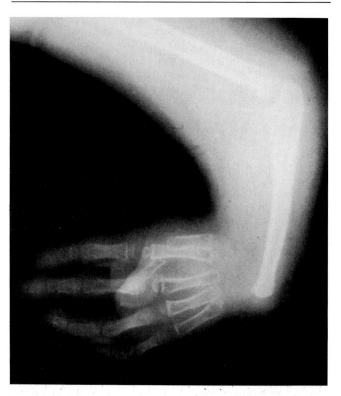

Fig. 3C-2 Radiograph of the patient in Figure 3C-1 shows an absent radius and lack of skeletal support. The carpal bones are angled and displaced radially with respect to the distal end of the ulna.

tions for (1) radial club hand, (2) aplastic thenar muscles, and (3) an absent or nonfunctioning thumb.

Radial Club Hand

Appearance

The predominant characteristics of radial club hand are defects of the radius, carpal bones, and first metacarpal of the forearm and hand. There is general hypoplasia of the upper extremity, shortening and bowing of the forearm, radial angulation, and radial displacement of the carpus with respect to the distal ulna.[10] The thumb may be absent or hypoplastic.

The clubbed appearance of the hand may be the re-

sult of various skeletal abnormalities. In most patients, the radius is partially or completely absent with a notable deficiency at the distal end, giving the forearm the appearance of a J-shaped club (Fig. 3C-1). The clubbed appearance reflects both radial displacement and radial angulation and is secondary to a lack of radial skeletal support (Fig. 3C-2). Clubbing can also occur along with a hypoplastic radius, which again provides insufficient radial skeletal support (Fig. 3C-3). Proximal radial defects with dislocation and migration of the radius are rare and are usually associated with minimal clubbing[11] (Fig. 3C-4). Significant clubbing can occur with a radius of normal length (Fig. 3C-5), but this is also extremely rare; in this situation, clubbing is thought to be secondary to underdeveloped radial carpal bones and contracted radial soft-tissue structures. A severely bowed ulna can contribute significantly to the clubbed appearance (Figs. 3C-6 and 3C-7). There is insignificant angulation or displacement of the hand, but clubbing secondary to the pronounced bowing is seen on clinical examination.

Function

Although children who have radial club hand deformities adapt adequately to their anomalous condition, there are obvious functional deficits that limit their

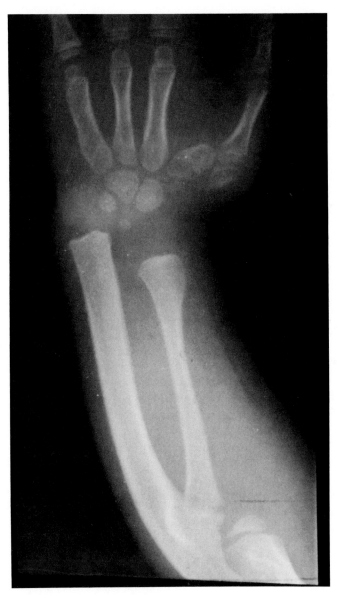

Fig. 3C–3   Radiograph of a patient who has a hypoplastic radius and club hand deformity. Note that the patient has had index finger pollicization.

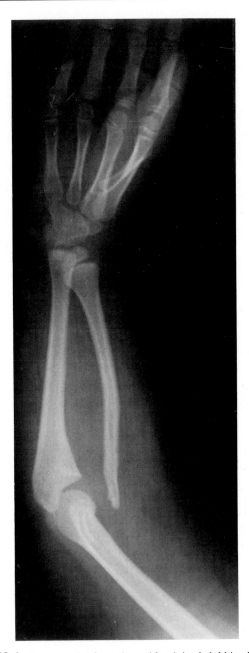

Fig. 3C–4   Radiograph of a patient with minimal clubbing because of proximal radial deficiency and proximal migration of the radius.

activities. Decreased motion is occasionally noted in the elbow joint, or the joint can be fixed in a position of extension. Wrist and finger motion may be limited, with decreased digital motion progressing in severity from the index to the small fingers.[12] The factors contributing to the restricted motion are unclear but undoubtedly include defects in the articular surface and contracted capsular and ligamentous tissue.

Two-handed activities are difficult when a normal hand must be brought to meet the shorter extremity. This discrepancy in forearm length becomes more apparent as the extremity grows, even though the percentage of deficit remains constant. When both the extremities are involved, activities are significantly impaired by the reduced length. In the presence of a severe radial deviation deformity, the fingers are located nearly in the antecubital fossa, and objects are grasped in this fossa between the fingers and the arm.

The carpus and hand of patients who have radial club hand deformities are unsupported on the radial side. As the wrist and fingers are flexed, the force of the flexor mass results in radial deviation of the hand and volar displacement of the carpus; thus, the power available for finger flexion is dissipated by an increase in the deviation deformity.

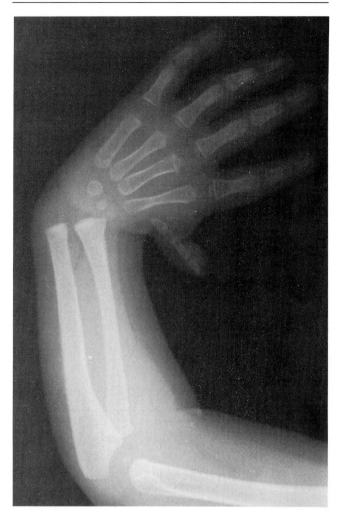

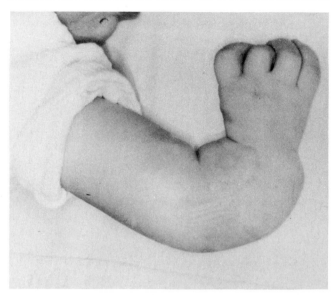

Fig. 3C–6　Photograph of patient who has apparent radial club hand deformity secondary to severe ulnar bowing. (Reproduced with permission from Manske PR, McCarroll HR Jr, Swanson K: Centralization of the radial club hand: An ulnar surgical approach. *J Hand Surg* 1981;6:423–433.)

Fig. 3C–5　Radiograph of a patient with evidence of club hand deformity and a radius and ulna of equal length. Note that the radial carpal bones have not yet ossified, but are presumed to be hypoplastic. Note also the rudimentary thumb.

Patients with a radial club hand frequently have a hypoplastic or aplastic thumb. They often develop a side-to-side pinch mechanism that is useful for handling small objects but is ineffective for grasping large objects.

Since the radial club hand anomaly was described by Petit[13] in 1733, there has been considerable interest in its surgical correction. However, surgical reconstruction of this deformity is not universally accepted. It has been suggested that the results of surgical treatment are poor and not substantially better than the preoperative condition, and that attempts to improve the deformity by surgery are ill-advised.[14] It is generally accepted that children adapt quite well to congenital deformities, and develop activity patterns that are functional. Lamb[12] documented little functional loss in the patient with unilateral radial club hand.

Objectives of Surgical Treatment

A primary objective of surgical treatment is to improve the appearance of the upper limb. Particularly in the adult, the appearance of the deformity is unsightly and attracts considerable attention. There are also several functional objectives of surgical treatment: (1) Correction of the angled position and stabilization of the carpus on the forearm improve the mechanical advantage of the forearm flexor musculature. Surgical correction decreases the abnormal radial moment of the flexor muscle mass and minimizes the power lost to radial deviation of the unstable wrist. Theoretically, this improved mechanical advantage is manifest as increased digital motion or grip strength. (2) Realignment of the hand in the direct line of the distal forearm can effectively lengthen the shortened upper extremity. (3) Reconstruction of a hypoplastic thumb or index finger pollicization is hindered by the close proximity of the hand in the clubbed position to the radial side of the forearm or the antecubital fossa. By repositioning the hand, such reconstructive procedures are more easily and effectively accomplished.

Not all of the manifestations of the radial dysplastic condition are correctable by surgery. Both the surgeon and the parents of the patient must understand that the appearance and function of the postoperative limb

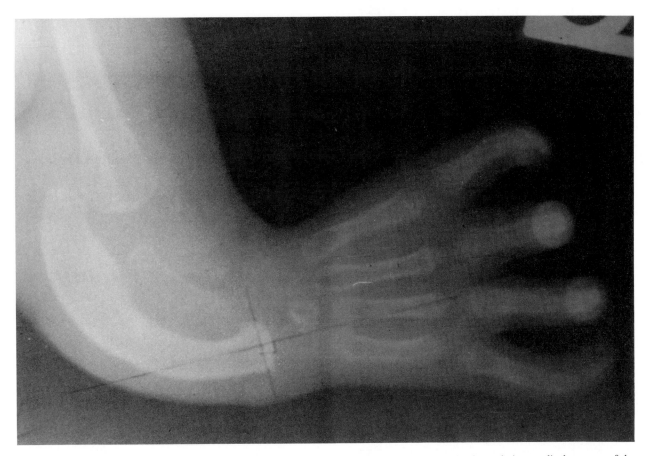

Fig. 3C-7   Radiograph of the patient in Figure 3C-6 showing severe ulnar bowing with minimal angulation or displacement of the hand with respect to the distal ulna. (Reproduced with permission from Manske PR, McCarroll HR Jr, Swanson K: Centralization of the radial club hand: An ulnar surgical approach. *J Hand Surg* 1981;6:423–433.)

will have some residual deformity. The extremity will always be relatively shortened, joint motion will be limited, grip strength will be diminished, and residual hand-forearm angulation may continue. However, the majority opinion is that surgical treatment by an experienced surgeon will considerably improve the function and appearance of the hand.

Minimal Clubbing

Minimal clubbing of less than 10 to 15 degrees may be seen with a hypoplastic radius or a proximal radial deficiency (Fig. 3C-4). This clubbing is not significant clinically and does not require surgical correction. The decision to operate is based on the clinical appearance rather than the radiographic findings, because a significant radial deficiency can be associated with minimal clubbing.

Clubbing Associated With Partial or Complete Absence of the Radius

Surgical procedures have been used most frequently to correct the radial club hand deformity associated with complete or significant distal deficiency of the ra-

dius. Many authors[15-17] suggest a preoperative period of serial casting to stretch the tight soft-tissue structures on the radial side of the forearm. The casting corrects the abnormal angulation, not the abnormal position of the carpus with respect to the distal ulna. Consequently, preoperative casting is not necessary when the clubbed hand can be passively placed in the neutral position (Fig. 3C-8).

The sensation and movement of an unencumbered hand is important to infant growth and development; therefore, if preoperative casting is used to obtain mechanical correction, it is recommended that: (1) corrective casting be postponed if surgery on the hand is to be delayed, (2) digits be left as free and mobile as possible in the corrective casts, (3) casts or splints be applied alternately rather than simultaneously in the case of bilateral radial club hand, and (4) removable splints rather than plaster casts be used to maintain a cast-corrected position.

Realignment and Stabilization of the Carpal Bones Historically, there have been several general surgical methods

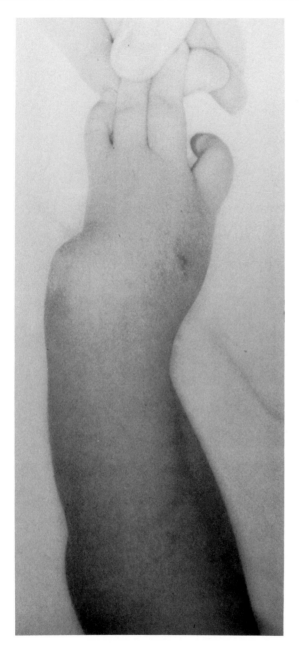

Fig. 3C-8   Patient with absent radius whose angulation deformity was easily corrected to the neutral position without serial casting. Note that although the angulation has been corrected, the carpus remains radially positioned with respect to the prominent distal ulna.

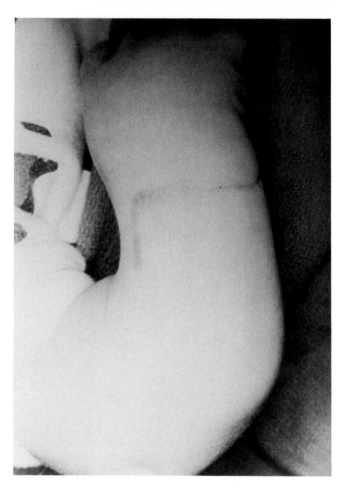

Fig. 3C-9   Postoperative photograph showing the incision I prefer for centralization. The transverse ulnar component allows excision of the excess skin and subcutaneous tissue, and the longitudinal extension on the radial side allows release of any tight or contracted tissue.

to realign and stabilize the carpal bones on the forearm. Early surgical treatment of clubbing consisted primarily of soft-tissue releases and various types of ulnar osteotomy.[15,18–20] Results of these procedures are temporary, and recurrence of the deformity is frequently noted. Several surgeons have attempted to construct an osseous support to replace the absent radius, using a free fibular graft,[21] a portion of the distal ulna,[22–24] or the proximal fibula.[25] The principle of providing a radial support is mechanically sound; however, these proce-

dures have failed primarily because the grafted component does not grow. Recent attempts to provide radial osseous support have used the proximal fibular epiphysis in experimental animals and microvascular surgical techniques.[26,27] The long-term results are not yet available. Arthrodesis of the carpal bones to the distal ulna improves the cosmetic appearance and stabilizes the wrist; however, this procedure is infrequently used by most surgeons except as a salvage procedure in the skeletally mature patient.

Centralization of the carpal bones on the distal ulna was one of the earliest described procedures and, at present, is the principal operation used to treat radial club hand. In 1893, Sayre[15] placed a sharpened distal ulna into a notch created in the carpus by excising the lunate and capitate. The paring down of the distal ulnar epiphysis must be done with caution to avoid interfering with the physeal growth plate. The procedure has been modified by several authors.[10,12,28–30]

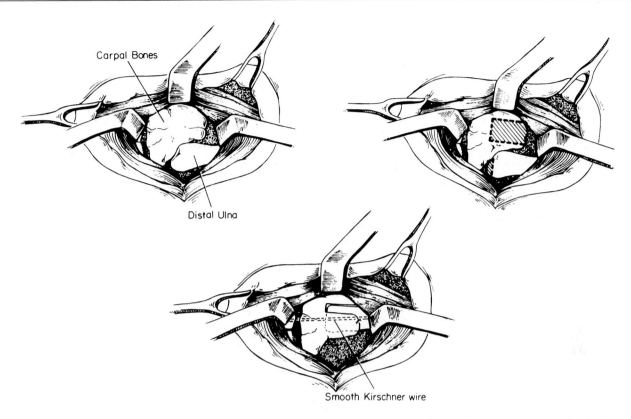

Carpal Bones

Distal Ulna

Smooth Kirschner wire

Fig. 3C–10 Diagram of a centralization procedure using an ulnar approach. (Reproduced with permission from Manske PR, McCarroll HR Jr, Swanson K: Centralization of the radial club hand: An ulnar surgical approach. *J Hand Surg* 1981;6:423–433.)

The traditional surgical approach to the wrist is through a dorsal-radial incision that enables the surgeon to release the contracted soft tissue on the radial side of the wrist. However, an ulnar incision (Fig. 3C–9) provides an easier approach to excising the mass of excess ulnar soft tissues and stabilizing the ulnar side of the wrist by capsulodesis or tendon transfers.[10]

Centralization is usually accomplished by excising a segment of the central carpal bones and placing the distal ulna in the resultant notch (Fig. 3C–10). The removal of a segment of carpal bones is in effect a reduction osteotomy, which may help to accommodate the tight radial soft-tissue structures. The distal ulna may be quite large and surrounded by adherent fibrous tissue that prevents its placement into the carpal notch. The ulna must be carefully dissected free of this tissue and reduced in size by paring down the cartilage; the surgeon must be careful to preserve the distal ulnar growth plate. Centralization has also been accomplished by placing the carpus on the distal ulna without forming a carpal notch.[31] In my experience, this results in instability and recurrence of the deformity unless the ulna is positioned radial to the carpus, as suggested by Buck-Gramcko.[29] The hand is overcorrected and ulnarly oriented; the longer ulna acts as a lever and is thought to improve the biomechanical stability of the

wrist. Most surgeons advocate temporary stabilization of the carpus on the distal ulna with a Kirschner wire that is removed at approximately two to three months.

Tendon Transfers The extensor carpi ulnaris is the principal tendon advanced to provide an ulnar and dorsiflexion vector to the wrist and hand.[3,10,16,30] The flexor carpi ulnaris,[16] flexor digitorum sublimis,[27] flexor carpi radialis,[12,32] and the common mass of radial flexor and extensor muscles[29] have also been used to contribute to the stability of the centralization procedure. The importance of these transfers to the stability and function of the centralized hand should be emphasized. However, because of the variety of anomalous conditions, the ideal tendons are not always available for transfer.

Ulnar Bowing It is uncertain whether ulnar bowing is a progressive[12,16] or a static[10,28] deformity. The ulnar bow can be corrected by single or multiple closing wedge osteotomies at the time of centralization[3,12,16,29]; as many as three osteotomies may be needed to obtain a straight ulna. The procedure is most easily performed when the radius is absent or present as a rudimentary fragment. Although this procedure straightens the forearm, the closing wedges result in reduction in the ulnar length. If length reduction is insufficient, tethering and tight-

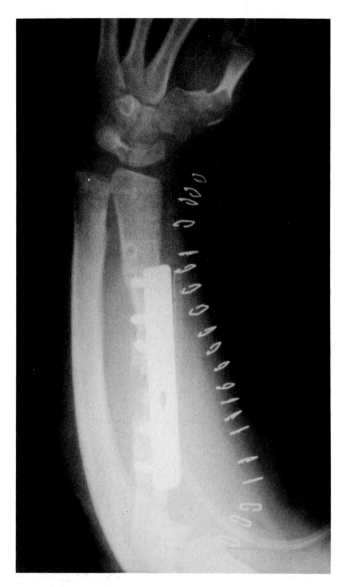

Fig. 3C–11 Radiograph of the patient shown in Figure 3C–3 after osteotomy and placement of a lengthening device. When an adequate distraction gap was obtained, the defect was filled with bone graft and maintained with plate and screws. The defect was subsequently bridged by callous and osseous union was obtained.

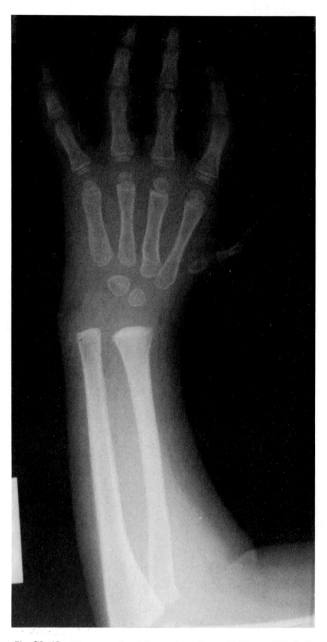

Fig. 3C–12 Photograph of the patient shown in Figure 3C–5 after release of the tight ulnar capsule, transfer of extensor carpi radialis to the distal stump of the extensor carpi ulnaris, and transfer of the extensor carpi ulnaris to the base of the third metacarpal. The radial deviation and active wrist dorsiflexion have been corrected.

ening of the radial soft-tissue structures results. It is my experience that if the osteotomies are performed as a second-stage procedure, the tightened radial structures result in recurrent radial deviation of the hand. Corrective osteotomies should be performed at the time of centralization prior to the placement of the carpus on the distal ulna, rather than subsequent to this placement.

Clubbing Associated With Shortened Distal Radius

In a small number of radial club hands, the distal radius is 1 to 2 cm shorter than the distal ulna (Fig. 3C–3). Little has been written about this deformity. I have treated several of these patients by radial length-

ening (Fig. 3C–11), using an osteotomy of the mid-shaft of the radius and applying an external fixator that is advanced as tolerated (up to 1 mm/day). After a distraction gap of 15 to 20 mm is achieved, the defect is filled with bone graft and maintained with plate and screw fixation. Although the clubbing can be significantly improved with this technique, recurrence of the deformity has made it necessary to repeat the bone lengthening procedure after several years; this is probably because of the decreased growth at the distal radius.

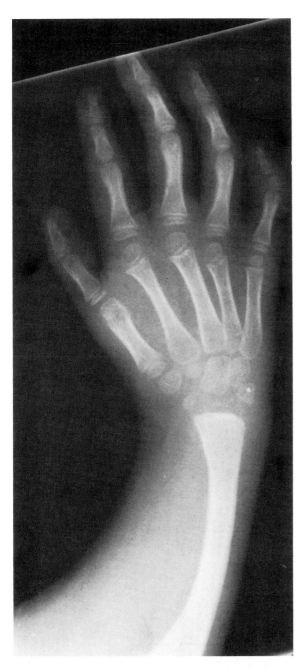

Fig. 3C–13 Radiograph of a patient five years after centralization of radial club hand. Note the corrected angulation and position of the wrist and hand with respect to a widened distal ulna.

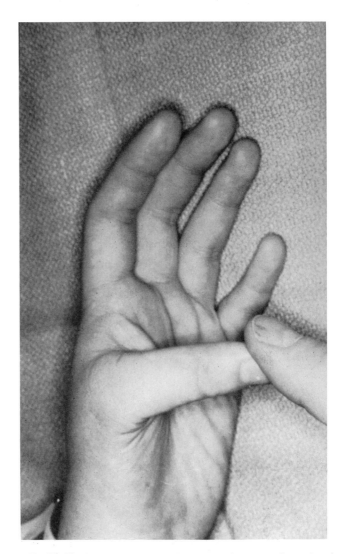

Fig. 3C–14 Patient with absent thenar muscle mass and associated laxity of the ulnar collateral ligament of the metacarpophalangeal joint of the thumb.

Clubbing Not Associated With Longitudinal Radial Deficiency

Rarely, clubbing is associated with a radius and ulna of equal lengths (Fig. 3C–5). Although the carpal bones of the patient shown in Figure 3C–5 are not yet ossified, those on the radial side are likely to be underdeveloped. The radial capsular structures were also tight in this patient, preventing ulnar deviation. Treatment consisted of only soft-tissue procedures. The tight radial capsule and soft-tissue structures were surgically released. The extensor carpi radialis was transferred to the distal insertional stump of the extensor carpi ulnaris to facilitate ulnar deviation, and the extensor carpi ulnaris was transferred to the base of the third metacarpal to improve wrist dorsiflexion. This procedure corrects the clubbing and provides dorsiflexion of the wrist (Fig. 3C–12).

Results of Surgery

Most authors agree that the appearance of the deformed upper extremity is improved by surgery (Fig. 3C–13), although few have quantitated their results. Lamb[12] observed a quantitative improvement from a preoperative radial deviation angle of 78 degrees to a postoperative angle of 22 degrees after centralization. McCarroll and I[10] noted an improvement of 26 degrees in the radial angulation and an improved carpal position from 10 mm radial to 12 mm ulnar to the longitudinal axis of the distal ulna. Buck-Gramcko[29] reported postoperative wrist extension from neutral to 20 de-

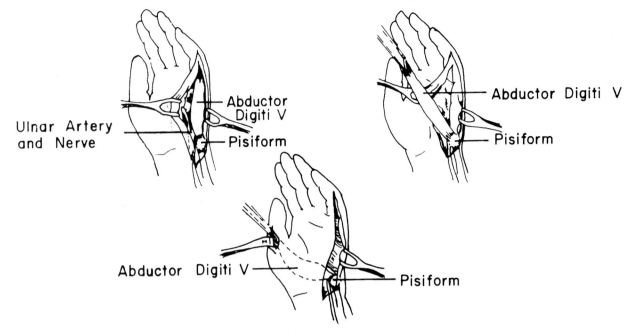

Fig. 3C-15   Diagram of abductor digiti minimi opponensplasty.

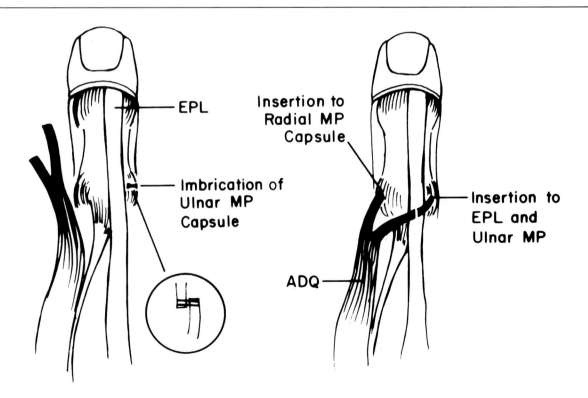

Fig. 3C-16   Diagram demonstrating imbrication of the ulnar capsule of the metacarpophalangeal joint and insertion of the two tendon ends to obtain ulnar capsular stability at that joint. (Reproduced with permission from Manske PR, McCarroll HR Jr: Abductor digiti minimi opponensplasty in congenital radial dysplasia. *J Hand Surg* 1978;3:552–559.)

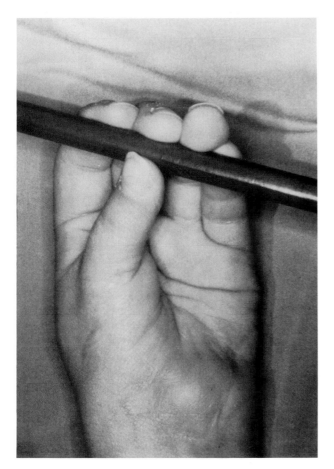

Fig. 3C-17 Patient with absent thenar musculature treated with abductor digiti minimi opponensplasty. Note that the abductor digiti quinti at the base of the palm pulls the thumb into opposition for improved pinch.

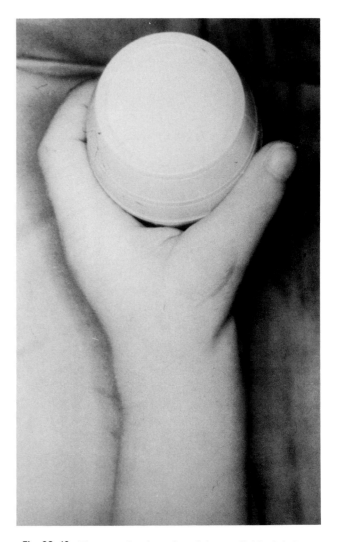

Fig. 3C-18 Photograph taken after abductor digiti minimi opponensplasty and stabilization of the ulnar collateral ligament of the metacarpophalangeal joint.

grees and postoperative wrist flexion from 40 to 90 degrees. Bora and associates[17] noted digital motion in postcentralization patients to be 54% of normal compared with 27% of normal in patients who did not have surgery.

Postcentralization improvement of specific functional activities is difficult to document in a growing child, because children generally adapt well to the limitations of congenital deformities. Lamb[12] noted no deterioration of functional activities with the centralization procedure, and emphasized the functional benefits of surgery in patients with bilateral involvement.

The potential adverse effects of centralization have also been acknowledged. Bora and associates[28] noted unsatisfactory results in 28% of patients, primarily because of recurrence of the original radial deviation deformity. Retardation of growth at the distal ulna is associated with injury to the physeal plate at the time of surgery.[17,33] Lamb[12] indicated that this occurred only when the centralization procedure was performed in children over 8 years of age.

Thenar Muscle Deficiency

Congenital absence or hypoplasia of the thenar muscles is a subtle manifestation of radial dysplasia. It is frequently unrecognized by parents, pediatricians, and treating surgeons (Fig. 3C–14). The deficiency is confined to the median innervated abductor pollicis brevis and opponens pollicis muscles, which are essential to thumb opposition. I have not noted congenital absence of the adductor pollicis and flexor pollicis brevis muscles in association with radial dysplasia. An associated component of thenar muscle deficiency is laxity and instability of the ulnar collateral ligament at the metacarpophalangeal joint. In rare cases, both the radial and ulnar collateral ligaments are unstable.

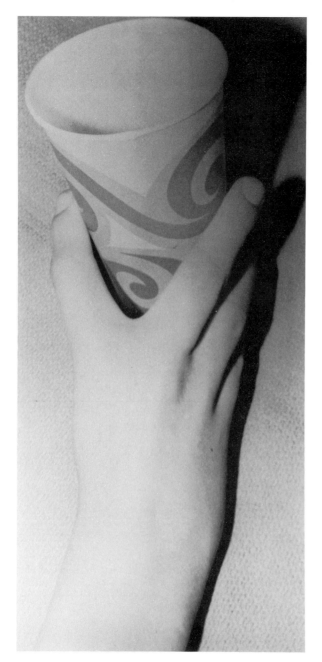

Fig. 3C–19 Patient with absent thumb demonstrating difficulty in grasping large objects.

Weakness of opposition and instability of the collateral ligaments at the metacarpophalangeal joint constitute a significant functional disability, because it interferes with the child's ability to rotate the thumb in front of the fingers and stabilize the thumb for effective pinch activities. Numerous opponensplasty procedures have been described. I prefer using the abductor digiti quinti muscle transfer[34,35] (Fig. 3C–15) described originally by Huber[36] and Nicholaysen[37] for median nerve injury and poliomyelitis. The transferred abductor digiti quinti is the same length, of similar strength, and

pulls in the correct direction with respect to the deficient muscles of opposition. Cosmetically, it adds muscle mass in the thenar eminence.

Stabilization of the metacarpophalangeal joint at the time of opponensplasty is also essential to the restoration of thumb function. In the younger child, this can usually be accomplished by imbricating the ulnar capsule at the metacarpophalangeal joint and reinforcing it with the distal end of the abductor digiti quinti tendon used in the opponensplasty[34] (Fig. 3C–16). In the older child, the surgeon may choose to stabilize the metacarpophalangeal joint by arthrodesis. Infrequently, the radial collateral ligament is also deficient. In this case, capsular stabilization is difficult and arthrodesis is recommended.

Postoperative functional improvement in prehensile pinching activities has been noted consistently by patients and parents (Figs. 3C–17 and 3C–18). Postoperative fibrosis of the transferred muscle in two patients was the only complication I noted. This procedure is a muscle transfer, not a tendon transfer; consequently, a sufficiently large subcutaneous tunnel must be developed across the palm to accommodate the muscle mass. Additionally, recent studies in my laboratory have indicated that the muscle should not be detached from its origin on the pisiform bone at the time of transfer, because this osseous origin constitutes a significant source of vascularization to the muscle.

Absent or Nonfunctioning Thumb

Function

The child with the absent or nonfunctioning thumb adapts quite well, and becomes facile in using the remaining digits for picking up and grasping small objects by a side-to-side pinch. This usually involves a combination of the index and long fingers, but at times the interspaces between the long and ring fingers or the ring and small fingers are used. Children frequently develop a widened interdigital interspace and the ability to rotate the index finger 80 to 90 degrees (autopollicization). Functional difficulties arise primarily when attempting to handle large objects. Insufficient space between the digits and the absence of opposition results in a lack of power for grasping activities (Fig. 3C–19).

Concepts of Pollicization

The standard surgical treatment of an absent or nonfunctioning thumb is pollicization of the index finger[38–40] in a single-stage transfer on its neurovascular pedicle to a position of opposition. The procedure has three primary objectives: (1) to improve the grasp of large objects, (2) to improve the appearance of the hand (a thumb and three-fingered hand is a less noticeable abnormality than a four-fingered hand without a thumb), and (3) to facilitate handshake when the right hand is

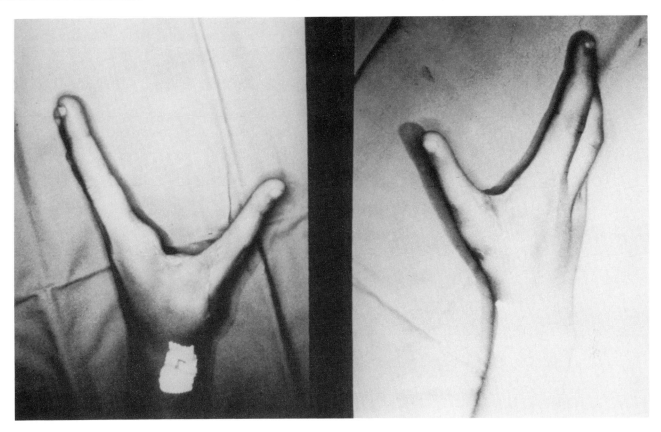

Fig. 3C-20 Photograph of patient with bilateral absent thumb after pollicization. Note that the pollicized digit on the left has the appearance of a finger projecting from the base of the palm, and the pollicized digit on the right has the appearance of a thumb. The difference results from placing the web space in a position to join the pollicized digit at the level of the proximal interphalangeal joint, rather than maintaining it in its normal position near the metacarpophalangeal joint.

involved. In my opinion, pollicization is indicated bilaterally when both hands are affected.

In contrast to traumatic thumb amputation, free tissue transfer of a toe is not usually regarded as an appropriate alternative to pollicization in the case of congenital deficiency.[41] Pollicization is preferred because the proximal musculotendinous and neurovascular structures necessary for toe transfer are usually absent in congenital thumb aplasia. In addition, the thumb-deficient child has no representation for the absent thumb on the cerebral cortex and, therefore, would not be likely to use the transferred toe for functional activities. In thumb agenesis, the index finger is cortically represented as the radial digit. Repositioning this finger to a position of opposition by surgical pollicization presents no problem in cortical recognition.

The timing of surgery is somewhat controversial. It has been advocated that pollicization be performed at 6 to 12 months of age,[40] because this is the time that the normal child develops awareness of the cortical representation of a normal thumb. However, in thumb agenesis, the index finger is cortically represented as the radial post, and the timing of the surgical repositioning of this digit should not be age-dependent.

McCarroll and I have performed the pollicization procedure[42] on children from 9 months to 16 years old and have observed no age-related difference in the initiation of voluntary activity or the cortical recognition of the transposed digit as a thumb. Patients usually initiate motion and functional use of the hand by three to four months after surgery, but this can be delayed as long as two years postoperatively. The longest functional delay in my experience occurred in a 2-year-old child. Early surgery is encouraged for social reasons related to restoring a more normal appearance to the hand, not for enhancing the cortical representation of the digit as the thumb or improving function.

For a child with a hypoplastic thumb, the surgeon must decide whether to attempt reconstruction of the hypoplastic ray by skeletal stabilization, tendon transfers, and deepening of the thumb-index web space, or whether it is more appropriate to ablate the hypoplastic digit and pollicize the index finger. This decision is most appropriately made by observing the child during activities. If the child attempts to use the thumb during activity, then reconstruction is appropriate. However, if the child ignores the thumb, ablation and index finger pollicization is preferable to reconstruction no matter

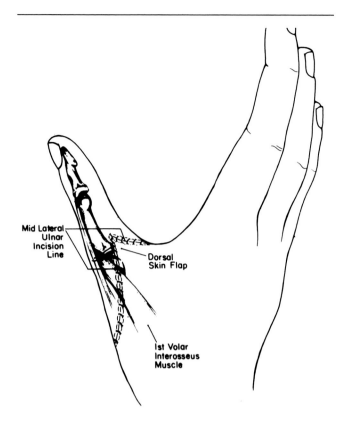

Mid Lateral
Ulnar
Incision
Line

Dorsal
Skin Flap

Ist Volar
Interosseus
Muscle

Fig. 3C-21 Drawing of the ulnar side of the transposed digit shows the ulnar midlateral incision through which the palmar interosseous muscle was attached; the incision was not closed, but was allowed to gap open, forming an inverted V. The dorsal skin was tailored to fit into the inverted V. (Reproduced with permission from Manske PR, McCarroll HR Jr: Index finger pollicization for a congenitally absent or nonfunctioning thumb. *J Hand Surg* 1985;10A:606–613.)

how large the thumb appears. A surgical procedure will facilitate the function of an already useful digit, but it will not reprogram the cerebral cortex to use an ignored digit. This concept is obviously not applicable in cultures where social values dictate that a five-digit hand is more important than a functioning thumb.

The functional quality of the pollicized digit is related to the preoperative condition of the index finger, which has varying degrees of joint motion and tendon excursion. The index finger with very little motion preoperatively does not function as effectively after transposition as a finger with normal motion. The patient, parents, and surgeon must be aware that more extensive involvement limits improvement.

Surgical Procedure

The technical principles and concepts of pollicization have been well described and outlined.[38–40] These principles include skeletal shortening by reduction osteotomy of the metacarpal, repositioning of the digit proximally with 120-degree rotation, and intrinsic tendon transfers using the first dorsal and first volar interos-

seous muscle to function as the abductor pollicis brevis and the adductor pollicis, respectively. The surgeon should make the transposed digit resemble a thumb as much as possible, rather than a finger projecting from the base of the palm (Fig. 3C–20). In the normal hand, the web space joins the thumb on the ulnar side at the metacarpophalangeal joint. Therefore, the web space should also join the pollicized thumb at the metacarpophalangeal joint, which is actually the proximal interphalangeal joint of the transposed index finger. This can be accomplished by making a mid-lateral ulnar incision to reattach the volar interosseous muscle, which is then left open as an inverted V, and the resultant gap is filled in with dorsal skin[42] (Fig. 3C–21). This web-space attachment improves the appearance of the transposed digit so that it better resembles a thumb.

Subsequent surgical procedures may be needed to maximize the results of pollicization, including tenolysis, bone shortening, or scar revision.[43] In our study of 40 index finger pollicization procedures, McCarroll and I found that 20 required a subsequent operation and six required more than one additional procedure.[42] Subsequent surgical procedures were required most often in patients who had more notable manifestations of radial dysplasia preoperatively, such as radial club hand, presumably reflecting a more severely affected index finger. An abductor digiti quinti opponensplasty was necessary in 18 patients, even though the transferred first dorsal interosseous muscle was functioning after pollicization. The first dorsal interosseous muscle is often hypoplastic as a component of the radial dysplasia, and its origin from the base of the transposed digit is less biomechanically effective for functional opposition than a more ulnar origin. The abductor digiti quinti opponensplasty improved opposition and pinch in all patients. Extensor tendon shortening was not performed at the initial pollicization in this series of patients, and was necessary as a subsequent procedure in four patients. Arthrodesis of an unstable or deformed interphalangeal joint was performed in four patients.

The results of pollicization reported by numerous authors are positive.[38–40] In my series, there was no loss of a pollicized digit because of vascular insufficiency and no evidence of altered sensation. No patient rejected or avoided using the pollicized digit. All patients used the transposed digit to grasp large objects. All five patients who used the interspaces between the long and ring fingers or the ring and small fingers for grasping preoperatively continued to do so postoperatively when handling small objects; however, all five used the pollicized digit for grasping large objects. This suggests that the surgical procedure does not cause patients to alter previously established grasping patterns that are functioning effectively. Although the surgeon can reposition a digit to improve hand function, the procedure does not reprogram the central nervous system.

Summary

Radial deficiency has a spectrum of manifestations limited primarily to absent structures on the preaxial border of the forearm and hand. Surgical procedures treat the radial club hand, deficient thenar muscles, and the absent or nonfunctioning thumb and improve the appearance and function of the hand.

References

1. Beatty E: Upper limb tissue differentiation in the human embryo. *Hand Clin* 1985;1:391–403.
2. Pardini AG Jr: Radial dysplasia. *Clin Orthop* 1968;57:153–177.
3. Goldberg MJ, Meyn M: The radial clubhand. *Orthop Clin North Am* 1976;7:341–349.
4. Goldberg MJ, Bartoshesky LE: Congenital hand anomaly: Etiology and associated malformations. *Hand Clin* 1985;1:405–415.
5. Holt M, Oram S: Familial heart disease with skeletal malformations. *Br Heart J* 1960;22:236–242.
6. Schoenecker PL, Cohn AK, Sedgwick WG, et al: Dysplasia of the knee associated with the syndrome of thrombocytopenia and absent radius. *J Bone Joint Surg* 1984;66A:421–427.
7. Temtamy S, McKusick V: *The Genetics of Hand Malformations.* New York, Alan R Liss, 1978.
8. Fanconi G: Familial constitutional panmyelocytopathy, Fanconi's anemia (F.A.): I. Clinical aspects. *Semin Hematol* 1967;4:233–240.
9. Quan L, Smith DW: The VATER association: Vertebral defects, anal atresia, T-E fistula with esophageal atresia, radial and renal dysplasia. A spectrum of associated defects. *J Pediatr* 1973;82:104–107.
10. Manske PR, McCarroll HR Jr, Swanson K: Centralization of the radial club hand: An ulnar surgical approach. *J Hand Surg* 1981;6:423–433.
11. Skerick SK, Flatt AE: The anatomy of congenital radial dysplasia: Its surgical and functional implications. *Clin Orthop* 1969;66:125–143.
12. Lamb DW: Radial club hand: A continuing study of sixty-eight patients with one hundred and seventeen club hands. *J Bone Joint Surg* 1977;59A:1–13.
13. Petit JL: Remarques sur un enfant nouveau-né, dont les bras etaint difformes. *Mem Acad R Soc,* 1733, p 17.
14. Lloyd-Roberts GC: *Orthopaedics in Infancy and Childhood.* New York, Appleton-Century-Crofts, 1971.
15. Sayre RH: A contribution to the study of club-hand. *Trans Am Orthop Assoc* 1893;6:208–216.
16. Bayne LG: Radial club hand (radial deficiencies), in Green DP (ed): *Operative Hand Surgery,* ed 2. New York, Churchill Livingstone, 1988, vol 1, pp 261–275.
17. Bora FW Jr, Osterman AL, Kaneda RR, et al: Radial club-hand deformity: Long-term follow-up. *J Bone Joint Surg* 1981;63A:741–745.
18. Bardenheuer B: Vorstellung von 4 Patienten, an welchen die totale Resektion des ganzen Hüftgelenkes ausgeführt worden war. *Ber Verh Dtsch Ges Chir* 1894;23:105–107.
19. Hoffa A: *Lehrbuch der Orthopadischden Chirurgie,* ed 4. Stuttgart, Ferdinand Enke, 1902.
20. Romano C: Grave mano torta congenita: Raddrizzamento mercè osteoectomia segmentaria trapezoidale del cubito e tenotomia del muscolo grande palmare. *Arch Ortop* 1894;11:80–93.
21. Albee FH: Formation of radius congenitally absent: Condition seven years after implantation of bone graft. *Ann Surg* 1928;87:105–110.
22. Antonelli I: Su un caso macanza congenita bilaterale del radio. *Gazz Med Ital* 1904;55:501–513.

23. Ryerson EW, cited by Kato K: Congenital absence of the radius: With review of literature and report of three cases. *J Bone Joint Surg* 1924;6:589–626.
24. Define D: Treatment of congenital radial club hand. *Clin Orthop* 1970;73:153–159.
25. Starr DE: Congenital absence of the radius: A method of surgical correction. *J Bone Joint Surg* 1945;27:572–577.
26. Tsai TM: Free epiphyseal transfers. *Orthop Trans* 1985;9:409–410.
27. Yamauchi Y: Vascularized epiphyseal transfers: Animal experiments and some clinical experiences. *Orthop Trans* 1985;9:409.
28. Bora FW Jr, Nicholson JT, Cheema HM: Radial meromelia: The deformity and its treatment. *J Bone Joint Surg* 1970;52A:966–979.
29. Buck-Gramcko D: Radialization as a new treatment for radial club hand. *J Hand Surg* 1985;10A:964–968.
30. Lidge RT: Congenital radial deficient club hand. *J Bone Joint Surg* 1969;51A:1041–1042.
31. Watson HK, Beebe RD, Cruz NI: A centralization procedure for radial clubhand. *J Hand Surg* 1984;9A:541–547.
32. Snyder M, Faflik J: Leczenie wrodzonej reki koslawej. *Chir Narzadow Ruchu Ortop Pol* 1984;49:47–50.
33. Hippe P, Blauth W: Erfahrungen mit Klumphandoperationen. *Z Orthop* 1979;117:863–872.
34. Littler JW, Cooley SGE: Opposition of the thumb and its restoration by abductor digiti quinti transfer. *J Bone Joint Surg* 1963;45A:1389–1396.
35. Manske PR, McCarroll HR Jr: Abductor digiti minimi opponensplasty in congenital radial dysplasia. *J Hand Surg* 1978;3:552–559.
36. Huber E: Hilfsoperation bei Medianuslähmung. *Dtsch Z Chir* 1921;162:271–275.
37. Nicholaysen J: Nordisk Kirurgisk Forenung Fochandlingar. *Acta Chir Scand* 1923;55:183–184.
38. Littler JW: The neurovascular pedicle method of digital transposition for reconstruction of the thumb. *Plast Reconstr Surg* 1953;12:303–319.
39. Milford L: Amputations, in Crenshaw AH (ed): *Campbell's Operative Orthopaedics,* ed 7. St. Louis, CV Mosby, 1987, pp 291–323.
40. Buck-Gramcko D: Pollicization of the index finger: Method and results in aplasia and hypoplasia of the thumb. *J Bone Joint Surg* 1971;53A:1605–1617.
41. May JW Jr, Smith RJ, Peimer CA: Toe-to-hand free tissue transfer for thumb construction with multiple digit aplasia. *Plast Reconstr Surg* 1981;67:205–213.
42. Manske PR, McCarroll HR Jr: Index finger pollicization for a congenitally absent or nonfunctioning thumb. *J Hand Surg* 1985;10A:606–613.
43. Egloff DV, Verdan C: Pollicization of the index finger for reconstruction of the congenitally hypoplastic or absent thumb. *J Hand Surg* 1983;8:839–848.

P A R T   D

Ulnar Deficiency

Paul R. Manske, MD

Introduction

Congenital ulnar deficiency comprises a spectrum of developmental anomalies of the postaxial (ulnar) border of the upper limb. Although the abnormalities follow a longitudinal axis, ulnar deficiency is not the exact counterpart of radial deficiency. The hand anomalies in ulnar deficiency occur on both the ulnar and radial

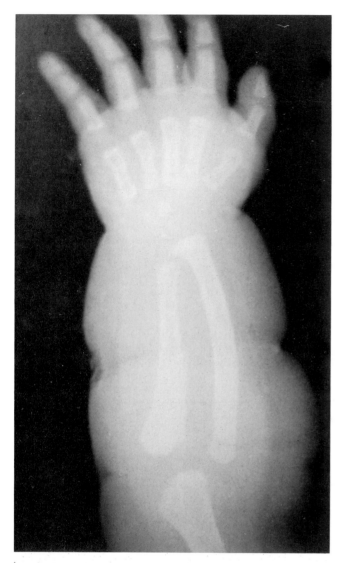

Fig. 3D-1   Ulnar deficiency as noted by hypoplasia of the ulna, in association with ulnar tilt of the distal radial epiphysis and probable radial head dislocation. Note the apparently normal appearance of the hand.

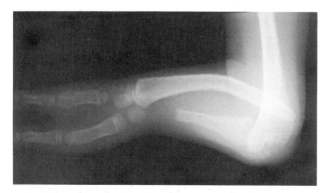

Fig. 3D-2   Ulnar deficiency with partial aplasia of the ulna. Note the bowed radius and dislocated radial head. The elbow has limited range of motion but is stable.

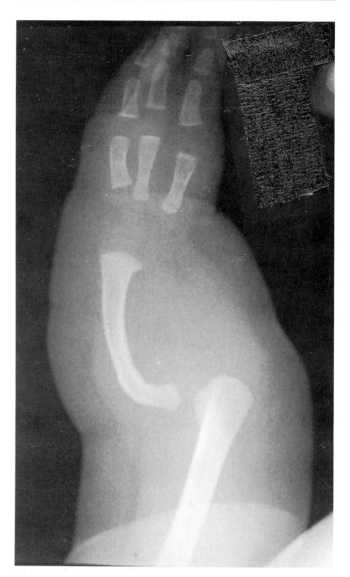

Fig. 3D-3   Ulnar deficiency with total absence of the ulna. Note the radial bow and dislocated radial head. The elbow is stable.

sides of the hand. Associated hematologic, cardiac, gastrointestinal, and genitourinary anomalies are unusual.

Ulnar deficiency is the least common manifestation of upper extremity failure of formation. A recent review by Johnson and Omer[1] identified only 185 reported cases. Their report collates the combined data excellently. Nearly one half of patients who have ulnar deficiency have an anomaly of the opposite hand, although not necessarily one of ulnar deficiency; almost one half have other musculoskeletal abnormalities.

Five different classification systems have been proposed,[2-7] based primarily on the radiologic status of the ulna. I prefer the classification suggested by Bayne[6]: type I, hypoplastic ulna (Fig. 3D-1); type II, partial ulnar aplasia (Fig. 3D-2); type III, total ulnar aplasia (Fig. 3D-3); and type IV, radial-humeral synostosis (Fig.

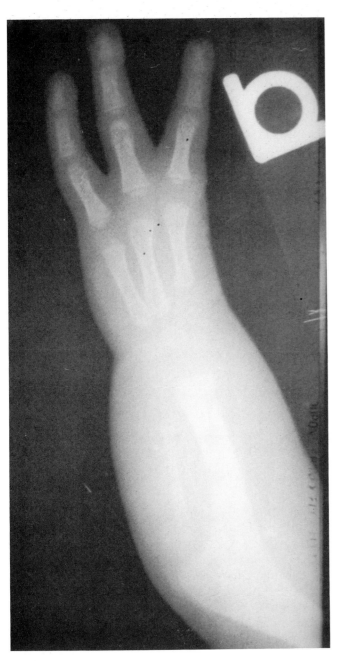

Fig. 3D–4   Radial-humeral synostosis. A rudimentary ulna persists. Note the three-digit hand with absence of a thumb ray.

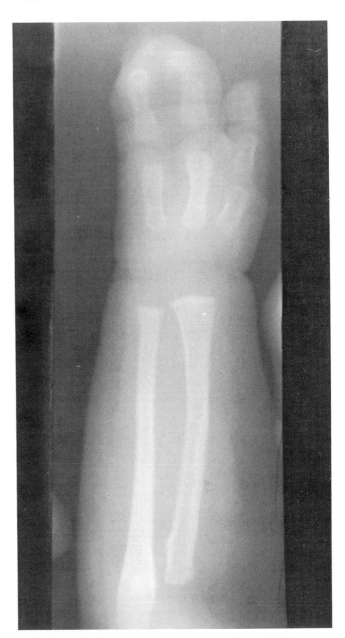

Fig. 3D–5   Radiograph of a patient with deficient ulnar rays in the hand but a normal ulna. The proposed classification systems currently in use do not consider this form of ulnar deficiency.

3D–4). None of the proposed classification systems correlate with specific hand abnormalities or with functional limitations of the upper extremity; therefore, they do not help to determine functional status or identify which patients will require surgical procedures. Furthermore, none of the classification systems includes the ulnar-deficient hand (a hand without fourth and fifth rays) with a normal ulna (Fig. 3D–5). This defect is the counterpart of the radial-deficient hand with an absent thumb and normal radius.

Skeletal Abnormalities

The entire upper extremity is somewhat hypoplastic in patients who have congenital ulnar deficiency and the most obvious abnormalities are located distal to the elbow in the forearm, wrist, and hand. The most significant abnormality proximal to the elbow is marked internal rotation and anterior bowing that orients the hand in a posterior direction (Figs. 3D–6 and 3D–7). This condition can occur in patients who have radial-humeral synostosis.

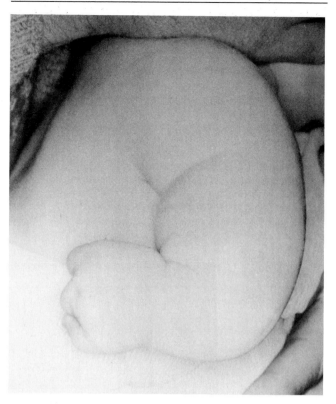

Fig. 3D–6 Lateral photograph of patient with radial-humeral synostosis, characterized by a severe anterior bow of the fused bones so that the hand is oriented posteriorly. (Note that the patient is facing to the right.)

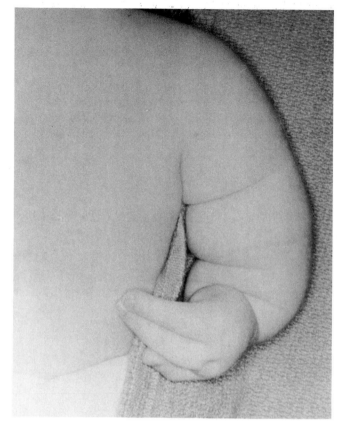

Fig. 3D–7 Posterior view of patient with radial-humeral synostosis and severe anterior bowing of the fused bone.

Elbow

The appearance and function of the elbow vary considerably depending on the position of the radial head. (1) The elbow may have normal or slightly limited range of motion and a reduced radial head. (2) The elbow may be stable but have a flexion contracture. This can occur with a distally deficient or completely absent ulna (Figs. 3D–2 and 3D–3). (3) Infrequently, the elbow may be unstable and the ulna completely absent. (4) The elbow may be in a fixed position when there is a radial-humeral synostosis; this is the most functionally limiting elbow deformity (Fig. 3D–4).

Forearm and Wrist

In congenital ulnar deficiency, the radius is always present, which provides a stable wrist articulation, but it is frequently bowed and characterized by an ulnar concavity. The ulna is completely absent in 22% of cases, partially absent in 61%, and hypoplastic in 16%. Even when the ulna is hypoplastic or only partially absent, radial growth and ulnar growth occur at relatively equal rates.[1]

The wrist is stable, but it may be in a position of ulnar deviation secondary to absent ulnar carpal bones and to ulnar tilt of the distal radial epiphysis. The appearance of ulnar deviation may be accentuated by the radial bowing. The ulnar deviation is thought to be nonprogressive, and rarely results in a functional disability.

A fibrous cartilaginous anlage connects the distal end of the rudimentary ulna to the distal radius and carpal bones.[3,8-11] Although the presence of the anlage is well accepted, its relationship to the various forearm and wrist deformities has not been established conclusively. The anlage may act as a static tether that may be responsible for decreased growth at the distal radial epiphysis, ulnar deviation of the wrist and hand, bowing of the radius, and dislocation of the radial head. This concept of tethering is appealing; however, other investigators[1,7,12,13] have noted that these deformities are relatively static, and think that the role of the anlage in their development is minimal or insignificant.

Hand

Hand abnormalities, such as hypoplasia, ectrodactyly, syndactyly, and digital malrotation, are frequently present and constitute the primary disability in patients who have ulnar deficiency. Syndactyly (Fig. 3D–8) occurs in 34% of patients; 89% of patients have one or more absent digits that are not restricted to the ulnar side of the hand (Fig. 3D–4). Thumb ray abnormalities

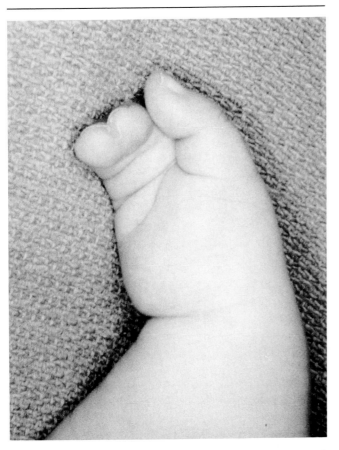

Fig. 3D-8 Patient with ulnar dysplasia characterized by absent ulnar rays and syndactyly of the remaining digits.

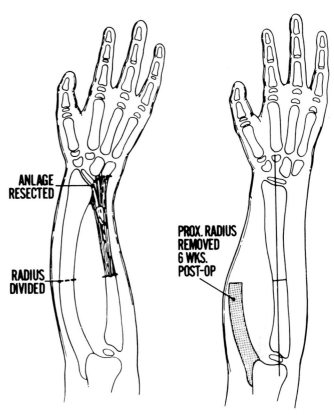

Fig. 3D-9 Drawing of surgical procedure creating a one-bone forearm using the radius and partially deficient ulna. The procedure is recommended only in the presence of an unstable forearm. (Reproduced with permission from Bayne LG: Ulnar club hand, in Green DP (ed). *Operative Hand Surgery*. New York, Churchill Livingstone, 1982, pp 25–257.)

occur in over half of the reported cases, an interesting fact from the viewpoint of developmental anatomy. This suggests that the early limb bud cells that develop into the thumb may be located near the postaxial border initially and migrate to the radial position as the five-digit hand evolves.

Surgical Treatment

Despite the obvious deformities, patients who have ulnar deficiency frequently have few functional limitations,[9,14] and these can be improved by surgery. Functionally, the most significant abnormalities occur in the hand. Several surgical procedures done proximal to the hand and wrist should be considered; however, these are performed infrequently. These procedures include radial-humeral osteotomy, radial head resection, and reconstruction of a one-bone forearm.

Radial-humeral synostosis is functionally limiting because elbow motion is not possible. Usually, the extremity is shortened and adequate wrist motion is present, so that the shortened arm can be used in conjunction with the opposite extremity or to hold objects against the body. Surgical correction is necessary

when there is a severe anterior bow that positions the hand posteriorly (Figs. 3D–6 and 3D–7). The hand and digits can be placed into a more functional position by using multiple closing wedge osteotomies.[7] Occasionally, rotational osteotomy must also be done to correct a severely supinated or pronated position.

Radial head resection[6,9] is infrequently necessary, because the elbow is usually stable and functions well despite the dislocated bone; it is unlikely that radial head resection alone would improve motion because of the other associated forearm abnormalities. Resection should be performed only when increased elbow motion is necessary and, preferably, at the time of skeletal maturity.

Reconstruction of a one-bone forearm[6,8,10,11] or establishing a proximal radial-ulnar synostosis[15] must also be considered in the unusual circumstance of forearm instability. I prefer the two-stage technique described by Bayne[6] (Fig. 3D–9).

Resection of the fibrocartilaginous anlage has been strongly recommended by some[3,9-11] on the premise that the anlage has a tethering action on the distal radius

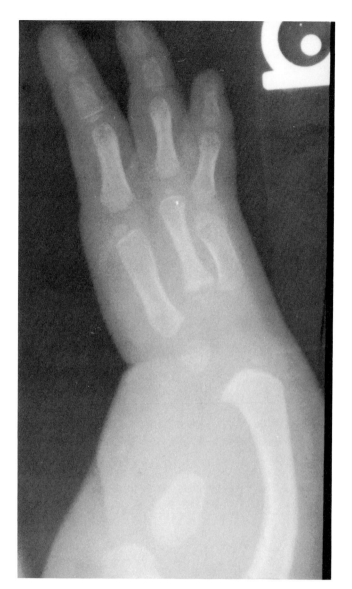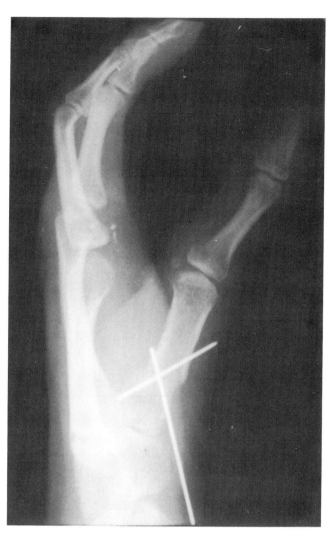

Fig. 3D-10 Absent ulnar rays. **Left:** Preoperative radiograph shows marked adduction of thumb. **Right:** Postoperative radiograph after deepening of the thumb-index web space and rotational osteotomy of the first metacarpal so that the thumb is now in opposition to the remaining digits.

and carpal bones and is responsible for the evolution of the deformities. More recent studies[1,7,12,13,16] have not documented a progression of deformity in patients whose anlage has not been resected, or they have noted insignificant functional improvement following surgery. Consequently, a more critical evaluation of this procedure is needed, and resection of the anlage is recommended only when progression of the deformity can be clearly documented.

The deformities of the hand are most improved by surgical procedures, especially those procedures that correct thumb abnormalities or syndactylized digits.

Release of syndactylized fingers using established techniques can increase the function of the limited number of digits that are present. Additionally, deepening of the thumb-index web space and rotational osteotomy of the first metacarpal (Fig. 3D–10), or pollicization (Fig. 3D–11) can provide more effective opposition for grasping. Significant improvement after correction of the hand deformities can be anticipated.[1,9]

Ulnar ray deficiency is an unusual manifestation of failure of formation. Despite the obvious deformities, patients usually function quite well. Surgical procedures principally involve the hand.

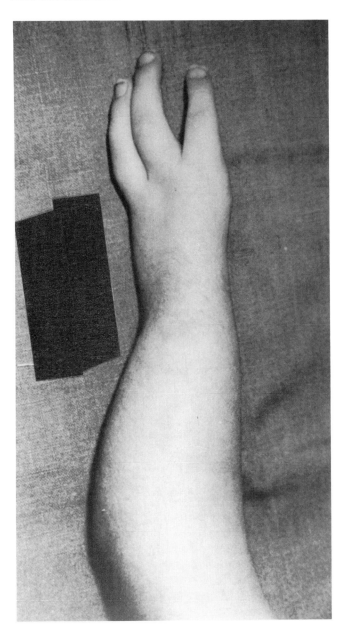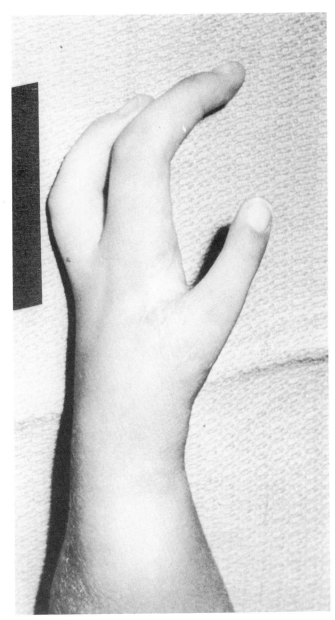

Fig. 3D-11 Absent thumb ray. **Left:** Preoperative photograph shows three digits and an absent thumb ray. **Right:** Postoperative photograph after pollicization.

References

1. Johnson J, Omer GE: Congenital ulnar deficiency, natural history and therapeutic implications. *Hand Clin* 1985;1:499–510.
2. Kummel W: *Die Missbildungen der Extremitäeten durch defekt, Verwachsung und Ueberzahl.* Kassel, Bibliotheca Medica, vol 3, 1895.
3. Ogden JA, Watson HK, Bohne W: Ulnar dysmelia. *J Bone Joint Surg* 1976;58A:467–475.
4. Swanson AB, Tada K, Yonenobu K: Ulnar ray deficiency: Its various manifestations. *J Hand Surg* 1984;9A:658–664.
5. Riordan DC: The upper limb, in Lovell WW, Winter RB (eds): *Pediatric Orthopaedics.* Philadelphia, JB Lippincott, 1978, vol 2, pp 685–719.
6. Bayne LG: Ulnar club hand (ulnar deficiencies), in Green DP (ed): *Operative Hand Surgery.* New York, Churchill Livingstone, 1982, vol 1, pp 245–257.
7. Miller JK, Wenner SM, Kruger LM: Ulnar deficiency. *J Hand Surg* 1986;11A:822–829.
8. Carroll RE, Bowers WH: Congenital deficiency of the ulna. *J Hand Surg* 1977;2:169–174.
9. Flatt AE: *The Care of Congenital Hand Anomalies.* St. Louis, CV Mosby, 1977, pp 328–341.
10. Riordan DC, Mills EH, Alldredge RH: Congenital absence of the ulna, abstract. *J Bone Joint Surg* 1961;43A:614.
11. Straub LR: Congenital absence of the ulna. *Am J Surg* 1965;109:300–305.
12. Broudy AS, Smith RJ: Deformities of the hand and wrist with ulna deficiency. *J Hand Surg* 1979;4:304–315.

13. Marcus NA, Omer GE Jr: Carpal deviation in congenital ulnar deficiency. *J Bone Joint Surg* 1984;66A:1003–1007.
14. Pardini AG Jr: Congenital absence of the ulna. *J Iowa Med Soc* 1967; 57:1106–1112.
15. Lloyd-Roberts GC: Treatment of defects of the ulna in children by establishing cross-union with the radius. *J Bone Joint Surg* 1973;55B:327–330.
16. Blair WF, Shurr DG, Buckwalter JA: Functional status in ulnar deficiency. *J Pediatr Orthop* 1983;3:37–40.

P A R T E

Central Deficiency

Paul R. Manske, MD

Central deficiency is characterized by failure of formation of one or more central rays of the hand. In contrast to radial and ulnar deficiency, there are usually no proximal wrist and forearm abnormalities. The deformity was first described in a 1770 report by the East India Trading Company on the status of its South American Dutch Guiana Colony.[1] This rather grotesque condition was described as "crawfish claw" and has subsequently been referred to as "lobster claw" or "split-hand." I prefer to use "cleft hand" as a more sensitive term to describe this anomaly of central ectrodactyly.

The defect always includes partial or complete

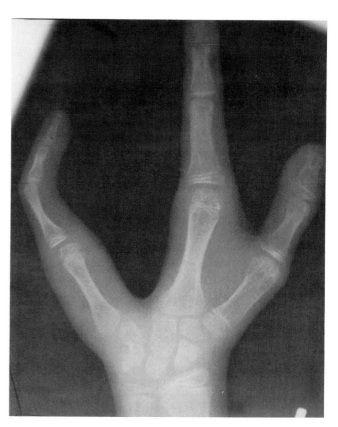

Fig. 3E–2 Radiograph of a patient who has a central defect that includes absent long and ring finger rays. Note the normal configuration of the carpal bones.

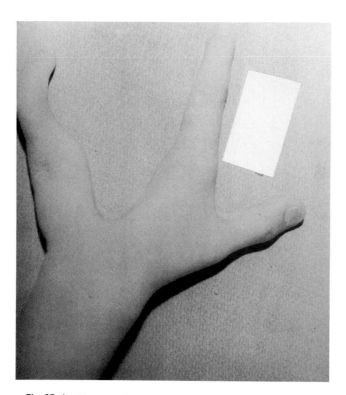

Fig. 3E–1 Photograph of a patient who has a severe central defect that includes absent long and ring finger rays.

suppression of formation of the middle ray, and involvement of the adjacent index and long finger rays varies. The border digits are usually present, at least in part. Although monodactylous hands have been considered a severe form,[2-4] they are not usually considered a central ray deficiency.[5-6] The defect has not been noted proximal to the wrist, although associated carpal coalescence and radial-ulnar synostosis have been reported.[7]

Classification

There have been several attempts to classify the central deformity, but the use of terminology varies. The simplest classification system categorizes the deformity by the digital rays present and the number of deficient bones in each ray.[5,8-10] Other systems distinguish between the typical and the atypical cleft hand. Although the terms are recognized by most investigators, the specific features of this classification are not universally accepted. The typical cleft hand is often inherited as an autosomal dominant trait and is characterized by partial or complete absence of one or more of the three central rays with border digits present (Figs. 3E–1 and

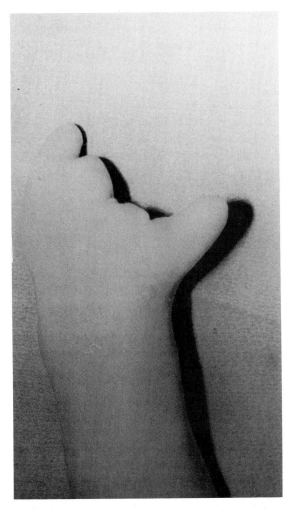

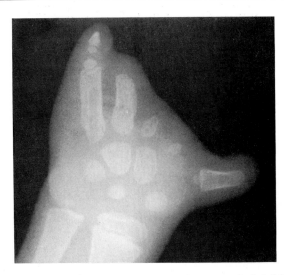

Fig. 3E–4 Radiograph of a patient who has an atypical cleft hand. Note the small border digits and the potential block to pinching by the rudimentary central metacarpals.

Fig. 3E–3 Photograph of a patient who has an atypical cleft hand. Note the hypoplastic border digits and the redundant skin in the central portion of the hand.

3E–2). It usually occurs bilaterally and is frequently associated with central ray defects of the feet.

The atypical cleft hand is characterized by absence of the three central rays and hypoplasia or partial absence of the border rays (Figs. 3E–3 and 3E–4). Although the atypical form might be considered a more extensive presentation of the typical cleft hand, this concept is probably not accurate. There are significant differences: the atypical cleft hand is usually unilateral, it is not associated with foot deformities, and there is no familial inheritance pattern. Flatt[11] and Buck-Gramcko[12] think that the atypical form is a manifestation of symbrachydactyly and should be categorized in another group of congenital malformations, rather than as a cleft hand.

The term atypical with reference to the cleft hand is further confused by the classification systems of Tada and associates[5] and Watari and Tsuge,[13] who used the term to designate central ray deficiency in association

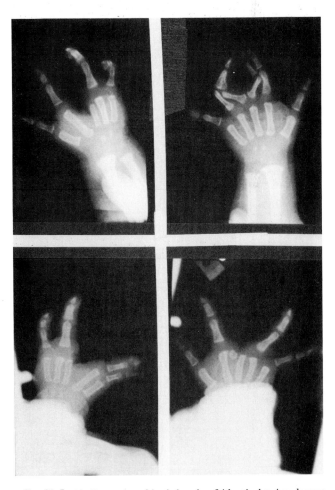

Fig. 3E–5 Radiographs of both hands of identical twins demonstrate a spectrum of anomalies including cleft hand, central polydactyly, and osseous syndactyly. (Reproduced with permission from Manske PR: Cleft hand and central polydactyly in identical twins: A case report. *J Hand Surg* 1983;8:906–908.)

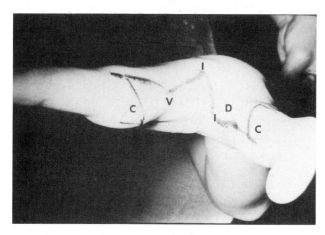

Fig. 3E-6 Preoperative photograph of the patient shown in Figure 3E-1 indicating the incisions used to create dorsal (D), volar (V), and commissural (C) flaps. The vertical incision (I) is at the base of the cleft.

with syndactyly and polydactyly. Although cleft hand is frequently associated with these other conditions, the term atypical is probably best reserved for the symbrachydactylous anomaly discussed above.

Cleft Hand, Polydactyly, and Syndactyly

Although it seems paradoxic, several investigators have noted a high association between cleft hand and syndactylized digits[14] or among cleft hand, central polydactyly, and syndactyly.[5,13,15,16] Ogino[17] supported this observation experimentally by administering a mutagenic agent to pregnant litter-mate female rats and produced this spectrum of central ray anomalies in the forepaws. I treated a human analogy to Ogino's study in identical twins who were born with a spectrum of central ray abnormalities in both hands, including a cleft defect, central polydactyly, and syndactyly[18] (Fig. 3E-5).

The polydactylous rays include bony, cartilaginous,

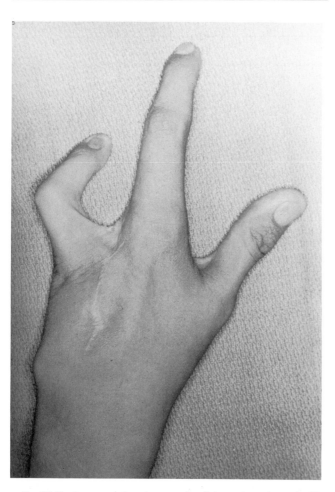

Fig. 3E-7 Postoperative photograph of the patient shown in Figure 3E-1 after the cleft was closed using the flaps outlined in Figure 3E-6.

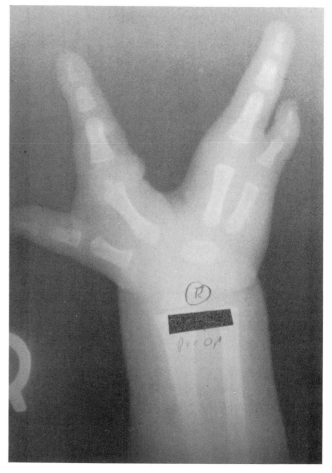

Fig. 3E-8 Preoperative radiograph of a patient who has a central defect and an absent middle finger ray. Note the widened space between the index and ring finger metacarpals.

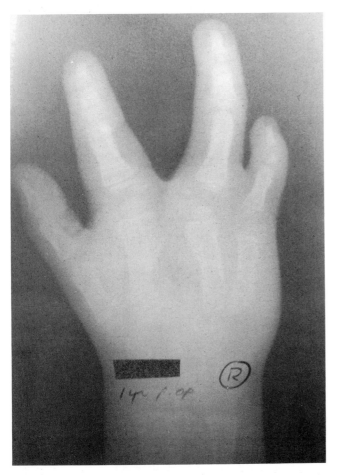

Fig. 3E–9   Postoperative radiograph of the patient shown in Figure 3E–8 after cleft closure and construction of a transverse metacarpal ligament using soft tissue dissected from the facing surfaces of the index and ring finger metacarpals. Note the narrowed space.

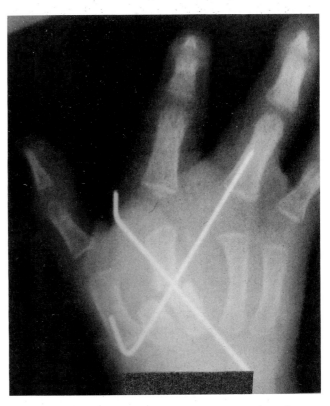

Fig. 3E-10   Postoperative photograph of a patient after cleft closure and ulnar transposition of the second metacarpal to the base of the third metacarpal. The immobilizing pins were removed after the osteotomy site healed.

and tendinous elements, and appeared to represent duplication of the middle ray. The osseous structures may be fused to the adjacent index and ring digits and form enlarged bones, representing an osseous syndactyly.

The manifestation of failure of formation, failure of differentiation, and formation of duplicated parts in genetically identical hands is at odds with the standard International Federation of Societies for Surgery of the Hand classification system.[19] This classification system distinguishes these as three separate and distinct kinds of congenital malformations; however, this system is primarily used to define treatment options and is not intended to define in utero developmental pathomechanics.

A common relationship among these anomalies can be postulated. At one end of this proposed spectrum, the polydactylous central rays form and retain their individual osseous identity. In the midportion of the spectrum, the duplicated bones unite with the index and ring fingers and the bones become enlarged, rep-

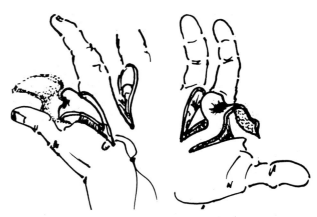

Fig. 3E-11   Drawing shows the release of an adducted thumb by transposing a volar-based pedicle flap from the cleft to the thumb-index web space. (Reproduced with permission from Snow JW, Littler JW: Surgical treatment of cleft hand, in Sanvenero-Rosselli G (ed): *Transactions of the Fourth International Congress of Plastic and Reconstructive Surgery, Rome, October 1967.* Amsterdam, Excerpta Medica Foundation, 1969, pp 888–893.)

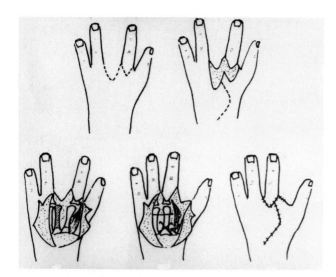

Fig. 3E-12 Diagram indicating the closure of a cleft and release of an adducted thumb by transposition of a dorsal pedicle flap from the cleft to the thumb-index web space. Note also the ulnar transposition of the index ray to the base of the third metacarpal. (Reproduced with permission from Miura T, Komada T: Simple method for reconstruction of the cleft hand with an adducted thumb. *Plast Reconstr Surg* 1979;64:65–67.)

resenting osseous and soft-tissue syndactyly; as the fusion of the duplicated middle rays with the adjacent rays becomes more complete, a central defect or cleft is formed. At the opposite end of the proposed spectrum, the duplicated central rays are incorporated completely into the adjacent long and ring finger rays, leaving a significant cleft.

Treatment of Typical Cleft Hand

As with most congenital deformities, children adapt well to their condition. However, the appearance of the cleft is so bizarre that the patient often becomes the subject of social curiosity, and surgical treatment is appropriate for cosmetic reasons alone.

The primary functional problem of the typical cleft hand is not related to the central hand defect, but to the narrowed thumb-index web space or the thumb-index syndactyly that occurs in a significant number of patients and can interfere with independent thumb function.

There are several surgical procedures related to the status of the thumb-index web space. If the web space

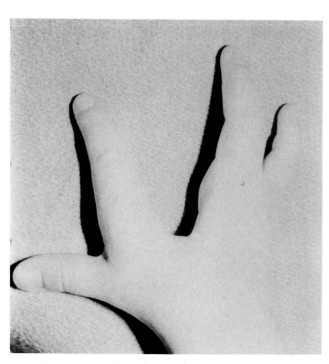

Fig. 3E-13 Preoperative photograph of a patient who has a severe cleft hand and an adducted thumb.

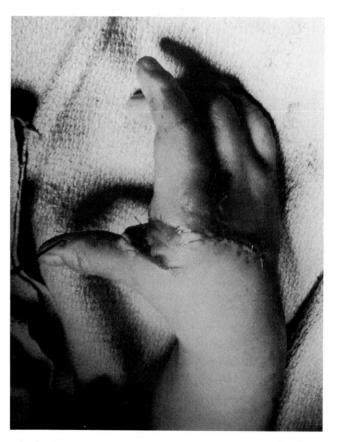

Fig. 3E-14 Photograph of the patient shown in Figure 3E-13 after cleft closure and transposition of the dorsal skin flap to the thumb-index web space to release the adducted thumb.

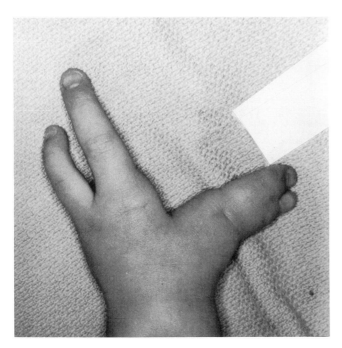

Fig. 3E-15 Preoperative photograph of a patient who has cleft hand and thumb-index syndactyly.

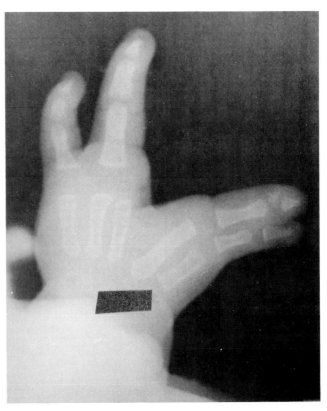

Fig. 3E-16 Preoperative radiograph of a patient who has a cleft hand and thumb-index syndactyly. Note the shortened index finger and the delta-shaped middle phalanx of the index finger.

is normal, closure of the cleft alone is sufficient. If the space is mildly narrowed, deepening of the space is accomplished by advancing local tissue. If there is severe adduction of the thumb, or a thumb-index syndactyly, skin must be transposed from the cleft into the thumb-index space.

Cleft Closure

Various skin incisions and local pedicle flaps have been proposed[10,11,20]; common to all is the elevation of dorsal and palmar skin to close the major portion of the cleft and the formation of commissural flaps from the skin at the distal end of the cleft to form an interdigital commissure. I prefer to use the incision outlined in Figure 3E–6, because of the improved appearance usually obtained (Fig. 3E–7).

A somewhat radical approach has been proposed by Streli,[21] who not only closes the palmar cleft but extends the closure to the distal end of the index and ring fingers, thereby converting the cleft hand into an index-ring finger syndactyly. Although good function may result, the hand is not as attractive as one with closure of the cleft alone.

When the cleft is deep, closure of the skin alone is insufficient; the surgeon must also narrow the palm by constructing a transverse metacarpal ligament between the index and ring fingers (Figs. 3E–8 and 3E–9), or transposing the index metacarpal in an ulnar direction to the rudimentary base of the third metacarpal (Fig. 3E–10). If the distal metacarpals are not stabilized, the

digits will, in time, diverge and the deformity will recur within the closed skin envelope. I prefer to construct a transverse metacarpal ligament using soft-tissue flaps dissected from the index and ring metacarpals. An alternative procedure is to pass a strip of tendon or fascia lata around the circumference of the metacarpal necks and suture the strip to itself. Merely placing sutures through transverse drill holes in the bone[10] is considered inadequate stabilization.[7]

Web-Space Deepening

Many standard techniques are used to widen the thumb-index web space, including the standard Z-plasty, or the four-or five-flap web plasties.[22,23] I have no preference.

Release of the Adducted Thumb

When there is insufficient local tissue in the thumb-index web space, skin must be transposed from the cleft to the web space itself. Fibrous bands and even a rudimentary transverse carpal ligament are often present between the thumb and index metacarpals and must be released also. Snow and Littler[24] (Fig. 3E–11) have made popular the transposition of a volar pedicle flap from the cleft to the thumb-index space. I prefer to transpose

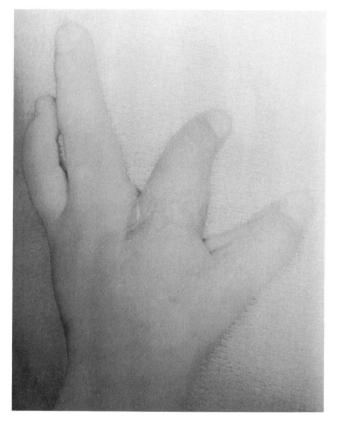

Fig. 3E-17 Postoperative photograph of the patient shown in Figure 3E-15 after transposition of a volar-based pedicle flap[21] and a dorsal rotational flap from the base of the index finger. Note the short index finger that has a radial tilt toward the thumb.

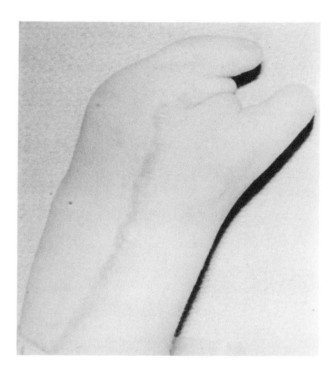

Fig. 3E-18 Postoperative photograph of the patient in Figure 3E-3 after excision of the central metacarpals and redundant skin, which facilitates a pincer mechanism.

dorsal skin, as advocated by Miura and Komada[25] (Fig. 3E-12) because I think it is more important to have pliable skin on the dorsal aspect of the web space than on the palmar side (Figs. 3E-13 and 3E-14). Ulnar transposition of the index metacarpal to the rudimentary third metacarpal base facilitates deepening and widening of the thumb-index web space.

Release of Thumb-Index Syndactyly

Thumb-index syndactyly is the most difficult presentation of central deficiency to treat. It requires syndactyly separation, release of the adducted thumb, and closure of the cleft (Figs. 3E-15 and 3E-16). A staged operation has been proposed in which the syndactylized digits are released initially and the cleft is closed later[7]; however, I prefer to accomplish both at a single operation.

The syndactylized digits are released in a standard fashion, using additional skin grafts as necessary to fill in the uncovered areas. The thumb adduction deformity is usually so severe that both a palmarly based flap and a dorsal skin flap are necessary to create an adequate space; an additional split-thickness skin graft may

be necessary to fill in the defect on the index metacarpal (Fig. 3E-17). Both the extensor tendons and the flexor tendons may be joined together and must be separated proximally to allow independent thumb and index finger function. In addition, the middle phalanx of the index finger is usually delta-shaped, which creates an inclination of the index finger toward the thumb after syndactyly separation.

Despite the postoperative cosmetic improvement, there are persistent abnormalities, such as a short index finger that inclines toward the thumb because of the associated delta-shaped phalanx. Nevertheless, the surgical procedure is considered worthwhile because of the improved appearance of the hand.

Treatment of Atypical Cleft Hand

In the atypical cleft hand described by Lange[9] and Barsky,[10] the central digits are absent and only remnants of the thumb and small finger rays on the radial and ulnar border are present. The ability of these remnants to function together as pincers may be blocked by rudimentary metacarpals or skin folds (Figs. 3E-3 and 3E-4). The surgeon should consider resection of redundant skin and the central rudimentary metacarpals to facilitate function of the border rays; in effect, a deeper cleft is created. Although this is not more attractive, the procedure may result in improved function (Fig. 3E–18). The functional gains may be limited, because the patient usually has a normal opposite extremity.

Microvascular surgical techniques now make it possible to transfer toes onto the border digits or into the central defect; however, it has not been established that such procedures provide any significant cosmetic or functional benefit.

Summary

Cleft hand may be associated with central polydactyly and syndactyly of the central digits. Cleft closure usually entails construction of a transverse metacarpal ligament or ulnar transposition of the index ray. If the thumb is adducted toward or syndactylized to the index finger, it must be released.

References

1. Hartsinck JJ: *Beschryving van Guiana, of de wilde Kust in Zuid-America.* Amsterdam, Gerrit Tielenburg, 1770, vol 2, pp 811–812.
2. Henkel HL, Willert HG, Gressman C: Eine internationale Terminologie zur Klassifikation angeborener Gliedmassen fehlbildungen: Emptehlungen einer Arbeitsgruppe der International Society for Prosthetics and Orthotics. *Acta Orthop Trauma Surg* 1978;93:1–19.
3. Temtamy S, McKusick V: *The Genetics of Hand Malformations.* New York, Alan R Liss, 1978, pp 53–71.
4. Maisels DO: Lobster-claw deformities of the hands and feet. *Br J Plast Surg* 1970;23:269–282.
5. Tada K, Yonenobu K, Swanson AB: Congenital central ray deficiency in the hand: A survey of 59 cases and subclassification. *J Hand Surg* 1981;6:434–441.
6. David TJ: The differential diagnosis of the cleft hand and cleft foot malformations. *Hand* 1974;6:58–61.
7. Green DP (ed): *Operative Hand Surgery,* ed 2. New York, Churchill Livingstone, 1988, pp 275–291.
8. Nutt JN III, Flatt AE: Congenital central hand deficit. *J Hand Surg* 1981;6:48–60.
9. Lange M: Grundsätzliches über die Beurteilung der Entstehung und Bewertung atypischer Hand-und Fussmisbildungen. *Z Ortop* 1937;66(suppl):80–87.
10. Barsky AJ: Cleft hand: Classification, incidence, and treatment. Review of the literature and report of nineteen cases. *J Bone Joint Surg* 1964;46A:1707–1720.
11. Flatt AE: *The Care of Congenital Hand Anomalies.* St. Louis, CV Mosby, 1977, pp 265–285.
12. Buck-Gramcko D: Cleft hands: Classification and treatment. Symposium on congenital deformities of the hand. *Hand Clin* 1985;1:467–473.
13. Watari S, Tsuge K: A classification of cleft hands, based on clinical findings: Theory of developmental mechanism. *Plast Reconstr Surg* 1979;64:381–389.
14. Miura T: Syndactyly and split hand. *Hand* 1976;8:125–130.
15. Pokorny L: Zur Klinik und Ätiologie der Spalthand. *Fortschr Geb Röentgenstr Nuklearmed* 1924;32:274–280.
16. Egawa T, Horiki A, Senrui H, et al: Charakteristische anatomische Befunde der Spalthand-ihre Bedeutung und ihre Klassifikation. *Handchirurgie* 1978;10:3–8.
17. Ogino T: A clinical and experimental study on teratogenic mechanism of cleft hand, polydactyly and syndactyly. *Nippon Seikeigeka Gakkai Zasshi* 1979;53:535–543.
18. Manske PR: Cleft hand and central polydactyly in identical twins: A case report. *J Hand Surg* 1983;8:906–908.
19. Swanson AB: A classification for congenital limb malformations. *J Hand Surg* 1976;1:8–22.
20. Kelikian H: *Congenital Deformities of the Hand and Forearm.* Philadelphia, WB Saunders, 1974, pp 467–489.
21. Streli R: Behandlung der Spalthand durch Syndaktylisierung, eine neue einfache Methode. *Handchirurgie* 1969;2:104–107.
22. Woolf RM, Broadbent TR: The four-flap Z-plasty. *Plast Reconstr Surg* 1972;49:48–51.
23. Hirshowitz B, Karev A, Rousso M: Combined double Z-plasty and Y-V advancement for thumb web contracture. *Hand* 1975;7:291–293.
24. Snow JW, Littler JW: Surgical treatment of cleft hand, in Sanvenero-Rosselli G (ed): *Transactions of the Fourth International Congress of Plastic and Reconstructive Surgery, Rome, October 1967.* Amsterdam, Excerpta Medica Foundation, 1969, pp 888–893.
25. Miura T, Komada T: Simple method for reconstruction of the cleft hand with an adducted thumb. *Plast Reconstr Surg* 1979;64:65–67.

Evaluation of Impairment of Hand and Upper Extremity Function

PART A

Foreword

Sidney J. Blair, MD

It is important to understand the approved definitions of disability, impairment, and handicapped. Impairment means an alteration in an individual's health status assessed by medical means. It is the loss of use or derangement of any body part, system, or function. Disability is defined as an alteration in an individual's capacity to meet personal, social, or occupational demands, or statutory or regulatory requirements. It is the gap between what an individual can do and what the individual needs or wants to do. The handicapped, as defined under federal law, are individuals who have impairment that substantially limits one or more life activities, including work, and where there is a record of an impairment.

Many different systems for rating physical impairment and disability have been recommended, including a number in Russia and in Germany that go back to the turn of the century. In 1924, a standard permanent disability schedule was published by the United States Department of Labor. In 1936, Earl McBride wrote a textbook, *Disability Evaluation and Treatment*, that became the basis of much of the thinking on the subject. During World War II, Sterling Bunnell emphasized the importance of separating anatomic from functional disability. In 1946, Donald Slocum presented his rating system to the American Society for Surgery of the Hand. His system was based on the hand's functional components of hook, pinch, and grasp.

The American Academy of Orthopaedic Surgeons first presented an Instructional Course on impairment evaluation in 1949. A number of courses have been given since that time. The American Medical Association created a committee on medical rating of impairment and published the *AMA Guide* in 1958. Republished in 1971 and 1984, the *AMA Guides* were revised again in 1988. Dr. Henry Kessler was very active in both the Academy and the AMA. Dr. Joseph Boyes also participated in the writing of the *AMA Guides*. Beginning in 1960, Dr. Alfred Swanson offered his teaching and writing on the subject. In 1963, a committee of the American Society for Surgery of the Hand, which included Daniel Riordan, John Adams, and Swanson, presented a report to the Society. In 1966, Swanson was appointed chairman of a committee of the Inter-national Federation of Societies for Surgery of the Hand charged to research a system of impairment evaluation that could be used throughout the world. This was done in conjunction with other hand surgeons around the world and was officially accepted by the Federation in 1980. This system is included in the *AMA Guides* published in 1988. It is strongly recommended that certain standards and methods for evaluating anatomic impairment be widely accepted and understood by those working in the field. Continued research is needed for functional impairment, which is less understood.

PART B

Evaluation of Impairment

Alfred B. Swanson, MD
Genevieve de Groot Swanson, MD

Physicians interested in treating disabilities of the hand and upper extremity should accept the responsibility for accurate evaluation of the patient's physical condition, both local and general, and be able to compute the permanent medical impairment resulting from these deficiencies. This evaluation is usually limited to the analysis of the anatomic, functional, and cosmetic effect loss after optimal surgical and physical rehabilitation have been achieved. The physician is responsible for a medical evaluation of impairment, not a rating of disability.[1-3] The latter is a nonmedical administrative function that defines the patient's ability to engage in personal, social, and occupational activities related to earning capacity and social and economic standard of living.

Accurate and complete records are essential for determination of treatment programs and proper evaluation of results. Furthermore, records are increasingly under review by insurance companies, law courts, and other judicial bodies who evaluate the effects of trauma or diseases of the hand and upper extremity.

Proper rating of impairment in the upper extremity presumes a sound knowledge of the normal functional anatomy. It requires an appraisal of the loss of function as it relates to the activities of daily living and work and the more specialized activities of the hand. It is usually a determination of loss of structure, limitation or loss of motion, strength, presence of pain, and/or loss of sensibility, as compared with the opposite normal limb; if both are impaired, comparison with an average limb is made.

Table 4–1
Severity index classifying common deformities*

Deformity	Severity		
	Mild	Moderate	Severe
Swan-neck			
Thumb, flexion limit of MCP	ROM, +10° to 50°	ROM, +20° to 30°	ROM, +30° to 10°
Finger, flexion limit of PIP	ROM, +10° to 50°	ROM, +20° to 30°	ROM, +30° to 10°
Boutonniere			
Thumb, extension limit of MCP	−5° to −20°	−20° to −40°	>−40°
Finger, extension limit of PIP	−5° to −10°	−10° to −30°	>−30°
Instability, excess passive mediolateral motion	<10°	10° to 20°	>20°
Subluxation to dislocation	Complete reduction manually	Incomplete reduction manually	Cannot be reduced
Deviation			
Radial or ulnar	<10°	10° to 30°	>30°
Lateral, wrist or elbow	<20°	20° to 30°	>30°
Rotational, fingers	<15°	15° to 30°	>30°
Crepitation with motion	Inconstant during active ROM	Constant during active ROM	Constant during passive ROM
Joint swelling from synovial hypertrophy	Visually apparent	Palpably apparent	>10% increase
Constrictive tenosynovitis	Inconstant triggering on active ROM	Constant triggering on active ROM	Constant triggering on passive ROM
Intrinsic tightness with MCP extended	PIP flexion, 80° to 60°	PIP flexion, 61° to 20°	PIP flexion, <20°
Extensor tendon subluxation	Subluxates on MCP flexion	Reducible subluxation in IMC groove	Nonreducible subluxation in IMC groove
Painful joint with motion	On active motion	On active motion, interferes with activity	At rest, prevents activity

*MCP, metacarpophalangeal joint; PIP, proximal interphalangeal joint; ROM, range of motion; IMC, intermetacarpal.

In 1966, a special committee of the International Federation of Societies for Surgery of the Hand was charged to develop a system for evaluation of physical impairment in the hand and upper extremity that would be reliable and easy to use. We brought together systems of medical societies and classic works, and with the participation of many hand surgeons, we have refined and extended the evaluation methods of physical impairment of the hand and upper extremity.[4-6] The system developed has been tested and used by many hand surgeons around the world and was approved for international application by the International Federation of Societies for Surgery of the Hand at their first Congress held in Rotterdam, Holland, in 1980. It has been recently approved by the American Medical Association for national usage and has been included in their *Guide to the Evaluation of Permanent Impairment of the Extremities and Back.*

Evaluation Methods

Evaluation of the upper extremity can be arbitrarily divided into anatomic, cosmetic, and functional cate-gories. A combination of these methods is necessary to show an accurate profile of the patient's condition. Their effect on the patient's psychologic, sociologic, environmental, and economic status must also be considered. The *physical evaluation* is necessary to determine the anatomic impairment for preoperative and postoperative surgical considerations. It is based on the history and a detailed examination of the upper extremity and patient. The *cosmetic evaluation* concerns the patient's and society's reaction to the impairment or the result of the surgical treatment. The *functional evaluation* is much more involved and is of great importance to the quality of function and the ability to perform the activities of daily living. Functional evaluation studies are becoming increasingly sophisticated and may add greatly to the evaluation process.

A complete and detailed examination of the upper extremity is facilitated by the use of a printed chart that lists the various tests and measurements in an orderly fashion. A sketch of the hand with dorsal and palmar views simplifies the description of loss of parts and the location of scars or other defects.[7] Examples of charts used for the evaluation of the hand are shown in Fig-

Table 4–2
Average hand strength in 100 subjects

Category	Strength (kg)			
	Men		Women	
	Dominant Hand	Nondominant Hand	Dominant Hand	Nondominant Hand
Unsupported Grip				
Occupation				
Skilled labor	47.0	45.4	26.8	24.4
Sedentary	47.2	44.1	23.1	21.1
Manual labor	48.5	44.6	24.2	22.0
Average	47.6	45.0	24.6	22.4
Grip				
Age (yrs)				
20	45.2	42.6	23.8	22.8
21 to 30	48.5	46.2	24.6	22.7
31 to 40	49.2	44.5	30.8	28.0
41 to 50	49.0	47.3	23.4	21.5
51 to 60	45.9	43.5	22.3	18.2
Chuck Pinch				
Occupation				
Skilled labor	7.3	7.2	5.4	4.6
Sedentary	8.4	7.3	4.2	4.0
Manual labor	8.5	7.6	6.1	5.6
Average	7.9	7.5	5.2	4.9
Pulp Pinch With Separate Digits				
Digit				
II	5.3	4.8	3.6	3.3
III	5.6	5.7	3.8	3.4
IV	3.8	3.6	2.5	2.4
V	2.3	2.2	1.7	1.6
Lateral Pinch				
Occupation				
Skilled labor	6.6	6.4	4.4	4.3
Sedentary	6.3	6.1	4.1	3.9
Manual labor	8.5	7.7	6.0	5.5
Average	7.5	7.1	4.9	4.7

ures 4–1 and 4–2. The evaluation record includes a checklist for the common information needed to record the history, type of disease, onset, duration, distribution of disease process, laboratory tests, and treatment. Organized columns are provided for recording the range of motion and strength of each joint, prehensile patterns, ability to perform the activities of daily living, and ambulatory status. Specific clinical abnormalities are recorded with a coded number system and are classified as mild, moderate, or severe (Table 4–1).

Principles and Methods of History-Taking

History-taking should include identification, vital statistics, diagnosis, and history of the disease. Additionally, in the case of trauma, it should narrate the accident, the mechanics and severity of the injury, and the time sequence of treatment in regard to emergency care, definitive care, and postoperative therapy. The complaint of how the residual difficulty affects the pa-

tient's activities should be recorded in the patient's own words. Any history of previous difficulty in the same extremity and general conditions that would influence the patient's recovery are also noted.

As the examiner is taking the history and measuring the upper portion of the limb, the general posture of the hand, the position of its various joints, and the state of nutrition, color, moisture, swelling, or muscle weakness can be subtly checked without the patient's awareness. Malingering or psychogenic overlay may make it difficult to obtain an accurate estimation of impairment. The patient whose complaints are not justified by objective findings or whose response to testing varies widely from time to time should put the examiner on guard. It may be impossible to identify the malingerer without the help of evidence gathered outside the examining room when the patient is unaware of being observed.

RHEUMATOID ARTHRITIS EVALUATION RECORD
PREOPERATIVE

NAME _____ SEX: ☐ MALE ☐ FEMALE DATE_____ BIRTH DATE_____

ADDRESS _____

OCCUPATION _____ DOMINANT HAND: ☐ R ☐ L HOSPITAL_____ EXAMINER_____

DIAGNOSIS: ☐ JUVENILE RHEUMATOID ☐ ADULT RHEUMATOID ☐ EROSIVE DEGENERATIVE JOINT DISEASE ☐ PSORIATIC ARTHRITIS
☐ ANKYLOSING SPONDYLITIS ☐ SJORGREN'S SYNDROME ☐ SYSTEMIC LUPUS ERYTHEMATOSIS

ONSET DATE_____SEDIMENTATION RATE: ☐ WINTROBE ☐ WESTERGREN ☐ ROURKE_____RHEUMATOID TEST ☐ (+) ☐ (—)

ONSET DISTRIBUTION ☐ PERIPHERAL ☐ CENTRAL ☐ BOTH: REMISSION ☐ YES ☐ NO: ANEMIA ☐ YES ☐ NO: FAMILY HX ☐ (+) ☐ (—)

CHECK IF THE FOLLOWING HAS BEEN COMPLETED: ☐ X-RAYS ☐ PHOTOGRAPHS ☐ MOVIES ☐ CINERADIOGRAPHY

RANGE OF MOTION (ROM) USE NEUTRAL = ZERO METHOD OF AMERICAN ACADEMY OF ORTHOPEDIC SURGEONS 1965.

CODES 1-25 REPRESENT OBSERVED AND MEASURED ABNORMALITIES. USE AS INDICATED IN APPROPRIATE SECTIONS.

SEVERITY INDICES MILD, MODERATE AND SEVERE ARE REPRESENTED BY a, b, & c AND FURTHER CATEGORIZE CODES 1-25.

THE CODE 1-25 IS BELOW ON THIS SHEET. SEVERITY INDICES ARE ON SEPARATE DETACHABLE SHEET.

THIS EVALUATION RECORD HAS BEEN DESIGNED FOR COMPUTER ANALYSIS. RESPONSES MUST BE COMPLETE.

CODES TO USE FOR THUMB 1, 2, 3, 9-14, 19, & 22

THUMB	CODE R	CODE L	JOINTS		ROM R	ROM L
			MC	Abd		
			See	Add		
			above	Opp		
			MP			
			IP			

FINGER CODES 3-15, 19, 22-25 — ROM

	R	L		R	L
INDEX			MP		
			PIP		
			DIP		
FLEX DIP CREASE TO PALMAR CREASE (cm.)					
MIDDLE			MP		
			PIP		
			DIP		
FLEX DIP CREASE TO PALMAR CREASE (cm.)					
RING			MP		
			PIP		
			DIP		
FLEX DIP CREASE TO PALMAR CREASE (cm.)					
LITTLE			MP		
			PIP		
			DIP		
FLEX DIP CREASE TO PALMAR CREASE (cm.)					

CODES 3,7-14, 19, 20, 22, 23

WRIST			
FLEX			
EXT			
U. DEV			
R. DEV			

PREHENSILE PATTERNS: Check if able to perform

GRASP:

		R	L
CYLINDERS	1 INCH		
	2 INCH		
	3 INCH		
	4 INCH		
SPHERES	2 INCH		
	3 INCH		
	4 INCH		
	5 INCH		

STRENGTH: ☐ Lb ☐ Kg ☐ mm. Hg.

PULP PINCH		R	L
	INDEX		
	MIDDLE		
	RING		
	LITTLE		
LATERAL OR KEY PINCH			
GRIP			

ADL: I = Independent A = Assisted U = Unable

DRESSING	I	A	U	HYGIENE	I	A	U
UPPER EXT				TEETH			
TRUNK				HAIR			
LOWER EXT				SHAVE			
BATH				PICK UP COIN			
SHOWER				TURN KEY			
EATING				DOOR KNOB			
TOILET				CAR DOOR			
TELEPHONE				SCREW TOP JAR			
TYPEWRITE				AEROSOL CAN			
WRITE							

AMBULATORY STATUS:
☐ INDEPENDENT ☐ WHEELCHAIR WITH PARTIAL WALKING
☐ ASSISTED WALK ☐ BEDFAST

CODE FOR CLINICAL ABNORMALITY

1 — THUMB SWAN NECK
2 — THUMB BOUTONNIERE
3 — SUBLUXATION — DISLOCATION
4 — SWAN NECK, FINGER
5 — BOUTONNIERE, FINGER
6 — INTRINSIC TIGHTNESS
7 — ULNAR DRIFT
8 — RADIAL DRIFT
9 — ANKYLOSIS
10 — INSTABILITY
11 — TENDON RUPTURE
12 — CONSTRICTIVE TENOSYNOVITIS
13 — SYNOVIAL HYPERTROPHY
14 — CREPITATION WITH MOTION
15 — EXTENSOR TENDON SUBLUXATION
16 — VARUS ANGLE

17 — VALGUS ANGLE
18 — ROTATIONAL DEFORMITY
19 — EROSIONS
20 — JOINT NARROWING
21 — SUBCHONDRAL SCLEROSIS
22 — PAINFUL JOINT WITH MOTION
23 — NERVE COMPRESSION — M.U.R.
24 — VASCULITIS
25 — NODULES

SEVERITY INDEX

a — Mild
b — Moderate
c — Severe

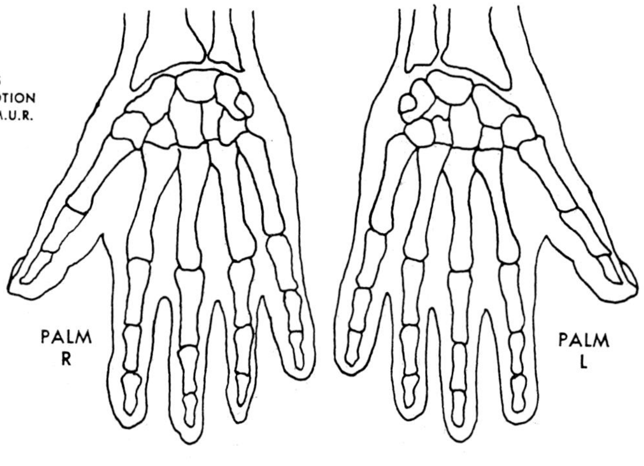

PALM R

PALM L

Fig. 4-1 Preoperative evaluation record. Form designed for evaluation of rheumatoid and arthritic hands. (Reproduced with permission from Swanson AB: *Flexible Implant Resection Arthroplasty in the Hand and Extremities.* St. Louis, CV Mosby, 1973, p 97.)

HAND EVALUATION RECORD

261.

Name _____ Age _____ Date _____ Major Hand _____
Occupation _____ X-Rays _____ Photographs _____
History:

Shoulder:	L.	R.	Wrist:			Circ:		
For ____ ____			DF ____ ____			Biceps ____ ____		
Back ____ ____			PF ____ ____			Forearm ____ ____		
Abd ____ ____			RD ____ ____			Grip: L ____ ____		
Add ____ ____			UD ____ ____			R ____ ____		
Rotation Int ____ ____			Elbow: Ext ____ ____			Forearm: Pro ____ ____		
Ext ____ ____			Flex ____ ____			Sup ____ ____		

		MP	IP				% Impair.
Thumb	Ext			Abd			
	Flex			Add			
	Ankylosis			Opp			
		MP	PIP	DIP	Flex Pulp to Mid-palmar Crease		
Index	Ext						
	Flex						
	Ankylosis						
Middle	Ext						
	Flex						
	Ankylosis						
Ring	Ext						
	Flex						
	Ankylosis						
Little	Ext						
	Flex						
	Ankylosis						

Chart:
1) Amputations
2) Scars
3) Skin-Subcut, Loss
4) Nail Bed Injury
5) Major Nerve Loss: R,M,U.
6) Digital Bundle Loss
7) Neuroma
8) Pain and Tenderness
9) Bone Damage
10) Joint Damage
11) Flexor Tendon Loss
12) Extensor Tendon Loss
13) Ligament Injury
14) Sensibility-pick up
 two point
 ninhydrin
15) Prehension:
 Grasp-small
 large
 Pinch-pulp
 tip
 lateral
 Hook-distal
 proximal
 Scoop-
16) Maximum Improvement
17) Rehabilitation Needed
18) Further Treatment
19) Classification
NOTE: Degrees of motion
 recorded as left/right.

Total %

Dorsum R Hand
or
Palmar L Hand

Dorsum L Hand
or
Palmar R Hand

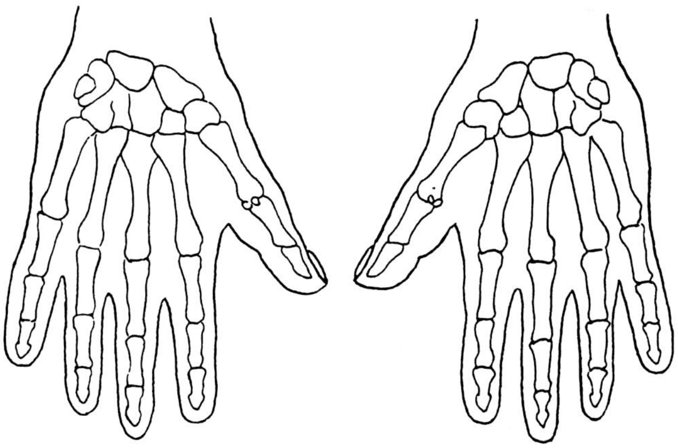

Fig. 4-2 Form designed for posttraumatic conditions and other disorders of the hand. (Reproduced with permission from Swanson AB: *Flexible Implant Resection Arthroplasty in the Hand and Extremities.* St. Louis, CV Mosby, 1973, p 33.)

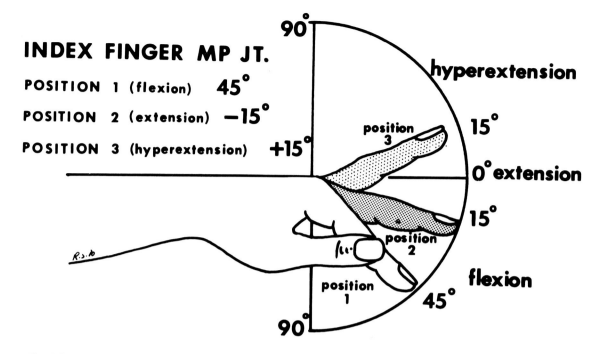

INDEX FINGER MP JT.

POSITION 1 (flexion)   **45°**

POSITION 2 (extension)   **–15°**

POSITION 3 (hyperextension)   **+15°**

Fig. 4-3   Range of motion of index finger. Measure hyperextension as plus value, extension lag as minus value, and neutral position as 0 degrees.[10]

Photographic Record

A set of standard position photographs of the hand is an essential part of the record. Suggested sequences should include views of the hand from various positions while the patient performs flexion-extension of the fingers and the functions of grasp and pinch. Film sequences may also be used to evaluate the patient's adaptation to the needs of daily living—manipulating buttons and safety pins, threading a needle, turning the screw-top lid of a jar, writing, picking up and releasing objects, and turning a nut on and off a bolt, are but a few of the activities.

Radiologic Evaluation

A standard series of roentgenograms, including anterior, posterior, lateral, and oblique views of the hand and wrist, should be part of the record. Radiographs of other joints of the upper extremity may also be included as needed. These should be taken without jewelry or other items about the extremity. The anatomic extended position is desired but must not be forced so that the degree of deformity can also be evaluated on the radiographs. Cineradiography can help show the range of motion of the digits and wrist.

Anatomic Evaluation

The hand is primarily a grasping or prehensile organ. The action of the shoulder, elbow, and wrist joints enables the hand to be placed at almost any area of the body or to be pulled toward or pushed away from the

body. It is obvious, therefore, that every examination should include an evaluation of the entire limb. The condition of all the structures of the extremity, including skin, nails, neurovascular and musculotendinous structures, and bones and joints should be appraised. Circumferential measurement of the extremity, compared with that of the opposite extremity, should be recorded.

The cutaneous coverage of the limb should be evaluated for scars, abnormal pigmentation, redundancy, ulcerations, loss of subcutaneous tissues, and adhesions or contractures, and their effect on function. Temperature, color, swelling, texture, and tenderness should be noted as well as nail-bed deformities.

For each joint, the range of motion or position of ankylosis, the presence and degree of synovitis, instability, subluxation, lateral deviation, and rotation should be measured and recorded. Circumferential measurements of individual joints should be measured in centimeters, and angulation and rotation should be measured in degrees. The status of the musculotendinous system is evaluated by stating the presence or absence of tendon ruptures, constrictive tenosynovitis, extensor tendon subluxations, and intrinsic tightness. Description of the thumb also includes length, mobility, stability, and capacity for placement to the rest of the hand. Flexibility and depth of the thumb web are noted.

Intrinsic tightness in the hand may be demonstrated by a test described by Bunnell.[8] Hyperextension of the metacarpophalangeal joint in a normal hand still allows

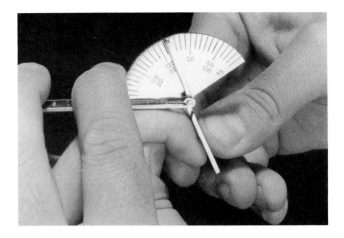

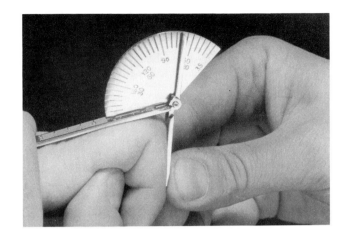

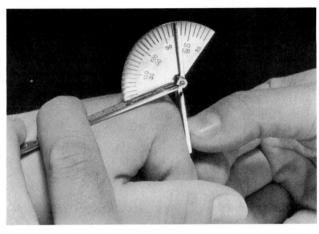

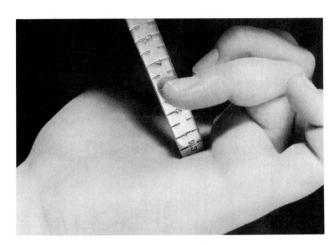

Fig. 4–4 Techniques for measuring digital joints. **Top left:** Distal interphalangeal joint. **Top right:** Proximal interphalangeal joint. **Bottom left:** Metacarpophalangeal joint. **Bottom right:** Maximal flexion distance measured by Boyes' method as distance pulp of finger lacks to distal palmar crease.

passive flexion of the proximal interphalangeal joint. If the intrinsic muscles are tight or contracted, the available stretch of these muscles is taken up by the hyperextended position of the metacarpophalangeal joint, and passive flexion of the proximal interphalangeal joint will be difficult.

It is important to describe the posture of the hand as it relates to the normal arches. Any disturbance of the normal carpal and metacarpal transverse arches and of the longitudinal arches of the digital rays is noted. Collapse deformities from joint instability, skeletal malalignment, or muscle imbalance contribute to the loss of function. The thumb ray on one side and the ring and little finger rays on the other side normally move widely around the firmly fixed, stable axis of the index and middle metacarpals. The normal longitudinal arch of each digital ray is especially necessary for prehension of small objects.

A complete anatomic evaluation also includes measurement of the range of motion of individual joints, strength of pinch and grasp, muscle testing, sensory evaluation, and assessment of pain.

Important tools for a good examination include a goniometer, dynamometer, pinch meter, ruler, sensory testing devices, a two-point compass, familiar objects for tactile identification and the pickup test, and cylinders of various sizes to measure effective grasp.

Prehension and Strength Measurements

Measurements of strength of pinch and grasp can be made by comparing the force with that of the examiner and measuring the size of the arms, forearms, and hands for estimating atrophy. Properly gauged mechanical devices provide more accurate measurements. The mechanical dynamometer may be inadequate to measure grasp in a weak hand. To record grips of lesser power, a sphygmomanometer can be rolled to 5 cm in diameter and inflated to 50 mm Hg; the cuff is then squeezed and the change in millimeters of mercury from 50 mm Hg is recorded as the power of grip. An electronic

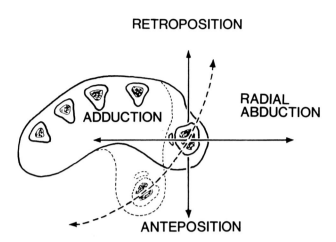

RETROPOSITION

RADIAL ABDUCTION

ADDUCTION

ANTEPOSITION

Fig. 4–5 Movements of thumb are adduction and radial abduction, anteposition or palmar abduction, and retroposition. Opposition (dotted line) is accomplished by movements of axial rotation, abduction, and flexion of all three joints of the thumb, resulting in rotation of thumb in position to present its palmar pad to the pad of any finger. (Adapted with permission from Tubiana R, Valentin P: Opposition of the thumb. *Surg Clin North Am* 1968;48:967–977.)

pinch meter based on the strain-gauge principle can be used to measure the strength of pinch in pounds or kilograms of pressure.

Many factors, including fatigue, handedness, time of day, age, state of nutrition, pain, and cooperation of the patient, can influence strength measurements. Tests repeated at intervals during the examination are reliable if there is less than a 20% variation in the readings; otherwise, one can assume that the patient is not exerting full effort. The test is usually repeated three times with each hand at different times during the examination and then recorded and later compared.

A baseline of normal grip and pinch strength was studied in our clinic by testing a group of 100 healthy persons.[9] The strength was recorded as applied in basic hand patterns: grasp, chuck, pinch (three-digit pinch), pulp pinch with separate fingers, and lateral pinch. Measurements were expressed in kilograms of force units.

The strength of the grip was measured with the ad-justable handle of a Jamar dynamometer spaced at 6 cm. Most subjects were comfortable at this breadth of grip and could apply maximal force when tested. The grip measurement ranged from 30.4 to 70.4 kg in the male group and 14 to 38.6 kg in the female group. The average strength of grip, listed by occupation and measured with the extremity unsupported, and the average strength of grip listed by age, are shown in Table 4–2. It has been demonstrated that approximately 4 kg of force is needed for a grip adequate to perform 90% of the activities of daily living.

Pinch strength was measured with an electronic pinch meter based on the strain-gauge principle; however, similar findings were obtained with a standard pinch meter. The majority of subjects preferred chuck pinch to any other type of pinch for applying the most force. The interphalangeal joint of the thumb was hyperextended in most cases when maximal force of chuck pinch was applied. Table 4–2 shows the average strength of chuck pinch and pulp pinch with separate fingers. A tendency to hyperextend either the proximal interphalangeal or the distal interphalangeal joints was evident when maximal pinch force was applied. For the proximal interphalangeal joint, this tendency increased from the radial to the ulnar sides of the hand. Lateral pinch may be an important adaptation in the disabled hand and may provide very useful function when pulp pinch is lost (Table 4–2).

In comparing dominant and nondominant hands, the dominant hand was usually stronger in those doing heavy manual work; however, the nondominant hand may be stronger in a significant percentage of other individuals tested. The grip strength of the nondominant hand was weaker in 5.4% of men and 8.9% of women. The pinch strength of the nondominant hand was weaker by only 4% in men and 6% in women. These results indicated that there is less difference in strength between the dominant and nondominant hands than has generally been thought.

Muscle Testing

Muscle testing may be an important part of evaluating impairment in the hand disabled by paralysis or paresis resulting from a proximal or peripheral nerve lesion. Manual muscle testing is based on the ability to

Table 4–3
Cosmetic results*

Cosmetic Improvement	Examiner		Patient	
	Rest	Activity	Rest	Activity
Minimum (1 point)	—	—	—	—
Moderate (2 points)	—	2	—	—
Marked (3 points)	3	—	3	3

*In this sample, the hand received 11 out of a possible 12 points.

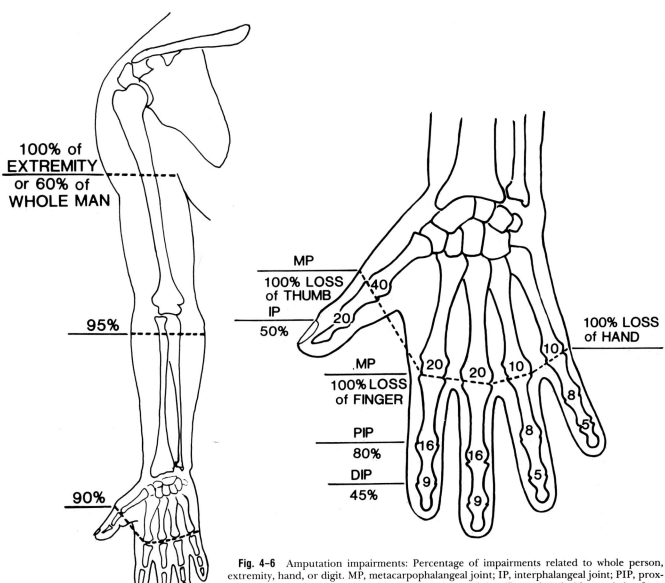

Fig. 4-6 Amputation impairments: Percentage of impairments related to whole person, extremity, hand, or digit. MP, metacarpophalangeal joint; IP, interphalangeal joint; PIP, proximal interphalangeal joint; DIP, distal interphalangeal joint. (Reproduced with permission from Swanson AB: Evaluation of impairment of function in the hand. *Surg Clin North Am* 1964;44:925–940.)

Table 4-4
Impairment relative values

Segment	Impairment to Upper Extremity (%)	
	Lost Function	Amputation
Hand	90	90
Wrist	60	90
Elbow	70	95
Shoulder	60	100

raise the distal part through its range of motion against gravity and holding the part against resistance. Muscle strength can be classified as (1) normal (0% impairment of strength), with complete range of motion against gravity with full resistance; (2) good (1% to 25% impairment of strength), with complete range of motion against gravity with some resistance; (3) fair (26% to 50% impairment of strength), with complete range of motion against gravity without resistance; (4) poor (51% to 75% impairment of strength), with complete range of motion with gravity eliminated; (5) trace (76% to 99% impairment of strength), with evidence of slight contractility and no joint motion; or (6) zero (100% impairment of strength), with no evidence of contractility.

When evaluating impairment for paralysis or paresis and associated sensory defects, impairment values for loss of motion or ankylosis of parts are not included as this would result in a duplication of impairment rating.

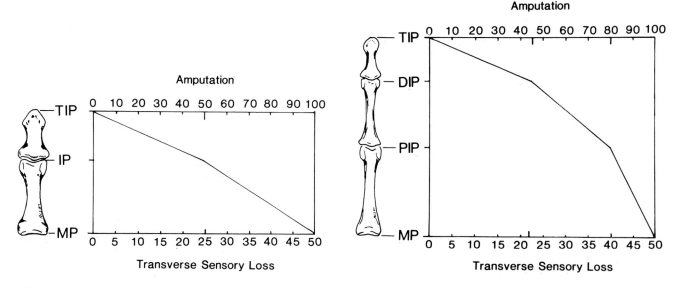

Fig. 4–7 Percentages of impairment to digit in thumb **(left)** and finger **(right)**. The scales at the top show the amputation impairment scale (up to 100%). The scales at the bottom represent the transverse sensory loss impairment (up to 50%), which represents one-half the amputation value.

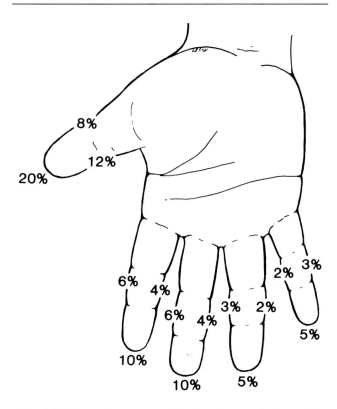

Fig. 4–8 Sensory impairment. Relative value to whole hand for total sensory loss of digit and comparative loss of radial and ulnar sides. Sensory loss is calculated as 50% that of amputation.

Range of Motion

As illustrated in Figure 4–3, the range of motion is recorded on the principle that neutral position equals 0 degrees.[10] In this method all motions of the joint are measured from defined zero as the starting position. The "extended anatomic position" of an extremity is therefore accepted as 0 degrees rather than 180 degrees. The degree of motion of a joint is added in the direction the joint moves from the zero starting position. Active motion is that motion obtained at the joints with full flexion or extension muscle force. Passive motion is the motion measured after normal soft-tissue resistance to movement is overcome; in the finger joints this is approximately 0.5 kg of force.

A distinction should be made between the terms "extension" and "hyperextension." The term "extension" is used for motions opposite to that of flexion to the zero or neutral starting position. If motion opposite to flexion exceeds the zero or neutral starting position, such as seen at the metacarpophalangeal, elbow, or knee joints, it is referred to as "hyperextension," and is given a "plus" (+) value. Incomplete motion of extension from a flexed position to the zero starting position is reported as a negative or "minus" (−) degree from zero. As an example, finger joint flexion contracture of 15 degrees with flexion to 45 degrees is recorded as a joint motion of −15 to 45 degrees. This refers to a lack of extension of 15 degrees to the zero position. A finger joint that has 15 degrees of hyperextension to 45 degrees of flexion would be recorded as a joint motion of +15 to 45 degrees.

Proximal joints should be in neutral or straight-line

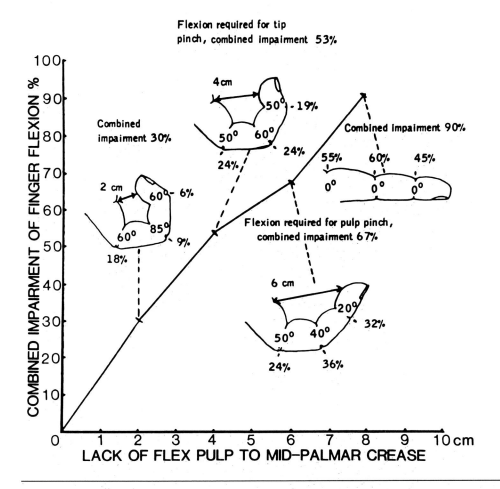

Fig. 4–9 Boyes'[11] linear measurement of distance between finger pulp and middle palmar crease is the simplest method of rating finger flexion capacity. Several common functional postures of fingers are noted. The impairment values to digit for loss of flexion of each joint in these positions are shown. Combined impairment values for each posture are also represented and were calculated from the formula: A% + B% (100% – A%) = combined impairment value for finger. This illustration correlates Boyes' linear measurements with combined angular measurement of finger flexion. For example, linear measurement of 6 cm lack of flexion from fingertip to palmar crease corresponds to 67% impairment according to Boyes' linear chart. For the same position, ankylosis impairment can be obtained for each joint (24% for the metacarpophalangeal joint at 50 degrees, 37% for the proximal interphalangeal joint at 40 degrees, and 32% for the distal interphalangeal joint at 20 degrees). These values combined according to the above formula: 24% + 36% (100% – 24%) = 51%, 51% + 32% (100% – 51%) = 67%. Note that there is a good correlation between linear and angular measurements of impairment. (Reproduced with permission from Swanson AB: Evaluation of impairment of function in the hand. *Surg Clin North Am* 1964;44:925–940.)

position when the distal joints are measured (Fig. 4–4). Active motion or ankylosis is recorded. Digits are named rather than numbered, that is, thumb, index, middle (long), ring, and little fingers. The spread of the fingers and its strength are measured. The method, described by Boyes,[11] of measuring maximal finger flexion by noting the distance that the pulp of the finger lacks in touching the distal palmar crease is included in the evaluation of finger flexion (Fig. 4–4, *bottom right*). Description of the thumb includes a measurement of radial abduction, adduction, opposition, anteposition (palmar abduction), retroposition, and flexion-extension of the metacarpophalangeal and interphalangeal joints (Fig. 4–5).[12]

The motion of the wrist in dorsal and palmar flexion, and radial and ulnar deviations are measured. Elbow flexion, extension, pronation, and supination are noted. Shoulder motion in flexion, extension, abduction, adduction, and internal and external rotation is recorded.

Neurologic Examination

The presence of peripheral nerve disorders, including those of the nerve roots and brachial plexus, radial, ulnar, and median nerve palsies, as evidenced by motor and sensory disturbances in the hand, is noted. Digital nerve loss and the presence and localization of neuromas are evaluated. Tenderness, sensitivity, and painful states such as the causalgias and other sympathetic dystrophies are appraised. A complete sensory examination is performed.[13]

The Ninhydrin test for sudomotor function can be a useful method for documenting the interruption of the digital nerves. However, it has limitations in evaluating the "recovering" nerve, because there is no direct relationship between return of sudomotor function and return of tactile gnosis. A two-point discrimination test can help determine functional loss of tactile gnosis. More than 18 to 20 mm in two-point discrimination testing is considered a total loss of this function. Functional isolation of the finger, as noted in the blindfolded pickup test, will aid the examiner in determining the presence or absence of any useful sensation in the digit.

Pain Evaluation

Pain can be defined as a disagreeable sensation that has as its basis a highly variable complex made up of afferent nerve stimuli interacting with the emotional

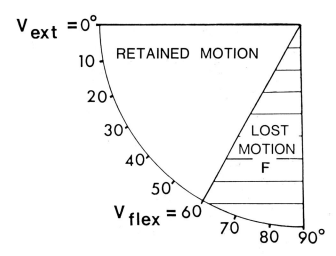

Fig. 4-10 Example of metacarpophalangeal joint presenting motion from 0 degrees of extension to 60 degrees of flexion; lost flexion, F, is equal to theoretically largest possible angle of flexion (90 degrees) minus measured flexion angle (V_{flex} = 60 degrees), or F = 90 degrees – 60 degrees, or 30 degrees. (Reproduced with permission from Swanson AB: Evaluation of impairment of hand function, in Hunter JM, Schneider LH, Mackin EJ, et al (eds): *Rehabilitation of the Hand*, ed 2. St. Louis, CV Mosby, 1984.)

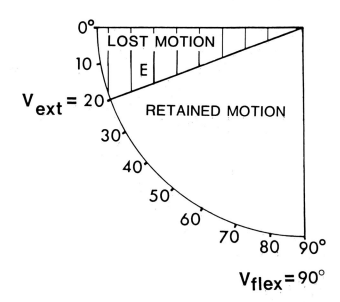

Fig. 4-11 Example of metacarpophalangeal joint presenting motion from 20 degrees of extension lag to 90 degrees of flexion; lost extension, E, is equal to measured extension angle (V_{ext} = 20 degrees) minus theoretically smallest possible extension angle (0 degrees), or E = 20 degrees. (Reproduced with permission from Swanson AB: Evaluation of impairment of hand function, in Hunter JM, Schneider LH, Mackin EJ, et al (eds): *Rehabilitation of the Hand*, ed 2. St. Louis, CV Mosby, 1984.)

state of the individual and modified by past experience, motivation, and state of mind. It is difficult to evaluate because it is a subjective symptom. Pain may be verified and its intensity evaluated in a thorough physical examination. Pretended pain may be detected by tests that confuse the patient into responding with signs that contradict the usual clinical findings. Examination can further demonstrate whether the pain has an anatomic background or if it is associated with other signs of nerve dysfunction. Permanent loss of function because of pain or discomfort is described as a condition that exists after optimum physiologic adjustment and maximum medical rehabilitation have been administered. Subjective complaints of pain that cannot be substantiated along these lines should not be considered for impairment.

It is important to have an impairment classification for pain and discomfort to clarify subjective symptoms that interfere with the patient's activities. Such a classification must be set on arbitrary baselines. Pain associated with peripheral spinal nerve disorders can be classified according to how the pain interferes with the individual's performance of activities: (1) minimal—it is annoying (0% to 25%); (2) slight—it interferes with activity (26% to 50%); (3) moderate—it prevents activity (51% to 75%); (4) severe—it prevents activity and also causes distress (76% to 100%). The percentage of impairment of the part caused by pain or discomfort can be calculated on the same principles used when evaluating amputation of a part (for example, in severe causalgia there may be 100% loss of usefulness of the

extremity). Partial impairment can be taken as a percentage of the whole part, by using the amputation tables to obtain the relative value of each part to the larger part.

Cosmetic Effect

The cosmetic effect implies both a passive and an active element.[4-6] The *passive* cosmetic effect of a normal hand at rest may be simulated by certain artificial hands now available; however, the postures and slight movements that a hand normally assumes during motion are absent, and the hand loses some of its cosmetic effect. The *active* cosmetic effect concerns movements characteristic of a normal hand during performance that provide a pleasant grace and elegance to the hand. These movements may compensate for other losses in the hand.

The cosmetic effect can be evaluated according to the general appearance of the hand at rest and during activity, including the aspect of scars, stiffness, residual joint imbalance, rotational deformities, and coordination. Using the cosmetic improvement "point system," the number of points for the degree of cosmetic improvement at rest and during activity are rated from both the patient's and the examiner's point of view. The maximum possible points are 12 (Table 4–3).

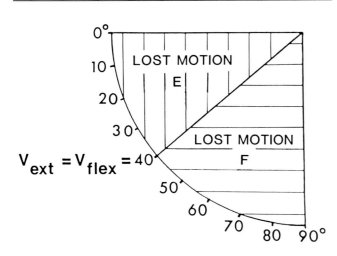

Fig. 4–12 When no motion is retained, there is ankylosis—in this example at 40 degrees. Total motion lost to ankylosis (A) is equal to 40 degrees of lack of extension (E) plus 50 degrees of lack of flexion (F), or A = 40 degrees + 50 degrees, or 90 degrees. (Reproduced with permission from Swanson AB: Evaluation of impairment of hand function, in Hunter JM, Schneider LH, Mackin EJ, et al (eds): *Rehabilitation of the Hand*, ed 2. St. Louis, CV Mosby, 1984.)

Functional Evaluation and Measurements

Evaluation of an accurate profile of a patient's condition requires an appraisal of the resultant loss of function as it relates to the activities of daily living and the more specialized activities of the hand common to all persons. In evaluating the functional capacity of a patient, it is important to determine the ambulatory status and the ability to perform certain basic activities in an independent or an assisted fashion, or not at all, as listed in Figure 4–1. The functional evaluation of the hand includes mainly functional tests for the activities of daily living and the motion-time measurements.

The use of graduated sizes of cylinders and spheres to determine the ability to open the hand and grasp and hold these objects can be a very helpful method for measuring grasp functions and evaluating the patient's functional ability. The end of the cylinder can be used to simulate the shape of the sphere. The examination should include the ability of the patient to perform small and large grasp, pulp, tip, and lateral pinch, distal and proximal hook, and scoop functions.

Functional Evaluation Systems

Most systems for evaluation of physical impairment attempt to establish a numerical deficit from normality by weighing factors such as missing or nonfunctional portions of the body. The resultant figure provides an index of anatomic impairment. However, this does not provide sophisticated insight into the effect of the impairment on the individual patient. Most commonly, the physician is asked to judge physical impairment in

Table 4–5
Impairment percentage resulting from loss of metacarpophalangeal joint flexion from a neutral position (0°)*

Degrees of Flexion	Degrees of Lost Motion (Flexion)	% Impairment
0	90	55
10	80	49
20	70	43
30	60	37
40	50	31
50	40	24
60	30	18
70	20	12
80	10	6
90	0	0

*These figures are taken from the AMA *Guide*.[1]

Table 4–6
Impairment resulting from metacarpophalangeal joint ankylosis*

Degrees of Joint Ankylosis	% Impairment of Finger Function
0	55
10	52
20	48
30	45
40	54
50	63
60	72
70	82
80	91
90	100

*These figures are taken from the AMA *Guide*.[1]

order to permit a nonphysician or third-party judicial body to rate the patient's disability. The disability index should also be a measure of performance, which can change as motivation, fatigue, pain, coordination, and strength change. As only the output is measured, it can have an important place in the evaluation of the patient's ability. In a way, the anatomic impairment evaluation is what the patient is able to put into a functional situation. The evaluation of disability should hinge to a certain degree on a measure of the patient's motor performance in accomplishing functional activities.

Industrial engineers have been evaluating the normal motor performance in the industrial setting for many years. A person's condition can be analyzed according to the ability to perform a given task composed of any given type of motion element and by matching the performance at a selected performance level. Therefore, from a synthetic test of performance ability, performance in an industrial setting may be predicted. A performance index may be described for specific tasks. An example of how a disabled person might perform certain activities would be a pianist who has lost the left upper extremity and is severely disabled as a pianist but who would be essentially nondisabled as a radio an-

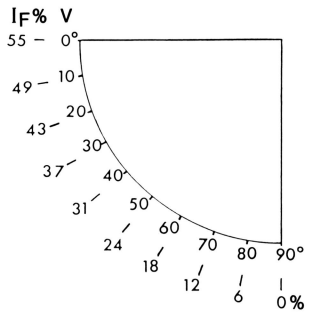

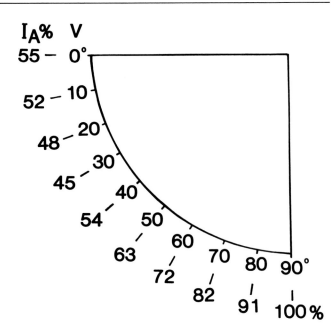

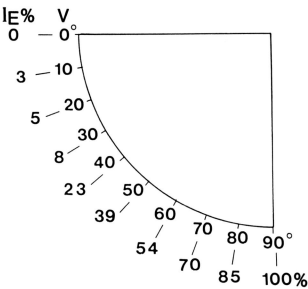

Fig. 4-13 *Percentage impairment of finger function.* **Top left:** Lack of flexion (F) is expressed as I_F. AMA values[1] (Table 4–5) have been transposed to arc of motion. If V_{flex} = 40 degrees, F is 50 degrees and corresponds to I_F = 31%. Note that I_F is a function of V_{flex} and reaches 0% when V_{flex} equals 90 degrees or F reaches 0 degrees. **Top right:** Ankylosis (A) is expressed as I_A. AMA values[1] (Table 4–6) have been transposed to arc of motion. If joint is ankylosed at 40 degrees, A = E (40 degrees) + F (50 degrees), or 90 degrees, and I_A = 54%. **Bottom:** Value of I_E can be derived for each angle from the formula: $I_A = I_E + I_F$, or $I_E = I_A - I_F$. When a metacarpophalangeal joint presents an extension lag of 40 degrees, I_E = 54% (I_A) – 31% (I_F) = 23%. I_E is a function of V_{ext} and reaches 0% when V_{ext} equals 0 degrees or E reaches 0 degrees. (Reproduced with permission from Swanson AB: Evaluation of impairment of hand function, in Hunter JM, Schneider LH, Mackin EJ, et al (eds): *Rehabilitation of the Hand*, ed 2. St. Louis, CV Mosby, 1984.)

nouncer. However, most injuries and vocational situations are less clear. It would be very useful to be able to indicate that an injured worker could perform at 10% of normal on job A and at 90% of normal on job B. It should also be possible to analyze job A to determine how that task could be altered to take advantage of the worker's abilities, while minimizing the disabilities, thereby improving work performance.

The system of analysis of motor performance, motion-time measurements, is concerned with the physical aspect of disability. It basically allows evaluation of general manual dexterity and helps predict specific skills. The ideal evaluation should include a representation of all skills required by specific, available jobs and a

determination of all the significant manual skills possessed by the patient being tested. This method is contained in a predetermined motion-time system and is used widely in industry in the improvement, analysis, and timing of industrial work.

Sophisticated derivatives of motion-time study have been developed that are capable of (1) defining the subunits of the elements of motion that compose virtually any test performance, (2) timing the performance of these motion elements, and (3) relating the timed individual performance of these motion elements to the established "norms" of performance. One of these systems is the methods-time measurement (MTM) system. This is a procedure that analyzes any manual operation

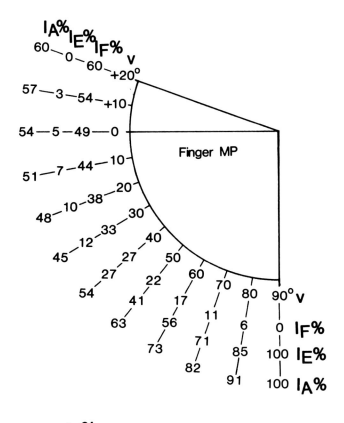

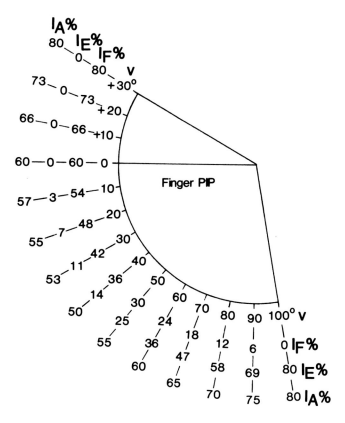

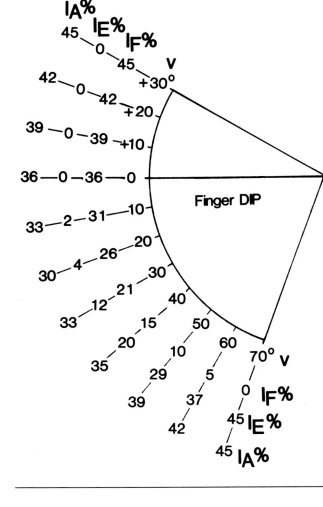

Fig. 4-14 Impairment of finger function. **Top left:** Metacarpophalangeal joint. I_A represents ankylosis impairment, I_F represents flexion impairment, and I_E represents extension impairment. Since the position of function is 30 degrees, I_A is lowest, or 45%, at this angle. Impairment values for hyperextension deformities are included. Relative value of the joint to finger is 100%, the same as amputation through the joint. **Top right:** Proximal interphalangeal joint. Since the position of function is 40 degrees, I_A is lowest, or 50%, at this angle. Values for hyperextension deformities are included. Relative value of the joint to finger is 80%, the same as amputation through the joint. **Bottom:** Distal interphalangeal joint. Since the position of function is 20 degrees, I_A is lowest, or 30%, at this angle. Relative value of the joint to finger is 45%, the same as amputation through the joint. (Reproduced with permission from Swanson AB: Evaluation of impairment of hand function, in Hunter JM, Schneider LH, Mackin EJ, et al (eds): *Rehabilitation of the Hand*, ed 2. St. Louis, CV Mosby, 1984.)

Table 4-7
Combined values for impairment increments of 1%*

	1	2	3	4	5	6	7	8	9	10	11	12	13	14	15	16	17	18	19	20	21	22	23	24	25	26	27	28	29	30
1	2	3	4	5	6	7	8	9	10	11	12	13	14	15	16	17	18	19	20	21	22	23	24	25	26	27	28	29	30	31
2	3	4	5	6	7	8	9	10	11	12	13	14	15	16	17	18	19	20	21	22	23	24	25	26	27	27	28	29	30	31
3	4	5	6	7	8	9	10	11	12	13	14	15	16	17	18	19	19	20	21	22	23	24	25	26	27	28	29	30	31	32
4	5	6	7	8	9	10	11	12	13	14	15	16	16	17	18	19	20	21	22	23	24	25	26	27	28	29	30	31	32	33
5	6	7	8	9	10	11	12	13	14	15	15	16	17	18	19	20	21	22	23	24	25	26	27	28	29	30	31	32	33	34
6	7	8	9	10	11	12	13	14	14	15	16	17	18	19	20	21	22	23	24	25	26	27	28	29	30	30	31	32	33	34
7	8	9	10	11	12	13	14	14	15	16	17	18	19	20	21	22	23	24	25	26	27	27	28	29	30	31	32	33	34	35
8	9	10	11	12	13	14	14	15	16	17	18	19	20	21	22	23	24	25	25	26	27	28	29	30	31	32	33	34	35	36
9	10	11	12	13	14	14	15	16	17	18	19	20	21	22	23	24	24	25	26	27	28	29	30	31	32	33	34	34	35	36
10	11	12	13	14	15	16	16	17	18	19	20	21	22	23	24	24	25	26	27	28	29	30	31	32	33	33	34	35	36	37
11	12	13	14	15	15	16	17	18	19	20	21	22	23	23	24	25	26	27	28	29	30	31	31	32	33	34	35	36	37	38
12	13	14	15	16	16	17	18	19	20	21	22	23	23	24	25	26	27	28	29	30	30	31	32	33	34	35	36	37	38	38
13	14	15	16	16	17	18	19	20	21	22	23	23	24	25	26	27	28	29	30	30	31	32	33	34	35	36	36	37	38	39
14	15	16	17	17	18	19	20	21	22	23	23	24	25	26	27	28	29	29	30	31	32	33	34	35	36	36	37	38	39	40
15	16	17	18	18	19	20	21	22	23	24	24	25	26	27	28	29	29	30	31	32	33	34	35	35	36	37	38	39	40	41
16	17	18	19	19	20	21	22	23	24	24	25	26	27	28	29	29	30	31	32	33	34	34	35	36	37	38	39	40	40	41
17	18	19	19	20	21	22	23	24	24	25	26	27	28	29	29	30	31	32	33	34	34	35	36	37	38	39	39	40	41	42
18	19	20	20	21	22	23	24	25	25	26	27	28	29	29	30	31	32	33	34	34	35	36	37	38	39	39	40	41	42	43
19	20	21	21	22	23	24	25	25	26	27	28	29	30	30	31	32	33	34	34	35	36	37	38	38	39	40	41	42	42	43
20	21	22	22	23	24	25	26	26	27	28	29	30	30	31	32	33	34	34	35	36	37	38	38	39	40	41	42	42	43	44
21	22	23	23	24	25	26	27	27	28	29	30	30	31	32	33	34	34	35	36	37	38	38	39	40	41	42	42	43	44	45
22	23	24	24	25	26	27	27	28	29	30	31	31	32	33	34	34	35	36	37	38	38	39	40	41	42	42	43	44	45	45
23	24	25	25	26	27	28	28	29	30	31	31	32	33	34	35	35	36	37	38	38	39	40	41	41	42	43	44	45	45	46
24	25	26	26	27	28	29	29	30	31	32	32	33	34	35	35	36	37	38	38	39	40	41	41	42	43	44	45	45	46	47
25	26	27	27	28	29	30	30	31	32	33	33	34	35	36	36	37	38	39	39	40	41	42	42	43	44	45	45	46	47	48
26	27	27	28	29	30	30	31	32	33	33	34	35	36	36	37	38	39	39	40	41	42	42	43	44	45	45	46	47	47	48
27	28	28	29	30	31	31	32	33	34	34	35	36	36	37	38	39	39	40	41	42	42	43	44	45	45	46	47	47	48	49
28	29	29	30	31	32	32	33	34	34	35	36	37	37	38	39	40	40	41	42	42	43	44	45	45	46	47	47	48	49	50
29	30	30	31	32	33	33	34	35	35	36	37	38	38	39	40	40	41	42	42	43	44	45	45	46	47	47	48	49	50	50
30	31	31	32	33	34	34	35	36	36	37	38	38	39	40	41	41	42	43	43	44	45	45	46	47	48	48	49	50	50	51

*Based on the formula: A% + B% (100% − A%) = the combined values of A% + B%. If three or more values are to be combined, two may be selected and their combined value found. This combined value and the third value are combined to give the total figure. This process can be repeated indefinitely with the value obtained in each case being a combination of all the previous values. After having the two values, one enters the table at one value horizontally and at the other value vertically, and the combined value will be read at intersections. This combined value must then be combined with the third value to give a final combined value; for example, 30% impairment to DIP, 20% impairment to PIP, and 25% impairment to MP: this would add as follows on this chart: 30% DIP + 20% PIP = 44% to the digit. The following step is calculated on Table 4–8: 44% digit + 25% MP = 59% combined impairment to digit.

or method into the basic motion elements required to perform it and assigns to each motion element a predetermined time standard determined by the nature of the motion and the conditions under which it is made. The system implies that the time involved in task performance is meaningless unless a manner of task performance is defined. The principal elements employed in the methods-time-measurements system are various degrees and purposes of reaching, grasping, moving, turning, applying pressure, and positioning. For complex analyses, there are guides for motion that can or cannot be performed simultaneously by two hands as well as eye-travel time, eye-focus time, principal gross body movements, walking, side-stepping, and so on. An index of disability, a numerical figure that allows the disabled person to be compared with a normal person,

can be obtained. The use of these elements should make it possible to evaluate the hand impaired by trauma or disease and to give it some index of impairment of function, which, combined with the physical impairment, can more fairly attest to the patient's true disability. Further work and research are needed in this area to develop the necessary methods and personnel requirements to use the well-established methods-time-measurements system in disability evaluation.

Principles and Methods of Impairment Evaluation

The most practical and useful approach to the evaluation of digit impairment is through comparison of the loss of function found to be present with that re-

Table 4–8
Combined impairment values representing increments of 5%

	5	10	15	20	25	30	35	40	45	50	55	60	65	70	75	80	85	90	95
5	10	15	19	24	29	34	38	43	48	52	57	62	67	72	76	81	86	91	95
10	15	19	24	28	33	37	42	46	51	55	60	64	69	73	78	82	87	91	96
15	19	24	28	32	36	41	45	49	53	58	62	66	70	75	79	83	87	92	96
20	24	28	32	36	40	44	48	52	56	60	64	68	72	76	80	84	88	92	96
25	29	33	36	40	44	48	51	55	59	63	66	70	73	78	81	85	89	93	96
30	34	37	41	44	48	51	55	58	62	65	69	72	76	79	83	86	90	93	97
35	38	42	45	48	51	55	58	61	64	68	71	74	77	81	84	87	90	94	97
40	43	46	49	52	55	58	61	64	67	70	73	76	79	82	85	88	91	94	97
45	48	51	53	56	59	62	64	67	70	73	75	78	81	84	86	89	92	95	97
50	52	55	58	60	63	65	68	70	73	75	78	80	83	85	88	90	93	95	98
55	57	60	62	64	66	69	71	73	75	78	80	82	84	87	89	91	93	96	98
60	62	64	66	68	70	72	74	76	78	80	82	84	86	88	90	92	94	96	98
65	67	69	70	72	73	76	77	79	81	83	84	86	88	90	91	93	95	97	98
70	72	73	75	76	78	79	81	82	84	85	87	88	90	91	93	94	96	97	99
75	76	78	79	80	81	83	84	85	86	88	89	90	91	93	94	95	96	98	99
80	81	82	83	84	85	86	87	88	89	90	91	92	93	94	95	96	97	98	99
85	86	87	87	88	89	90	90	91	92	93	93	94	95	96	96	97	98	99	99
90	91	91	92	92	93	93	94	94	95	95	96	96	97	97	98	98	99	99	100
95	95	96	96	96	96	97	97	97	97	98	98	98	98	99	99	99	99	100	100

sulting from amputation. Most schedules of evaluation consider the upper limb as a unit of the whole person and divide it into hand, wrist, elbow, and shoulder. The hand is further separated into digits and their parts.

Total loss of motion of a digit, total loss of sensation, and ankylosis and severe malposition that render the digit essentially useless are considered about the same as amputation of the part. Ankylosis in the optimum functional position of joints is given the least disability on the charts. The great majority of functional activities of the hand require a 5-cm opening in the fingers and thumb, and therefore this degree of opening should be considered favorably in the impairment charts. The ability to flex the fingers to within 1 or 2 cm of the distal palmar crease is indicative of a useful range of motion and should also be considered favorably.

Amputation Impairment Evaluation

Amputation of the entire extremity or 100% loss of the limb is considered 60% impairment of the whole person. Amputations at levels below the elbow, distal to the biceps insertion and proximal to the metacarpophalangeal level are considered a 95% loss of the total limb (Fig. 4–6). Amputation of the fingers and thumb through the metacarpophalangeal joint removes the most essential functional parts and is considered 100% impairment of the hand or 90% impairment of the total limb. Since loss of the entire limb equals 60% impairment of the whole person, 90% impairment of the limb equals 54% impairment of the person. Using this principle of progressive multiplication of percentage values, the impairment of each digit or portion thereof can be related to the hand, the upper limb, and eventually to the whole person (Table 4–4).

The digits represent five coordinated units into which all hand function is unequally divided. In evaluating the impaired function of the whole hand, each finger and the thumb are evaluated separately according to the 100% scale in relation to the entire digit; each digit is then weighed according to its respective value to the total hand as follows: thumb 40%, index and middle finger 20% each, and ring and little finger 10% each (Fig. 4–6). Any portion of the digit is taken as a percentage of the whole digit (Fig. 4–7). Amputation through the metacarpophalangeal joint equals 100% loss of the digit; amputation through the proximal interphalangeal joint equals 80% loss to the finger; amputation through the distal interphalangeal joint equals 45% loss to the finger; and amputation through the interphalangeal joint of the thumb equals 50% loss to the thumb. The value of each portion of a digit can be related to the whole hand by multiplying it by the digit's relative value to the hand; for example, amputation through the proximal interphalangeal joint of the index finger represents 80% loss of this finger or 80% × 20% = 16% loss to the hand. The values relating the loss of each part of each digit to the whole hand have been calculated as above and are shown in Figure 4–6. When amputation of multiple digits or parts of digits is present, the hand impairment is calculated by adding the hand impairments derived from each digit. Since the hand represents 90% to the upper extremity, the hand impairment value is multiplied by 90% to obtain upper extremity impairment, and then by 60% to obtain the impairment of the whole person. For example, amputation of the entire thumb (40% hand impairment) with amputation through the distal interphalangeal joint of the index finger (9% hand impairment) equals 49% impairment of the whole hand; 49% × 90% = 44% im-

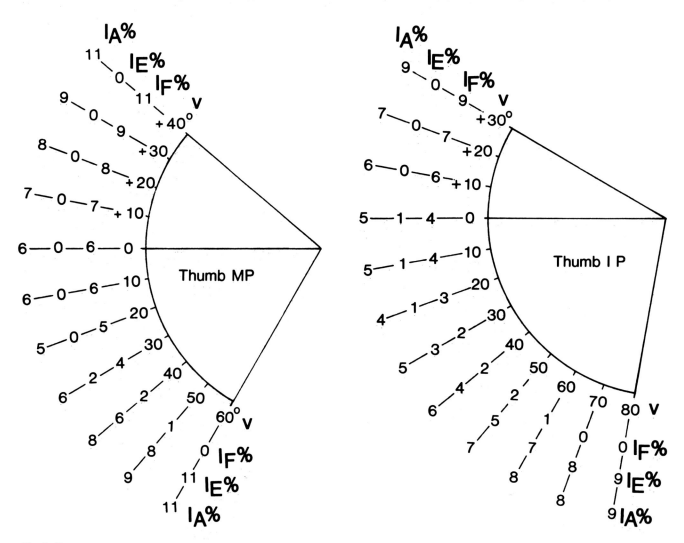

Fig. 4–15 Impairment percentages to thumb for loss of flexion and extension and for ankylosis. Functional position is 20 degrees of flexion at the interphalangeal and metacarpophalangeal joints. Thumb flexion-extension represents 20% of motion units. Of this, a value of 11% is given to the metacarpophalangeal joint (**left**) and a value of 9% to the interphalangeal joint (**right**).

pairment of the upper extremity; and 44% × 60% = 26% impairment of the whole person.

Sensory Impairment Evaluation

Any loss resulting from sensory deficit, pain, or discomfort that contributes to permanent impairment must be unequivocal and permanent. Loss of sensation on the dorsal surface of the fingers is not considered disabling. Sensation on the palmar surface of the distal segment contributes to the function of the digit. Sensory loss on the least-often opposed surfaces of the fingers and thumb should be given less value than the more important surfaces used in the usual pinch-and-grasp activities.

Complete loss of palmar sensation is considered as a 50% deficit of functional capacity. Its value is calculated, therefore, as 50% that of an amputation; for example, loss of both digital nerves of the thumb is considered one half of its amputation value, or half of 40%, or 20% hand impairment. Complete loss of sensation of the index or middle fingers equals 10% hand impairment each, and complete loss of sensation of the ring and little fingers equals 5% hand impairment each (Fig. 4–8).

Partial transverse sensory loss is calculated as a percentage value of a portion of the digit; for example, sensory loss of the distal phalanx of the thumb equals one half the value assigned for amputation through the interphalangeal joint, or 25% thumb impairment and 10% hand impairment. The values for each transverse level of sensory loss can be calculated from the amputation values, as shown in Figures 4–6 and 4–7.

Partial longitudinal sensory loss is based on the relative importance of the side of the digit for sensory function. Loss of sensation on the radial half of the thumb is

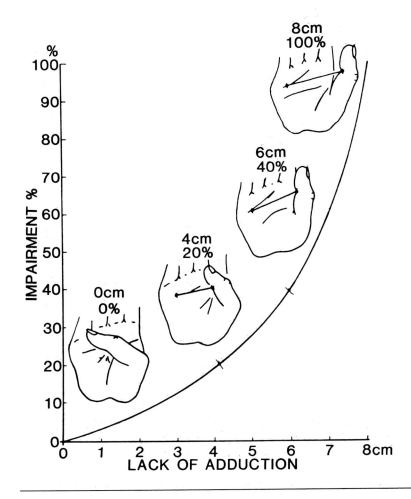

Fig. 4-16 Adduction is measured (linear measurement) as the distance between the flexor crease of the interphalangeal joint of thumb to the distal palmar crease over the metacarpophalangeal joint of fifth finger. Graph represents percentage value for lack of adduction relative to this function and not to whole thumb function. Adduction contributes 20% to thumb function and impairments shown must be multiplied by 20% to obtain impairment percentages to entire thumb function, as shown in Table 4–9. (Reproduced with permission from Swanson AB: Evaluation of impairment of hand function, in Hunter JM, Schneider LH, Mackin EJ, et al (eds): *Rehabilitation of the Hand*, ed 2. St. Louis, CV Mosby, 1984.)

rated as 40% thumb sensory impairment; loss on the ulnar half is rated as 60%. Sensory loss on the ulnar half of the fingers is rated as 40% finger sensory impairment; loss on the radial half is rated as 60%, except for the little finger where sensation on the ulnar border is more important. The impairment value for longitudinal sensory deficit of each digit is converted to hand impairment by multiplying it by the digit's sensory relative value to the hand (half of its amputation relative value to the hand). For example, 100% loss of thumb sensation corresponds to a 20% hand impairment; longitudinal sensory loss on the ulnar side of the thumb represents a 60% thumb sensory impairment or 12% hand impairment (40% × 50% = 20%; 20% × 60% = 12%). The values for radial and ulnar longitudinal sensory impairment to the hand for each digit are shown in Figure 4–8.

Finger Motion Impairment Evaluation

A variety of methods have been proposed for evaluation of flexor tendon repair. The method suggested by Boyes[11] of *a linear measurement* from the fingertip to the distal palmar crease has been used by many. Litch-

man and Paslay[14] have attempted to give values for impairment of the finger function related to a linear distance from fingertip to distal palmar crease. Van't Hof and Heiple[15] proposed a method for evaluation of lack of extension as a linear measurement from the rim of the nail to the point to which the nail is expected to reach in case of full extension. White used a numeric sum of the angles in maximum flexion of the three finger joints (K. White, personal communication, 1965). Swanson[4] in 1964 proposed a method for evaluating impairment caused by loss of flexion motion based on a *combined angular measurement principle*. The individual values for impairment of finger function caused by ankylosis and lack of flexion were obtained from the AMA's *Guide to the Evaluation of Permanent Impairment of the Extremities and Back*.[1] A system based on the formula A% + B% (100% – A%) = the combined values of A% + B% was developed and used to add the combined values of impairment. Swanson also correlated the *combined angular measurement with the linear measurement of Boyes* and developed charts that could be used for everyday clinical practice[4] (Fig. 4–9). The Committee on Impairment Evaluation of the American Medical Associ-

Table 4-9
Thumb impairment

Impairment*	Thumb Impairment (%)	
	Lost Motion	Ankylosis
Lack of adduction (cm)		
0	0	20
1	0	19
2	1	17
3	3	15
4	4	10
5	6	15
6	8	17
7	13	19
8	20	20
Radial abduction (degrees)		
50	0	10
40	1	10
30	3	10
20	7	10
10	9	10
0	10	10
Measured opposition (cm)		
0	50	50
1	35	45
2	25	40
3	15	35
4	10	30
5	6	25
6	3	27
7	1	30
8	0	32

*Taking into consideration that adduction contributes 20% to thumb function, radial abduction contributes 10%, and opposition contributes 50%.

ation had proposed the use of combining joint angles. Tubiana and associates[16] proposed methods of evaluation of results after operations for Dupuytren's contracture.

"A = E + F" Method of Finger Impairment Evaluation

The evaluation of impaired joint motion presented here is based on the American Medical Association *Guide*[1] and the work of Swanson.[4] In these studies, values for ankylosis and impaired flexion are calculated on the assumption that the normal extension for the metacarpophalangeal and interphalangeal joints is 0 degrees. Previously, impairment values for lack of extension were not adequately taken into consideration, and for that reason a method for rating the lack of extension impairment has been worked out and is presented here.

The range of motion of a joint is the total number of degrees of movement traced by an arc from maximum extension to maximum flexion. To determine the range of motion, the two angles of extreme motion are measured and are represented by a "V" as follows:

$$\text{Flexion V } (V_{flex}) =$$
largest possible angle to achieve by flexion
$$\text{Extension V } (V_{ext}) =$$
smallest possible angle to achieve by extension

Assuming a metacarpophalangeal joint has a normal range of motion from 0 to 90 degrees, the largest possible angle to achieve by flexion is 90 degrees, and the smallest possible angle to achieve by extension is 0 degrees. When V_{flex} equals 90 degrees and V_{ext} equals 0 degrees, there is no impairment of joint motion. Considerations for normal hyperextension of the metacarpophalangeal joints are discussed later.

Assuming a decrease of joint flexion from 90 to 60 degrees while extension remains unchanged at 0 degrees, V_{flex} now equals 60 degrees and V_{ext} equals 0 degrees (Fig. 4-10). The lost flexion is represented by F and is equal to the theoretically largest V_{flex} minus the measured value of V_{flex}. For a metacarpophalangeal joint extending from 0 to 60 degrees of flexion, the lack of flexion can be expressed as follows:

$$F = 90° (V_{flex} \text{ largest}) - 60° (V_{flex} \text{ measured}) = 30°$$

Assuming there is a lack of extension of 20 degrees, V_{ext} equals 20 degrees (Fig. 4-11). The lost motion of extension is represented by E and is equal to the measured value of V_{ext} minus the theoretically smallest value of V_{ext}. For a metacarpophalangeal joint lacking 20 degrees of extension, the lost extension can be expressed as follows:

$$E = 20° (V_{ext} \text{ measured}) - 0° (V_{ext} \text{ smallest}) = 20°$$

With decreased flexion there is a decrease in V_{flex}, and with impaired extension there is an increase of V_{ext}; these two values will finally meet each other and be located at the same point of the arc, or V_{flex} equals V_{ext} (Fig. 4-12). This situation represents ankylosis. The total loss of joint motion is represented by A. This does not refer to the angle of the arc of motion at which a joint is ankylosed but to the sum of the lack of extension (E) and the lack of flexion (F) resulting from this ankylosis. The total loss of joint motion can be expressed as A = E + F. If the joint is ankylosed at 40 degrees, as shown in Figure 4-12:

$$V_{ext} = V_{flex} = 40°$$
$$E \text{ (extension loss)} = 40°$$
$$F \text{ (flexion loss)} = 90° - 40° = 50°$$
$$A \text{ (total motion loss)} = 40° + 50° = 90°$$

The value A represents total loss of joint motion and is always equal to the same number of degrees as the normal full range of motion of that joint. For a metacarpophalangeal joint, A always equals 90 degrees, no matter where in the arc of motion the ankylosis has occurred. For example:

Ankylosis at 30°: A = 30° (E) + 60° (F) = 90°
Ankylosis at 80°: A = 80° (E) + 10° (F) = 90°

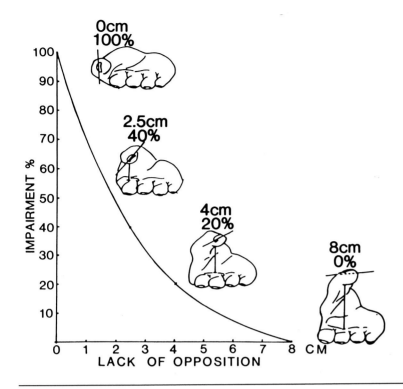

Fig. 4-17 Opposition is measured as largest possible distance from flexor crease of interphalangeal joint to distal palmar crease over third metacarpophalangeal joint. Impairment value curve for lack of opposition is shown relative to this function. Opposition contributes 50% to entire thumb function, and values of impairment shown must be multiplied by 50% to obtain impairment percentage to entire thumb function, as shown in Table 4-9. (Reproduced with permission from Swanson AB: Evaluation of impairment of hand function, in Hunter JM, Schneider LH, Mackin EJ, et al (eds): *Rehabilitation of the Hand*, ed 2. St. Louis, CV Mosby, 1984.)

The above formula is of basic importance in the discussion of impaired function and its evaluation. Impairment of finger function may be caused by lack of extension (E) with or without lack of flexion (F) or ankylosis (A). The motion impairment of finger function may then be called I_E, I_F, and I_A, respectively. These are functions of V, the angle measured at examination. More specifically, the percentage of impairment can be expressed in the following way:

I_E is a function of V_{ext} (smallest angle measured for extension) and goes to 0% when V_{ext} reaches its theoretically smallest value (for example, 0 degrees for the metacarpophalangeal joint).

I_F is a function of V_{flex} (largest angle measured for flexion) and goes to 0% when V_{flex} reaches its theoretically largest value (for example, 90 degrees for the metacarpophalangeal joint).

I_A is a function of V when V_{ext} equals V_{flex} and similarly $I_A = I_E + I_F$.

The function impairment is expressed as a percentage relating the loss of function (for example, flexion) to the part affected (for example, the finger) on the 100% scale. Percentage values for impairment of the metacarpophalangeal joint from lack of flexion from 0 to 90 degrees and from ankylosis are available from the AMA *Guide* (Tables 4–5 and 4–6).[1] These can be expressed as shown in Figure 4–13, *top left and right*. According to the formula previously described, $I_A = I_E +$

I_F, which can also be written, $I_E = I_A - I_F$, we can derive the value for extension impairment, I_E, at each given angle. For example, at an angle of 30 degrees, if I_A equals 45% and I_F equals 37%, the value I_E can be derived as follows: 45% (I_A) – 37% (I_F) = 8% (I_E). This same process can be applied to each angle of the arc of motion to derive the values of I_E (Fig. 4–13, *bottom*). However, the AMA *Guide*[1] does not take into account values for hyperextension; therefore, we have slightly modified the values for I_F to account for hyperextension values for the metacarpophalangeal joint up to 20 degrees, which can be considered normal. These modified impairment values are shown for the metacarpophalangeal joint in Figure 4–14, *top left*.

The derivation of I_E is of fundamental importance for adequate evaluation of functional impairment resulting from limitation of joint motion. Values for both I_E and I_F are now available to estimate the percentage of impairment relating not only to the number of degrees of lost movement but, importantly, to their location in the arc of finger motion. The maximum motion impairment value at the metacarpophalangeal joint reaches 100% or the same as the relative value of the metacarpophalangeal joint to the finger.

Assuming a metacarpophalangeal joint has 30 degrees of retained motion, the impairment is not as severe when the preserved motion occurs from 10 degrees of extension lag to 40 degrees of flexion as it would be if the motion took place between 50 degrees

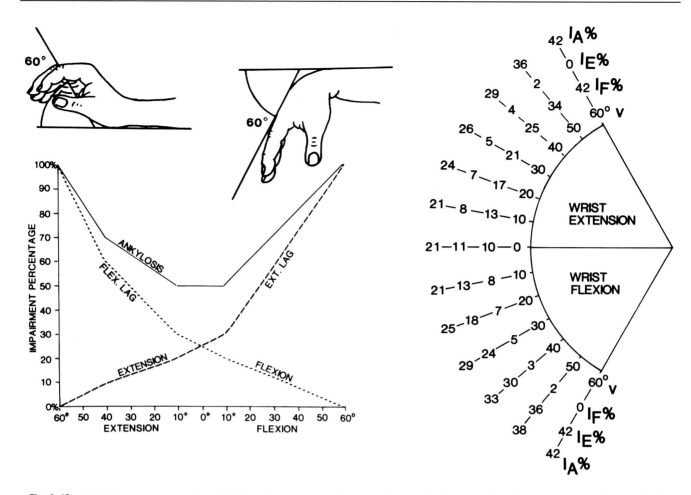

Fig. 4-18   Wrist flexion and extension. **Left:** Impairment curves shown relative to this function. Note that usual range of motion is from 60 degrees of dorsiflexion to 60 degrees of palmar flexion; position of function is from 10 degrees of dorsiflexion to 10 degrees of palmar flexion. Values for impairment ankylosis reach their lowest between these two angles (I_A = 50%). (Reproduced with permission from Swanson AB: Evaluation of impairment of hand function, in Hunter JM, Schneider LH, Mackin EJ, et al (eds): *Rehabilitation of the Hand*, ed 2. St. Louis, CV Mosby, 1984.) **Right:** Impairments in upper extremity values. Flexion-extension contributes 70% to the wrist's functional value and the wrist contributes 60% to the upper extremity function; therefore, the conversion factor for the curve shown on the left is 70% × 60%, or 42% upper extremity impairment.

of extension lag and 80 degrees of flexion. For a metacarpophalangeal joint extending from −10 degrees and flexing to 40 degrees, I_E equals 7% and I_F equals 27%, for a total impairment of 7% + 27%, or 34%. For a metacarpophalangeal joint extending from −50 degrees to 80 degrees, I_E equals 41% and I_F equals 6%, for a total impairment of 41% + 6%, or 47%. Ankylosis of the metacarpophalangeal joint at 30 degrees, or the position of function, equals 45% or the lowest value for I_A (Fig. 4–14, *top left*).

Impairment values for loss of function of the fingers, thumb, wrist, elbow, and shoulder have been derived from the basic formula discussed above. The principle for combining multiple impairments of a finger or of various segments of the extremity needs to be detailed.

Impairment Estimation for Combined Values

When multiple impairments involve the whole finger, the principle of relating the smaller part of the next larger part to obtain a combined value is useful. The method of combining various impairments is based on the principle that each impairment acts not on the whole part (for example, the whole finger) but on the portion that remains (for example, the proximal interphalangeal joint and proximally) after the preceding impairment has acted (for example, on the distal interphalangeal joint). When there is more than one impairment to a given part, these impairments must be combined before the conversion to a larger part is made. The combined values determination is based on the formula:

$$A\% + B\% (100\% - A\%) =$$
the combined values of A% + B%

When this formula is used, all percentages combined must be expressed on a common denominator. For example, multiple impairments of a finger are combined

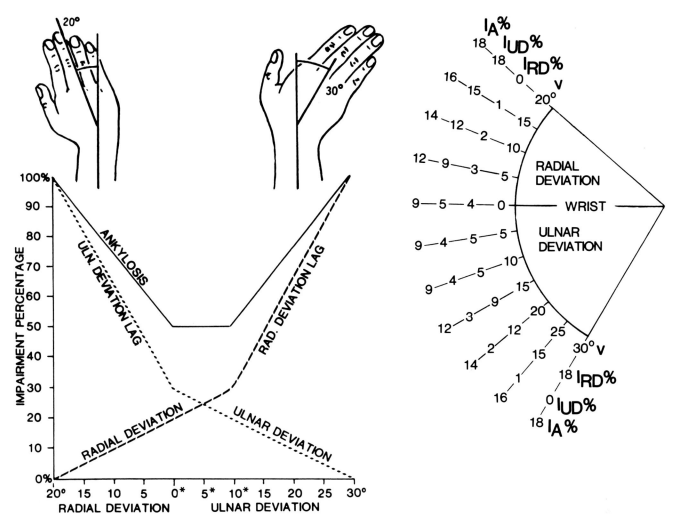

Fig. 4-19 Wrist radial and ulnar deviation. **Left:** Impairment curves shown relative to this function. Note that usual range of motion is from 20 degrees of radial deviation to 30 degrees of ulnar deviation; position of function is from 0 to 10 degrees of ulnar deviation. Ankylosis impairment values reach their lowest point between these angles (50%). (Reproduced with permission from Swanson AB: Evaluation of impairment of hand function, in Hunter JM, Schneider LH, Mackin EJ, et al (eds): *Rehabilitation of the Hand*, ed 2. St. Louis, CV Mosby, 1984.) **Right:** Impairments in upper extremity values. Radial-ulnar deviation contributes 30% to the wrist's functional value and the wrist contributes 60% to the upper extremity function; therefore, the conversion factor for the curve shown on the left is 30% × 60%, or 18% upper extremity impairment.

as expressed on the 100% relative value of the finger. The combined value is rounded to the nearest 5% and converted to the next larger part, for example, the hand. If three or more values are to be combined, two may be selected and their combined value found. This combined value and the third value are combined to give the total value. This procedure can be repeated indefinitely, with the value obtained in each case being a combination of all the previous values. Combined value tables for ease of determination are provided in Tables 4–7 and 4–8; combined values can, in turn, be related to the finger, the hand, the extremity, and the whole person.

For example, an index finger presents an amputation at the distal interphalangeal joint and ankylosis of the proximal interphalangeal joint at 90 degrees; the combined impairment to the index finger can be computed according to the formula: amputation of the distal interphalangeal joint represents a 45% impairment of the finger (Fig. 4–6), and ankylosis of the proximal interphalangeal joint at 90 degrees represents a 75% impairment of the finger; the combined impairment of the finger is:

$$45\% + 75\% \ (100\% - 45\%) = 45\% + 75\% \ (55\%) = 45\% + 41\% = 86\%$$

The index finger represents 20% to the hand; therefore this impairment represents a 86% × 20%, or 17% impairment of the hand. The combined impairment value of the above example can also be found quickly in Table

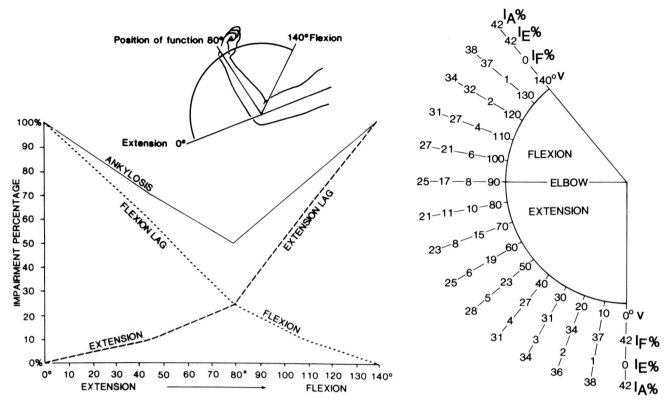

Fig. 4–20 Elbow flexion-extension. **Left:** Impairment curves shown relative to this function. Range of motion of elbow is usually from 0 degrees of extension to 140 degrees of flexion; position of function is 80 degrees of flexion. Note that impairment ankylosis percentage is lowest for position of function (50%). (Reproduced with permission from Swanson AB: Evaluation of impairment of hand function, in Hunter JM, Schneider LH, Mackin EJ, et al (eds): *Rehabilitation of the Hand*, ed 2. St. Louis, CV Mosby, 1984.) **Right:** Impairments in upper extremity values. Flexion-extension contributes 60% to the elbow's functional value and the elbow contributes 70% to upper extremity function; therefore, the conversion factor for the curve shown on the left is 60% × 70%, or 42% upper extremity impairment.

4–8 at the intersection of the vertical and horizontal coordinates represented by 45% and 75% = 86% finger impairment.

Impairment Evaluation Tables and How To Use Them

Finger Impairment

Motion and ankylosis impairment values for the metacarpophalangeal, proximal interphalangeal, and distal interphalangeal joints are given in Figure 4–14. I_A gives the impairment of finger function attributable to ankylosis at any angle; I_E and I_F give the impairment of finger function attributable to lack of extension and lack of flexion, respectively. In a normal hand, the metacarpophalangeal joint can usefully hyperextend to 20 degrees. A very small percentage of impairment (5%) has been assigned to loss of this normal hyperextension. The proximal and distal interphalangeal joints normally extend to 0 degrees, and I_E equals 0% at this angle. Between 0 and +30 degrees, impairment values for these joints are given for lack of flexion and not for hyper-

extension. However, consideration for hyperextension angles now allows us to rate impairment of flexion when ankylosis in a hyperextended position occurs; for example, proximal interphalangeal joint ankylosis at +30 degrees equals 80% impairment. Note that for each joint the percentage of impairment ankylosis, or I_A, is at its lowest at the angle of position of function; I_A at 30 degrees equals 45% for the metacarpophalangeal joint, I_A at 40 degrees equals 50% for the proximal interphalangeal joint, and I_A at 20 degrees equals 30% for the distal interphalangeal joint. The maximum percentage of motion impairment given to each joint is the same as their amputation value: 100% for the metacarpophalangeal joint; 80% for the proximal interphalangeal joint; and 45% for the distal interphalangeal joint.

These diagrams are used in the following way: measure the range of motion, for example, 20 degrees of extension lag to 60 degrees of flexion for the metacarpophalangeal joint. The extension impairment is found under I_E, or 10% impairment at 20 degrees of extension lag, and the flexion impairment is found un-

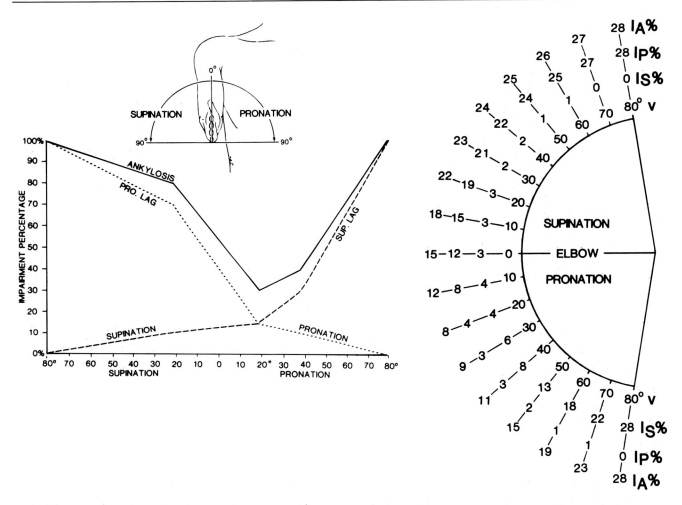

Fig. 4-21 Rotation of forearm. **Left:** Impairment curves shown relative to this function. Usual range of rotation is from 80 degrees of supination to 80 degrees of pronation; position of function is 20 degrees of pronation. Note that impairment ankylosis percentage is lowest for position of function (30%). **Right:** Impairments in upper extremity values. Pronation-supination contributes 40% to the elbow's functional value and the elbow contributes 70% to upper extremity function; therefore, the conversion factor for the curve shown on the left is 40% × 70%, or 28% upper extremity impairment.

der the row headed I_F, or 17% at 60 degrees of flexion. The metacarpophalangeal joint impairment resulting from the above range of motion totals 10% + 17%, or 27%.

When more than one joint is impaired in a finger, the motion impairment of the finger is found by using the combined values formula. For example, 30% motion impairment of the distal interphalangeal joint, 50% motion impairment of the proximal interphalangeal joint, and 40% motion impairment of the metacarpophalangeal joint are combined as follows: 30% + 50% (100% − 30%) = 65%; 65% + 40% (100% −65%) = 79% finger impairment. The finger impairment is converted to hand impairment by multiplying it by the conversion factor for the specific finger involved, for example, 79% impairment of the index finger represents 79% × 20%, or 16% hand impairment; 79% impairment of the little finger represents 79% × 10%, or 8% hand impairment (Fig. 4–6).

Thumb Impairment

The thumb represents 40% of the whole hand; it is considered to have four different functional units, each of which contributes to its total motion function: (1) flexion-extension of the metacarpophalangeal and interphalangeal joints, (2) adduction, (3) radial abduction, and (4) opposition. Adduction is measured as the smallest possible distance in centimeters from the flexor crease of the interphalangeal joint of the thumb to the distal palmar crease at the level of the fifth metacarpophalangeal joint. Radial abduction is measured as the largest possible angle in degrees formed by the first and second metacarpals during maximum active radial abduction. Opposition is measured in centimeters as the largest distance possible to achieve between the flexor crease at the interphalangeal joint of the thumb to the distal palmar crease over the third metacarpophalangeal joint.

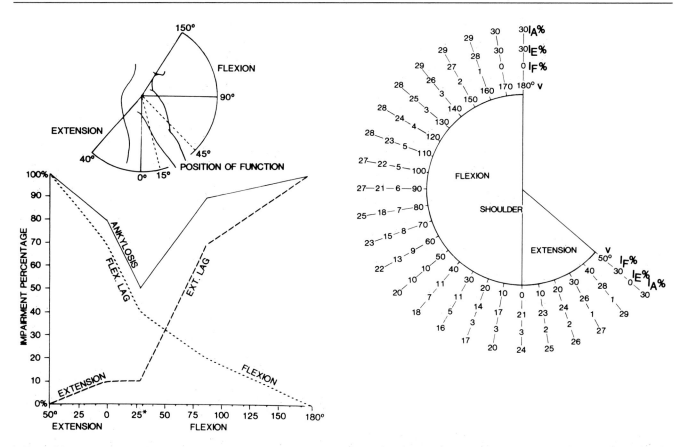

Fig. 4-22 Shoulder flexion-extension. **Left:** Impairment curves shown relative to this function. Position of function has been established at 25 degrees of flexion. **Right:** Impairments in upper extremity values. Extension contributes 10% and flexion 40% to the shoulder's functional value, or 50% for the combined motion, and the shoulder contributes 60% to upper extremity function; therefore, the conversion factor for the curve shown on the left is 50% × 60%, or 30% upper extremity impairment.

Combined flexion-extension of the metacarpophalangeal and interphalangeal joints contribute 20% to thumb function. On the 100% scale, the relative functional value of the metacarpophalangeal joint is 55%, and that of the interphalangeal joint 45%. This is equivalent to 55% × 20% or 11% relative value for metacarpophalangeal joint motion and 45% × 20% or 9% relative value for interphalangeal joint motion. These values have been taken into consideration in the Thumb Motion Impairment Charts (Fig. 4–15). Note that the functional position of the metacarpophalangeal and interphalangeal joints is 20 degrees; thus, the I_A values are the lowest at this angle. For example, thumb metacarpophalangeal ankylosis at 20 degrees of flexion equals 5% impairment ankylosis (I_A), and interphalangeal ankylosis at 20 degrees of flexion equals 4% impairment ankylosis (I_A).

Adduction contributes 20% to thumb function and impairment values have been calculated taking this factor into account. The adduction impairment curve is shown in Figure 4–16. For example, adduction to 4 cm represents a 20% impairment of adduction (Fig. 4–16), or 20% × 20%, or 4% impairment of the entire thumb (Table 4–9).

Radial abduction contributes 10% to the thumb motion value, and impairment values have been calculated taking this factor into consideration (Table 4–9). Note that ankylosis in any position of radial abduction corresponds to a complete impairment of this function, since prehension is not possible without some opposition component.

Opposition contributes 50% to the thumb function. Its impairment curve and calculated values for loss of motion or ankylosis are shown in Figure 4–17 and Table 4–9.

The values derived for each thumb motion impairment are added numerically to obtain the total motion impairment of the thumb. The combined table is not used. Hand impairment values are obtained by multiplying the thumb values by the thumb's relative value to the hand (40%).

Wrist Impairment

Dorsal and palmar flexion are given a 70% relative value to the total wrist motion, and radial and ulnar deviation are given a 30% value. The usual range of motion of the wrist is from 60 degrees of dorsiflexion

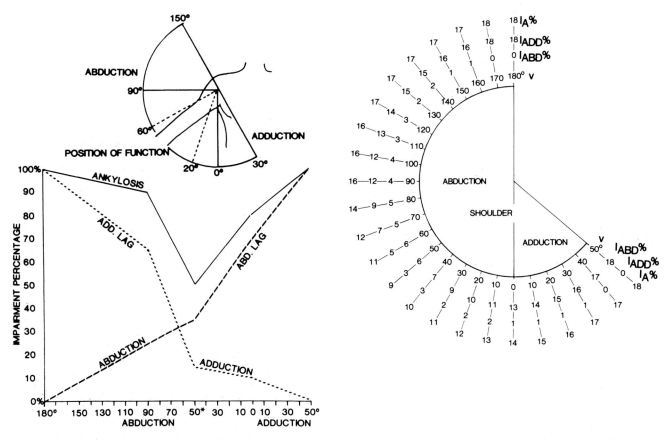

Fig. 4–23 Shoulder abduction-adduction. **Left:** Impairment curves shown relative to this function. Position of function is 50 degrees of abduction. **Right:** Impairments in upper extremity values. Abduction contributes 20% and adduction 10% to the shoulder's functional value, or 30% for the combined motion, and the shoulder contributes 60% to upper extremity function; therefore, the conversion factor for the curve shown on the left is 30% × 60%, or 18% upper extremity impairment.

to 60 degrees of palmar flexion; the position of function is from 10 degrees of palmar flexion to 10 degrees of dorsiflexion. The usual range of lateral motion of the wrist is from 20 degrees of radial deviation to 30 degrees of ulnar deviation; the position of function in lateral deviation is from 0 to 10 degrees of ulnar deviation.

The dorsiflexion-palmar flexion impairment curve is shown in Figure 4–18, *left*. These values were converted to upper extremity impairment values, taking into consideration that this motion contributes 70% to the wrist function and that wrist function contributes 60% to upper extremity impairment. The conversion factor for this curve is 70% × 60%, or 42% upper extremity impairment (Fig. 4–18, *right*).

The lateral deviation motion impairment curve is shown in Figure 4–19, *left*. These values were converted to upper extremity impairment values taking into consideration that this motion contributes 30% to wrist function. The conversion factor for this curve is 30% × 60%, or 18% upper extremity impairment (Fig. 4–19, *right*).

Upper extremity impairment caused by loss of wrist

motion is calculated by adding the flexion-extension and lateral deviation percentages. For example, wrist motion of 20 degrees of extension, 30 degrees of flexion, 5 degrees of radial deviation, 15 degrees of ulnar deviations result in an upper extremity impairment of:

$$I_E\ (7\%) + I_F\ (5\%) + I_{RD}\ (5\%) + I_{UD}\ (3\%) = 20\%$$

Elbow Impairment

The elbow functional unit represents 70% to the upper extremity. On a scale of 100%, elbow flexion-extension is given 60% of this value and pronation-supination is given 40%. The conversion factor for the flexion-extension curve is 60% × 70%, or 42% upper extremity impairment (Fig. 4–20). The conversion factor for the pronation-supination curve is 40% × 70%, or 28% upper extremity impairment (Fig. 4–21).

The average normal range of motion in the elbow is assumed to be from 0 to 140 degrees of flexion-extension. The position of function is 80 degrees of flexion. The most useful range of motion from the functional point of view is considered to be from 45 to 110 degrees of flexion. Lack of extension less than 45 degrees and

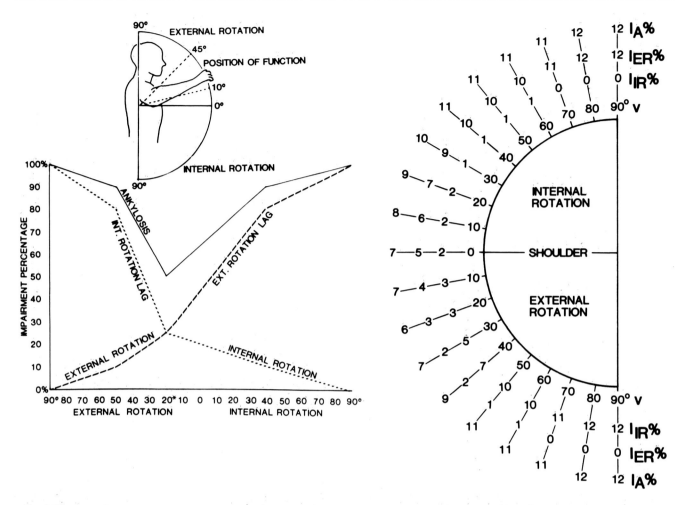

Fig. 4-24 Shoulder internal-external rotation. **Left:** Impairment curves shown relative to this function. Position of function is 20 degrees of external rotation. **Right:** Impairments in upper extremity values. Rotation motion contributes 20% to the shoulder's functional value and the shoulder contributes 60% to upper extremity function; therefore, the conversion factor for the curve shown on the left is 20% × 60%, or 12% upper extremity impairment.

lack of flexion from 110 to 140 degrees are therefore considered to give a relatively small impairment of function. The usual range of rotation is from 80 degrees of supination to 80 degrees of pronation. The position of function is considered to be 20 degrees of pronation.

Upper extremity impairment from loss of elbow motion is calculated by adding the flexion-extension and pronation-supination percentages. For example, elbow motion of −30 degrees of extension, 110 degrees of flexion, 60 degrees of pronation, and 40 degrees of supination results in an upper extremity impairment of:

$$I_E\ (3\%) + I_F\ (4\%) + I_P\ (1\%) + I_S\ (2\%) = 10\%$$

Shoulder Impairment

The shoulder functional unit represents 60% to the upper extremity. The motion units and their relative value to shoulder function on a 100% scale are flexion, 40%; extension, 10%; abduction, 20%; adduction, 10%; and internal-external rotation, 20%. The conversion factor for the flexion-extension curve is 50% × 60%, or 30% upper extremity impairment (Fig. 4-22). The conversion factor for the abduction-adduction curve is 30% × 60%, or 18% upper extremity impairment (Fig. 4-23). The conversion factor for the rotation curve is 20% × 60%, or 12% upper extremity impairment (Fig. 4-24).

For each of these three functions, the position of function was chosen according to recommendations in the literature concerning arthrodesis of the glenohumeral joint,[17,18] even though motions of different joints are involved in each function (glenohumeral joint, acromioclavicular joint, sternoclavicular joint, and the movement between the scapula and the chest wall).

The average normal range of shoulder motion is assumed to be from 50 degrees of extension to 180 degrees of flexion; the position of function is 25 degrees of flexion. Ankylosis in the position of function gives 50% impairment of function, ankylosis in 0 degrees of flexion gives 80% impairment, and ankylosis in 90 degrees of flexion gives 90% impairment (Fig. 4–22, *left*). The most important range of flexion is from 0 degrees to the position of function with a decrease of impairment from 70% at 0 degrees to 40% at 25 degrees. From there, the flexion curve becomes relatively more flat to end at 0% of impairment at 180 degrees of flexion. The most important range of extension is to bring the arm from 90 degrees of flexion to the position of function; the impairment consequently decreases from 70% at 90 degrees to 10% at 25 degrees. Extension from the position of function to 50 degrees is of less importance, and the extension curve becomes relatively flat within this range.

The average normal range of shoulder motion is considered to be from 50 degrees of adduction to 180 degrees of abduction; the position of function is 50 degrees of abduction. Ankylosis in the position of function gives 50% impairment, ankylosis in 0 degrees of abduction gives 80% impairment, and ankylosis in 90 degrees of abduction gives 90% impairment (Fig. 4–23, *left*). Abduction from 0 degrees to the position of function is considered to be the most important part of abduction, with a decrease of impairment from 70% at 0 degrees to 35% at the position of function (Fig. 4–23, *left*). From there, the abduction curve becomes relatively more flat to 0% impairment at 180 degrees of abduction. The most important range of adduction is from 90 degrees of abduction down to the position of function; thus, the impairment decreases from 65% at 90 degrees to 15% at 50 degrees. Adduction from the position of function to 50 degrees of adduction is considered to be of less importance, and the adduction curve becomes relatively flat within this range.

The average normal range of shoulder motion is assumed to be 90 degrees of internal rotation and 90 degrees of external rotation; the position of function is 20 degrees of external rotation. Ankylosis in the position of function gives 50% impairment; ankylosis in 50 degrees of external rotation and 40 degrees of internal rotation gives the same impairment, or 90% (Fig. 4–24, *left*). The most important range of external rotation is from 40 degrees of internal rotation to the position of function, with a decrease of impairment from 80% to 20%. The most important range of internal rotation is from 50 degrees of external rotation to the position of function, with a decrease of the impairment from 80% to 25%.

Upper extremity impairment caused by loss of shoulder motion is calculated by adding flexion-extension, abduction-adduction, and rotation percentages. For example, shoulder flexion 110 degrees, extension 20 degrees, abduction 70 degrees, adduction 40 degrees, internal rotation 20 degrees, and external rotation 10 degrees results in an upper extremity impairment of:

$$I_F (5\%) + I_E (2\%) + I_{ABD} (5\%) + I_{ADD} (0\%) + I_{IR} (2\%) + I_{ER} (4\%) = 18\%$$

How To Combine Upper Extremity Impairment

For each level of involvement, impairments from amputation, motion loss, sensory loss, pain, strength loss, and other derangements must be expressed in the same denominator before combining their value with the combined values principle (Tables 4–7 and 4–8).

When multiple joints or multiple impairments are present in a finger, they are combined with the combined values principles. Thumb functional impairments at the level of the carpometacarpal, metacarpophalangeal, and interphalangeal joints are added directly together because the relative value of each thumb level has been figured on a 100% scale to the thumb (80% for the carpometacarpal joint, 11% for the metacarpophalangeal joint, and 9% for the interphalangeal joint). Note that these values differ from the thumb amputation values (100% for the metacarpophalangeal joint and 50% for the interphalangeal joint, as shown in Figure 4–6).

When multiple digits are involved, each digit impairment is expressed in terms of hand impairment by multiplying it by the relative value of the digit to the hand. The relative value of each digit has been figured on a 100% scale to the hand (40% for the thumb, 20% for the index finger, 20% for the middle finger, and 10% for the ring and little fingers, as shown in Figure 4–6). Therefore, hand impairment values derived for each digit are added directly together.

When there is involvement at multiple levels of the extremity, for example, hand, wrist, elbow, or shoulder, the impairment percentage for each level is converted into upper extremity impairment values. These are then combined by means of the combined values principle.

Discussion of Impairment Evaluation Methods

Although in the diagrams the impairments have been given a linear configuration that is of practical benefit, it might have been more accurate to note greater changes of impairment immediately around the positions of function for the various joints discussed. It should be observed that the angle of ankylosis has its lowest impairment at the position of function; we have used the values recommended by the American Medical Association[1] of 30 degrees for the metacarpophalangeal joint, 40 degrees for the proximal interphalangeal joint, and 20 degrees for the distal interphalangeal joint in reference to their respective positions of function.

Values for hyperextension of the finger joints have been calculated and included in the charts presented here. We consider about 20 degrees of hyperextension of the metacarpophalangeal joint to be normal and of some functional importance in opening the hand completely. Lack of this hyperextension in the metacarpophalangeal joint, therefore, is considered to give some impairment. The linear function representing ankylosis, I_A, has simply been extended to include 20 degrees of hyperextension. Hyperextension of the proximal and distal interphalangeal joints is, however, considered unnatural, or at least without importance functionally. Lack of hyperextension in these joints, therefore, does not produce any impairment. We consider ankylosis or severely limited flexion within this sector, as occurs in severe swan-neck deformity, to produce a more pronounced impairment and we have therefore drawn the functions more steeply within this sector.

References

1. Committee on Medical Rating of Physical Impairment: *A Guide to the Evaluation of Permanent Impairment of the Extremities and Back.* Chicago, American Medical Association, 1958.
2. McBride ED: *Disability Evaluation: Principles of Treatment of Compensable Injuries*, ed 6. Philadelphia, JB Lippincott, 1963.
3. Smith WC: *Principles of Disability Evaluation.* Philadelphia, JB Lippincott, 1959.
4. Swanson AB: Evaluation of impairment of function in the hand. *Surg Clin North Am* 1964;44:925–940.
5. Swanson AB, Göran-Hagert C, de Groot Swanson G: Evaluation of impairment of hand function, in Hunter JM, Schneider LH, Mackin EJ, et al (eds): *Rehabilitation of the Hand.* St. Louis, CV Mosby, 1978, pp 31–69.
6. Swanson AB, Göran-Hagert C, de Groot Swanson G: Evaluation of impairment of hand function. *J Hand Surg* 1983;8:709–722.
7. Swanson AB, Mays JD, Yamauchi Y: A rheumatoid arthritis evaluation record for the upper extremity. *Surg Clin North Am* 1968;48:1003–1013.
8. Bunnell S: The management of the non-functional hand: Reconstruction vs prosthesis. *Artif Limbs* 1957;4:76–102.
9. Swanson AB, Matev IB, de Groot Swanson G: The strength of the hand. *Bull Prosthet Res*, 1970, pp 145–153.
10. *Joint Motion, Method of Measuring and Recording.* Park Ridge, IL, American Academy of Orthopaedic Surgeons, 1965. (This book is out of print and is no longer being distributed by the Academy.)
11. Boyes JH: *Bunnell's Surgery of the Hand*, ed 5. Philadelphia, JB Lippincott, 1970.
12. Tubiana R, Valentin P: Opposition of the thumb. *Surg Clin North Am* 1968;48:967–977.
13. Moberg E: Objective methods for determining the functional value of sensibility in the hand: Detailed study of relation of tactile gnosis and sudomotor function. *J Bone Joint Surg* 1958;40B:454–476.
14. Litchman NM, Paslay PR: Determination of finger-motion impairment by linear measurement: Description of method and comparison with angular measurement. *J Bone Joint Surg* 1974;56A:85–91.
15. Van't Hof A, Heiple KG: Flexor-tendon injuries of the fingers and thumb: A comparative study. A report on sixty primary tendon repairs by the authors, to which reports of other series have been added to furnish statistics on 310 cases. *J Bone Joint Surg* 1958;40A:256–262.
16. Tubiana R, Michon J, Thomine JM: Scheme for the assessment of deformities in Dupuytren's disease. *Surg Clin North Am* 1968;48:979–984.
17. Crenshaw AH (ed): *Campbell's Operative Orthopaedics*, ed 5. St. Louis, CV Mosby, 1971.
18. dePalma AF: *Surgery of the Shoulder*, ed 2. Philadelphia, JB Lippincott, 1973.

The Spine

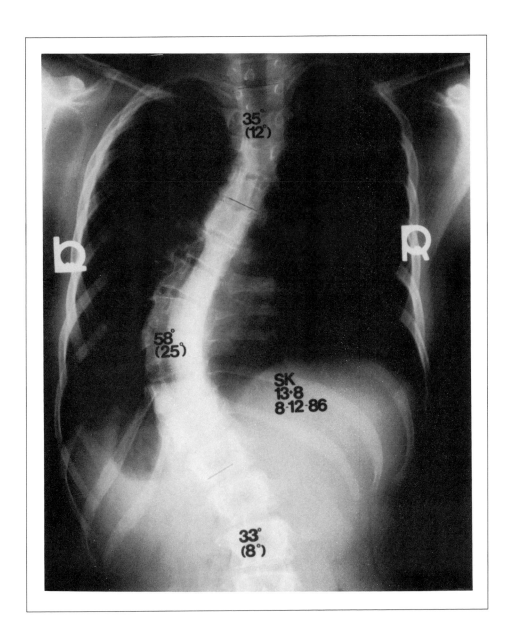

Adolescent Idiopathic Scoliosis: Screening and Diagnosis

John E. Lonstein, MD

Scoliosis in adolescents is rarely associated with pain; thus, it is the discovery of back asymmetry that prompts evaluation by a family physician or pediatrician. The most common means of detection today is by school screening programs, but asymmetry can be noted first by parents or at a routine physical examination by the family physician. If the family physician confirms the asymmetry, a radiograph is taken and the child is referred to an orthopaedic surgeon for further evaluation and treatment.

School Screening

School screening, conducted in most states and in many foreign countries, is the most common method today for the early detection of spinal deformities in adolescence.[1-7] In many areas, school screening is a mandated program.

Screening is defined by the Commission on Chronic Illness as "the presumptive identification of unrecognized disease or defect by applications of tests, examination or other procedures which can be applied rapidly." Scoliosis screening fulfills these criteria, but epidemiologists have raised the following questions about school screening: (1) Has the effectiveness of the screening program been demonstrated in a randomized trial? (2) Are effective treatments available for the screened cases? (3) Does the current burden of suffering from the screened condition warrant screening? (4) Is there a good screening test? (5) Does the screening reach the persons for whom it is intended? (6) Can the health system cope with the screening program? A question has also been raised about the role of nonsurgical treatment in altering the natural history of idiopathic scoliosis. These questions have no clear answers. We should seek the answers while we continue screening, and, in this way, aim for a modified, more effective screening program.

Organizing a Program

School screening for scoliosis is set up initially on a community or district basis and later expands to involve part of a state or the whole state. Parents, school personnel, school or county nurses, and physicians who are interested in organizing a program meet to plan the program. Then they must interest individual schools or school districts in the screening program, as this is where the children are screened. The program planning includes screening staff, organizing workshops, the screening and referral process, and setting up a reporting system. In most cases the screening staff is the school staff (nurses and physical education teachers) aided by outside individuals, such as parents and county or state nurses. Workshops are held to educate the screening staff about spinal deformities and their treatment, the screening process, making referrals and establishing a reporting system. Educational material for the children and their parents is also made available. Yearly workshops provide a refresher course for trained screeners and instruction for new screeners.

Screening

Screening tests detect back asymmetry, an early sign of spinal curvature. The most common test is a visual examination using the forward-bending test. (This test is described later in the section on Physical Examination.) Minimal asymmetry is normal.[8] Thus, only a definite asymmetry is considered a positive finding. The difference in symmetry can be quantified using a scoliometer; a difference of 5 to 7 degrees or more is a positive finding.[9] The optimal screening test is carried out by two people: one at the head, and one at the side, with the latter recording the findings and checking for structural kyphosis. Other screening tests are available, such as Moire topography[7] and thermography.[10] These tests are more time-consuming and expensive.

The children screened, ages 11 to 14 (grades 5 through 9), are those considered at risk. Screening is performed on an annual basis. The best time to screen is early in the school year in a physical education class. Because of a high false-positive referral, that is, children referred who do not have a curve and only minimal asymmetry, the screening should be repeated. All children with asymmetries are rechecked by the screening staff on another day. Only after this second screening detects a positive finding is the child referred to a pediatrician or family practitioner. This physician evaluates the asymmetry with the forward-bending test, and, if it is confirmed, orders a standing posteroanterior radiograph to be taken. Once scoliosis is confirmed, further referral depends on the system in that community. This second referral, of either the radiograph or the child, is to an orthopaedic surgeon who is interested in and knowledgeable about scoliosis.

Problems

In the many years of screening in Minnesota, problems have been encountered. These include compliance, education, staffing, physician referral, and reporting.[4]

Persuading schools to establish a screening program and maintaining involvement are both time-consuming. The school administration has many projects to organize, and school screening, in many cases, gets low priority. In addition, with budget cutbacks, the school nurse is often one of the first to be laid off. Alternative screeners, such as physical education staff, aides, and parents, must be involved to overcome staffing problems.

Education is an important part of the program. In addition to the screening staff, administrators, parents, and students should all be made knowledgeable about spinal deformities. Information about the back can be included in the health curriculum to achieve this education.

The physician who examines the child must be aware of the screening program and must examine the child and confirm the physical finding before ordering a radiograph. The advice of the examining physician regarding scoliosis and follow-up can be incorrect; therefore, education of the primary care physician is essential. This education is achieved with articles in state medical journals and presentations to medical staff meetings.

The best way to assess the screening program is to record accurate data that monitor the program and its effects. Even in an organized program with a reporting mechanism, only 50% of schools submit data regarding the screening.

Costs

The actual cost of screening can be kept low if existing school staff and volunteers are used. Additional costs are those for organizing the program and the workshops. Minnesota employs a part-time state coordinator, whose salary plus mailing costs, workshops, and printing expenses is $20,000 per year. In Minnesota, the cost is approximately 8 cents per child screened. There are indirect costs related to the referral. These include the cost for radiographs, the physician visit, travel, and time off work for parents. These costs can be reduced if only appropriate cases are referred and followed up and unnecessary radiography is eliminated.

Results

In the United States, more than 18 states have mandated screening programs, and over 3 million children

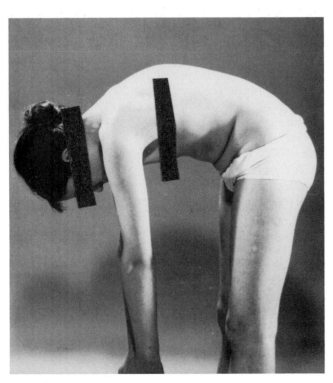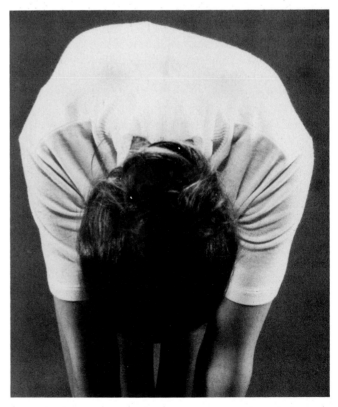

Fig. 5-1 Forward-bending test. **Left:** A side view of a child in the test position. (Reproduced with permission from Bradford DS, Lonstein JE, Ogilvie SW, et al: *Moe's Textbook of Scoliosis and Other Spinal Deformities.* Philadelphia, WB Saunders, 1987, p 51.) **Right:** This view of the child shows an obvious asymmetry in the thoracic area.

are screened annually.[4] Minnesota has had a statewide program for 14 years, and approximately 250,000 children are screened each year. Of those screened, 3.2% are referred and 1% to 1.2% are diagnosed as having scoliosis. Approximately three to six per 1,000 require treatment, of whom two thirds require bracing and one third surgery. In Minnesota and in Gothenburg, Sweden, it was reported that with screening the rate of surgery decreased[4,11]; however, recent figures from these centers suggest an increase in the surgery rate.

Should screening be discontinued because of the questions and controversy surrounding both screening and its results? The best approach is to proceed with screening while collecting data to answer the epidemiologic questions regarding screening, and gain more knowledge about the natural history of idiopathic scoliosis and nonsurgical treatment. The program is organized and strengthened as more information is generated. Education reduces unnecessary referral and leads to appropriate radiographs and follow-up. With these improvements and more knowledge of the natural history and nonsurgical treatment results, screening programs for scoliosis can be modified, if necessary.

Evaluation of Spinal Deformities

Once a child is referred to a physician, the evaluation should identify the deformity, its etiology, and treatment recommendations. To accomplish this, an adequate history, physical examination, and appropriate radiographs are necessary. The objective of the evaluation is to exclude unusual causes of spinal deformity, and the evaluation should result in appropriate decision-making and recommendations.[12]

History

The history gathers information on how the curve was detected, if any progression was noted, and accompanying complaints. A family history identifies familial conditions and notes other immediate family members with scoliosis. The general health of the child is noted, including previous illness or operations. The level of physical maturity attained by the child is important to ascertain. By history, the growth rate is obtained. In addition, in girls the onset of menarche is ascertained. At the onset of menarche, the growth spurt is usually two-thirds complete, and curve progression is less likely.

Physical Examination

The physical examination assesses the deformity and helps establish the etiology. It is important to examine the back, perform a neurologic evaluation, assess maturity, and evaluate any associated conditions. All findings must be well-documented to form a baseline for subsequent evaluations.

The back is observed first for any obvious deformi-

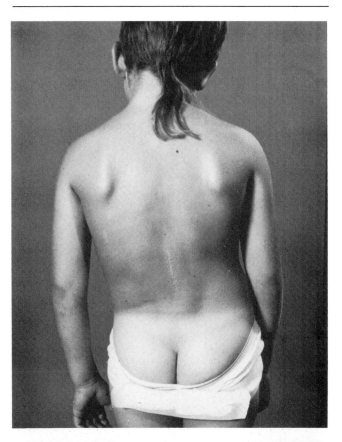

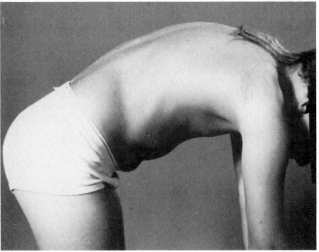

Fig. 5-2 Views of a boy, who was 7 years 8 months old, who had a three-year history of waking up at night with back pain in the thoracic area that had become more frequent and persistent. He stands tilted to the right (top) and forward bending shows marked back spasm without deviation (bottom). Neurologic findings were completely normal (see Figure 5–5).

ties. Any imbalance of the shoulders, neckline, waistline, and thoracopelvic relationship is noted and, where possible, measured; for example, shoulder levels by the deviation from a plumb line dropped from the seventh cervical vertebra. The forward-bending test should be performed. The child stands with feet together and

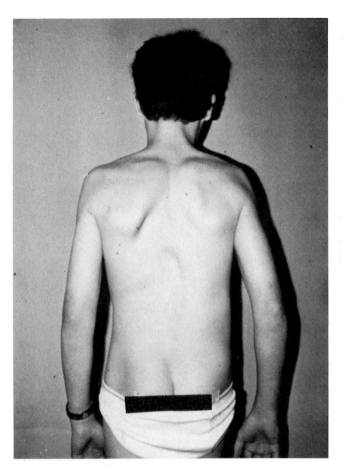

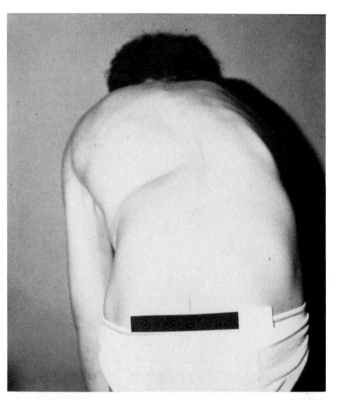

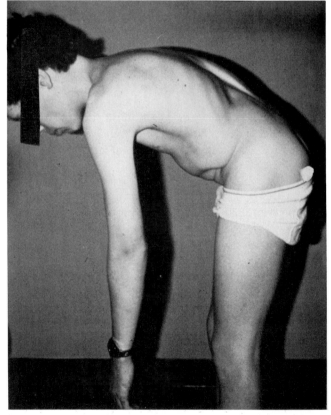

Fig. 5–3   Views of a boy, who was 14 years 4 months old. **Top left:** A view of the patient's back. His curve was detected two years before these views were taken and he had been treated with exercises. He had no back pain. Physical findings were completely normal except for persistent deviation to the left on forward bending **(top right)** and restriction of forward bending **(bottom).** A myelogram revealed an intraspinal tumor from the occiput to the conus that was found to be an ependymoma.

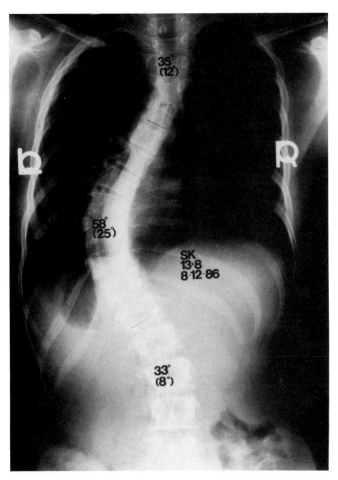

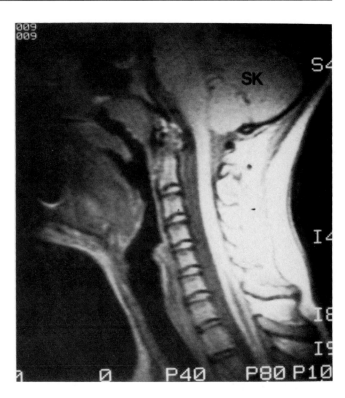

Fig. 5–4 Views of a patient, who was 13 years 8 months old, who had been treated for idiopathic scoliosis with a Milwaukee brace since the age of 6 years. After initial improvement in the brace, the curve progressed. Neurologic findings were normal. A standing posteroanterior radiograph showed a 58-degree left thoracic curve. Figures in parentheses show flexibility of curves on side bending **(left)**. A magnetic resonance imaging scan showed a syrinx at the cervicothoracic area **(right)**. The diagnosis was scoliosis resulting from syringomyelia and not idiopathic scoliosis.

knees straight and bends forward at the waist with arms hanging and palms together (Fig. 5–1). The examiner should view the back from the patient's head, comparing the two sides for symmetry and examining the upper thoracic area, thoracic area, thoracolumbar area, and lumbar area. Any difference in height is noted and measured with a spirit level or a scoliometer.

The manner in which the child bends forward during the forward-bending test is important. Normally, the child bends forward without deviation and flexes approximately 90 degrees. In some cases, the child is unable to bend forward, as, for example, with tight hamstrings in spondylolisthesis. Also, the child may consistently deviate to one side on forward flexion. This can indicate an irritative lesion, such as osteoid osteoma, spinal cord lesion, or herniated disk. In these cases, additional radiographic evaluation is necessary (Figs. 5–2 and 5–3).

The spine is also viewed from the side in the forward-bending position to evaluate the contour of the back and to diagnose an acute area of angulation, which is the hallmark of a structural kyphosis.

A brief neurologic examination is performed to evaluate muscle strength and reflexes in the lower extremities. Any foot deformity is noted, especially a cavus foot. When any neurologic abnormality is found, a complete neurologic examination is essential.

During the general evaluation, the physician should look for other conditions, for example, Marfan's syndrome, or neurofibromatosis. An important part of the general examination is evaluation of physical maturity by assessing breast development in girls, pubic hair development in both sexes, and genital development in boys. These are all rated using the Tanner grading system.[13]

Radiographic Evaluation

Radiographs form the basis of evaluating spinal deformities. With the initial radiographs, a determination is made of the site and magnitude of the scoliosis, the etiology, and the child's maturity. The radiographs necessary for adequate initial assessment depend on the type of deformity and treatment plan. A standing posteroanterior view is necessary for the initial evaluation. A lateral view is taken only if hyperkyphosis is present. Flexibility films are taken only when active treatment (nonsurgical or surgical) is planned, and are *not* part of a routine initial evaluation.

A radiograph uses radiation to produce an image, and thus exposes the patient to higher than normal amounts of radiation. The areas of concern are breast and gonadal doses.[14-16] The breast is especially sensitive to radiation in its formative years. Radiographic techniques, therefore, must minimize radiation and reduce organ dosage as much as possible.[17-20] The most important way to reduce radiation is to reduce the number of radiographs taken. Each examination should be tailored to the patient's needs. A radiograph should be ordered only if the view will give information that may affect or alter the diagnosis or treatment.

The radiographic technique should minimize the radiation dosage. Faster radiographic film reduces the exposure with slight loss in detail. The radiographic beam should be collimated to the body to reduce scatter. Beam filtration reduces unnecessary radiation and gives a more uniform density to the radiograph. Intensifying screens (for example, Quanta rare-earth screens) reduce the exposure by converting roentgen photons to light, which exposes the film.

The gonads are shielded with a lead shield. The use of the posteroanterior position further reduces breast irradiation.[14,16,18] In the anteroposterior position, breast shields or a lead stole can be used to reduce breast dosage.[20]

The upright standing posteroanterior film is taken at a distance of 6 feet (2 m), preferably on a 14 × 36-inch (36 × 91-cm) cassette that will show the whole spine on one film. If this cassette is not available, a 14 × 17-inch (36 × 43-cm) film can be used. This film is positioned with its lower end at the level of the anterosuperior iliac spines, which allows the thoracic and lumbar spine to be viewed on a single radiograph. The cervical and upper thoracic spine is missed on this smaller film.

The initial film is evaluated and the site and direction of the curves are noted. The most common finding in idiopathic scoliosis is a right thoracic and left lumbar curve, either as a single- or a double-curve pattern. A left thoracic curve is unusual and may be neuromuscular in origin, necessitating additional tests (described below). Vertebral and rib anatomy is evaluated to exclude congenital deformities and neurofibromatosis. The pedicles and interpediculate distance are also studied. The ossification of the iliac apophysis is noted and graded using the Risser scale.[21]

The curve or curves are measured using the Cobb-Lippman technique.[22] The upper and lower end vertebrae of the curve, that is, vertebrae maximally tilted from the horizontal apical vertebra, are identified. The angle formed by the intersection of the lines perpendicular to the end vertebral lines (at end-plate or pedicle level) is measured for each curve. This measurement of curve magnitude is important in decision-making.

Additional Radiographic Tests Additional radiographs are occasionally necessary for the initial evaluation of a child's spinal deformity. These radiographs can be either additional views or special imaging tests. An upright lateral view of the spine is taken to evaluate the presence of kyphosis. A supine anteroposterior view is used to delineate bony detail, such as congenital anomalies. Supine bending views to determine flexibility are used when surgical or nonsurgical (bracing or electrical stimulation) treatment is indicated, because it helps decide which curves need treatment. They should *not* be a routine part of the initial evaluation of scoliosis.

Spot lateral standing lumbosacral and/or supine oblique views of the lumbosacral joint are indicated when spondylolysis or spondylolisthesis is suspected. Spondylolysis or spondylolisthesis may be associated with lumbosacral pain, an abnormal restriction of forward bending, or an abnormal curve on the initial posteroanterior view caused by a decompensated lumbar spine

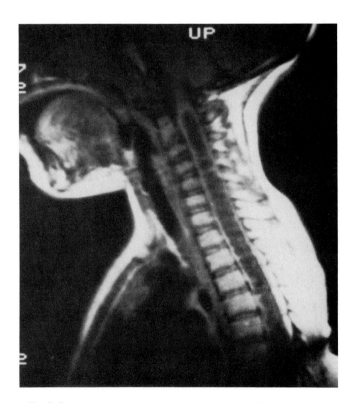

Fig. 5–5 A magnetic resonance imaging scan of the patient seen in Figure 5–2 shows a large syrinx extending the length of the cervical and thoracic cord.

with maximum vertebral rotation at the lumbosacral junction.

Additional imaging techniques are needed occasionally. A bone scan is ordered when there is pain with scoliosis and a bone tumor or infection is suspected. A magnetic resonance imaging scan is obtained in special cases in which a cord tumor or intraspinal pathology is suspected, for example: left thoracic curve (syringomyelia, Arnold-Chiari malformation), shown in Figure 5–4; painful scoliosis (cord tumor, syringomyelia) shown in Figure 5–5; abnormal deviation on forward bending (cord tumor); abnormal physical finding, shown in Figure 5–6, or disk protrusion. A computed axial tomographic scan is an alternative test in cases of suspected disk protrusion.

A diagnosis is made by the above techniques, and curve magnitude and patient maturity are evaluated. Causes other than idiopathic scoliosis are identified and treated with the appropriate regimens.

Decision-Making

After idiopathic scoliosis is diagnosed, a treatment decision is made. The three choices of treatment are observation, nonsurgical treatment (orthosis or stimulator), and surgical treatment.

The two most important factors in treatment decisions are the magnitude of the curve and the growth potential of the child. Growth potential is assessed by determining where the child's growth is in relation to the adolescent growth spurt. In general, the onset of the growth spurt coincides with the appearance of secondary sex characteristics: pubic hair development in both sexes and breast budding in girls.[23] Menarche in girls and the appearance of axillary hair in boys occur in the decreased-growth phase. At this time, approximately 18 months of growth remain. This phase coincides with a Risser grade of 2 or more. For convenience, the growth can be divided into the rapid, active phase that precedes menarche in girls or axillary hair appearance in boys and the decreased-growth phase after this point.

The other factor to evaluate in making a treatment decision is curve magnitude. Curve magnitude is classified as follows: less than 19 degrees, 20 to 29 degrees, 30 to 39 degrees, and over 40 degrees. The decision-making process is summarized in Table 5–1. For a curve

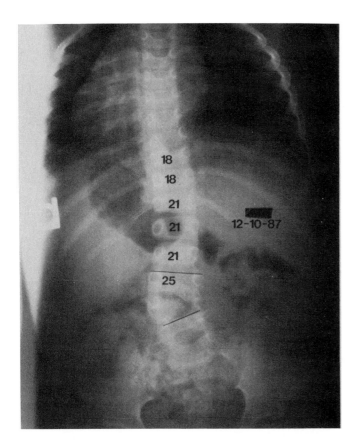
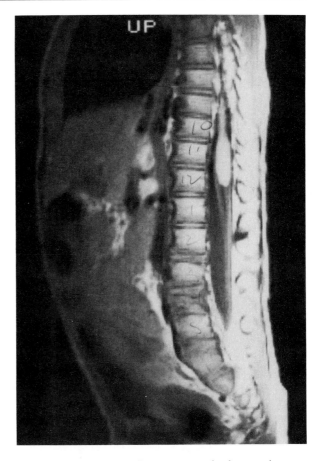

Fig. 5–6 Radiographic views of a boy, who was 3 years 8 months old, who had congenital scoliosis. Findings were completely normal except for tight heelcords bilaterally. The anteroposterior spinal view shows that the fourth lumbar vertebra is a left hemivertebra **(left)**. The interpediculate distance is normal. A magnetic resonance imaging scan was taken because of a possible spinal dysraphism or tethered cord. A sagittal cut **(right)** shows a spinal cord tumor in the distal cord. An astrocytoma was found.

Table 5–1
Summary of treatment decisions in adolescent idiopathic scoliosis

Curve Magnitude (degrees)	Treatment	
	Active Growth	No Active Growth
>40	Surgical	Surgical or observation
30 to 39	Nonsurgical	Observation
20 to 29	Observation, or nonsurgical if progressive	Observation
<19	Observation	Observation (discharge)

of more than 40 degrees in an actively growing child, the choice is for surgical treatment. In a child not in the active growth phase, the choice is surgical treatment for larger curves and observation for smaller curves.

For a curve of 30 to 39 degrees in an actively growing child, the choice is for nonsurgical treatment. In a child who is not actively growing, the treatment choice is usually observation. Curves of less than 30 degrees are the ones more commonly referred from a screening program. For curves of 20 to 29 degrees in an actively growing child, nonsurgical treatment is used when progression is documented. Thus, if a prior radiograph shows that progression has occurred, nonsurgical treatment is indicated. With no prior radiograph, observation is indicated. In a child with a 20- to 29-degree curve who is not actively growing, the treatment choice is observation. A curve of less than 19 degrees is observed in all children and more mature children do not require further follow-up.

Observation of these children for curve progression is an important treatment option. Two questions arise: (1) What is progression? (2) How often should the curve be reevaluated? The error in curve measurement is ± 3 degrees.[24-26] Thus, a minimum change of 5 degrees is significant. I define curve progression in an initial curve of less than 19 degrees as a curve that increases by 10 degrees and results in a curve of more than 20 degrees, for example, a curve of 15 degrees that progresses to 25 degrees. By this definition, a curve of 8 degrees is not classified as progressive unless it becomes greater than 20 degrees. An initial curve of 20 to 29 degrees must increase 5 degrees or more to be classed as progressive.

The frequency of follow-up visits for observation depends on the treatment choices. If the choice is between observation or surgery, as in a more mature child with a slower growth rate, a one-year follow-up period is sufficient. In addition, the progression must be confirmed, and thus a return in one year is appropriate. If the choice is between observation and nonsurgical treatment, as in an actively growing child, more frequent follow-up visits are necessary. In smaller curves

in which a 10-degree difference indicates treatment, a return visit in six to eight months is appropriate. In curves of over 20 degrees in which a 5-degree change is being monitored, a return visit in three to four months is necessary. In both of these examples, if no change occurs in a rapidly growing child after a few follow-up visits, then a slightly more extended follow-up period is permissible.

A baseline for treatment or follow-up is established with adequate initial assessment of a child, confirmation of the diagnosis of idiopathic scoliosis, and exclusion of other causes in rare cases. Thoughtful decision-making and analysis of each case will eliminate automatic or routine treatment choices. Individual treatment plans will provide the best care to each child, minimize radiographic exposure, and reduce the cost of care for minimal scoliosis. Ongoing studies will continue and will answer the epidemiologic questions about scoliosis screening, natural history, and nonsurgical treatment.

References

1. Ascani E, Salsano V, Giglio G: The incidence and early detection of spinal deformities: A study based on the screening of 16,104 school children. *Ital J Orthop Traumatol* 1977;3:111–117.
2. Asher M, Green P, Orrick J: A six-year report: Spinal deformity screening in Kansas school children. *J Kansas Med Soc* 1980;81:568–571.
3. Hensinger RN, Cowell HR, MacEwen GD, et al: Orthopaedic screening of school age children: Review of a 10 year experience. *Orthop Rev* 1975;4:23–28.
4. Lonstein JE, Bjorklund S, Wanninger MH, et al: Voluntary school screening for scoliosis in Minnesota. *J Bone Joint Surg* 1982;64A:481–488.
5. Segil CM: The incidence of idiopathic scoliosis in the Bantu and white population groups in Johannesburg. *J Bone Joint Surg* 1974;56B:393.
6. Span Y, Robin G, Makin M: Incidence of scoliosis in school children in Jerusalem. *J Bone Joint Surg* 1976;58B:379.
7. Takemitsu Y, Harada Y, Ando M, et al: Incidence of scoliosis in Japan by mass screening examination of school children. Presented at the annual meeting of the Scoliosis Research Society, Chicago, September 1980.
8. Burwell RG, James NJ, Johnson F, et al: Standardised trunk asymmetry scores: A study of back contour in healthy school children. *J Bone Joint Surg* 1983;65B:452–463.
9. Bunnell WP: An objective criterion for scoliosis screening. *J Bone Joint Surg* 1984;66A:1381–1387.
10. Cooke ED, Carter LM, Pilcher MF: Identifying scoliosis in the adolescent with thermography: A preliminary study. *Clin Orthop* 1980;148:172–176.
11. Torell G, Nordwall A, Nachemson A: The changing pattern of scoliosis treatment due to effective screening. *J Bone Joint Surg* 1981;63A:337–341.
12. Lonstein JE: Patient evaluation, in Bradford DS, Lonstein JE, Moe JH, et al (eds): *Moe's Textbook of Scoliosis and Other Spinal Deformities,* ed 2. Philadelphia, WB Saunders, 1987, pp 47–88.
13. Tanner JM: Growth and endocrinology of the adolescent, in Gardner L (ed): *Endocrine and Genetic Diseases of Childhood.* Philadelphia, WB Saunders, 1975, p 14.
14. Drummond D, Ranallo F, Lonstein J, et al: Radiation hazards in scoliosis management. *Spine* 1983;8:741–748.

15. Gregg EC: Radiation risks with diagnostic X-rays. *Radiology* 1977;123:447–453.

16. Nash CL Jr, Gregg EC, Brown RH, et al: Risks of exposure to X-rays in patients undergoing long-term treatment for scoliosis. *J Bone Joint Surg* 1979;61A:371–374.

17. Andersen PE Jr, Andersen PE, van der Kooy P: Dose reduction in radiography of the spine in scoliosis. *Acta Radiol Diag* 1982;23:251–253.

18. De Smet AA, Fritz SL, Asher MA: A method for minimizing the radiation exposure from scoliosis radiographs. *J Bone Joint Surg* 1981;63A:156–161.

19. Gray JE, Hoffman AD, Peterson HA: Reduction of radiation exposure during radiography for scoliosis. *J Bone Joint Surg* 1983;65A:5–12.

20. Raia TJ, Kilfoyle RM: Minimizing radiation exposure in scoliosis screening. *Appl Radiol* 1982;11:45–55.

21. Risser JC: The iliac apophysis: An invaluable sign in the management of scoliosis. *Clin Orthop* 1958;11:111–119.

22. Cobb JR: Outline for the study of scoliosis, in Blount WP (ed): American Academy of Orthopaedic Surgeons *Instructional Course Lectures, V.* Ann Arbor, JW Edwards, 1948.

23. Anderson M, Hwang S-C, Green WT: Growth of the normal trunk in boys and girls during the second decade of life. *J Bone Joint Surg* 1965;47A:1554–1564.

24. Gross C, Gross M, Kuschner S: Error analysis of scoliosis curvature measurement. *Bull Hosp Joint Dis Orthop Inst* 1983;43:171–177.

25. Kittleson AC, Lim LW: Measurement of scoliosis. *AJR* 1970;108:775–777.

26. McAlister WH, Shackelford GD: Measurement of spinal curvatures. *Radiol Clin North Am* 1975;13:113–121.

Adolescent Idiopathic Scoliosis: Prevalence and Natural History

Stuart L. Weinstein, MD

Treatment decisions for patients with adolescent idiopathic scoliosis (AIS) require a thorough knowledge of the disorder and its implications for patients. With modern orthoses and the development of spinal instrumentation devices enabling better surgical correction of a deformity, it is imperative that physicians treating patients with scoliosis have a thorough knowledge of the natural course of this condition to offer treatment options that alter the natural history of the disorder in a positive way.

By definition, AIS is a structural lateral curvature of the spine that occurs at or near the onset of puberty and for which no cause is established.[1,2] AIS is suspected when the patient has body asymmetries in the standing position and in the forward-bending test (see the section on physical examination in Chapter 5). The diagnosis is confirmed by an upright roentgenogram of the spine. The entire spine and the iliac crests must be included on the roentgenograms to assess skeletal maturity. The minimum curvature required to make a diagnosis of AIS is 10 degrees as measured by the Cobb method (Fig. 6–1).[1]

The prevalence of AIS in the population at risk, with curves of more than 10 degrees and an upper age limit of 16 years, is approximately 2% to 3%.[1,3-20] In larger curves, the prevalence decreases (Table 6–1).

The overall female-to-male prevalence for AIS is 3.6 to 1. However, in small curves of approximately 10 degrees, the male and female prevalence is equal. With increasing curve severity, there is an increasing female predominance (Table 6–1).[4,5,10,14,16,20-27]

Epidemiologic and natural history studies indicate that less than 1% of the screened population and fewer than 10% (range, 3% to 9%) of positively screened patients (curve greater than 10 degrees) will require active treatment (Table 6–2).[3-5,14,24,27] This small group of patients is the focus of this chapter.

The four main curve patterns seen in patients with AIS are thoracic, lumbar, thoracolumbar, and double major (usually right thoracic, left lumbar components) (Figs. 6–2 to 6–5). Other less common curve patterns include cervicothoracic, double thoracic, and thoracicthoracolumbar. Each curve pattern has a unique natural history.[28-35]

Natural History in Skeletally Immature Patients

The main area of concern in the skeletally immature patient is the probability of curve progression. Back

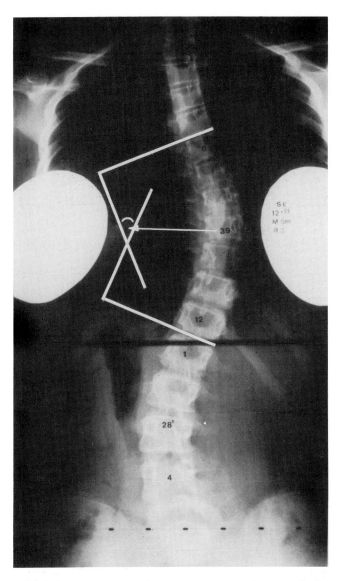

Fig. 6–1 Cobb method of curve measurement. A perpendicular is erected from the end plate of the most caudal vertebra, whose inferior end plate tilts maximally to the concavity of the curve (inferior end vertebra). A perpendicular is erected from the end plate of the most cephalad vertebra, whose superior end plate tilts maximally to the concavity of the curve (superior end vertebra). The curve value is the number of degrees formed by the angle of intersection of these perpendicular measures (arrow shows a curve angle of 39 degrees; compensatory lumbar curve measures are 28 degrees).

pain and pulmonary symptoms are unusual in these patients. The relationship of spinal growth to the events of maturity (Fig. 6–6) must be evaluated in the skeletally

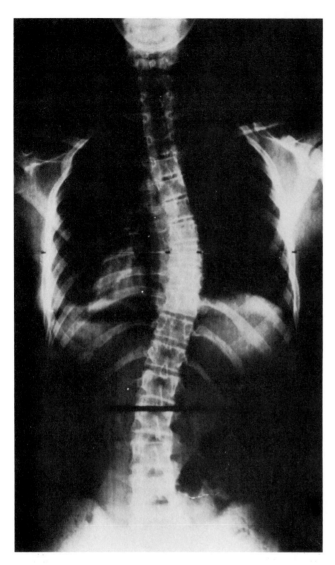

Fig. 6-2 Thoracic curve. Ninety percent right convexity involving an average of six vertebrae: apex T8, T9; upper end vertebrae T5, T6; lower end vertebrae T11, T12.

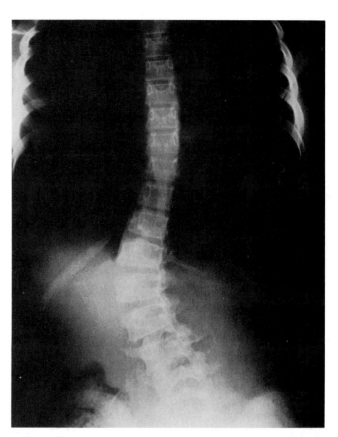

Fig. 6-3 Lumbar curve. Seventy percent left convexity involving an average of five vertebrae: apex L1, L2; upper end vertebrae T11, T12; lower end vertebrae L3, L4.

immature patient.[36] These events affect the course of AIS in the skeletally immature patient and determine the risks of curve progression.

The majority of information available on curve pro-

gression is from studies of females, particularly those with thoracic curves. There are six main factors that influence the probability of progression in the skeletally immature patient: (1) Double-curve patterns have a greater tendency for curve progression than single-curve patterns. (2) The younger the patient at the time of diagnosis, the greater the risk of curve progression. (3) There is a significantly greater risk of curve progression prior to the onset of menarche than after menarche. (4) The lower the Risser grade at curve detection the greater the risk of progression. (5) Larger-magnitude curves at detection have a greater risk of progression. (6) The risk of curve progression in males is approxi-

Table 6-1
Prevalence of adolescent idiopathic scoliosis (ages 10 to 16 years)

Cobb Angle (degrees)	Prevalence	
	At-Risk Population (%)	Female to Male
>10	2.0 to 3.0	1.4 to 2:1
>20	0.3 to 0.5	5.4 to 1
>30	0.1 to 0.3	10 to 1
>40	<0.1	

Table 6-2
Incidence of patients requiring treatment

Screened Population*	% Requiring Treatment
Total	0.6%
Girls	1.0%
Boys	0.1%

*Aged 10 to 16 years.

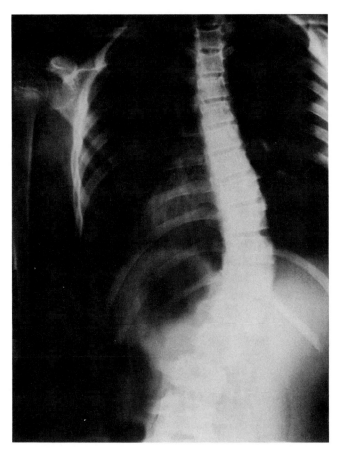

Fig. 6–4 Thoracolumbar curve. Eighty percent right convexity involving an average of six to eight vertebrae: apex T11, T12; upper end vertebrae T6, T7; lower end vertebrae L1, L2.

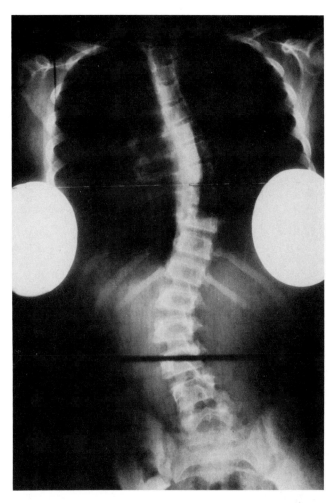

Fig. 6–5 Double curve. Ninety percent right thoracic convexity and left lumbar convexity. Thoracic component, average five vertebrae: apex T7, upper end vertebrae T5, T6; lower end vertebrae T10. Lumbar component, average five vertebrae: apex L2, upper end vertebra T11; lower end vertebra L4.

mately one tenth that of females with comparable curves.[2,3,14,19,24,26,27,30,35,37–41]

In 1982, Nachemson and associates[39] calculated the probabilities of progression prior to skeletal maturity based on all of the known prognostic factors at that time (Table 6–3). Lonstein and Carlson[24] evaluated the probabilities of progression based on the Risser grade (Table 6–4). These studies showed that the risks of curve progression decrease with increasing skeletal maturity. However, with larger-magnitude curvatures, there may be considerable risk of progression despite maturity.

Another key factor that has not been calculated into the probability of progression is the effect of loss of thoracic kyphosis (hypokyphosis). Dickson and associates[42] and Perdriolle and Vidal[43] have demonstrated the importance of loss of thoracic kyphosis in AIS. Loss of thoracic kyphosis affects orthotic treatment of patients.[44] In addition, the loss of thoracic kyphosis may require adjustment of the surgical treatment techniques used.[45,46] The loss of thoracic kyphosis increases the loss of pulmonary function associated with curve severity.[47]

Natural History in Adults

There are five considerations in the natural history of untreated AIS: back pain, pulmonary function, psychosocial effects, mortality, and curve progression.[19,40,48]

Back Pain

The generally accepted incidence of backache in the general population is approximately 60%.[19,28,49–54] The incidence reported in the literature, however, varies widely.[52] The reported incidence of back pain is questionnaire-dependent. Jackson and associates[53] reported the incidence of back pain in the general population to be 80%, while Kostuik and Bentivoglio[50] reported a 60% incidence. Horal,[51] in an epidemiologic study of back pain in Gothenburg, Sweden, found that 81% of

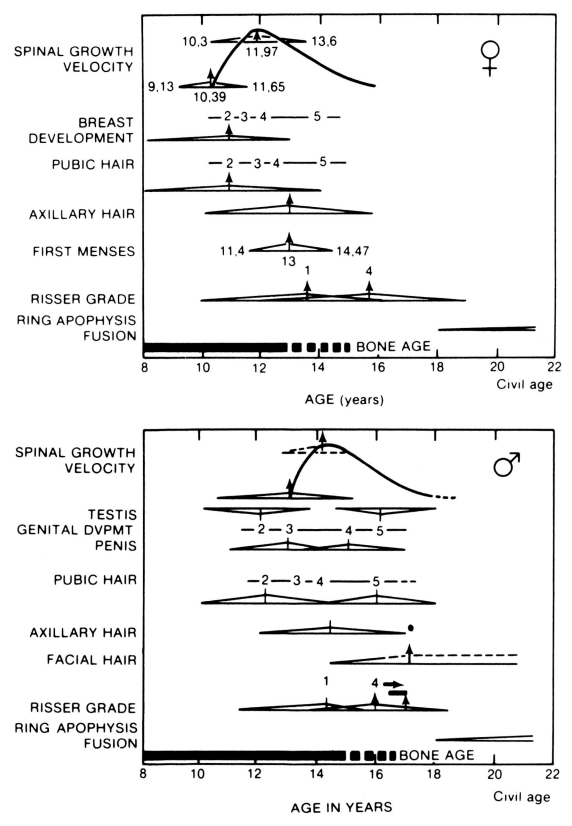

Fig. 6-6 The relationship of spinal growth velocity to maturity landmarks and the events of puberty in girls (**top**) and boys (**bottom**). Numbers above breast development, pubic hair, axillary hair, and genital development refer to Tanner stages. (Modified with permission from Terver S, Kleinman R, Bleck EE: Growth landmarks and the evolution of scoliosis: A review of pertinent studies on their usefulness. *Dev Med Child Neurol* 1980;22:675–684.)

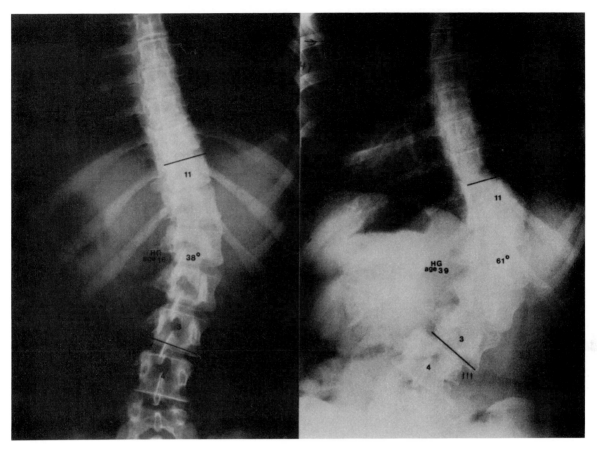

Fig. 6-7 Sixteen-year-old girl with a 38-degree right lumbar curve from T11 to L3 (**left**). Her skeletal maturity is assessed as grade 5 on the Risser scale. At age 39, her right lumbar curve has increased to 61 degrees (**right**). Note the translatory shift of L3 on L4 (arrows). (Reproduced with permission from Weinstein SL: The natural history of scoliosis in the skeletally mature patient, in Dickson JH (ed): *Spinal Deformities*. Philadelphia, Hanley & Belfus, 1987, vol 1, pp 195–212.)

patients had some spinal pain, with 66% complaining of lumbar pain. Bjure and Nachemson[28] reported a 60% incidence of back pain in the general population, and Frymoyer and associates[52] reported a 67% incidence in 292 subjects in a randomly selected group of 1,221 men, with 21% of these individuals having severe pain.

The incidence of back pain in patients with scoliosis is comparable to the incidence of back pain in the general population. In the Iowa long-term follow-up study (average follow-up of 40 years) of 161 living patients with AIS, 80% of the scoliotic patients complained of

some backache.[19] In a control group of 100 patients who were age- and sex-matched and screened as not having scoliosis, 86% reported backache. Twenty-four percent of the patients with scoliosis had been to a doctor because of back pain, while 6% had been hospitalized for backache. In the control group, 30% had been to a physician for backache and 16% had required hospitalization (Table 6–5).[19] The incidence of frequent or daily backache was slightly higher in the scoliosis

Table 6–3
Probabilities of progression based on curve magnitude and age[39]

Curve Magnitude at Detection (degrees)	Age (yrs)		
	10–12	13–15	16
<19	25%	10%	0%
20 to 29	60%	40%	10%
30 to 59	90%	70%	30%
>60	100%	90%	70%

Table 6–4
Probabilities of progression based on Risser grade and curve magnitude at detection*

Risser Grade	Curve Magnitude (degrees)	
	5 to 19	20 to 29
0 to 1	22 %	68%
2 to 4	1.6%	23%

*Reproduced with permission from Lonstein JE, Carlson, JM: The prediction of curve progression in untreated idiopathic scoliosis during growth. *J Bone Joint Surg* 1984;66A:1061–1071.

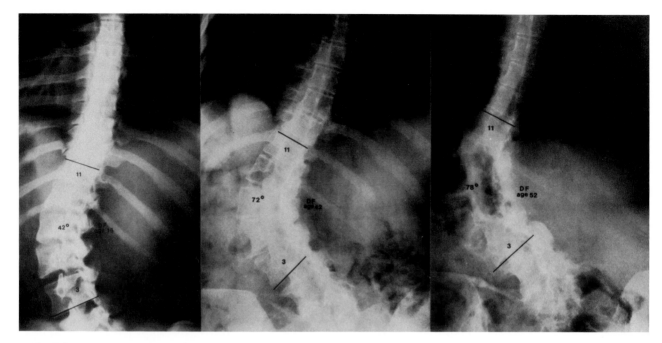

Fig. 6–8 Fifteen-year-old girl (Risser grade 4) with a 42-degree left lumbar curve from T11 to L3 (**left**). At age 42 (**center**), the patient's curve has increased 30 degrees, to 72 degrees. At age 52 (**right**), the patient's curve has increased 6 degrees, to 78 degrees. Patient never had backache. (Reproduced with permission from Weinstein SL: The natural history of scoliosis in the skeletally mature patient, in Dickson JH (ed): *Spinal Deformities*. Philadelphia, Hanley & Belfus, 1987, vol 1, pp 195–212.)

group (37%) compared with the control group (25%). Patients with lumbar or thoracolumbar curves, particularly those with translatory shifts at the lower end of their curves, tended to have a slightly greater incidence of backache than did patients with other curve patterns. The presence of translatory shifts in these curves (Fig. 6–7) is associated with backache.[48]

An estimated 1% of patients with scoliosis will require surgery specifically for backache, an incidence similar to that for the general population.[49,55] Horal[51] showed that scoliosis cases did not represent a disproportionate number of disability pensions. Three Swedish long-term follow-up studies of AIS, all with follow-ups longer than 30 years and all with more than 90% of the patients traced, demonstrated that low back pain was not a significant problem in scoliotic patients.[33,56,57] In the Iowa scoliosis series, patients' symptoms varied from mild to severe. Most commonly, patients complained of mild backache at the end of a strenuous day or after unusual activities, with the pain relieved promptly by rest. The location of pain was variable and generally unrelated to the location of the curve or its magnitude.[19] The pain was also unrelated to the severity of osteoarthritic changes, except in areas of translatory shifts in thoracolumbar and lumbar curves (Figs. 6–8 and 6–9).

Thirty-eight percent of the patients in my study[40] had radiographic evidence of degenerative joint disease (Fig. 6–8). These changes ranged from minimal osteophyte formation and mild narrowing of the intervertebral disk space to moderate facet joint sclerosis, and, rarely, to spontaneous fusion on the curve concavity. The severity of these changes was unrelated to the degree and location of the spinal curvature.[19,39] Back pain may develop in the compensatory curves below lumbar and thoracolumbar curves.[49,53,55]

Kostuik and Bentivoglio[50] and Robin and associates[58] demonstrated that lumbar or thoracolumbar curves may arise *de novo* in adult life. This "degenerative" scoliosis may progress and cause severe pain and discomfort that requires treatment (Fig. 6–10). This type of scoliosis and its related problems should not be confused with the natural history of untreated AIS. The cause of the back pain in the adult scoliotic patient is unknown but may be spondylogenic or diskogenic in origin.[50]

Pulmonary Function

Only in thoracic curves is pulmonary function affected.[19,32,47,59–66] In thoracic curves, there is a direct correlation between decreasing vital capacity and increasing curve severity. The same relationship exists with the forced expiratory volume in one second (FEV_1). In all other curve patterns there is no correlation between curve severity and a decrease in pulmonary function. The same correlation also applies to Pao_2. Nonsmoking patients with thoracic curves all have restrictive

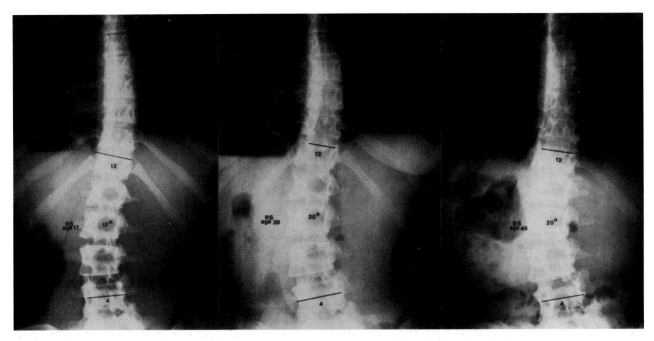

Fig. 6-9 Seventeen-year-old girl (Risser grade 5) with a 17-degree left lumbar curve from T12 to L4 (**left**). At age 39 (**center**), the patient's curve has increased 3 degrees, to 20 degrees. At age 49 (**right**), the patient's curve remains stable at 20 degrees. The patient reports daily low backache for as long as she can remember. (Reproduced with permission from Weinstein SL: The natural history of scoliosis in the skeletally mature patient, in Dickson JH (ed): *Spinal Deformities*. Philadelphia, Hanley & Belfus, 1987, vol 1, pp 195–212.)

Table 6-5
Back pain in scoliotic patients*

Clinical Findings	Back Pain	
	Scoliotic Patients (No. = 161)	Control Group (No. = 100)
Never	20%	14%
Rarely (one to five times in life)	19% ⎫	25% ⎫
Occasionally (few days/year)	24% ⎪	36% ⎪
Frequently (few days/month)	20% ⎬ 80%	19% ⎬ 86%
Daily	17% ⎭	6% ⎭
Visited doctor for back pain	24%	30%
Hospitalized for back pain	6%	16%

*Reproduced with permission from Weinstein SL: The natural history of scoliosis in the skeletally mature patient, in Dickson JH (ed): *Spinal Deformities*. Philadelphia, Hanley & Belfus, 1987, vol 1, pp 195–212.

lung disease. Smokers have more severe restrictive lung disease than nonsmokers. Significant limitation in the forced vital capacity (FVC) of nonsmokers does not occur until the curve approaches 100 to 120 degrees (Fig. 6–11).[19] As discussed earlier, thoracic hypokyphosis increases the loss of pulmonary function associated with curve severity.[47]

Mortality

The mortality rate for AIS is comparable to that in the general population.[39,67] Kolind-Sørensen[56] reported

that the mortality rate in patients with curves in the range of 40 to 100 degrees was comparable to that in the general population, but in those whose curves were greater than 100 degrees, the mortality rate doubled. Thus, it is only in AIS patients with thoracic curves of more than 100 degrees that there is an increased risk of death from cor pulmonale and right ventricular failure. In the Iowa long-term series, the mortality rate was 15%,[19] and in only one case was cor pulmonale secondary to scoliosis implicated as the cause of death. Actuarial data for patients born in the same years as

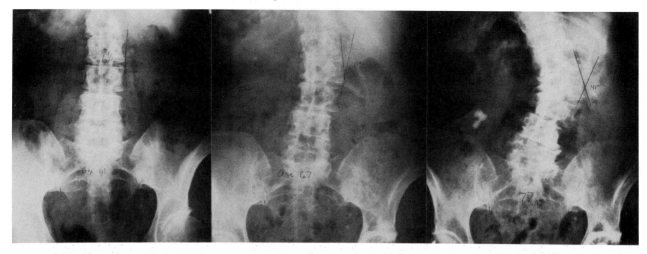

Fig. 6-10   Degenerative scoliosis at age 61 (**left**), age 67 (**center**), and age 77 (**right**). Note the development of a severe lumbar curve with marked degenerative changes. Clinically, the patient reported increasing back pain. (Reproduced with permission from Weinstein SL: The natural history of scoliosis in the skeletally mature patient, in Dickson JH (ed): *Spinal Deformities*. Philadelphia, Hanley & Belfus, 1987, vol 1, pp 195–212.)

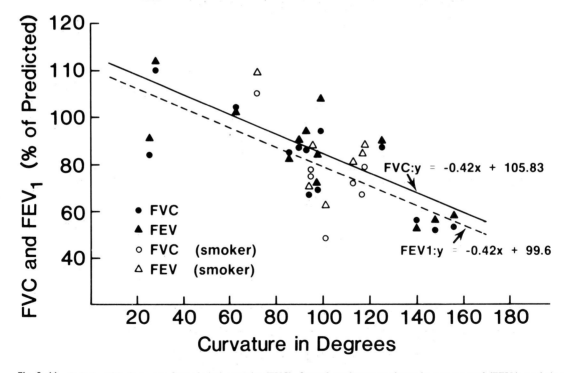

Fig. 6-11   Relationship between forced vital capacity (FVC), forced expiratory volume in one second (FEV₁), and size of the curve in 20 patients with thoracic scoliosis, using a line of regression. (Reproduced with permission from Weinstein SL, Zavala DC, Ponseti IV: Idiopathic scoliosis: Long-term follow-up and prognosis in untreated patients. *J Bone Joint Surg* 1981;63A:702–712.)

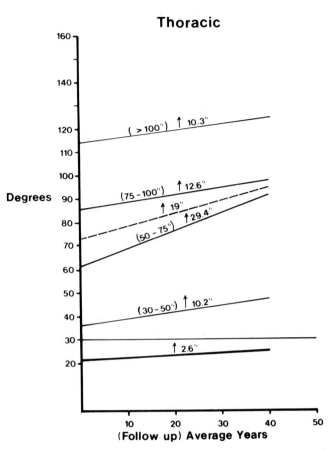

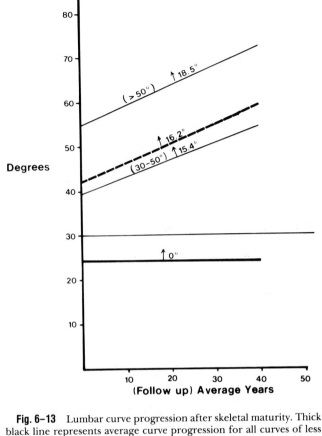

Fig. 6-12 Thoracic curve progression after skeletal maturity. Thick black line represents average curve progression for all curves of less than 30 degrees at skeletal maturity. Thick dashed line represents average curve progression for all curves of more than 30 degrees at skeletal maturity. Thin black lines represent average curve progression for each range in parentheses. Progression is not necessarily linear. Lines connect average values at maturity and at average 40-year follow-up. Based on data from Weinstein and Ponseti.[48] (Reproduced with permission from Weinstein SL: The natural history of scoliosis in the skeletally mature patient, in Dickson JH (ed): *Spinal Deformities.* Philadelphia, Hanley & Belfus, 1987, vol 1, pp 195–212.)

Fig. 6-13 Lumbar curve progression after skeletal maturity. Thick black line represents average curve progression for all curves of less than 30 degrees at skeletal maturity. Thick dashed line represents average curve progression for all curves of more than 30 degrees at skeletal maturity. Thin black lines represent average curve progression for each range in parentheses. Progression is not necessarily linear. Lines connect average values at maturity and at average 40-year follow-up. Based on data from Weinstein and Ponseti.[48] (Reproduced with permission from Weinstein SL: The natural history of scoliosis in the skeletally mature patient, in Dickson JH (ed): *Spinal Deformities.* Philadelphia, Hanley & Belfus, 1987, vol 1, pp 195–212.)

this scoliosis group indicate an expected mortality rate of 17%.[68]

Psychosocial Effects

Scoliosis causes a cosmetic deformity that may result in severe psychosocial problems, particularly in adolescents. The psychosocial effects of scoliosis appear to be better tolerated by middle-aged patients than by teenagers. Some adults, however, with a moderate to severe deformity may become mentally disabled by the deformity.[28] There is no correlation between the location or degree of curvature and the extent of psychosocial effect.[19] Many patients with minimal curvatures have severe limitations psychosocially. This limitation is often expressed in buying clothing to try to hide the deformity. Other patients with severe de-

formities express little psychosocial limitation and are more accepting of their deformity. This is an area in great need of clinical research. There are many studies on the psychologic effects, but most conclusions are based on clinical judgment rather than empirical data.[28,69]

Curve Progression

It was once thought that when the patient reached skeletal maturity there would be no further curve progression.[70,71] However, the study of Duriez[38] and two subsequent studies[31,48] demonstrated that curves may continue to progress throughout life. In a review of 102 patients followed for an average of 40 years at the University of Iowa, 68% of the curves progressed after maturity.[19,48] From this group of patients, prognostic

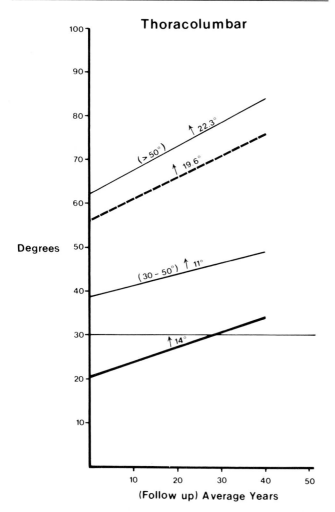

Fig. 6–14 Thoracolumbar curve progression after skeletal maturity. Thick black line represents average curve progression for all curves of less than 30 degrees at skeletal maturity. Thick dashed line represents average curve progression for all curves of more than 30 degrees at skeletal maturity. Thin black lines represent average curve progression for each range in parentheses. Progression is not necessarily linear. Lines connect average values at maturity and at average 40-year follow-up.[48] (Reproduced with permission from Weinstein SL: The natural history of scoliosis in the skeletally mature patient, in Dickson JH (ed): *Spinal Deformities.* Philadelphia, Hanley & Belfus, 1987, vol 1, pp 195–212.)

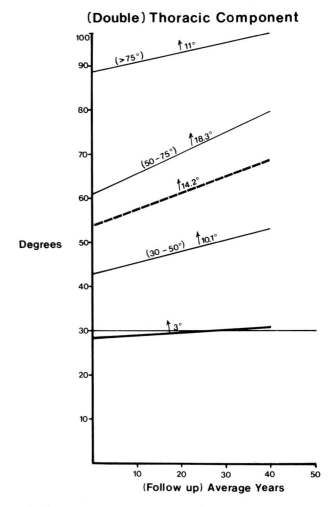

Fig. 6–15 Thoracic component of double (combined) curve progression after skeletal maturity. Thick dashed line represents average curve progression for all curves of more than 30 degrees at skeletal maturity. Thin black lines represent average curve progression for each range in parentheses. Progression is not necessarily linear. Lines connect average values at maturity and at average 40-year follow-up. Based on data from Weinstein and Ponseti.[48] (Reproduced with permission from Weinstein SL: The natural history of scoliosis in the skeletally mature patient, in Dickson JH (ed): *Spinal Deformities.* Philadelphia, Hanley & Belfus, 1987, vol 1, pp 195–212.)

factors associated with curve progression in each curve pattern were elucidated.

In the thoracic curve pattern, those patients with curves of less than 30 degrees at maturity[70] tended to have apical vertebral rotations of less than 20%[72] and Mehta angles[73] of less than 20 degrees; these curves did not progress. Curves of more than 30 degrees at maturity progressed an average of 19 degrees during the 40-year follow-up. The most marked progression was noted in curves between 50 and 75 degrees at skeletal maturity; these continued to progress at 0.75 to 1 degree per year during the follow-up period (Fig. 6–12). All of these patients had a Mehta angle greater than

20 degrees and an apical vertebral rotation of more than 30%.[40,48] Thus, in the thoracic curve pattern, the Cobb angle, Mehta angle, and apical vertebral rotation are important factors in curve progression after maturity.

In the lumbar curve pattern, curves of less than 30 degrees did not tend to progress after skeletal maturity (Fig. 6–13). In only one patient did a lumbar curve of less than 30 degrees progress from 24 degrees at 18 years to 45 degrees at 54 years. This patient had an apical vertebral rotation of more than 33% and a high-riding fifth lumbar vertebra (that is, the intercrest line passed through the body of the fifth lumbar vertebra).[74]

A translatory vertebral shift of the third lumbar vertebra on the fourth developed, with lateral tilting of the fourth lumbar vertebra on the fifth. Farfan and associates[75] demonstrated that the anulus fails in torsion. MacGibbon and Farfan[74] demonstrated that a high intercrest line (an intercrest line falling at or above the fourth to fifth disk space) is an antitorsional device. When the anulus fails in patients with a high-riding fifth lumbar vertebra and a high degree of apical rotation, lateral translatory shift and significant curve progression result.[48] These translatory shifts are usually at the third to fourth lumbar vertebrae but occasionally occur at the fourth to fifth lumbar vertebrae. In addition to translatory shifts, there is lateral tilting of the fourth lumbar vertebra on the fifth toward the curve convexity, especially in cases in which the fifth lumbar vertebra is not well seated (Fig. 6–7).

All lumbar curves of more than 30 degrees at maturity had an apical vertebral rotation of more than 33%. All but four of these curves progressed; no progression was seen in two patients in whom the fifth lumbar vertebra was deeply seated or in two other patients in whom the fifth lumbar vertebra was sacralized. These four curves were the only ones that did not develop translatory shifts at follow-up. Thus, in lumbar curves, the factors leading to progression are curves of more than 30 degrees at maturity, particularly those with apical vertebral rotation of more than 33%. If the fifth lumbar vertebra is high-riding, translatory shifts of the third lumbar vertebra on the fourth tend to develop, with lateral tilting of the fourth lumbar vertebra on the fifth. Right lumbar curves tend to progress twice as often as left lumbar curves. The reasons for this could not be determined.[40,48]

The thoracolumbar curve pattern manifested the most significant amount of apical vertebral rotation (40% to 65%) of any curve pattern (Fig. 6–14). This rotation increased with increasing curve severity. As with lumbar curves, patients with the thoracolumbar curve pattern developed translatory shifts at the lower end of their curve. The marked vertebral rotation in combination with translatory shifts at the lower end of the curve led to significant curve progression.[40,48]

In double (combined) curves, there were no correlative factors with curve progression after maturity. The percent of apical vertebral rotation tended to be less than in thoracolumbar curves. The ribs remained level in the thoracic component; therefore, the Mehta angle was usually low. There was no prognostic value in the relationship of the fifth lumbar vertebra to the intercrest line in combined curves (Figs. 6–15 and 6–16).[40,48]

At maturity, the thoracic curves tended to be larger than the lumbar curves, but there was selectively greater progression over time in the lumbar component of the double major curve,[48] which resulted in more balanced curves at follow-up. Similarly, increases in compensa-

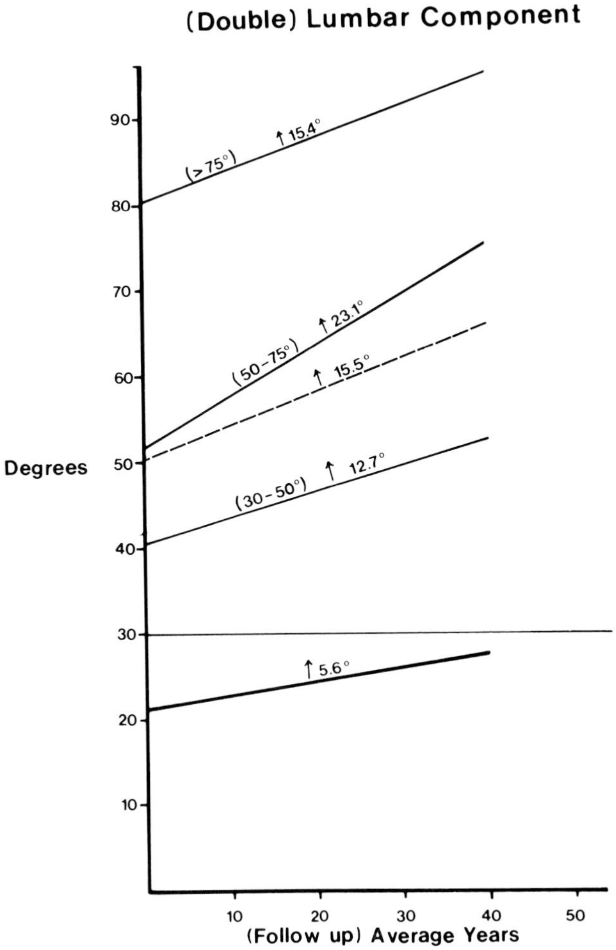

Fig. 6–16 Lumbar component of double (combined) curve progression after skeletal maturity. Thick dashed line represents average curve progression for all curves of more than 30 degrees at skeletal maturity. Thin black lines represent average curve progression for each range in parentheses. Progression is not necessarily linear. Lines connect average values at maturity and at average 40-year follow-up. Based on data from Weinstein and Ponseti.[48] (Reproduced with permission from Weinstein SL: The natural history of scoliosis in the skeletally mature patient, in Dickson JH (ed): *Spinal Deformities*. Philadelphia, Hanley & Belfus, 1987, vol 1, pp 195–212.)

tory curves in all curve patterns developed to balance the spine better.[40,48]

Ascani and associates[3] published the results of a multicenter Italian study of 187 patients followed for 34 years. The results of this study and the Iowa study[19,40,48] are similar concerning the amount of progression during the follow-up period for each specific curve pattern (Table 6–6).

Thus, in considering post-maturity curve progression, curves of less than 30 degrees at skeletal maturity do not tend to progress in adult life regardless of curve pattern. Many curves, however, continue to progress throughout life, particularly thoracic curves between 50 and 80 degrees.[48]

Table 6–6
Average curve progression after maturity*

Pattern	Progression (degrees)	
	Iowa City Group[†]	Italian Group[‡]
Thoracic	17	17
Lumbar	10	16
Thoracolumbar	18	14
Double thoracic	14	13
Lumbar	14	16
All patterns	13	15

*Reproduced with permission from Weinstein SL: The natural history of scoliosis in the skeletally mature patient, in Dickson JH (ed): *Spinal Deformities*. Philadelphia, Hanley & Belfus, 1987, vol 1, pp 195–212.
[†]A total of 102 patients; average curve is 50 degrees; average follow-up is 40 years.
[‡]Multicenter; 187 patients; average follow-up is 34 years.

Table 6–7
Treatment indications for the skeletally immature patient

Initial Curve (degrees)	Progression*
<19	At least 10 degrees with progression to a curve of ≥25 degrees
20 to 29	At least 5 degrees
≥30	No progression documentation needed

*In general, an indication for treatment is a progressive curvature of ≥25 degrees in a skeletally immature child.

Pregnancy and Scoliosis

The effect of pregnancy on scoliosis is unknown. Nachemson and associates[76] and MacGibbon and Farfan[74] demonstrated a statistically significant effect on curve progression in patients who had multiple pregnancies prior to the age of 23 years. They recommended avoidance of pregnancy in the early 20s, particularly in brace-treated patients. Blount and Mellencamp[77] and Berman and associates[78] also demonstrated that scoliosis progressed as a result of pregnancy. Blount and Mellencamp[77] related this effect to the stability of the curve. Bunnell,[37] on the other hand, was unable to detect any deleterious effect of pregnancy on scoliosis in his natural history study group. In the Iowa series,[19,40] there were only two women who required cesarean sections. Significant complications during pregnancy or delivery were subjectively attributed to their spinal deformity.[17] No conclusions can be drawn about the effect of pregnancy on the natural history of curve progression, but, from the obstetric point of view, scoliosis has no adverse effects on pregnancy.

Summary

The natural history presented in this chapter applies only to AIS. Other types of scoliosis have their own natural history and associated problems that may significantly affect the ability of the patient to meet the demands of daily life.[28,29,45]

Increased public awareness and screening clinics have resulted in an increased number of children referred for orthopaedic opinion, less severe curve magnitude at initial detection, and earlier institution of treatment.

Treatment of each patient must be individualized, taking into consideration the probability of curve progression based on curve magnitude, skeletal maturity, sexual maturity, and age (Table 6–7). Overdiagnosis and unnecessary treatment must be avoided.

As our knowledge of the natural history of AIS expands, treatment decisions can be based on objective rather than subjective data. Any proposed treatment of this condition must have a reasonable chance of altering the natural history in a positive way. The information available on natural history has been accumulated on relatively small groups of patients and the conclusions presented represent generalities. There are probably many "natural histories" for AIS, especially with reference to curve progression; therefore, treatment decisions must be individualized. Long-term results of various treatments for scoliosis must take into consideration the natural history of the disorder.[79–86]

References

1. Kane WJ: Scoliosis prevalence: A call for a statement of terms. *Clin Orthop* 1977;126:43–46.
2. Weinstein SL: *Adolescent Idiopathic Scoliosis: Prevalence, Natural History, Treatment Indications.* Iowa City, University of Iowa Printing Service, 1985, pp 1–12.
3. Ascani E, Bartolozzi P, Logroscino CA, et al: Natural history of untreated idiopathic scoliosis after skeletal maturity. *Spine* 1986;11:784–789.
4. Brooks HL, Azen SP, Gerberg E, et al: Scoliosis: A prospective epidemiological study. *J Bone Joint Surg* 1975;57A:968–972.
5. Brooks HL: Current incidence of scoliosis in California, in Zorab PA, Siegler D (eds): *Scoliosis, 1979.* London, Academic Press, 1980, pp 7–12.
6. Bruszewski J, Kamza A: Czestosc wystepowania Skolioz na Podstawie Anacizy Zdec maxoobrakowych. *Chir Narzadow Ruchu Ortop Pol* 1957;22:115–116.
7. Burwell RG, James NJ, Johnson F, et al: Standardised trunk asymmetry scores: A study of back contour in healthy school children. *J Bone Joint Surg* 1983;65B:452–463.
8. Floman Y, Span Y, Makin M, et al: The prevalence of scoliosis in the Jerusalem school population. *Orthop Rev* 1980;9:73–77.
9. Fowles JV, Drummond DS, L'Ecuyer S, et al: Untreated scoliosis in the adult. *Clin Orthop* 1978;134:212–217.
10. Kane WJ, Moe JH: A scoliosis-prevalence survey in Minnesota. *Clin Orthop* 1970;69:216–218.
11. O'Brien JP: The incidence of scoliosis on Oswestry, in Zorab PA, Siegler D (eds): *Scoliosis, 1979.* London, Academic Press, 1980, pp 19–29.
12. Owen R, Taylor JF, McKendrick O, et al: Current incidence of scoliosis in school children in the city of Liverpool, in Zorab PA, Siegler D (eds): *Scoliosis, 1979.* London, Academic Press, 1980, pp 31–34.
13. Patynski J, Szczekot J, Szwaluk F: Boczne Skrywienie kregosyu-

paw swietle Statystyki. *Chir Narzadow Ruchu Ortop Pol* 1957;22:111–114.

14. Rogala EJ, Drummond DS, Gurr J: Scoliosis: Incidence and natural history. A prospective epidemiological study. *J Bone Joint Surg* 1978;60A:173–176.

15. Segil CM: The incidence of idiopathic scoliosis in the Bantu and white population groups in Johannesburg, abstract. *J Bone Joint Surg* 1974;56B:393.

16. Shands AR Jr, Eisberg HB: The incidence of scoliosis in the state of Delaware: A study of 50,000 minifilms of the chest made during a survey for tuberculosis. *J Bone Joint Surg* 1955;37A:1243–1249.

17. Skogland LB, Miller JAA: The incidence of scoliosis in northern Norway: A preliminary report, abstract. *Acta Orthop Scand* 1978;49:635.

18. Smyrnis PM, Valanis J, Voutsinas S, et al: Incidence of scoliosis in the Greek Islands, in Zorab PA, Siegler D (eds): *Scoliosis, 1979.* London, Academic Press, 1980.

19. Weinstein SL, Zavala DC, Ponseti IV: Idiopathic scoliosis: Long-term follow-up and prognosis in untreated patients. *J Bone Joint Surg* 1981;63A:702–712.

20. Wynne-Davies R: Familial (idiopathic) scoliosis: A family survey. *J Bone Joint Surg* 1968;50B:24–30.

21. Ascani E, Giglio GC, Salsano V: Scoliosis screening in Rome, in Zorab PA, Siegler D (eds): *Scoliosis, 1979.* London, Academic Press, 1980, pp 39–44.

22. Burwell RG, James NJ, Johnson F, et al: The rib hump score: A guide to referral and prognosis?, abstract. *J Bone Joint Surg* 1982;64B:248.

23. Lonstein JE, Bjorklund S, Wanninger MH, et al: Voluntary school screening for scoliosis in Minnesota. *J Bone Joint Surg* 1982;64A:481–488.

24. Lonstein JE, Carlson JM: The prediction of curve progression in untreated idiopathic scoliosis during growth. *J Bone Joint Surg* 1984;66A:1061–1071.

25. Torell G, Nordwall A, Nachemson A: The changing pattern of scoliosis treatment due to effective screening. *J Bone Joint Surg* 1981;63A:337–341.

26. Zaoussis AL, James JIP: The iliac apophysis and the evolution of curves in scoliosis. *J Bone Joint Surg* 1958;40B:442–453.

27. Willner S, Udén A: A prospective prevalence study of scoliosis in Southern Sweden. *Acta Orthop Scand* 1982;53:233–237.

28. Bjure J, Nachemson A: Non-treated scoliosis. *Clin Orthop* 1973;93:44–52.

29. Chapman EM, Dill DB, Graybiel A: The decrease in functional capacity of the lungs and heart resulting from deformities of the chest: Pulmonocardiac failure. *Medicine* 1939;18:167–202.

30. Clarisse P: *Pronostic Evolutif des Scolioses Idiopathiques Mineures de 10° à 29°, en Période de Croissance,* thesis. Lyon, 1974.

31. Collis DK, Ponseti IV: Long-term follow-up of patients with idiopathic scoliosis not treated surgically. *J Bone Joint Surg* 1969;51A:425–445.

32. Lindh M, Bjure J: Lung volumes in scoliosis before and after correction by the Harrington instrumentation method. *Acta Orthop Scand* 1975;46:934–948.

33. Nachemson A: A long term follow-up study of non-treated scoliosis. *Acta Orthop Scand* 1968;39:466–476.

34. Ponseti IV, Friedman B: Prognosis in idiopathic scoliosis. *J Bone Joint Surg* 1950;32A:381–395.

35. Weinstein SL: Idiopathic scoliosis: Natural history. *Spine* 1986;11:780–783.

36. Terver S, Kleinman R, Bleck EE: Growth landmarks and the evolution of scoliosis: A review of pertinent studies on their usefulness. *Dev Med Child Neurol* 1980;22:675–684.

37. Bunnell WP: The natural history of idiopathic scoliosis before skeletal maturity. *Spine* 1986;11:773–776.

38. Duriez J: Évolution de la scoliose idiopathique chez l'adulte. *Acta Orthop Belg* 1967;33:547–550.

39. Nachemson A, Lonstein J, Weinstein S: *Report of the Prevalence and Natural History Committee 1982.* Denver, Scoliosis Research Society, 1982.

40. Weinstein SL: The natural history of scoliosis in the skeletally mature patient, in Dickson JH (ed): *Spinal Deformities.* Philadelphia, Hanley & Belfus, 1987, vol 1, pp 195–212.)

41. Scott MM, Piggott H: A short-term follow-up of patients with mild scoliosis. *J Bone Joint Surg* 1981;63B:523–525.

42. Dickson RA, Lawton JO, Archer IA, et al: Combined median and coronal plane asymmetry: The essential lesion of progressive idiopathic scoliosis, abstract. *J Bone Joint Surg* 1983;65B:368.

43. Perdriolle R, Vidal J: Étude de la courbure scoliotique: Importance de l'extension et de la rotation vertébrale. *Rev Chir Orthop* 1981;67:25–34.

44. Winter RB, Carlson JM: Modern orthotics for spinal deformities. *Clin Orthop* 1977;126:74–86.

45. Moe JH, Winter RB, Bradford D, et al: *Scoliosis and Other Spinal Deformities.* Philadelphia, WB Saunders, 1978, pp 429–433.

46. Shufflebarger HL, King WF: Composite measurement of scoliosis: A new method of analysis of the deformity. *Spine* 1987;12:228–232.

47. Winter RB, Lovell WW, Moe JH: Excessive thoracic lordosis and loss of pulmonary function in patients with idiopathic scoliosis. *J Bone Joint Surg* 1975;57A:972–977.

48. Weinstein SL, Ponseti IV: Curve progression in idiopathic scoliosis. *J Bone Joint Surg* 1983;65A:447–455.

49. Dahlberg L, Nachemson A: The economic aspects of scoliosis treatment, in Zorab PA (ed): *Proceedings of the Fifth Symposium on Scoliosis.* London, Academic Press, 1977, pp 73–101.

50. Kostuik JP, Bentivoglio J: The incidence of low-back pain in adult scoliosis. *Spine* 1981;6:268–273.

51. Horal J: The clinical appearance of low back disorders in the city of Gothenburg, Sweden: Comparisons of incapacitated probands with matched controls. *Acta Orthop Scand* 1969;118 (suppl):1–109.

52. Frymoyer JW, Newberg A, Pope MH, et al: Spine radiographs in patients with low-back pain: An epidemiological study in men. *J Bone Joint Surg* 1984;66A:1048–1055.

53. Jackson RP, Simmons EH, Stripinis D: Incidence and severity of back pain in adult idiopathic scoliosis. *Spine* 1983;8:749–756.

54. Nagi SZ, Riley LE, Newby LG: A social epidemiology of back pain in a general population. *J Chron Dis* 1973;26:769–779.

55. Nachemson A: Adult scoliosis and back pain. *Spine* 1979;4:513–517.

56. Kolind-Sørensen V: A follow-up study of patients with idiopathic scoliosis. *Acta Orthop Scand* 1973;44:98.

57. Nilsonne U, Lundgren KD: Long-term prognosis in idiopathic scoliosis. *Acta Orthop Scand* 1968;39:456–465.

58. Robin GC, Span Y, Steinberg R, et al: Scoliosis in the elderly: A follow-up study. *Spine* 1982;7:355–359.

59. Bergofsky EH, Turino GM, Fishman AP: Cardiorespiratory failure in kyphoscoliosis. *Medicine* 1959;38:263–317.

60. Gazioglu K, Goldstein LA, Femi-Pearse D, et al: Pulmonary function in idiopathic scoliosis: Comparative evaluation before and after orthopaedic correction. *J Bone Joint Surg* 1968;50A:1391–1399.

61. Gucker T: Changes in vital capacity in scoliosis: Preliminary report on effects of treatment. *J Bone Joint Surg* 1962;44A:469–481.

62. Kafer ER: Respiratory and cardiovascular functions in scoliosis. *Bull Eur Physiopathol Respir* 1977;13:299–321.

63. Makley JT, Herndon CH, Inkley S, et al: Pulmonary function in paralytic and non-paralytic scoliosis before and after treatment: A study of sixty-three cases. *J Bone Joint Surg* 1968;50A:1379–1390.

64. Shannon DC, Riseborough EJ, Valenca LM, et al: The distribution of abnormal lung function in kyphoscoliosis. *J Bone Joint Surg* 1970;52A:131–144.

65. Zorab PA, Prime FJ, Harrison A: Lung function in young persons after spinal fusion for scoliosis. *Spine* 1979;4:22–28.

66. Westgate HD, Moe JH: Pulmonary function in kyphoscoliosis before and after correction by the Harrington instrumentation method. *J Bone Joint Surg* 1969;51A:935–946.

67. Edmonsson AS, Morris JT: Follow-up study of Milwaukee brace treatment in patients with idiopathic scoliosis. *Clin Orthop* 1977;126:58–61.

68. *Vital Statistics of the United States, II. Section 5: Life Tables.* Hyattsville, MD, Public Health Service National Center for Health Statistics, US Department of Health, Education and Welfare, 1978.

69. Eliason MJ, Richman LC: Psychological effects of idiopathic adolescent scoliosis. *Dev Behav Pediatr* 1984;5:169–172.

70. Cobb JR: Outline for the study of scoliosis, in Blount WP (ed): American Academy of Orthopaedic Surgeons *Instructional Course Lectures, V.* Ann Arbor, JW Edwards, 1948, p 261.

71. Risser JC, Ferguson AB: Scoliosis: Its prognosis. *J Bone Joint Surg* 1936;18:667–670.

72. Nash CL Jr, Moe JH: A study of vertebral rotation. *J Bone Joint Surg* 1969;51A:223–229.

73. Mehta MH: The rib-vertebra angle in the early diagnosis between resolving and progressive infantile scoliosis. *J Bone Joint Surg* 1972;54B:230–243.

74. MacGibbon B, Farfan HF: A radiologic survey of various configurations of the lumbar spine. *Spine* 1979;4:258–266.

75. Farfan HF, Cossette JW, Robertson GH, et al: The effects of torsion on the lumbar intervertebral joints: The role of torsion in the production of disc degeneration. *J Bone Joint Surg* 1970;52A:468–497.

76. Nachemson A, Cochran TP, Irstam L, et al: Pregnancy after scoliosis treatment. *Orthop Trans* 1982;6:5.

77. Blount WP, Mellencamp D: The effect of pregnancy on idiopathic scoliosis. *J Bone Joint Surg* 1980;62A:1083–1087.

78. Berman AT, Cohen DL, Schwentker EP: The effects of pregnancy on idiopathic scoliosis: A preliminary report on eight cases and a review of the literature. *Spine* 1982;7:76–77.

79. Carr WA, Moe JH, Winter RB, et al: Treatment of idiopathic scoliosis in the Milwaukee brace: Long-term results. *J Bone Joint Surg* 1980;62A:599–612.

80. Cochran T, Irstam C, Nachemson A: Long-term anatomic and functional changes in patients with adolescent idiopathic scoliosis treated by Harrington rod fusion. *Spine* 1983;8:576–584.

81. Emans JB, Kaelin A, Bancel P, et al: The Boston bracing system for idiopathic scoliosis: Follow-up results in 295 patients. *Spine* 1986;11:792–801.

82. Ginsburg HH, Goldstein LA, Chari DPK, et al: Longitudinal study of back pain in postoperative idiopathic scoliosis: Long term follow-up phases I, II, III. Presented at the annual meeting of the Scoliosis Research Society, Southampton, Bermuda, September 1986.

83. Mellencamp DD, Blount WP, Anderson AJ: Milwaukee brace treatment of idiopathic scoliosis: Late results. *Clin Orthop* 1977;126:47–57.

84. Keiser RP, Shufflebarger HL: The Milwaukee brace in idiopathic scoliosis: Evaluation of 123 completed cases. *Clin Orthop* 1976;118:19–24.

85. King HA, Moe JH, Bradford DS, et al: The selection of fusion levels in thoracic idiopathic scoliosis. *J Bone Joint Surg* 1983;65A:1302–1313.

86. Winter RB, Lonstein JE, Drogt J, et al: The effectiveness of bracing in the nonoperative treatment of idiopathic scoliosis. *Spine* 1986:11:790–791.

Nonoperative Treatment of Adolescent Idiopathic Scoliosis

Robert B. Keller, MD

Introduction

Spinal deformity and scoliosis were known in ancient medicine. Hippocrates recognized the deformity and devised a traction table, establishing a treatment principle that has continued to this day. Over the centuries many forms of bending and traction devices have been used. Old orthopaedic texts are filled with illustrations of complex and innovative braces and corsets that proved unsuccessful and were subsequently discarded. In the late 1800s, the advent of plaster casts led to their enthusiastic use by many physicians, again with limited success.

In 1941, a special committee of the American Orthopaedic Association[1] reviewed 425 cases of idiopathic scoliosis and found that 60% of the patients treated with braces had curve progression and the curves of the remaining patients were unchanged. Surgical results were equally disappointing. The committee concluded that all approaches to the treatment of scoliosis had failed.

It is against this backround of discouraging results that the modern era of nonoperative treatment began in the mid-1940s with the development of the Milwaukee brace by Blount and Schmidt.[2] Remarkable progress in this field occurred in the 40 years that followed. New treatment devices created interest and enthusiasm among treating physicians, and the development of new materials and technology stimulated continued research and development of new treatment concepts. A growing mass of knowledge about incidence, genetic patterns, neurophysiologic abnormalities, and the natural history of this deformity has been equally important in the development of nonoperative treatment.

Nonoperative treatment of adolescent idiopathic scoliosis is a continually developing and changing field, and one in which there is considerable debate among the experts. This chapter reviews and discusses the current treatment systems and guidelines in this field.

Treatment Methods

The Milwaukee Brace

Blount and Schmidt first demonstrated their brace at the Annual Meeting of the American Academy of Orthopaedic Surgeons in 1946. It was initially developed as a postoperative holding device but was soon recognized as being more effective in the nonoperative treatment of scoliosis. Early braces were beautifully constructed of leather and stainless steel. The principle of traction was considered important and, for some years, braces used a padded chin rest to which strong upward force was applied. In the 1960s, it was realized that this mandibular pressure produced significant facial deformity and the modern throat mold was developed. New materials and prefabricated pelvic girdles have resulted in a modern, aesthetically pleasing orthosis (Fig. 7–1).

Biomechanical principles have changed very little. Basic to the Milwaukee and all thoracolumbar orthoses is control of lumbar lordosis by producing a forward pelvic tilt in the pelvic girdle. The lateral lumbar curve is controlled by direct pressure from a molded lumbar pad built directly into modern braces. The adjustable metal uprights of the brace attach to the neck ring. The throat mold serves to maintain head position over the occipital pads. The patient gains active extension of the spine by levering against these pads. A molded thoracic pad attached to the upright on the convex side exerts pressure just below the curve apex. This passive force is augmented by the patient's ability to pull and rotate away from the pad. Occasionally, a flange or axillary sling device is added to treat high thoracic or cervicothoracic deformity.

The Milwaukee brace has also been used successfully to treat Scheuermann's disease.[3] Although very different from scoliosis, Scheuermann's disease (vertebral osteochondrosis, or juvenile roundback) is often encountered in the population at risk for idiopathic scoliosis. Children with this condition are frequently referred from screening programs and primary care physicians. As in scoliosis, the lumbar hyperlordosis common to this condition must be controlled by the pelvic girdle. A pad is fixed to each of the posterior uprights just below the apex of the kyphosis to permit active extension against the pressure exerted by the kyphosis.

Significant early curve correction using the Milwaukee brace led investigators to believe that permanent correction of the deformity would be obtained.[4,5] As long-term patient series have been published,[6,7] it has become clear that correction of the deformity gained during active treatment slowly degrades, with most curves returning to the original degree of deformity. This information has clarified the role of the Milwaukee brace. Because most curves return to their original form after brace treatment, there is no reason to embark on a bracing program for a patient whose curve is too

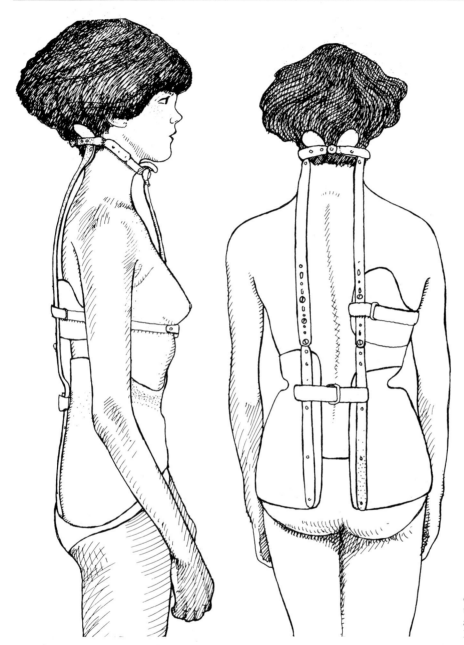

Fig. 7–1 Milwaukee brace fitting to show correction of lumbar lordosis, placement of thoracic pad, and adjustment of throat mold and occipital pads. **Left:** Lateral view. **Right:** Posterior view.

severe initially to accept as a final result. At the other end of the spectrum, natural history studies and large-scale school screening programs have taught us that many mild curves (up to 30 degrees) are not progressive and require no treatment. The result is that many fewer youngsters and their families are subjected to the rigors of nonoperative treatment than in the past.

The development of numerous underarm orthoses over the past 20 years has further limited the role of the Milwaukee brace. The improved comfort and more pleasing appearance of these later devices have made them more acceptable to patients. Thus, although the Milwaukee brace remains the benchmark for all other nonoperative treatment systems, it is prescribed rela-

tively infrequently. Its use is limited primarily to treatment of major thoracic curves with an apex above the level of the seventh thoracic vertebra and of high thoracic and cervicothoracic curve patterns. Simulator modeling studies indicate, however, that it may still be a more effective orthosis than its successors.[8]

Thoracolumbar Spinal Orthoses (Underarm Orthoses)

A large group of thoracolumbar spinal orthoses (TLSO) were developed for bracing during the 1960s and 1970s (Fig. 7–2). Their basic treatment concepts are similar. Devices using prefabricated pelvic girdles made on neutral models are less complex and can be produced more quickly.

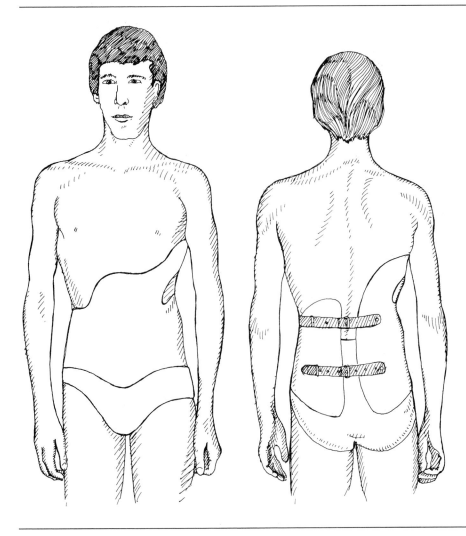

Fig. 7–2 Typical thoracolumbar spinal orthosis with built-in left lumbar pad and support for right thoracic curve. **Left:** Anterior view. **Right:** Posterior view.

Biomechanically, these braces are completely passive.[9] Lumbar lordosis is controlled by the pelvic girdle. A lumbar pad may be built into the brace. The thoracic curve is controlled by another built-in pad. Because the braces are circumferential to the curve, there is no possibility of active correction. Some of these orthoses have incorporated secondary superstructures of various types. TLSOs can be modified for treatment of kyphosis by using the principle of pelvic control and maintaining the anterior portion high on the chest with the posterior portion trimmed just below the apex of the deformity.

Published series on the short-term outcome of TLSO use in properly selected patients demonstrate satisfactory partial curve correction and stabilization.[10,11] As with the Milwaukee brace, long-term correction seems unlikely; therefore, TLSOs have a similar range of use. Patient acceptance and compliance is thought to be better for underarm orthoses than for the more cumbersome Milwaukee brace.

Using knowledge from long-term Milwaukee brace

studies, the role of TLSOs has been defined quickly. They are most effective in patients with thoracic curves that have an apex below the level of the seventh thoracic vertebra and those with thoracolumbar and lumbar curves.[9] These criteria include the large majority of patients who are candidates for brace treatment.

Electrospinal Stimulation

In 1856 in Paris, Seiler[12] applied galvanic current to treat deviations of the spine. Olsen and associates[13] produced and corrected spinal deformity in animals with implanted electrodes and, after doing animal studies, Bobechko and associates[14] developed an implantable system for human use. This system has never gained widespread acceptance, partly because of numerous technical problems.

Cutaneous electrical systems were developed by McCollough,[15] Axelgaard and Brown,[16] and Axelgaard and associates.[17] This method produces active contraction of trunk musculature on the convexity of the major scoliotic curve. Stimulation is applied through skin contact electrodes placed laterally at the upper and lower ends of the curve to be treated. The devices were designed to be used eight hours per day, usually at night. After extensive multicenter testing, they were approved by the Food and Drug Administration. Early reports indicated that curves were stabilized or slightly reduced but did not demonstrate the degree of correction seen with various orthoses. Proponents of the system believed that curve stabilization was a reasonable endpoint, because curve stability is the long-term outcome of successful orthotic treatment.

This treatment system, which could be used at night and did not require the use of an uncomfortable and potentially embarrassing brace, produced great enthusiasm among patients and physicians. Unfortunately, reports of poor compliance and treatment failures began to appear almost immediately. Failures, defined as those cases requiring brace therapy or surgery, were reported in up to 50% to 65% in some series.[18-20] Failure resulted from both poor patient compliance and curve progression during treatment. However, Mc-Collough[15] and Brown and Axelgaard[21] reported that 78% to 83% of their study group patients had stabilized curves at the end of treatment.

Although not completely dismissed as a treatment method, electrospinal stimulation has lost many proponents and its future is uncertain. Currently, it is recommended only for patients who are not mature (Risser grade 0 to 2), have thoracic or thoracolumbar curves of 25 to 35 degrees, and have 50% curve flexibility on side-bending radiographs.[18] Dual-channel units are also available for simultaneous treatment of double curves.

Electrospinal stimulation using the dual-channel unit has also been used to treat kyphosis by placing stimulator pads symmetrically above and below the curve apex near the midline of the spine.

Other Aspects of Nonoperative Treatment

Any assessment of treatment efficacy requires knowledge of patient compliance. Early reports classified patients as either compliant or noncompliant. Noncompliant patients were not considered in evaluating the success of a device and, thus, more favorable statistical results were produced. Also, investigators accepted patients' reports of brace use, exercise, and therapy. More recent articles have indicated that patients undergoing various methods of treatment may experience significant psychological problems, and compliance may be much lower than previously believed.[22,23] A series reported to the Scoliosis Research Society in 1984 indicated only 20% true compliance, with most patients wearing the brace no more than nine to 12 hours per day.[24]

A device called an E cell has been developed by Houghton and associates[25] for accurately measuring brace compliance. It consists of a pressure-sensitive switch built into the pelvic girdle. Hours of actual brace wear can be measured by a concealed timer without the patient's knowledge or cooperation. Actual time in the brace is significantly less than that recorded in patients' diaries of brace wear; it is usually only a few hours per day.

Thus, there are questions about whether or not we are accomplishing what we think we are in nonoperative therapy, and it is difficult to measure a treatment system if we are not sure how it is being used. Concern about compliance has led some experts to develop part-time bracing regimens. Green[26] reported a successful trial of 16-hour daily brace wear with curve improvement or stabilization in 95% of patients who complied with treatment. Riddick and Price[27] followed 62 patients who wore their braces 13 to 16 hours daily. Eighty percent of the curves stabilized or improved and 15% progressed 5 degrees or more but did not require a change in treatment.

If part-time brace wear is effective, what is the minimum number of hours that braces need to be worn? Further, if that number of hours continues to decrease, does the brace have any effect on the natural history of scoliosis? There are physicians who think that orthotic treatment is not a useful mode of therapy and that what is considered a favorable outcome from nonoperative therapy is simply the natural history of untreated scoliosis. Conversely, a 1984 symposium on the natural history of idiopathic scoliosis contained several papers that studied brace effectiveness under reasonably strict criteria.[28] Winter and associates[29] found that 84% of high-risk patients with 30- to 39-degree thoracic curves responded well to the Milwaukee brace: average 33-degree pretreatment curves were corrected to 31 degrees after one year of follow-up. Emans and associates[30] found that 88% of a group of 295 patients who met treatment criteria were successfully treated in TLSOs with best results in curves with an apex between the eighth thoracic and the second lumbar vertebrae.

Table 7-1
Treatment options by type of curve

Curve Type	Treatment*		
	MB	TLSO	ESS
Scoliosis			
Cervicothoracic	Yes	No	No
High thoracic	Yes	No	No
Thoracic	Yes	Yes	Yes
Thoracolumbar	Yes	Yes	Yes
Lumbar	Yes	Yes	Maybe
Kyphosis			
Apex above T6 to T7	Yes	No	No
Apex below T6 to T7	Yes	Yes	Maybe

*MB, Milwaukee brace; TLSO, thoracolumbar spinal orthosis; ESS, electrospinal stimulation.

The Scoliosis Research Society has initiated a multicenter prospective study that will follow up patients treated with various conventional methods and patients receiving no treatment to clarify questions regarding treatment effectiveness. It is hoped that this well-controlled study will provide definitive answers to these questions.

Physical therapy has long been thought essential. Blount and Schmidt[2] emphasized the importance of exercise in correcting the deformity. Currently, it is thought that the role of exercise is to maintain spinal flexibility and muscle tone. If patient compliance with brace wear programs is low, patient cooperation with exercise regimens may be limited as well. Roache and associates[31] found no difference in outcome in two similar groups of patients, one treated with and one without exercises. The question of whether or not patients follow therapy programs and the role of exercise in treatment remain unclear. There may be no harm in performing an exercise regimen, but if there is no benefit, the time, effort, and expense should not be expended. It is hoped that further studies will settle this issue.

Guidelines Based on Curve Pattern and Severity

The role of various forms of nonoperative treatment in specific patterns of scoliosis is outlined in Table 7–1. In general, the degree of deformity seen on initial radiographs represents the long-term result. Therefore, a curve deemed unacceptable at the time of diagnosis is probably best not treated by these techniques. There are exceptions to this principle. Small, immature patients or patients with juvenile scoliosis who will ultimately require surgery may be temporarily stabilized by bracing to permit further spinal growth. Other exceptions are those patients who refuse surgery and in whom nonoperative measures might limit curve progression. Such exceptions are infrequent. Most patients with deformities that are too severe for bracing are in the adolescent idiopathic group and definitive treatment need not be delayed.

Treatment recommendations are outlined by degree of curve severity (Cobb measurement) in Chart 7–1.

Idiopathic Scoliosis

Curves of 0 to 20 Degrees Curves in this category are treated by observation only. In the growing patient, periodic examination with curve assessment by a nonradiographic technique such as scoliosiometry is desirable. Excessive radiographs should be avoided and need be obtained only when the scoliosometer reading exceeds 10 degrees of trunk inclination. Most of these deformities will not progress.

Curves of 20 to 39 Degrees Curves in this range may not progress. In a large prospective series from Canada,

Rogala and associates[32] noted that curves did not progress in 21.2% of patients and treatment was not required. In the remaining 78.8% there was significant progression. Therefore, patients should not be treated until there is clear evidence of progression. Careful follow-up with radiographs at three- to six-month intervals is recommended. If a curve increase of 5 degrees or more occurs in a patient with a Risser grade of 3 or less, treatment should begin. Lonstein and Carlson[33] have defined the risk of progression in the following formula: Risk factor = [Cobb angle − 3× Risser grade] divided by the chronologic age. A factor of 1.6 or above indicates a 50% chance of progression. They stress that the risk of progression factor should be used to advise families as to the risk of curve increase and not as the sole basis for recommending treatment. Curves in the 30- to 39-degree range present a very different problem. There is a consensus that all immature youngsters in this category require prompt treatment. This group of patients is at high risk for progression and may rapidly develop deformity that is correctable only by surgery.

Although the Milwaukee brace is appropriate for all curves in the 20- to 39-degree range requiring treatment, it is generally used in patients with cervicothoracic, high thoracic, and thoracic curves with an apex above the seventh thoracic vertebra. The level of the seventh thoracic vertebra was chosen on clinical grounds because the lateral support of TLSO devices is limited to the axillary level. Thoracic curves below this apex and thoracolumbar and lumbar curves are usually treated with one of the many TLSO devices described previously.

Cutaneous electrical stimulation may be used in this group of patients, but its current role seems to be in the patient with a 25- to 35-degree curve, an immature spine (Risser grade 2 or less), and 50% side-bending flexibility. Curve progression of 5 degrees or more in these patients is an indication that orthotic treatment is needed.

Thoracic lordosis or hypokyphosis occurs occasionally in patients with 20- to 39-degree curves.[34] If orthotic treatment is contemplated, a lateral radiograph should be obtained to assess lateral spinal alignment. If hypokyphosis is present, orthotic treatment may not be indicated because the thoracic pressure pad tends to push the spine further forward into lordosis, potentially increasing the scoliotic deformity. These patients should be monitored carefully; if deformity progresses significantly, fusion is necessary.

Curves of 40 to 50 Degrees Currently, most experts think that curves in this category are in the surgical range. However, there may be instances when conservative treatment is useful, as in the patient who has a cosmetically acceptable double major curve. Carr and associates[7] have stated that brace therapy can be con-

Chart 7-1
Scoliosis treatment options by curve severity

Curve (degrees)	0 to 20	20 to 29*†	30 to 39*	40 to 49	≥50
Treatment‡	Observe	MB§	MB	MB*§	Surgery
		TLSO§	TLSO	TLSO*§	
		ESS§	ESS§	Surgery§	

*In immature spine (Risser grade 0 to 3).
†Treat if curve increases 5 degrees.
‡MB, Milwaukee brace; TLSO, thoracolumbar spinal orthosis; ESS, electrospinal stimulation.
§May be indicated.

sidered in such curves if there is 50% flexibility on the initial side-bending radiograph and 50% correction of the curve within one year of treatment. Specific types of orthoses are the same as recommended for lesser curves except that electrospinal stimulation is never indicated in this group.

Curves of More Than 50 Degrees Nonoperative treatment should not be used in patients who have these more severe deformities, and surgery is almost always needed. Occasionally, an orthosis may be prescribed as a temporary holding device in the immature patient awaiting surgery.

Scheuermann's Kyphosis

Patients who have Scheuermann's kyphosis can be treated successfully in the Milwaukee brace even with severe clinical deformity and kyphosis of more than 50 degrees. Permanent correction can be gained by brace treatment since there is a potential for healing vertebral end-plate defects and reconstituting vertebral height.[3] TLSOs are also thought to be effective in the treatment of Scheuermann's kyphosis. Electrospinal stimulation has been used and dual-channel units are available, but at present it is not a preferred treatment technique for this type of kyphosis.

Summary

Nonoperative treatment of spinal deformity will continue to change. In recent years, many long-held tenets regarding the natural history and response to various treatment methods have been challenged, and we do not yet have answers to many of the questions that have been raised. New orthotic devices and electrical stimulation have multiplied treatment approaches. From this array of options, the clinician must decide whom to treat and what method to use.

On the basis of the current consensus, patients who have significant, progressive deformity and an immature spine should be treated by one of the nonoperative techniques. The various TLSOs are most favored, although the Milwaukee brace still has a definite role in certain curve patterns and remains the standard of

braces. The role of electrical spinal stimulation is uncertain at present, and further research is necessary.

We have learned that only appropriate orthotic treatment of scoliosis produces long-term stabilization of deformity. Impressive initial curve correction does not signify the end result, and patients who have curves that are unacceptable when the patient is first seen should be considered for surgical treatment. Thus, while questions remain, the guidelines for treatment outlined in this chapter are appropriate for the present.

References

1. Shands AR Jr, Barr JS, Colonna PC, et al: End-result study of the treatment of idiopathic scoliosis: Report of the research committee of the American Orthopaedic Association. *J Bone Joint Surg* 1941;23:963–977.
2. Blount WP, Schmidt AC: The Milwaukee brace in the treatment of scoliosis, abstract. *J Bone Joint Surgery* 1957;39A:693.
3. Sachs B, Bradford D, Winter R, et al: Scheuermann kyphosis: Follow-up of Milwaukee-brace treatment. *J Bone Joint Surg* 1987;69A:50–57.
4. Edmonsson AS, Morris JT: Follow-up study of Milwaukee brace treatment in patients with idiopathic scoliosis. *Clin Orthop* 1977;126:58–61.
5. Moe JH, Kettleson DN: Idiopathic scoliosis: Analysis of curve patterns and the preliminary results of Milwaukee-brace treatment in one hundred sixty-nine patients. *J Bone Joint Surg* 1970;52A:1509–1533.
6. Mellencamp DD, Blount WB, Anderson AJ: Milwaukee brace treatment of idiopathic scoliosis: Late results. *Clin Orthop* 1977;126:47–57.
7. Carr WA, Moe JH, Winter RB, et al: Treatment of idiopathic scoliosis in the Milwaukee brace: Long-term results. *J Bone Joint Surg* 1980;62A:599–612.
8. Patwardhan AG, Dvonch VM, Bunch WH, et al: Orthotic stabilization of idiopathic scoliotic curve: A biomechanical comparison of low profile and Milwaukee braces. Presented at the annual meeting of the Scoliosis Research Society, Vancouver, Canada, Sept 15–19, 1987.
9. Wynarsky GT, Schultz AB, Green M, et al: Trunk muscle activities in braced scoliosis patients. Presented at the annual meeting of the Scoliosis Research Society, Vancouver, Canada, Sept 15–19, 1987.
10. Laurnen EL, Tupper JW, Mullen MP: The Boston brace in thoracic scoliosis: A preliminary report. *Spine* 1983;8:388–395.
11. Watts HG, Hall JE, Stanish W: The Boston brace system for the treatment of low thoracic and lumbar scoliosis by the use of a girdle without superstructure. *Clin Orthop* 1977;126:87–92.

12. Seiler X: Dilatation artificielle du thorax, et traitement des deviations de la colonne vertébrale, pour une nouvelle méthode d'appliquer le courant d'induction galvanique. *Bull Acad R Med Belg* 1856;16:69–74.
13. Olsen GA, Rosen H, Stoll S, et al: The use of muscle stimulation for inducing scoliotic curves: A preliminary report. *Clin Orthop* 1975;113:198–211.
14. Bobechko WP, Herbert MA, Friedman HG: Electrospinal instrumentation for scoliosis: Current status. *Orthop Clin North Am* 1979;10:927–941.
15. McCollough NC III: Nonoperative treatment of idiopathic scoliosis using surface electrical stimulation. *Spine* 1987;11:802–804.
16. Axelgaard J, Brown JC: Lateral electrical surface stimulation for the treatment of progressive idiopathic scoliosis. *Spine* 1983;8:242–260.
17. Axelgaard J, Nordwall A, Brown JC: Correction of spinal curvatures by transcutaneous electrical muscle stimulation. *Spine* 1983;8:463–481.
18. Davis RJ, Brown CW, Bunnell WP, et al: Efficacy of electrical surface stimulation versus bracing in the treatment of idiopathic scoliosis: A comparative study. *Orthop Trans* 1987;11:104.
19. Carr WA: Electrical stimulation for treatment of idiopathic scoliosis in a group of high risk progressive patients. Presented at the annual meeting of the Scoliosis Research Society, Vancouver, Canada, Sept 15–19, 1987.
20. O'Donnell CS, Bunnell WP, Betz RR, et al: Electrical stimulation in the treatment of idiopathic scoliosis. Presented at the annual meeting of the Scoliosis Research Society, Vancouver, Canada, Sept 15–19, 1987.
21. Brown JC, Axelgaard JA: Multi-center study of 1221 patients on LESS for idiopathic scoliosis. *Orthop Trans* 1985;10:3.
22. Green NE, MacLean WE: The psychological effects of brace wear on adolescent idiopathic scoliosis patients and their families. Presented at the annual meeting of the Scoliosis Research Society, Coronado, Calif, Sept 17–20, 1985.
23. Rowe DE: Comparison of patient acceptance to Scolitron and brace treatment of idiopathic scoliosis. *Orthop Trans* 1987;11:104.
24. DiRaimondo CV, Green NE, MacLean WE: Bracing compliance in adolescent idiopathic scoliosis. *Orthop Trans* 1985;9:109.
25. Houghton GR, McInerney A, Tew T: Monitoring true brace compliance. *Orthop Trans* 1987;11:105.
26. Green NE: Part-time bracing of adolescent idiopathic scoliosis. *J Bone Joint Surg* 1986;68A:738–742.
27. Riddick MF, Price CT: Time modified brace wear: An effective alternative treatment regimen. *Orthop Trans* 1985;9:109.
28. Lonstein JE (ed): Symposium: The natural history of idiopathic scoliosis. *Spine* 1986;11:771–808.
29. Winter RB, Lonstein JE, Drogt J, et al: The effectiveness of bracing in the nonoperative treatment of idiopathic scoliosis. *Spine* 1986;11:790–791.
30. Emans JB, Kaelin A, Bancel P, et al: The Boston bracing system for idiopathic scoliosis: Follow-up results in 295 patients. *Spine* 1986;11:792–801.
31. Roache JW, Herring JA, Wenger DR: The role of exercises in brace treatment of scoliosis. *Orthop Trans* 1984;8:149.
32. Rogala EJ, Drummond DS, Gurr J: Scoliosis: Incidence and natural history: A prospective epidemiological study. *J Bone Joint Surg* 1978;60A:173–176.
33. Lonstein JE, Carlson JH: The prediction of curve progression in untreated idiopathic scoliosis during growth. *J Bone Joint Surg* 1984;66A:1061–1071.
34. Winter RB, Lovell WW, Moe JH: Excessive thoracic lordosis and loss of pulmonary function in patients with idiopathic scoliosis. *J Bone Joint Surg* 1975;57A:972–977.

Preoperative and Intraoperative Considerations in Adolescent Idiopathic Scoliosis

Gordon L. Engler, MD

Preoperative Considerations

Once the decision for surgical correction of a spinal deformity has been made, certain preliminary precautions must be taken to ensure that the patient is properly prepared and examined before the scheduled procedure.

Medication

It is important to discontinue certain medications before any surgical procedure. Specifically, all aspirin-containing products and nonsteroidal anti-inflammatory medication must be avoided. These products may increase bleeding during surgery and, therefore, increase blood loss. Both prescription and nonprescription drugs of these types should be discontinued.

If pain medication is required during the two-week period prior to the scheduled surgery, acetaminophen may be substituted for an aspirin-containing product, if possible. Acetaminophen does not have the same blood-thinning effect and will not increase the amount of blood loss during the surgical procedure.

A patient should stop taking birth control pills, with a gynecologist's approval, at least one month prior to the surgery. These medications may increase blood clotting in the veins of the lower extremities and may lead to problems such as phlebitis in the postoperative period.

Other medications should be evaluated prior to hospital admission. Since corrective spinal surgery is usually an elective procedure, sufficient time is available to accomplish investigation of these medications and their appropriate alteration or cessation.

Radiographic Examination

As a routine procedure for hospital admission and surgical preparation, anteroposterior and lateral radiographs of the chest are usually required. In addition, certain radiographic examinations are required to determine the nature of the curve and its correctability at various levels of the spine and to rule out congenital or developmental problems that may alter the location of instrument placement and fusion limits. An erect posteroanterior radiograph of the entire spine must be obtained. It is best to have this view on one long cassette (34 inches) to determine the overall alignment and balance of the entire spine in one view. Spina bifida occulta must also be identified in order to avoid posterior hook placement on an incomplete lamina. Also, a full-length lateral view of the spine should be obtained on a long cassette. If thoracic lordosis is present, it may be evaluated using the lateral view, and the true anteroposterior dimension of the thorax may be determined prior to surgery. One must look for increased lumbar lordosis and spondylolisthesis, which may be an incidental finding.

To determine the exact placement of the anterior or posterior spinal instrumentation, the extent of spinal fusion, and the correctability and flexibility of the various segments of the spine, a radiographic evaluation must be made. The structural curve is usually less flexible and exhibits a greater degree of rotational deformation than the nonstructural curve. Both the supine anteroposterior projection and anteroposterior supine bending films will demonstrate the structural curve and the flexibility of the nonstructural segments. It is thought that the displacement of the nucleus pulposus toward the convexity of the structural curve prevents certain correctability of lateral side bending. Bending films must be taken with the patient in the supine position to avoid the patient's compensation by stance or pelvic obliquity. If necessary, a head halter and pelvic traction may be used to demonstrate the available correctability. The radiograph taken with the patient in this form of traction usually approximates the end result of the corrective spinal surgery. In severe cases, cast correction views may be necessary. The lateral side-bending films may exceed the correction obtainable by surgery, because the force exerted by the instrumentation to correct the spine is limited to that of the bone-metal interface. Osteoporotic bone cannot be manipulated excessively by instruments, although side-bending films may show marked correctability because of ligamentous laxity.

In general, the superior and inferior extent of the spinal instrumentation is determined by the last uncorrectable vertebral segment seen on lateral side-bend views. If the disk space beyond the end vertebral segment to be fused exhibits angulation reversal (presumed to indicate centralization of the nucleus pulposus and lack of structural change), it need not be included in the spinal fusion. It is necessary, however, to include all instrumented segments in the fusion mass. Occasionally, this level must be extended to achieve proper overall balance in both the frontal and sagittal planes. The need to extend the fusion level is determined by the method of spinal instrumentation and the configuration of the end-corrected spinal alignment.

Although preoperative traction has been used to increase spinal correction prior to surgery, overall, it has not been more effective than preoperative exercise programs.[1] If the patient has worn a brace prior to surgery, it is usually necessary to discontinue using the brace and allow the patient's spine to become more flexible preoperatively. An exercise program is prescribed to overcome the physiologic stiffening that has occurred because of prolonged use of the brace. A few degrees of progression may occur, but this is usually recovered because surgical correction is enhanced by the mobilization of the spinal segments.

Since the pelvis is the main site for bone-graft harvesting, an anteroposterior view of the pelvis should be obtained prior to surgery to ascertain whether or not the posterosuperior iliac crest is normal. Neoplastic or developmental changes may alter the decision to graft from this site. Although the pelvis is the prime location for harvesting bone grafts for all spinal fusions, it is sometimes necessary to augment the fusion with bank bone because of the occasional paucity of bone-graft material from the iliac crest. Cancellous and cortical morselized bits of bone are preferred for this augmentation. Augmentation will enhance the relative mass of the fusion and fill the void between the instrumentation and the spine to avoid potential space in this area.

Special radiographic techniques are often needed to rule out the existence of other pathologic findings. Computed axial tomography, magnetic resonance imaging, or myelography may be necessary to rule out syringomyelia, neurofibromatosis, diastematomyelia, or other lesions or deformities that are sometimes found with nonidiopathic scoliosis.

When the anterior approach is used, an intravenous pyelogram is needed to identify the urinary tract system. Since there is a slightly increased incidence of congenital urinary tract abnormalities in patients with scoliosis, it is essential to identify abnormally placed kidneys or ureters. A complete intravenous pyelogram is not usually necessary. A bolus injection of radiographic opaque fluid with one 15-minute "scout" film is usually sufficient. It is also necessary to determine if the patient has two functional kidneys in the event that one kidney or ureter is inadvertently injured.

Pulmonary Evaluation

A full pulmonary function study is usually done before surgery. Patients with idiopathic thoracic scoliosis often have an associated thoracic lordosis that causes some reduction in pulmonary function. The vital capacity and forced expiratory volume in one second (FEV_1) are often altered in these patients. Significant changes in pulmonary function should alert the anesthesiologist and surgeon to possible complications in the immediate postoperative period. Anesthetic agents and ventilation techniques may need to be revised as appropriate for these patients. If the anterior approach

planned involves transection of the diaphragm and subsequent chest tube installation, prolonged intubation in the postoperative period with gentle weaning on a ventilator may be required. If the preoperative pulmonary function studies do reflect a compromise in pulmonary function, preoperative aerobic exercises and pulmonary treatment are often requested. During the hospitalization, an incentive spirometer is used both in the preoperative period and for several months postoperatively for respiratory enhancement and to assist the patient in pulmonary care, such as coughing effectively to clear secretions. This is extremely important in those patients who will be confined postoperatively in a full body brace or cast in which thoracic expansion is limited.

Blood Transfusion

With the recent problem of the acquired immune deficiency syndrome (AIDS) and the long-standing fear of hepatitis from blood transfusions, two methods have been instituted in most hospitals to reduce the incidence of potential transmission of these diseases.

Preoperatively, one or two units of autologous blood are obtained from the patient two to three weeks prior to the surgical procedure. The protocol for collecting autologous blood is usually determined by the hospital blood bank facility. If the patient is very young, less than 100 lb, or in poor health, autologous blood may not be obtainable. In those situations, directed donors may be available from the patient's family or friends. These donors should have the same blood type as the patient. Even the directed donation blood is tested for both AIDS and hepatitis during the preliminary typing and screening of the blood-saving procedure.

In addition to the blood that is banked prior to the surgery, an intraoperative cell saver can be used for retransfusion of blood lost during the surgical procedure. One or two units of blood can be retransfused during the procedure by this method. With the intraoperative cell saver and one or two units of autologous blood, it is unlikely that additional blood will be needed during the patient's hospitalization for spinal surgery.

Laboratory Tests

Laboratory tests done prior to surgery can indicate the possibility of an undiagnosed or unsuspected problem. An elevated creatine phosphokinase level may indicate muscle disease. Muscle disease must be ruled out because of the possibility of malignant hyperthermia, especially in patients with a positive family history. The avoidance of succinylcholine in those patients is mandatory.

Prophylactic antibiotics are often given during the surgical procedure and for one or two days after surgery.

Intraoperative Considerations

Anesthetic

In each medical center or hospital, specific anesthetic techniques have been developed by the anesthesiology and orthopaedic staffs. Nevertheless, certain basic principles must be considered and used as guidelines in cases of scoliosis surgery.

Basic monitoring methods use an electrocardiogram, blood pressure cuff, and esophageal stethoscope for breath and heart sounds. An indwelling urinary catheter is used to ascertain urinary output. An arterial line monitors blood pressure and blood gases. A pulse oximeter is a useful adjunct to the arterial line. A rectal thermometer is often used; and a nerve stimulator can be used to assess the level of relaxation.

Proper positioning of the patient on the operating table is extremely important and is usually decided by the operating surgeon and the anesthesiologist. The prone position is used for the posterior approach. Pressure points should be carefully padded. An orthopaedic frame can be used to free the chest and abdomen from pressure that causes engorgement of the vertebral venous plexus and excessive bleeding. Lateral or semilateral positioning of the patient is necessary when the spine is approached anteriorly.

Patients with nonidiopathic scoliosis are more likely to require postoperative ventilation than patients with idiopathic scoliosis. Patients whose curves are greater than 65 degrees are more likely to have impaired pulmonary function. Therefore, the preoperative evaluation of pulmonary function and arterial blood gases is extremely important to establish a baseline for analysis of changes that occur during the surgical procedure.

With spinal cord monitoring using the technique of evoked potentials, it is best to avoid inhalation agents such as halothane and isoflurane. Diazepam and droperidol also should be avoided. It is best to use a balanced technique of nitrous oxide, narcotic (fentanyl citrate, sufentanil, morphine), and a muscle relaxant.[2,3] Endotracheal intubation and mechanical ventilation are necessary. Hypocarbia must be avoided, because it may reduce spinal cord blood flow.

Although hypotensive anesthesia is not a routinely accepted anesthetic principle, it has been used to reduce blood loss. Pretreatment with a beta-blocking agent and the use of a nitroprusside infusion can reduce the mean arterial pressure to slightly above 65 mm Hg. Arterial line monitoring is essential during this type of anesthesia, because reducing blood pressure during attenuation of a spinal artery may result in ischemia to the spinal cord. This ischemia is reflected in an alteration in the recorded somatosensory-evoked potentials.[4]

When the anterior approach is used, intubation with a double-lumen tube permits collapse of the nonde-pendent lung during the surgery. Both a high inspired oxygen concentration and occasional reinflation of the lung during surgery are necessary to maintain oxygenation. Both methods of increasing oxygenation are possible with the double-lumen tube.

When access to the anterior spine in the thoracic region is necessary, high-frequency jet ventilation through a single-lumen tube may offer certain advantages.[5] This ventilation technique allows the pericardium to be displaced and is especially useful when the surgeon is working in the anterior thoracic spine.

A technique for reduction of red cell mass is the acute normovolemic hemodilution method. Immediately before surgery, the patient may be bled to a hematocrit of approximately 20%. Blood is replaced by crystalloid or colloid to restore normovolemia and the patient is transfused during surgery as required. This technique and the autologous blood and the cell saver techniques have become popular in recent years.

Spinal Cord Monitoring

Three potential risks pertain to corrective spinal surgery. The incidence of infection is one risk that has been greatly reduced by the administration of prophylactic antibiotics. The second hazard of the procedure, postoperative pseudarthrosis of the spinal fusion, is usually insignificant in the adolescent because of enhanced bone healing in this age group. Nevertheless, if a pseudarthrosis is demonstrated, surgical correction is often required. The third potential hazard of corrective spinal surgery is alteration of the spinal cord within the spine and attenuation of the arterial blood supply to the spinal cord. If significant, this can result in paraplegia. Several methods have been devised to alert the surgeon to this hazard during the surgical procedure.

Perhaps the most common monitoring method involves the so-called Stagnara wake-up test.[6,7] The anesthesia is decreased after correcting the spinal deformity to bring the patient to a conscious level. The patient is asked to move both lower extremities before the surgical procedure is completed. Once movement is noted, anesthesia is returned to appropriate levels and the surgical procedure is completed. This test of motor function is commonly used only once during each procedure and may not indicate minor alterations of spinal cord transmission prior to spinal cord injury. Furthermore, it cannot be used in the presence of neuromuscular disease or weakness from other causes.

In order to alert the surgeon to evolving spinal cord injury, the somatosensory-evoked potential monitoring system has been used.[8] Stimulation of the distal sensory nerves while recording proximal to the surgical area can alert the surgeon to possible alteration of spinal cord transmission. Subsequent corrective measures might then avoid further hazard to the spinal cord and neurologic injury.

Table 8-1
Standard protocol for typical idiopathic scoliosis

Parameter	Setting
Hardware amplification	40,000 ×
Hardware filter	1.5 to 300 Hz
Stimulation	Both legs (unless there is a deficit in one)
Rate	2.3 per second
Randomization	±50%
Sweeps	200 samples
Epoch length	200 ms
Time window	0 to 200 ms
Software filter	20 to 250 Hz
Artifact level	20 to 30 μV
Screen scale	3 μV

The technique of evoked potential monitoring at New York University Medical Center is presently performed on a four-channel computerized monitoring device using signaling averaging. This system has a digital filter and multimodality capacity. The following standard leads are used for orthopaedic cases: (1) an FPZ as a surface reference electrode (placed on the forehead using pediatric electrocardiogram silver-silver chloride pads and leads); (2) a CZ as an active surface electrode (placed at the vertex using a silver cup electrode filled with calcium chloride electrode cream); and (3) a surface ground electrode (placed on the shoulder using pediatric electrocardiogram silver-silver chloride pads and leads). These electrodes are then connected to a preamplifier that is located near the patient's head. The active electrodes should be connected to the negative position and the reference electrode to the positive position on the preamplifier to obtain waveforms that have positive peaks.

The posterior tibial nerve at the level of the ankle is stimulated by a surface bipolar bar electrode placed on each leg. These electrodes are then connected to a stimulator that can be adjusted to a range of 0 to 40 mA with a pulse duration of either 0.1 or 0.5 ms. A 40-mA standard stimulation at a 0.5-ms duration is used. Both the stimulator and the preamplifier are connected to the monitoring system via long, insulated cables.

This type of monitoring system allows a wide array of options and flexibility in setting the protocol. Table 8-1 lists the standard protocol used for the typical idiopathic scoliosis patient. The system is a continuous monitor showing a sliding average that is updated to our standard protocol approximately every 10 ms throughout the procedure.

This evoked potential monitoring system has been used with some alteration over the past 12 years on all spinal operations that I have performed at New York University Medical Center. Although some false-positive results have occurred (an unobtainable somatosen-

sory-evoked potential tracing, for example, a flat line, in the presence of normal neurologic findings in the postoperative period), no neurologic deficits and no false-negative responses have resulted from its use.

Evoked potential monitoring has also been used with other protocols. Various stimulation and recording sites are now in use in many parts of the world. In addition, work is presently under way to establish a method of monitoring motor-evoked potentials for use in the operating field.[9] The future role of spinal cord monitoring is likely to involve a combination of motor-evoked potentials and sensory-evoked potentials to determine impending neurologic injury during the surgical procedure and in the immediate postoperative hours. If a neurologic problem is detected, the spinal instruments can be removed immediately to allow full restoration of the blood supply. In addition, exploration for hematoma or instrument impingement must be accomplished and any findings corrected. When these procedures are done during surgery or in the immediate postoperative period (within four hours), some neurologic recovery is usually obtainable.

Postoperative Management

The patient is usually confined to bed for the first few days postoperatively. Depending on the nature of the spinal instrumentation used, a cast or brace may be necessary. When Cotrel-Dubousset instrumentation is used, the patient may be positioned progressively upright after the third postoperative day, depending on the surgeon's protocol. When a cast or brace is used, the onset of postoperative immobilization will determine the date of upright activities. In general, the patient is confined to limited activities for the first four weeks after hospital discharge. If a cast or brace is used, it usually remains in place for four to six months, again depending on the protocol of the individual surgeon and the nature of the instrumentation used. Some surgeons now use a plastic body jacket that may be removed for short periods each day and for showering. When the internal fixation device is less secure, a full body cast may be necessary.

References

1. Nachemson A, Nordwall A: Effectiveness of preoperative Cotrel traction for correction of idiopathic scoliosis. *J Bone Joint Surg* 1977;59A:504–508.
2. Pathak KS, Brown RH, Nash CL Jr, et al: Continuous opioid infusion for scoliosis fusion surgery. *Anesth Analg* 1983;62:841–845.
3. Friedman WA, Grundy BL: Monitoring of sensory-evoked potentials is highly reliable and helpful in the operating room. *J Clin Monit* 1987;3:38–44.
4. Grundy BL, Nash CL Jr, Brown RH: Deliberate hypotension for

spinal fusion: Prospective randomized study with evoked potential monitoring. *Can Anaesth Soc J* 1982;29:452–462.

5. Howland SW, Carlon GC, Goldiner PL, et al: High-frequency jet ventilation during thoracic surgical procedures. *Anesthesiology* 1987;67:1009–1012.

6. Vauzelle C, Stagnara P, Jouvinroux P: Functional monitoring of spinal cord activity during spinal surgery. *Clin Orthop* 1973;93:173–178.

7. Hall JE, Levine CR, Sudhir KG: Intraoperative awakening to monitor spinal cord function during Harrington instrumentation and spine fusion: Description of procedure and report of three cases. *J Bone Joint Surg* 1978;60A:533–536.

8. Engler GL, Spielholz NJ, Bernhard WN, et al: Somatosensory evoked potentials during Harrington instrumentation for scoliosis. *J Bone Joint Surg* 1978;60A:528–532.

9. Levy WJ, York DH, McCaffrey M, et al: Motor-evoked potentials from transcranial stimulation of the motor cortex in man. *Neurosurgery* 1984;16:287–302.

Surgical Treatment of Adolescent Idiopathic Scoliosis

Vernon T. Tolo, MD

Although there are clear indications for surgical management of adolescent idiopathic scoliosis, the surgeon's decision to operate is multifaceted. Variables include the curve size, the bone age of the child, and the physical and psychological impact of the spinal and rib deformities. Of all age groups, adolescents are most sensitive to variations in body shape and size. Surgical treatment is often readily accepted by adolescents as a means to become "normal" again; therefore, the orthopaedist treating scoliosis must use scientifically accepted criteria when recommending surgical treatment.

It was once thought that scoliosis did not worsen after growth was complete; however, long-term follow-up studies have demonstrated that the curves of many adults do become worse. Patients whose standing spinal radiograph shows a thoracic curve greater than 50 degrees are most likely to have their curves become worse in adulthood. Spinal instrumentation and fusion is appropriate in these cases, since progression is expected to be approximately 1 degree per year. An adult with scoliosis requires surgery when serial, erect spinal radiographs, taken approximately three years apart, demonstrate worsening in the thoracic area. If a patient with thoracic scoliosis has a curve of less than 45 degrees at skeletal maturity, surgery is rarely needed and follow-up in five to ten years is appropriate.

As noted in Chapter 7, most thoracic curves of less than 45 degrees can be treated nonsurgically. However, if a 45-degree thoracic scoliosis is seen in a premenarchal child with one to two years of growth remaining, spinal instrumentation and fusion is acceptable. The principal reason to recommend instrumentation and fusion for a patient with thoracic scoliosis of less than 40 degrees is to prevent the increasing thoracic lordosis that may occur with orthotic treatment. Since progressive thoracic lordosis may compromise pulmonary function, surgery is prescribed when an increased lordosis is noted during the period of brace care. Pain is rarely an appropriate sole indication to recommend surgery for thoracic scoliosis, especially in the adolescent age group. If adolescents with scoliosis have pain, limitation of spinal mobility, or abnormal neurologic findings, further tests, such as a bone scan, magnetic resonance imaging, computed tomography/myelogram, erythrocyte sedimentation rate, complete blood cell count, and B-27 to screen for ankylosing spondylitis are needed before considering fusion.

Other considerations are required for lumbar scoliosis. Surgery is generally indicated for patients with idiopathic curves of more than 40 degrees, since these are expected to become worse even after skeletal maturity. If the trunk is decompensated to one side, continued progression is more likely, and more than 30% lumbar vertebral rotation has been correlated with an increased risk of progression. Adolescents who have lumbar idiopathic scoliosis with pain should be thoroughly examined for an underlying cause before surgery. Although low back pain with lumbar scoliosis is unusual in adolescents, those with curves of more than 40 degrees have an increased incidence of back pain during adult life.

After the decision to operate has been made, the levels of the spine to be fused and the type of spinal instrumentation to be used must be determined. Subfascial or subcutaneous rods can be used occasionally without fusion in the very young child; however, all instrumentation methods discussed in this chapter are accompanied by fusion of all instrumented levels. Like other mechanical devices, spinal instrumentation will fatigue and break or displace eventually in the absence of spinal fusion.

Fusion of one or two levels above the last rotated vertebra and two levels below the last rotated vertebra used to be recommended to prevent later progression above or below the instrumented area. The late effects of fusion to the low lumbar area are now recognized, however, so the area of fusion should include no more than all the rotated vertebrae. It is preferable to avoid fusion to the level of the fourth lumbar vertebra or below, but only if the scoliosis can be stabilized adequately.

Selecting posterior fusion levels is relatively simple with a single-curve pattern. However, if a double-curve pattern is present, it is important to consider selective fusion, in which only the more structural of the two curves is fused. King and associates[1] described the criteria for applying selective fusion. The following example illustrates their approach.

A 13-year-old patient had a 50-degree right thoracic, 42-degree left lumbar idiopathic scoliosis when first examined. Bending films showed thoracic correction to 27 degrees and lumbar correction to 9 degrees. Fusion of only the thoracic curve resulted in a final radiographic film showing a thoracic correction of 21 degrees and a lumbar correction of 18 degrees with excellent trunk balance (Fig. 9–1). In this example, the increased flexibility of the lumbar curve on lateral bending predicted that the lumbar curve would improve if the thoracic curve were significantly improved, and the final curve would be approximately of the magnitude necessary to balance the remaining thoracic curve. In this way, the lumbar spine was left more supple, decreasing the likelihood that the child will have low back pain as an adult. In this technique of selective fusion, the lower level of instrumentation should be at the "stable" vertebra, that is, the vertebra that is bisected by a line perpendicular to the mid-sacrum.

Although selective fusion has saved many children from too extensive instrumentation, a word of caution is needed: Do not compromise surgical goals by trying to save a level or two from fusion. The goal of spinal instrumentation and fusion is safe and lasting curve correction with restitution of trunk balance.

Posterior Spinal Instrumentation

Harrington Instrumentation

This system was developed in the 1950s by Dr. Paul Harrington of Houston, Texas.[2] It has been the most widely used type of spinal instrumentation. Originally applied to spinal deformities resulting from polio, this instrumentation system and technique was introduced to other scoliosis surgeons in the early 1960s and continues to be used world-wide today. By many, it is considered the standard by which the results of other newer methods of instrumentation should be judged.

Technique The basic Harrington instrumentation consists of ¼-inch stainless steel distraction rods, ⅛-inch flexible compression rods, and a wide array of numbered hooks through which these rods pass.[2] Initially, a distraction hook is placed under the lamina and inferior facet of the upper concave vertebra to be fused.

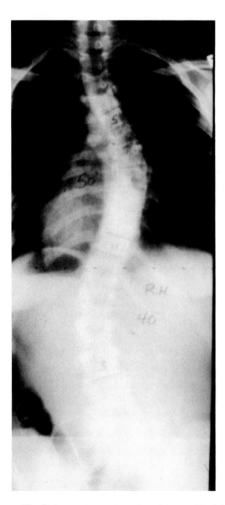
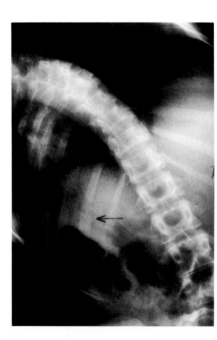
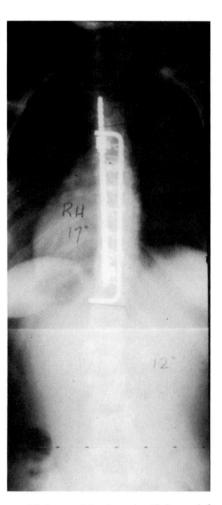

Fig. 9–1 Radiographs of a 13-year-old girl who had idiopathic scoliosis. **Left:** Radiograph shows a 50-degree right thoracic, 42-degree left lumbar idiopathic scoliosis. **Center:** A left lateral-bending radiograph showed lumbar curve correction from 42 to 9 degrees. (The thoracic curve had corrected from 50 to 27 degrees.) **Right:** Radiograph shows "selective fusion" of the less flexible curve. Excellent correction and good trunk balance were obtained for both curves.

A companion hook is placed over the superior lamina of the lowest concave vertebra to be fused. After facet joint excision and fusion has been completed, a smooth distraction rod with a 3-inch superior notched segment is placed between these two hooks. By means of a spreader, the upper hook is moved up to the notched portion of the rod. This lengthens the concavity of the scoliosis and draws the apex of the curve toward the midline. The hooks are held securely to the rod by tension and by tilting at the notched end.

Although a single distraction rod instrumentation is the most common form of Harrington instrumentation used, there may be some benefits gained from adding a compression rod on the convexity. The benefits for thoracic curves include increased stability of instrumentation and improvement in rib hump correction. In lumbar curves, preservation of lumbar lordosis is the main benefit. If a compression rod is used, it is applied before the distraction rod is placed. Contraindications to the use of the compression rod include the presence of (1) thoracic lordosis, which will worsen with compression rods, and (2) thoracic curves of more than 90 degrees, because a compression rod will limit correction otherwise possible by the distraction rod.

Because the Harrington rod or rods are not as securely fixed to the posterior elements as some other spinal instrumentation systems, a postoperative cast or brace is needed to protect the patient from hook displacement for about six months after surgery, at which time fusion is solid.

The results of Harrington instrumentation and fusion are very good.[1-4] In adolescent idiopathic scoliosis, the pseudarthrosis rate is 1% to 2% and reported curve correction varies from 40% to 55%. Despite a radiographic correction of about 50%, trunk balance is restored very well. Permanent rib hump correction varies. Approximately two thirds of the patients who appear much improved after cast removal lose some rib hump correction by four years postoperatively.[5]

Luque Instrumentation

Developed in the 1970s by Dr. Eduardo Luque of Mexico City,[6] the implants used in this system are simple, consisting of smooth, ¼-inch and 3/16-inch L-shaped rods and 16- or 18-gauge wire loops. This was the initial segmental spinal instrumentation system. The Luque system is now rarely used in idiopathic scoliosis; however, its introduction led to the development of other instrumentation systems that have segmental fixation as a primary consideration.

In general, Luque instrumentation requires more operating time and leads to more blood loss than Harrington instrumentation. After the posterior spine has been exposed, a window of ligamentum flavum is removed between each level to be fused, as well as one level above and below the fusion ends. Segmental wires are passed through the spinal canal into a sublaminar

position and double wires are passed beneath the end-vertebrae laminae. Two L-shaped rods are contoured to preserve thoracic kyphosis and lumbar lordosis and the sublaminar wires are tightened around the rods. The L-portion of the rod fits between spinous processes at the ends of the fusion to decrease rod migration. The rods are then wired together transversely to improve the construct stability. Because of the segmental fixation and stability, no postoperative cast or brace is usually needed.

The principal use of Luque instrumentation and fusion at the present time is in the treatment of neuromuscular scoliosis. There are a number of disadvantages to using the Luque technique in the treatment of adolescent idiopathic scoliosis. These include blood loss, risk of iatrogenic neural injury, difficulty in wire removal, and unknown long-term effects of wires in the spinal canal. The intraoperative blood loss is higher with the Luque technique because of the increased length of time generally needed to operate and the occasional problem of epidural venous bleeding during wire passage. The iatrogenic neural injury that has been reported primarily is lower-extremity paresthesia following surgery, although motor loss has been reported also.[7] Although these paresthesias are usually transient, their presence indicates dural irritation or nerve root stretch resulting from this procedure. Although rod and wire removal is not routinely indicated, when removal of sublaminar wires is needed, difficulties may result. In an animal model and in the human skeleton models, removal of a sublaminar wire leads to encroachment of the wire loop into the spinal canal and against the spinal cord. Recent reports, however, indicate sublaminar wire removal is safe because a fibrous sheath forms adjacent to the wire and prevents spinal cord injury. The long-term effects of sublaminar wires remain unknown, but animal models indicate that, in addition to the fibrosis adjacent to the wire, the dorsal columns of the spinal cord may develop neurolytic changes. This has not yet been reported to occur in humans.

In previously reported series using the Luque technique, the radiographic correction is 45% to 60%, with little rotational correction.[6,8] Instrumentation is technically more difficult with curves greater than approximately 70 degrees, as it is usually necessary to bend the rods in the frontal plane as well as the sagittal plane to allow stable wire fixation. In rigid, short curves, instrumentation contouring is also more challenging, and if the rods do not have good laminar contact at each level, loss of correction can be anticipated in the months after surgery.

Harrington Rod With Sublaminar Wires

A hybrid of the Harrington and Luque techniques, this approach was developed to take advantage of the distraction component of the Harrington system and the segmental fixation component of the Luque technique. The Harrington ¼-inch distraction rod is inserted in the usual way but is always contoured in the sagittal plane. This contouring necessitates a square-holed distal hook[9] to prevent rod rotation, which will always occur if a contoured rod is placed in a round-holed Harrington hook.

Segmental 16-gauge Luque wires are used wherever more fixation is required. Minimal wire placement would include an apical wire for transverse pull and end-vertebrae placement to stabilize the distraction rod hooks. Segmental wires are placed in a sublaminar position, as they are in the Luque technique. When tightening the wires, the surgeon must avoid lateral hook rotation of the upper hook. Some surgeons prefer to protect the instrumentation with a postoperative brace, especially if a minimum number of wires is used.

This technique is most useful to correct thoracic lordosis or hypokyphosis at the same time as the scoliosis is corrected.[10] Reported radiographic curve correction is 39% to 50%, with only minimal rotational correction. It is important not to use sublaminar wires with the ⅛-inch compression rod with laminar hooks, because spinal cord injury has been reported from the compression rod hooks lowering into the spinal canal after wire tightening.

Wisconsin Instrumentation (Spinous Process Wires)

This technique, developed by Dr. Denis Drummond and associates in the early 1980s,[11] was an attempt to preserve the concept of segmental fixation while eliminating some of the drawbacks inherent in the Luque technique. The implants used in this approach are a contoured, square-ended Harrington distraction rod, a contoured C-shaped ³⁄₁₆-inch Luque rod, and 18-gauge wires, each with a metal button. All spinous processes should be preserved at the time of posterior spine exposure. After facet joint removal, but prior to rod placement, holes are made laterally on each side of the base of each spinous process. One wire is passed through this hole from each side until the attached button contacts the spinous process, preventing the tightened wire from cutting through the bone. After wire passage is complete, each spinous process will have two wires, except the end vertebrae, at which a single wire is placed on the side opposite the hook at that level. After lateral decortication and fusion, the contoured square-ended distraction rod is inserted and initial correction is obtained. The wires on the side of the concavity are tightened to the square-ended distraction rod to gain further correction, although care must be taken not to rotate the hooks laterally during wire tightening. A C-shaped Luque rod is contoured sagittally and wired on the convexity of the curve. After segmental wire tightening is complete, the rods are linked together, again taking care not to rotate the distraction hooks laterally. For double-curve instrumentation, a crossover distraction rod is used initially, with a separate C-shaped Luque rod for each curve convexity. The resulting fixation is stable, and I use no cast or brace postoperatively.

Potential problems with this technique are relatively few. Reported radiographic curve correction is 50% to 60%. As with the other techniques described above, the rotational change is small; however, one can obtain modest improvement in thoracic lordosis. This technique is applicable to all idiopathic curves, particularly for single thoracic curves and all double-curve patterns (Figs. 9–2 and 9–3).

Cotrel-Dubousset Instrumentation

Cotrel and Dubousset developed the most current form of posterior instrumentation in France in the early 1980s.[12] Using segmental spinal fixation, the Cotrel-Dubousset system differs from other corrective systems. The scoliosis is corrected by a combination of initial longitudinally applied forces with subsequent vertebral rotation, converting the scoliosis to either thoracic kyphosis or lumbar lordosis.

The implants used to accomplish this correction are 7-mm rods with rough surfaces, open and closed pedicle and laminar hooks that fasten to the rod, and transverse linkage rods to increase implant stability. In selected instances, pedicle screws are used in the lumbar area, but pedicle screws are rarely used for adolescent idiopathic scoliosis.

Technique The Cotrel-Dubousset instrumentation technique begins before the patient is anesthetized. The hook sites to be used are carefully marked on the standing spinal radiograph and the type of hook is noted, whether it is a laminar or pedicle hook, as well as if the hooks are open or closed. In general, the end hooks on each rod are closed and the inner hooks open on one side to facilitate rod insertion. Laminar hooks are either thoracic (smaller) or lumbar (larger foot-piece), and pedicle hooks are used principally in the thoracic spine. Usually four or five hooks are used on each side for single curves and six or seven hooks on each side for double curves. After the hooks have been placed, decortication and fusion of the instrumented area is completed. A flexible rod of lead is used as a template and is bent to fit into the hooks on the side to be instrumented first, which is the concavity in the thoracic area and the convexity in the lumbar region. The rod is contoured to fit the residual scoliosis, and slight distraction (concave position) or compression (convex position) is applied to "set" the hooks. Distraction or compression to the degree used in the Harrington system, should be avoided, because rotation is difficult if too much initial longitudinal correction is attempted before rotation. Using C-rings, the surgeon can hold some tension on the hooks while allowing rotation of the rod within the hooks. As the contoured rod is rotated from a lateral curvature position to a contour in the sagittal plane, the scoliosis is corrected. The rod

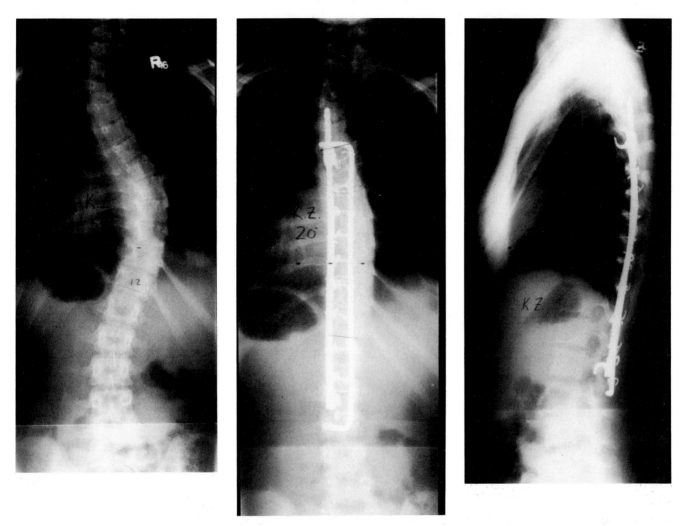

Fig. 9-2 Radiographs of a 15-year-old patient. **Left:** Posteroanterior erect radiograph shows a 54-degree right thoracic idiopathic scoliosis. **Center:** One year postoperatively erect posteroanterior radiograph demonstrates excellent correction by Wisconsin segmental instrumentation. Single wires are used at end vertebrae and double interspinous wires and buttons are used at each other level. The upper end of the C-rod is inserted ventral to the Harrington rod at the proximal end. No cast or brace is usually needed postoperatively. **Right:** Lateral standing radiograph one year after Wisconsin instrumentation demonstrates that sagittal plane contouring is possible. A square-ended Harrington rod must be used.

should appear straight when seen from posterior to anterior through the surgical wound after the rotation is completed. The set screw on each hook is tightened to hold the rod in this corrected position, but the screws are not broken off in case later readjustment is needed. The second rod is contoured in the sagittal plane and is inserted with little further scoliosis correction in most cases.

After the second rod is in place, two or three transverse linkage rods are applied between the larger rods to stabilize the system further. All hook positions are checked and, if satisfactory, all set screws are tightened until they break. Wound closure is routine. The patient is allowed out of bed in two or three days, because no cast or brace is generally used postoperatively.

The principal advantages of the Cotrel-Dubousset

system are versatility, ability to preserve sagittal alignment, and enhanced rotational correction. Although technically more difficult than the other systems, the ability to combine hook fixation with pedicle screw fixation along the same rod is useful, particularly when a laminectomy is needed or the posterior elements are deficient. Because of this versatility, Cotrel-Dubousset instrumentation can be used in any situation requiring internal spinal fixation.

The rotational correction seems superior to other posterior instrumentation systems because the reported correction is 39% in thoracic rotation and 22% in lumbar rotation. In addition, rod contouring by this method preserves the sagittal alignment better than the other systems. If, after instrumentation is completed, further sagittal correction is desired, in situ rod benders

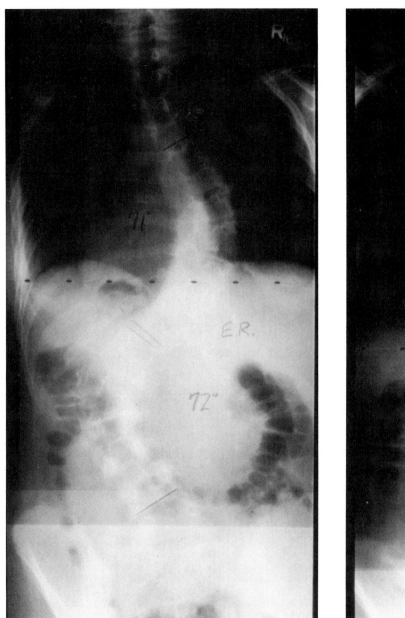
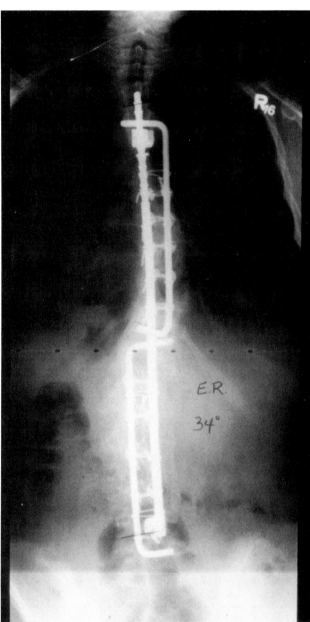

Fig. 9–3 Standing posteroanterior radiographs. **Left:** Radiograph shows a 14-year-old patient who had a 71-degree thoracic, 72-degree lumbar idiopathic scoliosis. **Right:** Radiograph taken one year following treatment using Wisconsin segmental instrumentation. For double curves, a single crossover Harrington distraction rod is used with a separate C-rod on the convexity of each curve.

are used to increase lumbar lordosis or thoracic kyphosis. In doing this, the end hooks must be observed and be prevented from cut-out or displacement. Radiographic correction of the scoliosis is 50% to 75%; the more flexible curves yield the higher correction rates.[13] It may be best to assess overall trunk correction using both frontal and sagittal radiographic measurements taken preoperatively and postoperatively.[14] When this technique of assessment is used, the results of Cotrel-Dubousset instrumentation and fusion appear to be

superior to those of the other systems, although no long-term studies are available (Fig. 9–4).

The primary drawback of the Cotrel-Dubousset system is that it is more technically difficult to insert correctly than the other posterior instrumentation systems available. Operating time is prolonged initially, especially when the surgeon is first learning the procedure. This system is widely applicable to spinal problems; however, it is not used easily in rigid curves or in curves of more than 75 degrees, as seen on standing radio-

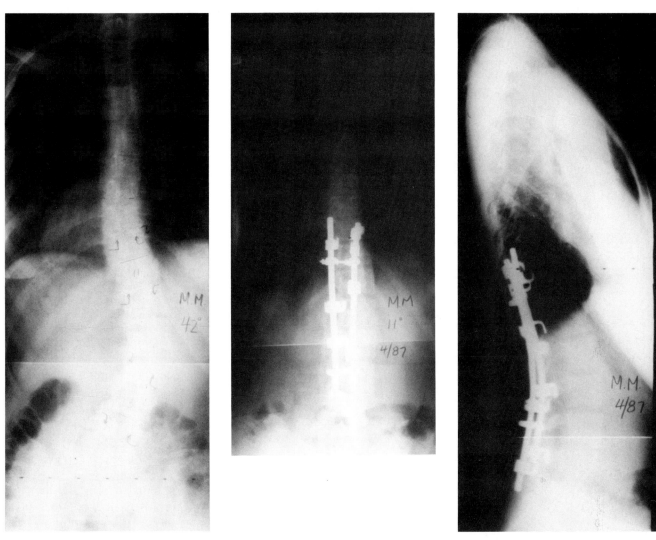

Fig. 9-4 Standing radiographs of a 17-year-old girl who had idiopathic scoliosis. **Left:** Posteroanterior radiograph shows a 42-degree right lumbar idiopathic scoliosis and trunk decompensation to the right. The arrows were placed on the radiograph preoperatively to indicate the type and position of the Cotrel-Dubousset hooks. **Center:** Posteroanterior radiograph one year following Cotrel-Dubousset instrumentation and fusion shows correction from 42 to 11 degrees and solid fusion. **Right:** Lateral radiograph shows excellent preservation of lumbar lordosis using Cotrel-Dubousset instrumentation. It is preferable to avoid instrumentation to the low lumbar region; however, the Cotrel-Dubousset system is best for maintenance of lordosis when instrumentation in this area is needed. Care must be taken to avoid displacement of the distal convex hook.

graphs. If the curve is rigid, rod rotation is not as easily obtained, even after anterior release and posterior facetectomy. If the curve is more than 75 degrees, the residual spinal curve is of such magnitude that it is difficult to contour a single rod into the desired sagittal curve position. More complex hook placement and use of an extra apical rod may be needed. For example, if the rod is contoured to fit a large scoliosis present in the prone position, when the rod is rotated, excessive thoracic kyphosis or lumbar lordosis will result or the apical hooks can come out. If lateral curves are also contoured into the rod, as may be needed with these severe curves, the contoured rod ends must be intersected by a perpendicular line drawn from the mid-

sacrum for good trunk balance after surgery. It may be difficult to judge this balance at the operating table.

Size and cost are two other considerations related to the implants. The hooks, when combined with the double rods and the transverse linkage rods, project posteriorly a significant distance. In the thin patient, these implants can be palpable through the skin, mainly at the mid-thoracic and low-lumbar levels, and primarily on the convex side of the scoliosis. The implants are very expensive, as is the instrumentation set. Separate instrumentation and implants are available for both regular and pediatric sizes. The cost of implants for a fifth thoracic to first lumbar vertebrae instrumentation and fusion is approximately nine times more than Harrington instrumentation and three times more than segmental interspinous spinal instrumentation.

Despite this expense, the Cotrel-Dubousset system is the most frequently used posterior spinal instrumentation system at the present time by members of the Scoliosis Research Society, constituting about 20% of the approximately 10,000 cases reported by members in 1987. No long-term studies are yet available, although the principal problem reported in the Morbidity Report of the Scoliosis Research Society in 1987 was neurologic in nature. The reported incidence of neurologic complication was three times that reported by those using other posterior instrumentation systems, although many of these problems were related to pedicle screw placement.

Summary of Posterior Spinal Instrumentation Systems

Harrington instrumentation is no longer the only posterior surgical treatment of adolescent idiopathic scoliosis. As detailed above, there are several posterior instrumentation systems now available, and the scoliosis surgeon must be familiar with the strengths and weaknesses of each technique. Table 9–1 lists my preferences for the use of each of these systems, and Table 9–2 lists the anticipated percentages of correction for each of these techniques. The combination of different techniques may be useful in complex situations.

Anterior Spinal Instrumentation

The principal uses of anterior spinal instrumentation and fusion with scoliosis treatment are (1) instrumentation of flexible thoracolumbar curves and (2) the initial stage of a two-stage anterior and posterior spinal instrumentation and fusion. Frequently, when a two-stage correction is planned, disk excision and anterior longitudinal ligament section is performed without anterior instrumentation, using halo-wheelchair traction for seven to ten days following this release, after which the posterior spinal instrumentation and fusion is completed.

The incision for the anterior approach to the spine is generally made on the convex side of the scoliosis. If severe kyphosis requiring placement of an anterior strut graft is also present, the concave approach is preferred. In the chest area, the incision should be along the rib leading to the superior vertebra to be fused. If the vertebrae to be fused are at the level of the tenth thoracic vertebra or above, a posterolateral thoracotomy is sufficient, but if the vertebral fusion level extends to between the 11th thoracic vertebra and the first lumbar vertebra the thoracotomy should be combined with a retroperitoneal approach and diaphragmatic detachment. The levels from the first to the fifth lumbar vertebra are reached readily by a retroperitoneal approach, either through or just below the 12th rib bed, although some surgeons prefer the transperitoneal approach for levels from the fourth lumbar to the first sacral vertebrae.

Dwyer Instrumentation

Developed in Australia in the 1960s by Dwyer, this instrumentation system was the first anterior system to be widely used.[15] At the present time, it is used sparingly for adolescent idiopathic scoliosis.[16]

The implants used in the Dwyer system are made of titanium and include staples that fit laterally on the vertebral body, screws that anchor the staples to the vertebral body, and a flexible cable that passes through the screw heads and connects the implants.

Technique The level of anterior approach is as noted in the preceding section. After the anterior spine is reached, each of the segmental vessels passing horizontally over each vertebral body is identified and ligated for all levels to be fused. It is important to ligate these vessels as close to the midline as possible to avoid neurologic injury from damaging the collateral circulation coursing more laterally. The anterior three fourths of each disk included in the fusion is removed. The levels of instrumentation should include all levels that have a wider disk space on the curve convexity as seen on preoperative bending radiographs. Staples are ap-

Table 9–1
Instrumentation systems*

Instrumentation	Single Thoracic		Double Thoracic	Thoracolumbar	Lumbar	Double Thoracic and Lumbar
	Lordosis	Kyphosis				
Harrington (D)	+	+	+	+	−	+
Harrington (C&D)	−	++	+	−	+	+
Luque	+	+	−	+	+	+
HRI/sublaminar	++	−	−	+	+	+
Wisconsin	++	++	++	++	+	++
C/D	++	++	−	+	++	++
Dwyer	−	−	−	++	+	−
Zielke	−	−	−	++	+	−

*As preferred by author; ++, most applicable; +, may be used; −, generally not used.

Table 9-2
Reported correction using instrumentation techniques selected in Table 9-1

Instrumentation	Curve Correction (%)	Rotation Change (%)	Postoperative Cast or Brace
Harrington	40 to 55	10	Yes
Luque	45 to 60	10	No
HRI/sublaminar	39 to 50	—	Yes
Wisconsin	50 to 60	—	No
Cotrel/Dubousset	50 to 75	40	No
Dwyer	60 to 80	20	Yes
Zielke	60 to 90	40	Yes

plied to the lateral vertebral body held in place by the vertebral screws that pass through both vertebral body cortices. The placement of the screws in a lateral or a more anterior position determines the rotational correction to be gained. Blocks of bone graft, either from the excised rib or from the iliac crest, are placed anteriorly in the excised disk beds to prevent local kyphosis from developing. The remaining disk bed is also bone grafted. The flexible cable is inserted between the screw heads and is tightened, beginning at one end, with the screw heads sequentially crimped to hold the correction obtained. Wound closure is routine. When a thoracotomy is performed, a chest tube is needed for two to three days after surgery. A brace or cast is usually needed postoperatively for approximately six months.

Although the Dwyer instrumentation is not widely used at the present time, this system corrects the scoliosis 60% to 80% radiographically, with an associated rotational correction of 20% to 30%. The principal advantage of Dwyer instrumentation over the posterior instrumentation systems is the possibility of fusing fewer segments than is necessary with a posterior approach. However, the Dwyer system can be recommended only for the thoracolumbar area. In the thoracic area, reported complications are high; and in the lumbar area, the anterior instrumentation excessively straightens the lumbar lordosis, leading to a "flat-back." Even in the thoracolumbar area, despite the use of anterior disk-space bone blocks, localized kyphosis remains a potential problem. In addition, even with a postoperative cast or brace, the pseudarthrosis rate is higher with the Dwyer technique than with posterior instrumentation and fusion.

Zielke Instrumentation

At the present time, the Zielke instrumentation system, developed in West Germany by Dr. Klaus Zielke in the 1970s, has largely replaced the Dwyer system when anterior instrumentation is used.[17]

The implants in the Zielke system include screws that are used to attach half-staples or washers to the vertebral body, and a 1/8-inch threaded solid rod fitted with

hexagonal nuts that passes through the screw heads to obtain and hold the correction.

Technique The level of the surgical incision is as noted in the general section on anterior spinal instrumentation. The segmental vertebral vessels are ligated and divided in the midline of each vertebral body included in the fusion. The disk is removed at each level that, as viewed on the preoperative bending radiograph, had a wider disk on the convex side of the curve. The vertebral screws are inserted sequentially in a line that will allow rotational correction but avoid angulation of more than 10 degrees when the rod linking the screw heads is applied. After placing the screws, the rod is inserted into the screw heads. Rib or iliac crest graft blocks are placed anteriorly in each of the excised disk beds to prevent localized kyphosis, and smaller pieces of bone graft fill the remaining disk bed. The derotation-tensioning device is applied when rotational correction is desired. After satisfactory correction has been obtained, the hexagonal nuts on the rod are tightened. A brace or cast is used for support postoperatively until fusion is solid.

Correction of scoliosis with the Zielke system has been excellent, with 60% to 90% improvement in the scoliosis and 40% to 50% correction in the rotational deformity.[9,18-20] The Zielke system is most applicable to single thoracolumbar curves, allowing fewer levels to be fused than if a posterior approach had been used. The primary potential problem, despite the use of anterior bone blocks, is localized kyphosis at the site of fusion resulting from disk removal and the subsequent shortening of the anterior spinal column from instrumentation and correction. Rod breakage has been reported mainly in obese individuals, and is usually reported only if a sharp angulation is present in the rod postoperatively because of inappropriate adjacent screw placement.[18] As with the Dwyer system, cases of retroperitoneal fibrosis with ureteral obstruction have been reported following the use of the Zielke technique, although this may be a complication of the anterior approach itself rather than of the instrumentation type.

Complications of Spinal Instrumentation

Early Complications

Neurologic Injury During Surgery The most feared intraoperative complication is iatrogenic neurologic injury. This may occur by inadvertent entry of surgical instruments into the spinal canal; however, neurologic injury is most likely to occur during the time of instrument correction of the scoliosis. Spinal cord monitoring, as discussed in Chapter 7, is essential to early detection of possible neurologic injury.

If, during spinal cord monitoring, the somatosensory-evoked potential recording changes markedly, especially with a marked increase in latency, the patient should be awakened to assess foot and leg movements. If awakening the patient will take more than a very short time, the rod should be removed and each hook site carefully inspected to see if there is spinal cord impingement. I give the patient a corticosteroid, such as dexamethasone, as soon as a potential neurologic injury is detected. If both feet move well and the evoked potential recordings have returned to normal when the patient is awakened intraoperatively, instrumentation is reinserted but with less correction than initially attempted. If there is any further alteration in either the wake-up test or the evoked potential recordings, the implants are left out at this time and fusion is performed without instrumentation. If the patient is unable to move the feet or legs when awakened during surgery, the implants are left out and fusion is performed. If neurologic recovery is apparent in the first few days postoperatively, instrumentation is performed about two weeks later, with careful monitoring.

Because rates of recovery from iatrogenic neurologic injury are better if the implants are removed within two to three hours of the onset of neurologic problems, spinal cord monitoring should lead to earlier detection of neurologic injury and an increased chance of reversibility. Some type of spinal cord monitoring should be used whenever spinal deformity correction is attempted.

Postoperative Wound Infection Prophylactic antibiotics should be given within an hour of the start of the surgical procedure and should be used for 24 to 48 hours to decrease the incidence of postoperative wound infections, which for idiopathic scoliosis patients should be less than 1%.

If a wound hematoma begins to drain postoperatively, a fascial defect is usually present that allows communication of this draining hematoma with the fusion area. Early irrigation and reclosure over the drain suffices for treatment of the draining hematoma, but if a draining hematoma is simply observed for several days, secondary infection generally will occur. A secondary infection will require more extensive surgical treatment and a more prolonged hospital stay.

If a wound infection is diagnosed, the wound is opened widely and thorough irrigation and debridement is performed. The implants and the majority of the bone graft are left in, and the wound is closed over subfascial and subcutaneous suction drains. I do not advocate suction with irrigation in most cases. Appropriate antibiotics are used for three to six weeks, depending on the severity of the infection. As soon as the infection is diagnosed, I prefer to begin hyperalimentation to improve the patient's healing capability.

If the infection recurs a few days after initial treatment, the wound may be packed open for prolonged periods, especially if a Harrington distraction rod instrumentation was used. However, if one of the segmental spinal instrumentation systems was used (Luque, Wisconsin, Cotrel-Dubousset), the wound may be very difficult to pack well, because the implants impede the dressing contact needed to promote granulation tissue and secondary wound closure. If the majority of the wound heals but the patient has a single draining sinus, local care and occasional antibiotics for several months are necessary to allow the fusion to heal. If drainage persists past six months, the fusion area is explored, the implants removed, fusion of pseudarthrosis levels is repeated without instrumentation, the sinus tract is excised, and the wound is closed over drains. Postoperative cast immobilization allows solid fusion to occur.

Malnutrition Although teenagers with idiopathic scoliosis are generally healthy individuals, those who require two-stage corrective procedures may become malnourished as a result of the limited oral caloric intake associated with closely spaced major surgical procedures. Since postoperative complications are more likely to occur in patients judged malnourished by indications such as low total lymphocyte count or low albumin level, I prefer to begin parenteral hyperalimentation immediately after the first procedure and to continue it until the patient has good oral caloric intake several days after the second surgical procedure.

Pneumothorax At the time of subperiosteal posterior spine exposure, the pleura may be opened inadvertently, especially in the area between adjacent thoracic spine transverse processes on the concave side of the scoliosis. If hooks are placed on the thoracic transverse processes or if rib grafts are obtained, the likelihood of pneumothorax is increased.

The patient should have a postoperative anteroposterior chest radiograph to rule out a pneumothorax. Observation is appropriate if the pneumothorax is less than 10% to 20%, but chest tube insertion is needed for a larger pneumothorax.

Dural Tear Dural tears may occur at the time of ligamentum flavum removal or at the time of hook or wire insertion into the spinal canal. Repair of all dural tears should be attempted using 5-0 or 6-0 silk suture. It is often necessary to enlarge the laminotomy to obtain the access needed to suture the dural tear. If the tear is large, freeze-dried dura or muscle augmentation can be used to facilitate repair. If dural tears are not repaired, drainage of cerebrospinal fluid through the wound may complicate the postoperative course.

Rod Malrotation Rod contouring to preserve the sagittal spinal alignment is widely accepted as an important component of spinal instrumentation. It is not possible to contour the original design of the Harrington rod effectively because of its round distal end. If this round-ended rod is contoured, the rod will rotate inappropriately when distraction is applied (Fig. 9–5). When the Harrington rod is used as a contoured implant, the square-holed hook must be placed at the distal hook site and a square-ended Harrington rod employed. When contouring the rod, the surgeon should remember that the distal hook is usually tilted laterally about 30 degrees when instrumentation is complete; therefore, allowance should be made for this tilt to achieve the best outcome.

Abnormal Sagittal Alignment ("Flat-Back") Careful attention to correct contouring is essential. Contouring of the thoracic kyphosis is usually adequate; however, it is common to overestimate the amount of lumbar lordosis that is bent into the rod, and postoperative films may show less lumbar lordosis than seemed present in the operating room. Failure to contour any lordosis into the instrumented lumbar area flattens the lumbar spine and places the pelvis in a tilted position, leading later to pain as well as an unsightly posture.

Incorrect Fusion Levels An error in achieving the correct fusion level can occur preoperatively when fusion level is selected radiographically, and intraoperatively when instrumentation is placed incorrectly. Fusion level selection has been discussed previously.

In the operating room, there are three methods to identify the correct vertebral levels for fusion: (1) identification of the lowest rib by palpation (used for thoracic curves), (2) identification of the sacrum by visual inspection (used for some lumbar curves), and (3) radiographic examination in the operating room using a marker on the vertebra to be identified (used for any curve). At least one of these methods must be used to identify the fusion level correctly.

Inappropriate Antidiuretic Hormone Secretion A high percentage of patients with adolescent idiopathic scoliosis will develop the syndrome of inappropriate antidiuretic hormone (SIADH) in the immediate postoperative period. This syndrome is characterized by a decline in urinary output, with the diminished urinary output maximal on the evening after surgery. The serum and urine osmolality should be checked before these patients are treated with a large volume of fluid replace-

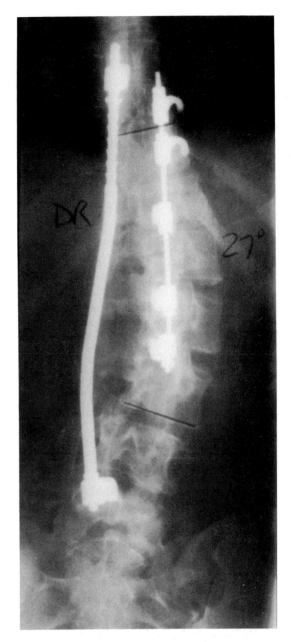

Fig. 9–5 Standing posteroanterior radiograph of a patient who underwent Harrington instrumentation for a 60-degree thoracolumbar idiopathic scoliosis. Although the Harrington distraction rod was contoured to preserve lumbar lordosis, a round-ended rod was used and the rod rotated in the immediate postoperative period, which led to flattening of the lumbar area. A square-ended rod must be used for sagittal plane contouring.

ment to improve urinary output. If the serum and urine osmolality are both elevated, the patient is likely to be hypovolemic, but if the serum osmolality is diminished and the urine osmolality elevated, SIADH should be diagnosed and fluid overload avoided. When SIADH is diagnosed and appropriately managed, the urinary output gradually increases in the two or three days following spinal surgery.[21]

Late Complications

Pseudarthrosis of Fusion In the teenager with idiopathic scoliosis, the pseudarthrosis rate is approximately 1%. This percentage is higher in adults with idiopathic scoliosis and is higher in children with neuromuscular scoliosis.

The most important factors in preventing pseudarthrosis are careful facet joint excision and fusion combined with stable spinal immobilization. The fusion should be solid by six months after surgery. If there is continued loss of correction after this time or if pain is present in the fusion area, a pseudarthrosis should be suspected. Bending radiographs may demonstrate a fusion defect, but with intact instrumentation, this is difficult to detect. A bone scan and fusion tomography may be useful adjuncts but, in my experience, both have on occasion shown what appeared to be pseudarthroses that were not present on fusion exploration. If a pseudarthrosis is identified, a second fusion with reinstrumentation of the nonunion site is generally necessary.

Breakage of Rod or Wire If the fusion over the entire instrumented area does not become solid, implant breakage can be expected. With the Harrington distraction rod, this failure usually occurs between one and two years after surgery; later breakage has been noted with the segmental spinal instrumentation methods.

If a rod breaks, the patient generally complains of back pain that often resolves over a few days. If pain persists or if loss of correction is noted, the broken rod should be removed. Over half of the broken Harrington rods do not have associated pseudarthroses, but, at the time of rod removal, the entire spinal fusion should be explored and refusion performed if a nonunion is found (Fig. 9–6).

The segmental spinal instrumentation implants are harder to remove than are the Harrington system implants. Broken sublaminar wires may project into the spinal canal. These wires should be extracted by winding them around a surgical instrument for safe removal. Often, the Drummond buttons are so enmeshed in the fusion mass that the only way to remove them partially is to cut the wire at the bone level. The Cotrel-Dubousset instrumentation also can be enmeshed in the fusion mass, and cutting the rods into several pieces may be the only means of allowing extraction of this instrumentation.

If the anterior spinal instrumentation breaks and a pseudarthrosis is diagnosed, the instruments are generally left in place. The pseudarthrosis is most easily treated by posterior spinal instrumentation and fusion at the same levels as those used for the initial anterior fusion.

Back Pain Because of the relatively high incidence of low back pain in adults without scoliosis, accurate projections regarding the increased risk of back pain after scoliosis surgery are difficult to ascertain. However, two major factors appear to lead to back pain: fusion below the level of the fourth lumbar vertebra and elimination of lumbar lordosis at the time of instrumentation and fusion. If the inferior fusion level is at the third lumbar vertebra or above, there is a 38% reported incidence of significant late back pain about 20 years after scoliosis surgery, and this incidence is 70% if the fusion level is to the fourth lumbar vertebra or below.[22] Because lumbar lordosis contouring was not routinely a part of the Harrington instrumentation when these instrumentations were performed, it is not known whether the late back pain results from a flattening of the lordosis or from the extent of fusion itself. Despite this uncertainty, it is currently accepted practice to avoid fusion below the fourth lumbar vertebra, if possible.

"Flat-Back" (Loss of Lumbar Lordosis) If spinal instrumentation and fusion eliminates the physiologic lumbar lordosis, disability and unsightly posture result. The patient stands with a forward trunk tilt and often complains of upper back pain resulting from persistent attempts to stand more upright by extending the upper thoracic area. Even if the fusion has been extended to the sacrum, low back and buttock pain with prolonged standing is a common complaint in this group. These patients often will bend their knees to allow better trunk position.

Prevention of this spinal malalignment is most important, but if present, the only treatment is extension osteotomy of the fusion mass, usually at the second or third lumbar vertebral level. The amount of extension correction should be at least equal to the amount of knee flexion needed to make the patient's trunk feel balanced when standing.

Kyphosis Above the Instrumentation (Luque System) Because the Luque sublaminar wire passage at the superior end of the instrumentation requires removal of the interspinous ligament and ligamentum flavum above the most superior level fused, late follow-up often reveals an acute kyphosis just above the fused and instrumented area.[23] This is a major problem if the instrumentation has been stopped in the mid-thoracic level but can also be seen in the higher thoracic sites. Although the Luque system is rarely used with idiopathic curves now, it is necessary to carry the fusion in neuromuscular curves to the first or second thoracic vertebra to avoid this problem, even if the scoliosis does not extend that high.

Summary

The surgical management of idiopathic scoliosis requires knowledge in several areas. In selecting patients for surgical care, it is necessary to know the natural

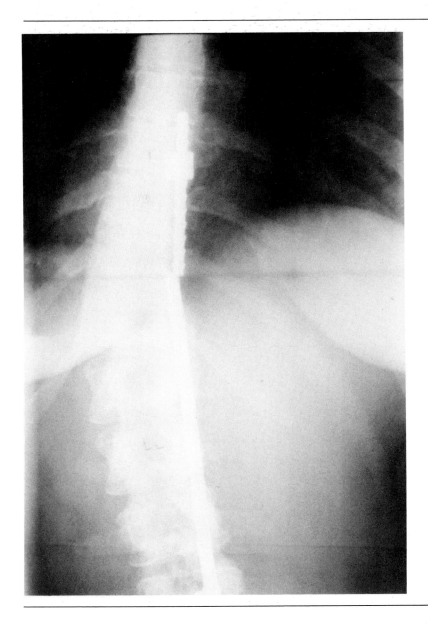

Fig. 9-6 Standing posteroanterior radiograph shows a broken Harrington distraction rod two years after surgical treatment. If fusion is not solid, this rod will break one to two years after instrumentation. If a rod breaks and the patient remains without pain or further curve progression, there is no need to remove the broken rod.

history for the type of curve present during the teenage years, as well as what can be expected of this type of curve during adult life. Preoperative evaluation must include screening for other than idiopathic causes before surgery is advised. Appropriate attention to preoperative radiographs, possible autologous blood utilization, and planning for spinal cord monitoring are essential. Finally, the ability to use a variety of techniques in spinal deformity surgery is needed, as is the knowledge of which technique or instrumentation is best in each situation.

Although the surgical care of spinal deformity has become more complex and requires attention in several areas, the advances in surgical care and in spinal instrumentation allow us to correct spinal deformity more safely and predictably in a more three-dimensional manner than was feasible even a decade ago.

References

1. King HA, Moe JH, Bradford DS, et al: The selection of fusion levels in thoracic idiopathic scoliosis. *J Bone Joint Surg* 1983;65A:1302–1313.
2. Harrington PR: Treatment of scoliosis: Correction and internal fixation by spine instrumentation. *J Bone Joint Surg* 1962;44A:591–610.
3. Lovallo JL, Banta JV, Renshaw TS: Adolescent idiopathic scoliosis treated by Harrington-rod distraction and fusion. *J Bone Joint Surg* 1986;68A:1326–1330.
4. Tolo V, Gillespie R: The use of shortened periods of rigid postoperative immobilization in the surgical treatment of idiopathic scoliosis. *J Bone Joint Surg* 1981;63A:1137–1145.
5. Weatherley CR, Draycott V, O'Brien JF, et al: The rib deformity in adolescent idiopathic scoliosis: A prospective study to evaluate changes after Harrington distraction and posterior fusion. *J Bone Joint Surg* 1987;69B:179–182.
6. Luque ER: Segmental spinal instrumentation for correction of scoliosis. *Clin Orthop* 1982;163:192–198.

7. Wilber RG, Thompson GH, Shaffer JW, et al: Postoperative neurological deficits in segmental spinal instrumentation: A study using spinal cord monitoring. *J Bone Joint Surg* 1984;66A:1178–1187.

8. Thompson GH, Wilber RG, Shaffer JW, et al: Segmental spinal instrumentation in idiopathic scoliosis: A preliminary report. *Spine* 1985;10:623–630.

9. Moe JH, Purcell GA, Bradford DS: Zielke instrumentation (VDS) for the correction of spinal curvature: Analysis of results in 66 patients. *Clin Orthop* 1983;180:133–153.

10. Winter RB, Lonstein JE, VandenBrink K, et al: Harrington rod with sublaminar wires in the treatment of adolescent idiopathic thoracic scoliosis: A study of sagittal plane correction. *Orthop Trans* 1987;11:89.

11. Drummond D, Guadagni J, Keene JS, et al: Interspinous process segmental spinal instrumentation. *J Pediatr Orthop* 1984;4:397–404.

12. Cotrel Y, Dubousset J, Guillaumat M: New universal instrumentation in spinal surgery. *Clin Orthop* 1988;227:10–23.

13. Shufflebarger HL, Clark C: Cotrel-Dubousset instrumentation in adolescent idiopathic scoliosis. *Orthop Trans* 1987;11:49–50.

14. Shufflebarger HL, King WF: Composite measurement of scoliosis. *Orthop Trans* 1986;10:26–27.

15. Hall JE: Dwyer instrumentation in anterior fusion of the spine. *J Bone Joint Surg* 1981;63A:1188–1190.

16. Hsu LC, Zucherman J, Tang SC, et al: Dwyer instrumentation in the treatment of adolescent idiopathic scoliosis. *J Bone Joint Surg* 1982;64B:536–541.

17. Hack H-P, Zielke K, Harms J: Spinal instrumentation and monitoring, in Bradford DS, Hensinger RM (eds): *The Pediatric Spine.* New York, Thieme Inc, 1985, pp 491–517.

18. Horton WC, Holt RT, Johnson JR, et al: Zielke instrumentation in idiopathic scoliosis. *Orthop Trans*, in press.

19. Kaneda K, Fujiya N, Satoh S: Results with Zielke instrumentation for idiopathic thoracolumbar and lumbar scoliosis. *Clin Orthop* 1986;205:195–203.

20. Ogiela DM, Chan DP: Ventral derotation spondylodesis: A review of 22 cases. *Spine* 1986;11:18–22.

21. Bell GR, Gurd AR, Orlowski JP, et al: The syndrome of inappropriate antidiuretic-hormone secretion following spinal fusion. *J Bone Joint Surg* 1986;68A:720–724.

22. Ginsburg HH, Goldstein LA, Robinson SC, et al: Back pain in postoperative idiopathic scoliosis: Long-term follow-up study, abstract. *Spine* 1979;4:518.

23. Kahn E, Brown JC, Swank SM: Postoperative thoracic kyphosis following Luque instrumentation. *Orthop Trans* 1987;11:88.

CHAPTER 10

Degenerative Spondylolisthesis

Michael J. Bolesta, MD

Henry H. Bohlman, MD, FACS

Introduction

Spondylolisthesis is derived from the Greek *spondylos*, meaning vertebra, and *olisthanein*, to slip.[1] It was coined by Kilian[2] in 1854, and refers to the ventral displacement of one vertebra relative to the subjacent one. The first description of this deformity is generally attributed to Herbinaux[3] in 1782, although the "hollow back" described by Andry[4] in 1743 may have been caused by spondylolisthesis.

In 1855, Robert[5] demonstrated that a normal fifth lumbar vertebra could not be translated relative to the first sacral vertebra, even after freeing all soft tissue, unless the neural arch was disrupted. Lambl[6] described such disruption of the pars interarticularis in some but not all cases. The inconsistent association between spondylolysis and spondylolisthesis generated confusion and controversy regarding the pathogenesis of spondylolisthesis.

In the 19th century, Lambl,[6] Neugebauer,[7] and Chiari[8] all described spondylolisthesis in patients who had an intact pars interarticularis. In describing 14 cases in Schmorl's collection, Junghanns[9] found the pars intact; therefore, he coined the phrase "pseudo-spondylolisthesis" and reserved spondylolisthesis for cases with concomitant spondylolysis. Macnab[10] thought that the term ignored the basic meaning of spondylolisthesis and proposed the phrase "spondylolisthesis with an intact neural arch." Most of the patients described by Macnab and Junghanns were female and middle-aged and older, who developed arthritis of the facet joints, with or without disk degeneration, and spondylolisthesis at the involved level, usually at the fourth to fifth lumbar vertebrae. Because this constellation is distinct from other instances of spondylolisthesis with an intact neural arch, degenerative spondylolisthesis, as proferred by Newman,[11] seems to be the best term for this form of slip. His five-part etiologic classification, based on careful analysis of 319 cases, has been revised and is widely accepted.[11,12]

Pathogenesis

Macnab[10] described the tendency of body weight, transmitted through the spine, to displace the lumbar vertebrae ventrally. Regardless of soft-tissue restraints, the facet joints would resist translatory forces in the coronal plane as they do at the lumbosacral level. This bony constraint does not apply when the joint plane is sagittal. Although lumbar facets are generally in a sagittal plane, Macnab noted that they are somewhat oblique and that there is an anterior-medial hook to the facet. That is, the facet hook is in the coronal plane and thus adds a bony block to slippage.

Junghanns[9] found that the plane of the inferior articular process relative to that of the pedicle of the superior vertebra approached 180 degrees in the sagittal plane, not 90 degrees. This would obviate the restraining effect of the bony facet anatomy. Junghanns postulated that the difference in orientation was the essential lesion of degenerative spondylolisthesis. Macnab[10] concurred with Junghanns and thought that the abnormal orientation was a congenital anomaly. He postulated that the forces of body weight would be borne by the disk, leading to premature degeneration and altered facet mechanics. These mechanical factors would explain the occurrence of hypertrophic arthritis of the facet joints as well as the spondylolisthesis.

Farfan[13] and Farfan and Sullivan[14] emphasized the interrelationship between the disk and facet joints, referred to as the "three-joint complex." Changes in the disk cause changes in the facet joints and vice versa. A cadaver study of degenerative spondylolisthesis by Farfan[15] showed disk degeneration in all 19 specimens, but it was lower-grade in 14. In contrast, there were moderate degenerative changes in the facet joint in all cases and 14 cases were high-grade. In all but two cases, apophyseal degeneration was more advanced than disk degeneration. Farfan found subluxation of the facet joint with marginal osteophytes. There was a neoarticulation with the subjacent posterosuperior lamina. Fourteen of the specimens had a rotary component to the spondylolisthesis averaging 6 degrees. In milder cases, the slip appeared to be the result of predominantly unilateral facet subluxation. The pedicle-facet angle described by Junghanns[9] was increased on the side of displacement in these cases. In cases of bilateral facet subluxation, the angle was increased on both sides. Farfan also thought that the joint on the side of greatest displacement moved medially, placing traction on the inferior nerve root. He did not think that there was significant central stenosis in his specimens; therefore, he postulated that the typical myelographic appearance was caused by this nerve-root traction and the incomplete root sleeve filling that resulted. Symptoms were also attributed to this presumed traction.

Kirkaldy-Willis and associates[16] described in detail the

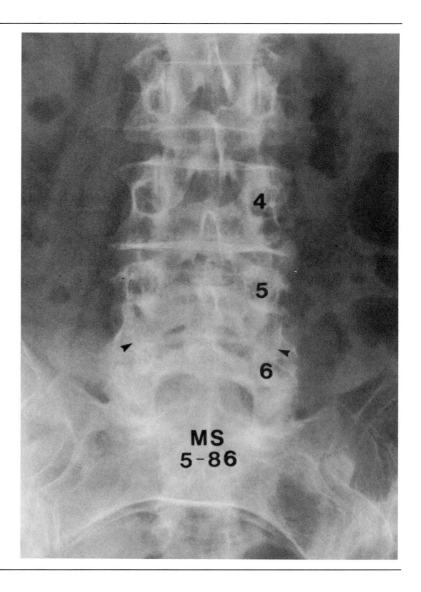

Fig. 10-1 Anteroposterior radiograph of a 56-year-old woman who has six lumbar vertebrae, and degenerative spondylolisthesis at the fourth to fifth and fifth to sixth lumbar vertebrae. Note the facet hypertrophy at both levels (arrows).

arthritic changes that occur with lumbar spondylosis and stenosis on the basis of 50 cadavers and 161 intraoperative observations. Although this material was not confined to degenerative spondylolisthesis, it is germane because it deals with degenerative spondylosis and stenosis. The facets were described as diarthrodial with articular cartilage, synovium, and capsule. The latter are conjoined anteromedially with the ligamentum flavum. Pathologic changes included synovitis, cartilage fibrillation, gross cartilage degeneration, osteophytes, articular process fracture, osteochondral loose bodies, and capsular laxity. With aging, the nucleus pulposus became dehydrated and fibrotic. The collagen fibers of the anulus fibrosis accrued disruptions that could coalesce into radial tears. In a complex interaction of biomechanical, biochemical, and possibly immunologic factors, internal disruption and resorption of the disk ensued.

Rosenberg[17] examined 20 skeletons culled from 2,000 in the Todd collection at Case Western Reserve University School of Medicine, as well as 200 consecutive clinical cases of degenerative spondylolisthesis. In the anatomic material, 18 of 20 slips occurred at the level of the fourth to fifth lumbar vertebrae and two at the third to fourth lumbar vertebrae. Slips were five to six times more common in skeletons of females than males, and three times more frequent in blacks than in whites. He noted profound arthritic changes in the facet joints. The posterior portion of the superior articular process of the inferior vertebra was eroded posteriorly, with hypertrophic bone formation anteriorly that encroached upon the lateral recesses. Rosenberg interpreted the increased angle of the inferior articular process to the pedicle, described by Junghanns in the slipped vertebra, as the result of remodeling. The consequence was articulation in the transverse plane. The osteophytes produced a bulbous articulation encompassing almost the entire articular process. The lamina of the inferior vertebra was dimpled to accommodate the tip of the inferior process

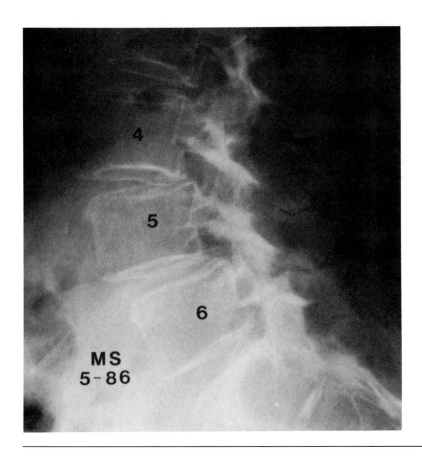

Fig. 10-2 Same patient shown in Figure 10-1. Lateral radiograph shows degenerative spondylolisthesis at both levels with concomitant disk degeneration.

of the superior vertebra. Slipping appeared to be arrested when the isthmus of the superior vertebra abutted the upper margin of the superior articular process of the lower vertebra.

Of Rosenberg's 200 patients,[17] 159 were female, and 190 had a single level involved: the fourth to fifth lumbar vertebrae in 159 patients, the fifth lumbar to first sacral vertebrae in 18, and the third to fourth lumbar vertebrae in 13. Six had concurrent spondylolisthesis at the fourth to fifth lumbar vertebrae and fifth lumbar to first sacral vertebrae. Four patients had spondylolisthesis at both the third to fourth and fourth to fifth lumbar vertebrae. The mean slip was 14% with a maximum slip of 30%. In most patients, advanced degenerative changes of facet joints were apparent radiographically at the time of diagnosis. Degenerative changes characteristic of degenerative disk disease were present in 139 patients, but these were not always at or restricted to the level of the slip. Sacralization was noted in 44 patients. Radiographs of Rosenberg's patients showed hypolordosis and mean lumbosacral angles of 145 degrees, which he compared to a published norm of 130 degrees. Rosenberg also compared his patients to a series of patients who had isthmic spondylolisthesis; these patients had a mean lumbosacral angle of less than 130 degrees. He noted increased height

of the posterior fifth lumbar vertebral body relative to its anterior height. Mild scoliosis occurred in 31 of these patients; in four this scoliosis appeared to be focused at the slip level because of asymmetric disk degeneration.

Although degenerative spondylolisthesis can result in slips of 30%, the majority are mild, and in Rosenberg's series averaged 14%.[17] Therefore, central canal stenosis is present but may not account for the neurologic symptoms. However, hypertrophic changes of the facet joints produce a significant lateral recess stenosis. In most cases, this stenosis affects the inferior nerve roots. For example, in a fourth to fifth lumbar spondylolisthesis, the fifth lumbar nerve roots are usually the most significantly involved. With higher-grade slips and more advanced facet arthritis, the superior nerve root (fourth lumbar in fourth to fifth lumbar slips) may be irritated. Several authors[17,18] have commented that symptoms do not correlate with the degree of slippage. Symptoms may correlate better with the degree of lateral recess stenosis demonstrated by computed tomography (CT) and magnetic resonance imaging (MRI). Another factor determining whether or not a patient has neurologic symptoms may be the vertebral level involved. Rosenberg[17] noted that minimal slips at the level of the third to fourth lumbar vertebrae could produce pro-

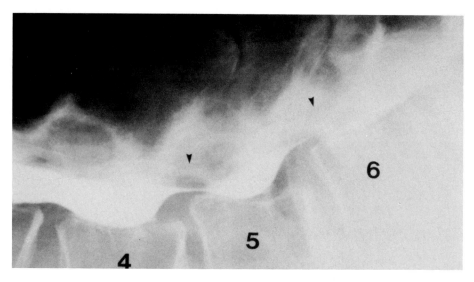

Fig. 10-3 Same patient shown in Figure 10–1. Lateral myelogram demonstrating the typical myelographic defect (arrows). At surgery, the radiolucency was found to be a ganglion originating in one of the facet joints (left arrow).

found symptoms, presumably because of the relatively small canal and foramina at this level.

Clinical Presentation

Symptoms

In the majority of Rosenberg's[17] patients, pain in the back, buttock, or thigh was the principal complaint, and 30% had distal pain. Symptoms included aching, pulling, weakness, heaviness, numbness, or burning. The onset of symptoms ranged from a few days to as long as 50 years before evaluation. Lower extremity symptoms could be unilateral, alternating, or bilateral. Neurogenic claudication was uncommon, but was relieved with rest. Urinary incontinence and perineal numbness were present in only 3.5% of the patients.

Cauchoix and associates[18] examined 26 patients who had symptoms of nerve root compression secondary to degenerative spondylolisthesis. Eighty percent had back pain, 46% chronic sciatica, 54% neurogenic claudication, and 4% (one patient) bladder incontinence. Reynolds and Wiltse[19] reported on 21 patients treated surgically for degenerative spondylolisthesis. Fifteen complained of sciatica and six of neurogenic claudication. Those patients who had sciatica tended to be older, and claudication was a complaint of the younger subset.

We compared the experience of Cauchoix and associates with 53 patients who had degenerative spondylolisthesis treated surgically. One half of these patients complained of significant back pain, one half had radicular symptoms, and approximately three fourths

complained of neurogenic claudication. Although the time from the onset of symptoms to seeking medical attention varied from one month to 40 years, most patients had had symptoms for six months to three years.

Signs

Rosenberg[17] observed that his patients were remarkably supple, and most were able to touch their toes. Significant tenderness and spasm were seen in only 10%. Forty-two percent had a neurologic deficit, most often at the level of the fifth lumbar vertebra. The deficit was noted as a decreased sensation to pin prick in the lateral thigh or the inability to walk on the heels. Atrophy occurred occasionally, and 20% had altered deep tendon reflexes. An offset of the spinous processes may be palpable.

Cauchoix and associates[18] found the results of the physical examination to be normal in 54% of the patients. Hypoesthesia was noted in 19%, and motor weakness occurred in 23% of the patients. Reynolds and Wiltse[19] did not describe their neurologic findings in detail. In our experience, one third had a sensory deficit and slightly more had mild motor weakness.

In degenerative spondylolisthesis, neurologic findings are normal in more than 50% of the patients. However, their symptoms may be significantly disabling.

In all of these patients, particularly those in whom claudication is a prominent complaint, clinical assessment of lower extremity vasculature is important. This is accomplished quickly and easily by examining the skin of the lower extremity for atrophic changes associated with peripheral vascular disease, palpating pulses, and auscultating for bruits. When a history and physical examination cannot differentiate vascular from neurogenic claudication, consultation with a vascular surgeon is indicated.

Diagnostic Evaluation

At the patient's first clinical examination, anteroposterior, lateral, and oblique radiographs will establish the diagnosis of degenerative spondylolisthesis. The most common finding on the anteroposterior view is facet hypertrophy (Fig. 10–1); disk narrowing and osteophyte formation are nonspecific findings associated with degenerative spondylolisthesis. The lateral view will also show facet disease and, in some cases, disk degeneration (Fig. 10–2). Because there is often a rotary component with degenerative spondylolisthesis, the amount of slip seen on radiographs may vary depending on the amount of minor rotation accompanying the lateral displacement. The oblique view will demonstrate the integrity of the pars interarticularis and may show the facet degenerative changes. The severity of symptoms does not appear to correlate with the amount of slip.[17,18]

Reynolds and Wiltse[19] used electromyography to examine patients for degenerative spondylolisthesis and found the results to be abnormal in 41% of those tested. Of this group, 80% showed involvement of the inferior nerve root. We have not used this modality routinely.

Myelography typically shows an hourglass constriction of the theca vertebralis at the level of the spondylolisthesis. Ventral constriction viewed on the lateral myelogram is sometimes interpreted as herniated nucleus pulposus, but this is not often corroborated at the time of surgery (Fig. 10–3). The anteroposterior (Fig. 10–4) and oblique views may show that the inferior and sometimes the superior nerve root sleeves are blunted. In more severe cases, redundant nerve root shadows may be seen. Newer, nonionic hydrophilic contrast media such as iohexol have greatly reduced the morbidity associated with this procedure.

Computed tomography demonstrates clearly the degenerative changes of the facet joint (Fig. 10–5). It enables the physician to assess the relative amounts of central and lateral stenosis. As with the myelogram, a diagnosis of herniated nucleus pulposus at the level of the slip must be made cautiously. A vacuum density seen on the CT scan, the "vacuum disk sign," is commonly associated with degenerative disk disease. Recently, a similar phenomenon was noted within the facet joint of a patient with degenerative spondylolisthesis.[20] It was postulated that the presence of gas or a vacuum density was an indirect sign of neural arch integrity. Although plain CT can delineate some of the pathologic changes, we recommend intrathecal contrast to delineate the neural elements. Improved patient tolerance of the contrast media has allowed for outpatient myelography followed by CT scanning.

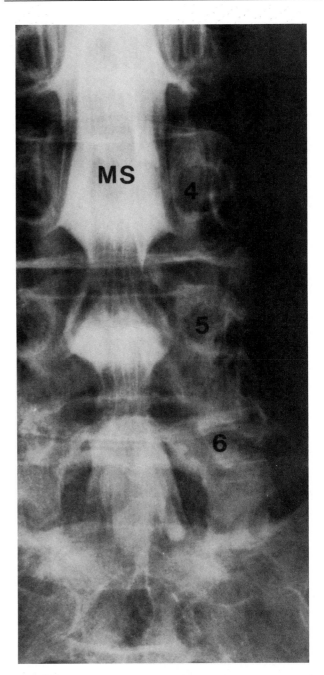

Fig. 10–4 Same patient shown in Figure 10–1. Anteroposterior myelogram shows an hourglass deformity. There is blunting of the fifth and sixth lumbar vertebrae root sleeves.

Magnetic resonance imaging can provide much the same information as myelography and CT without lumbar puncture or the use of ionizing radiation (Figs. 10–6 and 10–7). It provides direct sagittal and coronal images without reformatting. The foramina can be visualized well with a high-quality machine. The exquisite detail of the neural foramina is not available with CT unless thin contiguous slices are obtained followed by time-consuming reconstruction. We generally use MRI

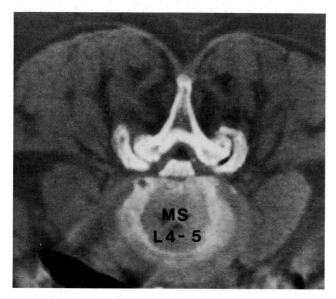 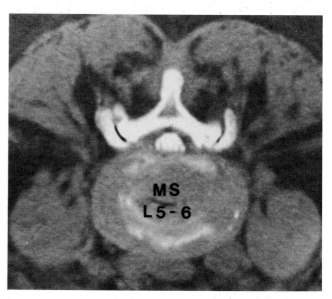

Fig. 10-5 Same patient shown in Figure 10-1. Computed tomography through the level of the slips, at the fourth to fifth **(left)** and at the fifth to sixth lumbar vertebrae **(right)**. Note the vacuum phenomena involving the disk and the facet joints. There is thickening of the ligamentum flavum and constriction of the theca.

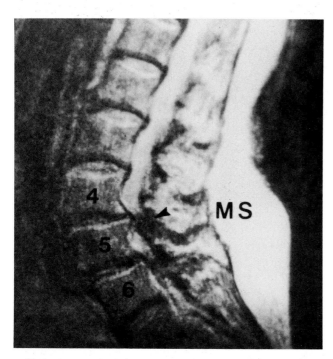

Fig. 10-6 Same patient shown in Figure 10-1. Magnetic resonance imaging in the sagittal plane demonstrating compression of the thecal sac (arrow).

as the first study after plain radiographs. Although we still rely on myelography and CT, further experience may show that these tests are unnecessary.

Overall evaluation of the patient is important; age, medical history, symptoms, and physical findings should be considered. Chest radiography, electrocardiography, complete blood cell count, serum chemistries, and urinalysis are routine. Special studies, such as serum protein electrophoresis, are obtained as indicated. In addition, we are investigating prospectively the use of somatosensory-evoked potentials in the management of these individuals.

Management

Nonsurgical Treatment

Eighty percent of Rosenberg's[17] patients never had incapacitating symptoms and required no specific treatment. Analgesic, ataractic, and anti-inflammatory medications, bedrest, bracing, exercises, traction, and heat were all unpredictable in their efficacy.

Of the remaining 39 patients, 15 improved with bedrest, traction, and medication while hospitalized. Seven of these, however, had to be rehospitalized. Twenty-nine were eventually offered surgery; of these, six refused, three went elsewhere, and one was found to have a tumor at the sixth thoracic vertebra.

The effectiveness of surgical modalities has not been demonstrated, but a trial period of conservative treatment is indicated in those patients who are minimally impaired, who have had symptoms for a short time, or who are seriously impaired by another condition that precludes surgical intervention. Age alone should not

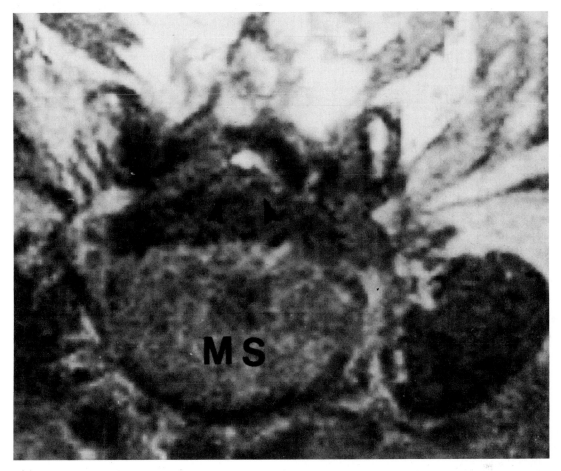

Fig. 10-7 Same patient shown in Figure 10–1. Magnetic resonance imaging in the transverse plane demonstrating severe thecal sac compression (arrows).

be considered a contraindication to surgery. We think that any patient active enough to exhibit neurologic symptoms should be offered decompression.

Surgical Treatment

Surgical management has two components: decompression and fusion. Decompression is indicated when nonsurgical, conservative treatment has failed and symptoms are incapacitating. Initially, Rosenberg[17] decompressed only the nerve roots on the symptomatic side but found better results with bilateral decompression. He did note an increased slip of up to 10% after decompression. Several authors have recommended fusion only if decompression results in an unstable spine, although few have presented firm guidelines for determining instability.[21-24] Others add the stipulation that the patient should be "young."[23,24] Still others fuse only after instability manifests as a progressive, symptomatic, postoperative slip.[18,25]

Although Brown and Lockwood[21] reported only a 5% incidence of increased spondylolisthesis postoperatively at the level of the decompression, Johnsson and associates[26] and White and Wiltse[27] reported a 65% incidence of increasing slip at the level of degenerative spondylolisthesis. However, all increasing slips are not symptomatic.[26] It is the risk of progression that prompts authors such as Macnab[10] and Newman[28] to recommend primary posterolateral fusion at the time of decompression. Two recent series[29,30] compared decompression with and without arthrodesis. These investigators thought that concurrent fusion yielded better results. This confirms our experience and we recommend posterolateral fusion at the time of decompression. Advanced age is not a contraindication to arthrodesis or to decompression.

There are advocates of internal fixation as an adjuvant to arthrodesis,[31,32] but it is not clear that internal fixation enhances the fusion rate or produces better long-term clinical results. The slip can progress despite instrumentation.[31] We cannot recommend routine spinal instrumentation for the surgical management of degenerative spondylolisthesis.

The patient should be mobile after the acute pain of surgery subsides, usually by the third postoperative day.

Corsets or orthoses are not usually necessary. Most patients can be released from the hospital after seven to ten days. Driving and strenuous activities are not advised until after the first checkup at six weeks, although general aerobic conditioning, such as walking, is encouraged. Flexibility exercises are started at six weeks. Radiographs are obtained at the six-week and three-month visits, and yearly thereafter. The fusion rate is 81% in these patients.

Results

Although disabling symptoms occur in patients who have degenerative spondylolisthesis, physical findings may not be directly associated with these symptoms. The symptoms reported do not correlate with the magnitude of the slip or amount of disk degeneration; it is, therefore, difficult to evaluate treatment results. Hence, reported results of therapy are subjective and vary from author to author. Successful outcome, defined as the reduction or elimination of symptoms, seems to occur in 50% to 90% of patients treated by decompression, with and without fusion.

Results can be optimized by careful evaluation and selection of appropriate candidates for surgery. A meticulous decompression must be obtained at the time of surgery, preserving the pars and facet joints whenever possible. We also recommend a concurrent posterolateral arthrodesis using autogenous bone from the iliac crest.

Summary

Degenerative spondylolisthesis is a unique form of spondylolisthesis that is characterized in most patients as a hypertrophic arthritis of the facet joint resulting in segmental instability predominantly in the sagittal plane. Disk degeneration is associated with degenerative spondylolisthesis to a varying degree. Joint involvement may not be uniform in all patients, and a rotary component, although small, is often present. The fourth to fifth lumbar level is most often involved, particularly in association with a relatively rigid lumbosacral segment. Degenerative spondylolisthesis is more common in females and in blacks, and it seldom occurs before the age of 40 years.

Symptoms are generally due to lateral stenosis that compromises the inferior nerve roots, usually at the level of the fifth lumbar vertebra. However, the superior nerve roots can be compressed in more advanced cases. Neurogenic claudication and radiculopathy are commonly reported symptoms at the time a patient is first examined. The findings of physical examination vary; less than half of the patients examined

exhibit a neurologic deficit. Rarely, a patient has cauda equina syndrome at the time of initial examination.

Mild cases can be successfully treated surgically, but significant neurologic symptoms can only be diminished by adequate decompression. We recommend posterolateral fusion because of the deformity's propensity to progress postoperatively.

References

1. *Dorland's Illustrated Medical Dictionary*, ed 26. Philadelphia, WB Saunders, 1981, p 1239.
2. Kilian HF: *Schilderungen neuer Beckenformen und ihres Verhaltens im Leben*. Mannheim, Verlag von Bassermann und Mathy, 1854.
3. Herbinaux G: *Traité sur divers accouchemens laborieux, et sur les polypes de la matrice*. Bruxelles, JL DeBoubers, 1782.
4. Andry N: *L'Orthopédie*. Paris, La Veuve Alix, 1743.
5. Robert, cited by Newman PH: The etiology of spondylolisthesis. *J Bone Joint Surg* 1963;45B:39–59.
6. Lambl W, cited by Newman PH: The etiology of spondylolisthesis. *J Bone Joint Surg* 1963;45B:39–59.
7. Neugebauer FL: A new contribution to the history and etiology of spondylolisthesis, in *The New Sydenham Society: Selected Monographs*. London, The New Sydenham Society, 1888.
8. Chiari H: Die Ätiologie und Genese der sogenannten Spondylolisthesis lumbo-sacralis: Eine pathologisch-anatomische Studie. *Z Heilkd* 1892;13:199–262.
9. Junghanns H: Spondylolisthesen ohne Spalt im Zwischengelenkstück ("Pseudospondylolisthesen"). *Arch Orthop Unfall-Chir* 1930;29:118–127.
10. Macnab I: Spondylolisthesis with an intact neural arch: The so-called pseudo-spondylolisthesis. *J Bone Joint Surg* 1950;32B:325–333.
11. Newman PH: The etiology of spondylolisthesis. *J Bone Joint Surg* 1963;45B;39–59.
12. Wiltse LL, Newman PH, Macnab I: Classification of spondylolisis and spondylolisthesis. *Clin Orthop* 1976;117:23–29.
13. Farfan HF: Effects of torsion on the intervertebral joints. *Can J Surg* 1969;12:336–341.
14. Farfan HF, Sullivan JB: The relation of facet orientation to intervertebral disc failure. *Can J Surg* 1967;10:179–185.
15. Farfan HF: The pathological anatomy of degenerative spondylolisthesis: A cadaver study. *Spine* 1980;5:412–418.
16. Kirkaldy-Willis WH, Wedge JH, Yong-Hing K, et al: Pathology and pathogenesis of lumbar spondylosis and stenosis. *Spine* 1978;3:319–328.
17. Rosenberg NJ: Degenerative spondylolisthesis: Predisposing factors. *J Bone Joint Surg* 1975;57A:467–474.
18. Cauchoix J, Benoist M, Chassaing V: Degenerative spondylolisthesis. *Clin Orthop* 1976;115:122–129.
19. Reynolds JB, Wiltse LL: Surgical treatment of degenerative spondylolisthesis: An abstract. *Spine* 1979;4:148–149.
20. Lefkowitz DM, Quencer RM: Vacuum facet phenomenon: A computed tomographic sign of degenerative spondylolisthesis. *Radiology* 1982;144:562.
21. Brown MD, Lockwood JM: Part III: Degenerative spondylolisthesis, in Evarts CM (ed): American Academy of Orthopaedic Surgeons *Instructional Course Lectures, XXXII*. St Louis, CV Mosby, 1983, pp 162–169.
22. Epstein NE, Epstein JA, Carras R, et al: Degenerative spondylolisthesis with an intact neural arch: A review of 60 cases with an analysis of clinical findings and the development of surgical management. *Neurosurgery* 1983;13:555–561.
23. Alexander E Jr, Kelly DL Jr, Davis CH Jr, et al: Intact arch

spondylolisthesis: A review of 50 cases and description of surgical treatment. *J Neurosurg* 1985;63:840–844.

24. Shiloni E, Wald U, Robin GC, et al: Degenerative lumbar spinal stenosis. *Isr J Med Sci* 1980;16:692–697.

25. Dall BE, Rowe DE: Degenerative spondylolisthesis: Its surgical management. *Spine* 1985;10:668–672.

26. Johnsson KE, Willner S, Johnsson K: Postoperative instability after decompression for lumbar spinal stenosis. *Spine* 1986;11:107–110.

27. White AH, Wiltse LL: Spondylolisthesis after extensive lumbar laminectomy, abstract. *J Bone Joint Surg* 1976;58A:727–728.

28. Newman PH: Surgical treatment for derangement of the lumbar spine. *J Bone Joint Surg* 1973;55B:7–19.

29. Feffer HL, Wiesel SW, Cuckler JM, et al: Degenerative spondylolisthesis: To fuse or not to fuse. *Spine* 1985;10:287–289.

30. Lombardi JS, Wiltse LL, Reynolds J, et al: Treatment of degenerative spondylolisthesis. *Spine* 1985;10:821–827.

31. Hanley EN Jr: Decompression and distraction-derotation arthrodesis for degenerative spondylolisthesis. *Spine* 1986;11:269–276.

32. Kaneda K, Kazama H, Satoh S, et al: Follow-up study of medial facetectomies and posterolateral fusion with instrumentation in unstable degenerative spondylolisthesis. *Clin Orthop* 1986;203:159–167.

The Shoulder

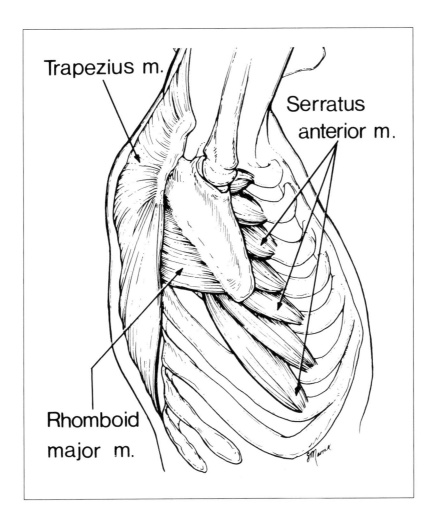

CHAPTER 11

Technique and Instrumentation for Shoulder Arthroscopy

Leslie S. Matthews, MD

Paul D. Fadale, MD

Introduction

Shoulder arthroscopy has gained acceptance as a valuable tool in the evaluation and treatment of various disorders affecting the shoulder.[1-10] Used appropriately, arthroscopy of the shoulder can enhance the surgeon's diagnostic and therapeutic capabilities.

Evaluation of the patient with shoulder problems should proceed systematically. The importance of a complete medical history and thorough and skillful physical examination cannot be overemphasized.[11-16] Various laboratory tests and radiographic studies can be invaluable in the evaluation of shoulder disorders.[17-19]

Shoulder arthroscopy may be considered under three broad categories: (1) as a definitive therapeutic treatment for a diagnosed condition, (2) as a confirming diagnostic procedure, and (3) as a diagnostic procedure for the patient who cannot be definitively or presumptively diagnosed by other means.

A thorough medical history and physical examination must be completed and all relative laboratory studies obtained prior to proceeding with arthroscopic shoulder surgery.

Technique

Diagnostic arthroscopy of the shoulder need not be difficult. With a standardized technique and some experience, it can be easier than arthroscopic evaluation of the knee. The approach presented here has been found effective at several centers and has evolved through a substantial amount of shared experience.[20-22]

Operating Room Setup

All equipment, except the sterile instrument table, should be positioned on the side of the operating table opposite the surgeon. The traction pole for the patient's upper extremity is also placed opposite the surgeon. Waterproof drapes are recommended. The assistant stands on the same side of the table as the surgeon in a position that allows manipulation of the arm and handling of instruments and equipment. The anesthesiologist's equipment should be anterior (not superior) to and somewhat removed from the patient to allow the surgeon access to the entire shoulder. The operating room setup for right shoulder arthroscopy is shown in Figure 11–1.

Anesthesia

General anesthesia and endotracheal intubation are mandatory in most cases of shoulder arthroscopy because of the need for muscle relaxation, lateral decubitus positioning, and placement of traction on the involved arm.

Position

After induction of general anesthesia and intubation, the patient is positioned in the lateral decubitus position with the involved side up. A slight posterior tilt in the shoulder position may help the arthroscopist by placing the glenoid articular surface parallel to the floor.[23] It is important to stabilize the patient adequately in this position. A beanbag is effective but kidney braces and wide adhesive tape also work well to secure the patient to the operating table.

Skin traction is applied to the forearm. The hand should be padded well. A sturdy, modified intravenous pole or traction pole with a pulley at the top is attached to the foot of the operating table opposite the surgeon. The patient's arm is suspended with traction at 45 to 60 degrees of abduction using 5 to 10 lb weights. The amount of weight used depends on the patient's size. Forward arm flexion of approximately 20 degrees is important to facilitate posterior entry into the shoulder joint and to reduce strain on the brachial plexus (Fig. 11–2). The traction pole should be affixed to the table rather than to the ceiling or floor so that the table can be moved without influencing the traction or applying dangerous stress to the arm. This traction should allow easy flexion, extension, abduction, adduction, and rotational changes to allow complete visualization of and access to pathologic structures.

Prepping and draping are done in a routine fashion. U-shaped waterproof drapes are placed above and below the shoulder, and the arm in traction is wrapped in a sterile drape.

Arthroscope Introduction

It is often helpful to outline bony landmarks with a sterile marking pen. The distal clavicle, acromioclavicular joint, acromion, and the coracoid process are outlined (Fig. 11–3). The course of the coracoacromial ligament may also be included. A posterior portal is generally the best site for initial introduction of the arthroscope. The surgeon should identify a point approximately 1 cm medial and 2 cm inferior to the posterolateral angle of the acromion. A 20-gauge spinal

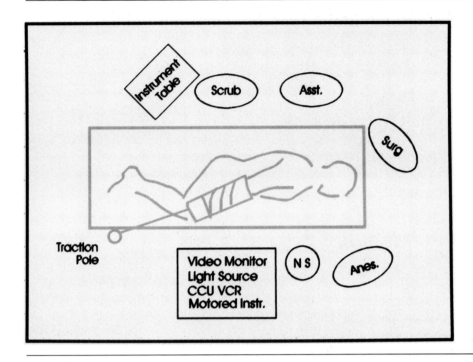

Fig. 11-1 Basic operating room setup for arthroscopy of the right shoulder.

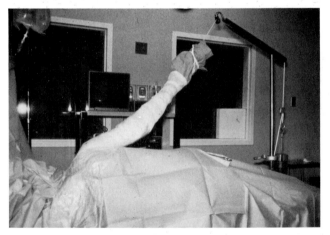

Fig. 11-2 The patient is positioned with the involved side up. The arm is suspended with 5 to 10 lb of weight, abducted 45 to 60 degrees, and forward flexed 20 degrees.

needle is introduced and directed slightly medially and inferiorly to enter the glenohumeral joint. The needle should be directed toward the tip of the coracoid process. As the needle pierces the posterior shoulder capsule, a definite yielding can be felt. A 50-ml syringe containing Ringer's lactate solution is placed into the spinal needle and a small amount of fluid is introduced. Then, the syringe is removed and the surgeon observes the shoulder joint for backflow of fluid. If there is no free return of fluid, the needle is not in an intra-articular position; therefore, the needle should be reposi-

tioned. It is important to confirm the intra-articular position before introducing the remaining amount of Ringer's lactate solution. When the needle is in the correct position, a total of 30 to 50 ml of Ringer's lactate solution is injected to distend the capsule. Often, the increasing pressure within the inflating capsule can be sensed as greater resistance to injection. After fluid has been injected into the joint, the syringe is removed from the needle and replaced with a 10-ml syringe containing a 0.5% solution of bupivacaine hydrochloride with epinephrine (as bitartrate) 1:200,000. This solution will aid in decreasing bleeding and reducing postoperative pain at the portal sites. The tract is injected as the needle is withdrawn.

A No. 11 blade is used to make a stab wound into the skin at the posterior portal. The arthroscope sleeve with a blunt trocar is introduced in the same direction previously defined by the spinal needle. The sleeve and trocar are advanced in a controlled manner through the posterior deltoid muscle, the infraspinatus muscle, the posterior capsule, and into the joint. Care must be taken to avoid injury to the articular surfaces from the penetrating trocar. In addition, a low entry site may injure the axillary nerve when the arm is in an abducted position.[24] One valve on the sleeve is left open so that, upon entering into the shoulder joint, fluid within the joint can be seen to leak from the cannula, reassuring the surgeon that the joint space has been entered. The trocar is removed and the arthroscope is introduced through the sleeve. A light cable, camera, and inflow and suction tubings are attached.

The intravenous pole holding the irrigation fluid

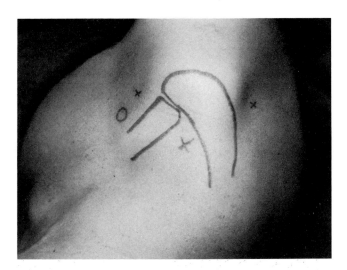

Fig. 11–3   Outline of bony landmarks, right shoulder.

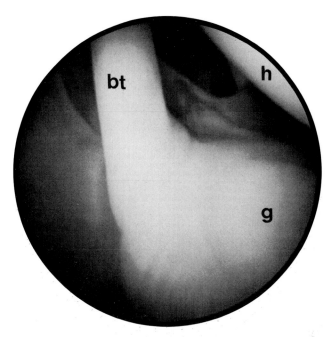

Fig. 11–4   Initial orienting view of the biceps tendon (bt), right shoulder.

should be elevated as high as possible. This elevation will provide hydrostatic pressure to distend the joint adequately, inhibit small vessel bleeding, and allow sufficient flow rate for the use of intra-articular shavers and other suction-requiring devices. Lactated Ringer's solution in 3-L bags is the irrigant of choice[25] unless electrosurgery is planned. Additional inflow cannulas can be used but are not necessary for routine diagnostic arthroscopy.

Diagnostic Arthroscopic Examination

The shoulder should be examined in a systematic fashion.[20,26] The biceps tendon is the best intra-articular landmark for initial orientation; therefore, it should be sought first after the scope is introduced. The subscapularis tendon is a substantial intra-articular structure, lying just inferior and anterior to the biceps tendon with which it can be confused. The following seven-area approach to diagnostic arthroscopy of the shoulder is recommended: (1) biceps tendon and bicipital groove, (2) rotator cuff, (3) glenoid articular surface and posterior glenoid labrum, (4) inferior recess, (5) humeral articular surface, (6) anterior glenoid labrum, and (7) anterior capsule and subscapularis bursa.

Biceps Tendon and Bicipital Groove

The biceps tendon is the best intra-articular landmark for gaining orientation. It is oriented approximately 10 to 15 degrees away from an imaginary vertical line to the glenoid. The tendon should be traced from its attachment on the superior aspect of the glenoid to where it enters the bicipital groove. The attachment of the biceps tendon to the glenoid is contiguous with the superior part of the glenoid labrum (Fig. 11–4). There

should be minimal instability at its insertion site and its surface should be free from tears or fraying.

Rotator Cuff

The intra-articular aspect of the rotator cuff tendons, particularly those of the supraspinatus and subscapularis, can be visualized well arthroscopically. From a position for viewing a supraglenoid attachment of the biceps tendon, rotation of the scope upward allows good visualization of the supraspinatus. Normally, the tendons, covered with capsule and synovium, appear smooth (Fig. 11–5). Tears are seen as fraying or rents within the tendon.

Glenoid Surface and Posterior Glenoid Labrum

Rotation of the scope posteriorly will allow visualization of the articular surface of the glenoid, which should appear smooth and white. The posterior labrum is similarly smooth, and the firmness of its attachment to the glenoid rim is variable (Fig. 11–6).

Inferior Recess

Continued rotation of the scope inferiorly reveals the inferior capsular reflection onto the humeral head. The humeral head can be visualized well and should be checked for loose bodies. This area corresponds to the axillary pouch of the inferior glenohumeral ligament (Fig. 11–7).

Humeral Head

From the posterior portal, all but the anterior aspect of the humeral head can be examined. The articular

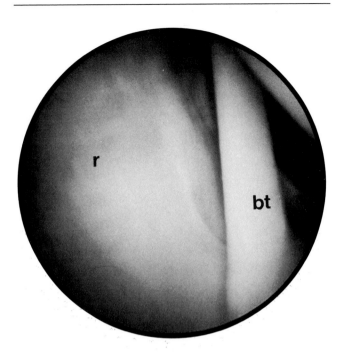

Fig. 11–5 The undersurface of the rotator cuff can be examined by rotating the arthroscope superiorly. Right shoulder, biceps tendon (bt), rotator cuff (r).

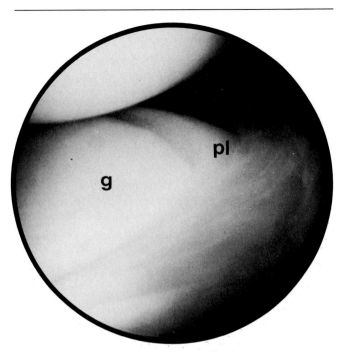

Fig. 11–6 By rotating the arthroscope posteriorly, the glenoid articular surface (g) and posterior glenoid labrum (pl) can be seen, right shoulder.

cartilage of the humeral head may not cover the entire intracapsular humerus. In particular, there may be an area of bare bone posteriorly between the articular surface and capsular insertion that should not be mistaken for a Hill-Sachs lesion (Fig. 11–8).

Anterior Glenoid Labrum

The anterior glenoid labrum should be smooth and firmly attached to the glenoid rim (Fig. 11–9). This is the most common site of arthroscopically identifiable pathology. A variety of tears can be visualized, ranging from degenerative fraying, flaps, and bucket handles to complete detachment with an obvious Bankart-type lesion. The condition of the anterior glenoid labrum can provide definitive evidence of subluxation or dislocation.

Anterior Capsule and Subscapularis Bursa

The subscapularis bursa opens into the joint just superior to the subscapularis tendon. It is near the center of the "intra-articular triangle" that is bounded by the humeral head, biceps tendon, and anterior glenoid rim (Fig. 11–10).

Accessory Portals

The posterior portal has become the standard location for introducing the arthroscope for routine diagnostic procedures about the shoulder. This portal

offers safe access to the shoulder and satisfactory visualization of the intra-articular structures. However, additional portals must be placed for the introduction of instruments to aid in the arthroscopic surgical procedures.

The best accessory instrument portal is the anterior site. Correct portal placement is mandatory because of the proximity of numerous important neurovascular structures and the fact that bleeding cannot be controlled with a tourniquet. The intra-articular triangle, shown in Figure 11–10, can be used as an excellent guide to safe and reproducible anterior portal placement. This has been confirmed by cadaver dissections and clinical experience.[27] The portals should pass through the anterior deltoid muscle and superolateral to the deltopectoral groove and cephalic vein. The coracoacromial ligament is at some risk of penetration.

Technique of Anterior Portal Placement

Routine diagnostic arthroscopy of the shoulder is performed using instruments placed into the shoulder joint posteriorly. Following this, the arthroscope is advanced with its angle directed upward into the intra-articular triangle. The arthroscope is advanced as far as possible so that its tip rests firmly against the anterior capsule. The light originating from the tip of the arthroscope transilluminates the skin, marking the anterior aspect of the shoulder through which the portal

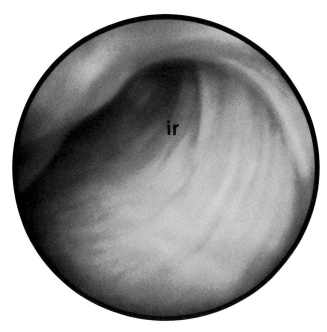

Fig. 11-7 Further inferior rotation of the arthroscope reveals the inferior recess (ir) from the inferior glenoid to the anatomic neck of the humerus, right shoulder.

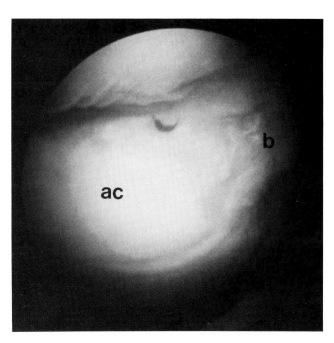

Fig. 11-8 Rotation of the arthroscope superiorly allows visualization of the humeral head. Gentle manipulation of the arm reveals more of the head, right shoulder. Note the articular cartilage (ac) and normal bare area (b).

will come. Temporarily dimming the operating room lights may aid in finding this spot. The surgeon places a finger on this point and then retracts the arthroscope until the borders of the triangle can be observed again. The arthroscopist then palpates the anterior aspect of the shoulder while confirming, by direct arthroscopic visualization, its location within the boundaries of the triangle. A 22-gauge spinal needle can be introduced from this anterior point to enter the joint in the center of the intra-articular triangle. The entrance point should be lateral and superior to the tip of the coracoid to avoid injury to the musculocutaneous nerve and other neurovascular structures beneath the coracoid process.

The trocar is removed from the needle and a solution of 0.5% bupivacaine hydrochloride with epinephrine 1:200,000 is infiltrated along the portal tract as the needle is removed. A No. 11 blade is used to make a stab wound through the skin only. Duplicating the angle created by the spinal needle, a blunt arthroscopic obturator is used to pierce the deltoid muscle and the rotator cuff and gain access into the anterior aspect of the shoulder, thus creating the anterior portal. This is done under direct arthroscopic visualization. The portal can be used for a probe or other arthroscopic surgical instruments to facilitate shoulder arthroscopy.

Johnson[1,5] has described an alternative method of anterior portal placement in which a long blunt rod is placed through the scope sleeve from the posterior direction to enter the intra-articular triangle. An incision is made over the tip of the rod to establish the portal. This is followed by introduction of a blunt obturator

into the anterior aspect of the shoulder. Once the anterior and posterior portals have been established, the arthroscope and instruments may be exchanged back and forth through both portals to allow for better visualization and access to the shoulder joint.

Technique of Superior Portal Placement

Caspari[4] has described the placement of a superior portal that is useful primarily for inflow cannula introduction. Landmarks for this approach are the junction of the apex of the clavicle and the scapula (Fig. 11-3). The sulcus of this junction can be palpated by the surgeon. A 22-gauge spinal needle can be introduced at this location and aimed toward the arthroscope. The position is easily confirmed by visualizing the needle as it enters the joint. A No. 11 blade is used to make a small skin incision, through which a blunt trocar pierces the joint. A portal so directed passes through the muscular portion of the supraspinatus rather than through its tendon. A distinct advantage of this portal is that it is located away from the portals used for surgical manipulation.

Technique for Lateral Portal Placement

Occasionally a lateral portal, approximately 2 cm inferior to the lateral portion of the acromion, may be

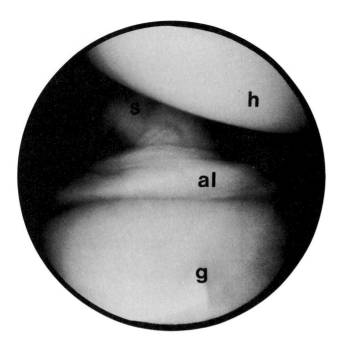

Fig. 11–9 Directing the arthroscope anteriorly brings the anterior glenoid into view. Note the anterior labrum (al), subscapularis tendon (s), humeral head (h), and glenoid (g), right shoulder.

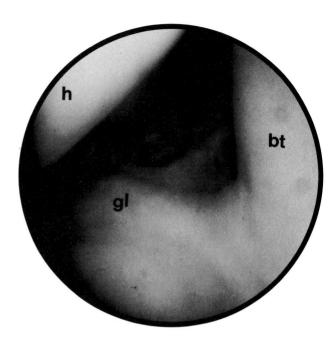

Fig. 11–10 The intra-articular triangle is bounded by the humeral head (h), the biceps tendon (bt), and the glenoid labrum (gl). The floor of the triangle is the anterior capsule, right shoulder.

used for instrumentation access. However, this portal is used most commonly to approach the subacromial space rather than the glenohumeral joint.

Subacromial Technique

The subacromial space is approached after complete glenohumeral joint evaluation. A blunt obturator is placed through the arthroscope sleeve into the original posterior skin incision for glenohumeral evaluation. The sleeve is redirected in a superior direction and aimed to pass immediately below the acromion. After penetrating the posterior soft tissue, the surgeon can use his free hand to feel the contact made by the obturator on the undersurface of the acromion. Then, the arthroscope is introduced. Inflow is obtained by redirecting a cannula through the anterior portal entrance site. A third or lateral portal is used for instrumentation. A 22-gauge spinal needle may be introduced approximately 2 cm below the lateral tip of the acromion, and the arthroscope is used to visualize the needle as it enters the subacromial space. A small incision is made and a blunt obturator can be used to gain access into the subacromial space via this posterolateral portal (Fig. 11–11). Care must be taken not to place this portal too distal; because, with the arm in abduction, the axillary nerve is moved into a more superior location.[24]

Instrumentation for Shoulder Arthroscopy

Surgeons who perform arthroscopy of the knee will be familiar with most of the instruments needed for arthroscopy of the shoulder. The basic knee arthroscopy setup with basket forceps, a probe, loose body graspers, and a motorized shaver are also the basic necessities for shoulder arthroscopy. Other instruments and equipment are not essential but can help the arthroscopist.

Arm Holder

Mobile arm holders are helpful for performing shoulder arthroscopy. Manual traction performed by an assistant may be difficult to hold in a constant position because of the assistant's fatigue. Traction with the arm tied to a fixed point should be avoided because, if the operating room table is moved, an excessive amount of traction could be placed on the arm. In addition, the amount of traction placed on the limb cannot be varied. The optimum method of traction is a system of pulleys suspended over the patient that can be attached directly to the operating table. This method allows for variation of both traction forces and arm position. An average of 10 lb of weight is used with this arm suspension system. Weights can be varied depending on the size of the patient treated.

Patient Support Device

After intubation, the patient should be placed in the lateral decubitus position. This is done most easily by the use of a beanbag. The patient should be secured on the operating room table before the extremity is connected to traction.

Cannulas

Some arthroscopists believe that a cannula system is essential for arthroscopy of the shoulder joint. The amount of tissue between the skin and the shoulder joint may be considerable and attempts to recreate a passage may be difficult when exchanging instruments, especially as swelling occurs.

A significant amount of swelling within the soft tissues about the shoulder is common during shoulder arthroscopy. This is the result of irrigation fluid extravasation into the soft tissues. The swelling may be reduced by avoiding multiple capsular punctures. Although no direct complications, such as compartment syndrome, have been encountered, swelling will make arthroscopy more difficult. In addition, swelling can make open shoulder surgery immediately following arthroscopy more difficult. Therefore, open shoulder surgery generally is not recommended after arthroscopy. Continuous irrigation is not used routinely for diagnostic arthroscopy. Suction and irrigation devices are attached to the arthroscope sleeve itself. If the joint becomes cloudy, it is suctioned and washed repeatedly with clear Ringer's solution. If the joint remains cloudy, an additional inflow cannula may be used, but this is rarely necessary.

Manual Instruments

Shoulder arthroscopy requires instrumentation similar to that used for the knee. The probe can be introduced into the anterior portal to allow for anterior palpation of intra-articular contents. Access to the inferior recess can be difficult with the probe in the anterior portal. If necessary, reversing the scope and probe can facilitate access to the inferior recess. Grasping forceps are a necessity for loose body removal. Basket forceps can be used to debride soft tissue. Curettes are important to debride large chondral defects or to roughen the bone in preparation for capsulorrhaphy.

Motorized Instruments

Serrated and full-radius resectors are also helpful for debridement of intra-articular pathology. Full-radius resectors are most helpful in performing synovectomy or lysis of small adhesions. Debridement of thicker tissue, such as the labrum, may necessitate the use of a serrated blade design. Although high-powered, aggressive meniscal resectors are available, they are rarely needed. Similarly, power instruments are helpful in arthroscopic subacromial decompression.

Technical Hints

Arthroscopy of the shoulder is not difficult but does require practice. With practice, it is easier than arthro-

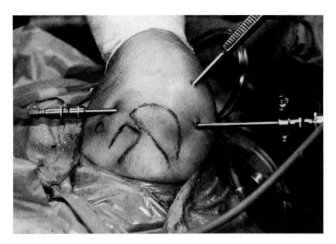

Fig. 11-11 The usual portal placement and instrumentation for subacromial surgery, right shoulder.

scopic evaluation of the knee. A systematic approach is essential to do the procedure with ease. The following section lists the most common problems encountered by the arthroscopist while evaluating the shoulder along with some possible solutions.

Difficulty with initial scope introduction may be frequent and frustrating. Arthroscopic introduction to the shoulder joint may be facilitated by identifying and using proper anatomic landmarks for the procedure. Predistention of the shoulder joint to enlarge the target is also very helpful. A valve of the arthroscope sleeve can be left open during the arthroscope's introduction to confirm proper positioning of the arthroscope by free backflow of fluid.

Loss of patient positioning during arthroscopy may occur if proper positioning details are not followed. The patient should be securely fixed in the lateral decubitus position using a beanbag, kidney braces, wide adhesive tape, or some combination of these devices. Only after the patient's body is secured should the arm be placed in traction and positioned appropriately. If these steps are followed, loss of patient positioning will not occur during the surgical procedure.

Bleeding can also be a problem for the shoulder arthroscopist. Dilutional effects may cause a small amount of bleeding to render visualization difficult and force premature termination of a procedure. Adequate hydrostatic pressure must be maintained throughout the arthroscopic procedure to control small vessel bleeding. Steps to maintain adequate hydrostatic pressure include the use of large-diameter inflow tubing and adequate elevation of inflow solution. Large-diameter inflow cannulas and inflow pumps may also be helpful to maintain hydrostatic pressure.

Arthroscopy of the shoulder joint may aid the orthopaedic surgeon in the diagnosis and treatment of shoulder disorders. As in knee arthroscopy, a systematic approach to arthroscope and portal placement and evaluation of normal and pathologic anatomy will give the surgeon a reproducible and helpful technique to deal with shoulder problems.

References

1. Johnson LL (ed): *Arthroscopic Surgery*, ed 3. St. Louis, CV Mosby, 1986.
2. Andrews JR, Carson WG Jr, McLeod WD: Glenoid labrum tears related to the long head of the biceps. *Am J Sports Med* 1985;13:337–341.
3. Andrews JR, Broussard TS, Carson WG: Arthroscopy of the shoulder in the management of partial tears of the rotator cuff: A preliminary report. *Arthroscopy* 1985;1:117–122.
4. Caspari RB: Shoulder arthroscopy: A review of the present state of the art. *Contemp Orthop* 1982;4:523–530.
5. Johnson LL: Arthroscopy of the shoulder. *Orthop Clin North Am* 1980;11:197–204.
6. Matthews LS, Ouieda SJ: Glenohumeral instability in athletes: Spectrum, diagnosis, and treatment. *Adv Orthop Surg* 1985;8:236–249.
7. Ha'eri GB, Maitland A: Arthroscopic findings in the frozen shoulder. *J Rheumatol* 1981;8:149–152.
8. McMaster WC: Anterior glenoid labrum damage: A painful lesion in swimmers. *Am J Sports Med* 1986;14:383–387.
9. Ogilvie-Harris DJ, Wiley AM: Arthroscopic surgery of the shoulder: A general appraisal. *J Bone Joint Surg* 1986;68B:201–207.
10. Dolk T, Gremark O: Arthroscopy and stability testing of the shoulder joint. *Arthroscopy* 1986;2:35–40.
11. Zarins B, Rowe CR: Current concepts in the diagnosis and treatment of shoulder instability in athletes. *Med Sci Sports Exerc* 1984;16:444–448.
12. Curran JF, Ellman MH, Brown NL: Rheumatologic aspects of painful conditions affecting the shoulder. *Clin Orthop* 1983;173:27–37.
13. Epps CH Jr: Painful hematologic conditions affecting the shoulder. *Clin Orthop* 1983;173:38–43.
14. Bateman JE: Neurologic painful conditions affecting the shoulder. *Clin Orthop* 1983;173:44–54.
15. Brown C: Compressive, invasive referred pain to the shoulder. *Clin Orthop* 1983;173:55–62.
16. Neviaser RJ: Painful conditions affecting the shoulder. *Clin Orthop* 1983;173:63–69.
17. Goldman AB, Ghelman B: The double-contrast shoulder arthrogram: A review of 158 studies. *Radiology* 1978;127:655–663.
18. Braunstein EM, O'Connor G: Double-contrast arthrotomography of the shoulder. *J Bone Joint Surg* 1982;64A:192–195.
19. Middleton WD, Reinus WR, Totty WG, et al: Ultrasonographic evaluation of the rotator cuff and biceps tendon. *J Bone Joint Surg* 1986;68A:440–450.
20. Matthews LS, Vetter WL, Helfet DL: Arthroscopic surgery of the shoulder. *Adv Orthop Surg* 1984;7:203–210.
21. Andrews JR, Carson WG Jr, Ortega K: Arthroscopy of the shoulder: Technique and normal anatomy. *Am J Sports Med* 1984;12:1–7.
22. Lilleby H: Shoulder arthroscopy. *Acta Orthop Scand* 1984;55:561–566.
23. Gross RM, Fitzgibbons TC: Shoulder arthroscopy: A modified approach. *Arthroscopy* 1985;1:156–159.
24. Bryan WJ, Schauder K, Tullos HS: The axillary nerve and its relationship to common sports medicine shoulder procedures. *Am J Sports Med* 1986;14:113–116.
25. Reagan BF, McInerny VK, Treadwell BV, et al: Irrigating solutions for arthroscopy: A metabolic study. *J Bone Joint Surg* 1983;65A:629–631.
26. Matthews LS, Terry G, Vetter WL: Shoulder anatomy for the arthroscopist. *Arthroscopy* 1985;1:83–91.
27. Matthews LS, Zarins B, Michael RH, et al: Anterior portal selection for shoulder arthroscopy. *Arthroscopy* 1985;1:33–39.

Arthroscopic Treatment of Impingement of the Shoulder

Harvard Ellman, MD

The indications, technique, and results of arthroscopic surgery in the treatment of the impingement syndrome will be described in this chapter. The role of the anterior acromion and coracoacromial ligament in the development of rotator cuff disease has been documented.[1-3] Anterior acromioplasty in the treatment of chronic impingement was originally described by Neer[1] in 1972, and subsequent reports have confirmed the efficacy of this procedure.[4,5] In 1983, I performed the first arthroscopic acromioplasty based on the criteria established by Neer. Preliminary reports by various investigators[6-10] indicate that the results of arthroscopic decompression compare favorably with the results achieved by open surgery.

Indications

The primary indication for arthroscopic subacromial decompression is advanced stage II impingement syndrome in patients who have failed to respond to conservative treatment for six months to one year, or more. Conservative management includes rest; the avoidance of repetitive overhead activity whenever possible; nonsteroidal anti-inflammatory medication; physical therapy modalities to decrease local inflammation; and therapeutic exercises in the subimpingement range. Steroid injections into the subacromial space are used sparingly and should be limited to a total of three injections over an extended period.

Arthroscopic subacromial decompression is also indicated in selected cases of partial- or full-thickness rotator cuff tear, and may be useful in the treatment of chronic calcific tendinitis. These indications will be discussed later in this chapter.

Equipment

Basic arthroscopic instrumentation is used to perform arthroscopic subacromial decompression. A powered synovial resector is used to debride the subacromial space and a large arthroplasty burr is required for the acromioplasty. Electrosurgical technique is used to cut the attachment of the coracoacromial ligament and is invaluable in obtaining hemostasis throughout the procedure. The operating room is set up with the television monitor at the head of the table. The position

of the anesthesiologist and power sources depends on whether surgery is to be performed on the right or left shoulder (Fig. 12–1).

Surgical Technique

The goals of arthroscopic subacromial decompression are to release the coracoacromial ligament, resect the anterior undersurface of the acromion, and perform a subtotal bursectomy within the subacromial space. Proper orientation and adequate visualization are essential to the performance of this procedure.

Positioning the Patient

The patient is intubated and placed on a suction-type beanbag in the lateral recumbent position. Kidney rests are used anteriorly and posteriorly for additional stabilization. Following routine preparation and draping, 10 to 15 lb of traction are applied with the arm abducted 15 to 20 degrees and flexed forward slightly. Further abduction will move the greater tuberosity closer to the acromion and obliterate the subacromial space.

Outlining Bony Landmarks

The posterolateral angle of the acromion is palpated and, from this point, a marking pencil is used to outline the acromion, the acromioclavicular joint, and the coracoid process. The coracoacromial ligament is also marked, from the end of the coracoid to the insertion on the anterior edge of the acromion. The arm should be placed in traction before these landmarks are outlined.

The posterior portal is marked approximately 2 cm medial and 2 cm distal to the posterolateral angle of the acromion. This spot corresponds to the posterior "soft spot" and may be used to enter the glenohumeral joint and the subacromial space. In nearly every case, I explore the glenohumeral joint prior to performing a subacromial decompression. From this posterior approach, the shoulder joint is distended with 30 ml of normal saline. When the joint accepts an unusually large quantity of fluid with relative ease, runoff may be occurring through a rotator cuff tear. With the table and patient angled about 20 degrees posteriorly, the glenoid approaches a horizontal position. This position facilitates entry into the joint with the arthroscope directed toward the tip of the coracoid. A routine

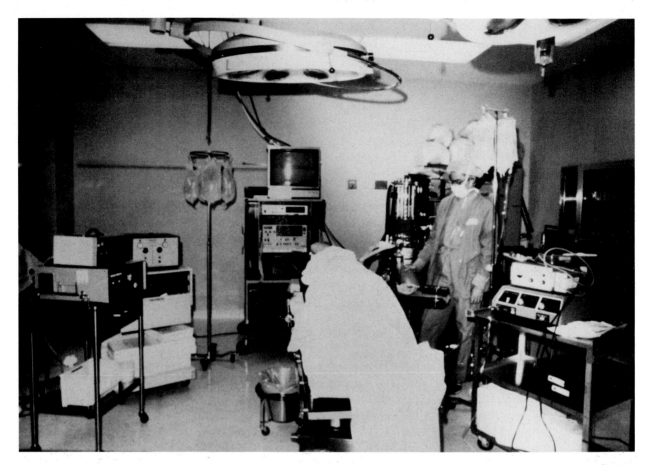

Fig. 12–1 Photograph showing the position of equipment in the operating room to be used for arthroscopic subacromial decompression.

glenohumeral inspection is done, with particular attention to the undersurface of the rotator cuff. Articular surface tears may be seen readily. Simple capsular fraying should be differentiated from partial-thickness tears, and, when necessary, a light debridement should be done to determine the depth of the tear. This differentiation requires the establishment of an anterior portal using a "switching stick." (The arthroscope is pressed against the anterior capsule just above the superior border of the subscapularis and inferior to the long head of biceps tendon. The switching stick is passed through the sheath of the arthroscope from back to front. Penetration should be lateral to the coracoid process to avoid injury to the axillary sheath.) The potential tear can also be investigated using a probe through the anterior portal. I avoid placing a superior portal when subacromial space surgery is anticipated. The additional fluid ingress required for suction shaving can be obtained by using a plastic shoulder cannula, with a diaphragm and right-angle fluid ingress arm, through the anterior portal. Glenohumeral inspection and manipulation should be as brief as possible to prevent overdistention of the area.

Surgery in the subacromial space requires additional portals. The arthroscope is removed from the posterior portal and an accessory metal cannula for fluids is introduced through this portal into the subacromial space. A second portal is marked just anterior to the posterolateral angle of the acromion and 2 cm inferiorly. The arthroscope is introduced through this portal in a line so that it will lie directly beneath the anterior margin of the acromion. Then, two 22-gauge lumbar puncture needles are used as marker pins to outline the attachment of the coracoacromial ligament. One pin is placed at the anterolateral margin of the acromion. The other is placed just anterior to the acromioclavicular joint. An anterolateral portal to be used for introducing surgical instruments is established by inserting a plastic cannula with a rubber diaphragm at a point no more than 3 cm from the edge of the acromion in a direct line with the two marker pins. If this portal is placed too far distal to the acromion in this line, injury to the axillary nerve may result. Figure 12–2 illustrates the position of marker pins and instruments for subacromial space arthroscopy. Figure 12–3 is a photograph of the surgery in progress.

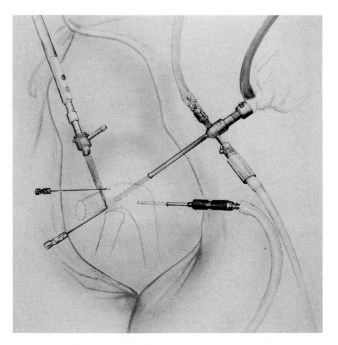

Fig. 12–2 The bony landmarks are outlined. Marker pins are placed at the medial and lateral margins of the coracoacromial ligament. The surgical cannula enters 6 cm from the lateral pin in direct line with the anterior acromion. The arthroscope is placed through the posterolateral portal, and the accessory fluid cannula is directed upward through the posterior "soft spot" portal to lie within the subacromial space. (Reproduced with permission from Ellman H: *Arthroscopic subacromial decompression*, in Parisien SS (ed): *Arthroscopic Surgery: Principles and Practice.* New York, McGraw-Hill, 1988.)

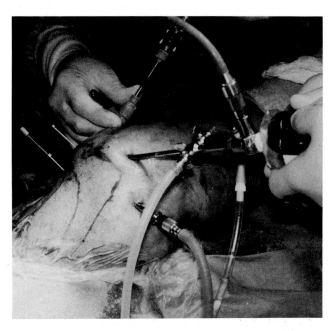

Fig. 12–3 Photograph of arthroscopic subacromial decompression.

Subtotal Bursectomy

The subacromial space of a patient with chronic impingement will be filled with hypertrophic tissue that obscures vision. The normal filmy, spiderweb-like strands of adventitious material are replaced by thick fibrous strands hung with clumps of fibrofatty-appearing matter. The frayed fibers of a superficially eroded or torn rotator cuff may obscure vision further. A preliminary debridement with the suction shaver must be carried out as the first step in visualization. I prefer the serrated shaver to the higher-speed, angled synovial resector. Frequently, I find it necessary to maneuver the shaver and scope to bring the initial efforts at shaving under direct vision in the midst of this jungle of strands.

The keys to visualization are debridement, distention, and traction. As the debridement proceeds, I check the traction routinely to be certain the pulleys are unobstructed and that the weight is not resting on the floor. Continuous distention requires an unobstructed fluid ingress cannula. The location of the tip of the cannula should be identified early in the procedure. The bags of fluid should be elevated on the intravenous stand, and empty bags should be replaced promptly to maintain adequate pressure. Debridement should proceed until the medial and lateral marker pins can be visu-

alized clearly. The undersurface of the coracoacromial ligament may be seen at times, but, more often, it is obscured by hypertrophic bursa. When properly positioned, the arthroscope makes it possible to visualize both the medial and lateral marker pins, which can be wiggled to aid in their identification.

Cutting the Coracoacromial Ligament

The coracoacromial ligament is released from its attachment using electrosurgical technique. I prefer a meniscal cutter with a right-angle tip that is covered with plastic material except at the very tip of the electrode. A trial passage of the electrode is done by passing it from the medial marker pin to the lateral pin (Fig. 12–4). Normal saline must be removed from the subacromial space and sterile distilled water, or some other nonconductive medium, must be introduced for the electrosurgical instrument to function. A Y-connector with tubing attached to each set of fluid bags is most efficient for this transfer of fluids. Clamps to control each type of fluid are clearly marked so that the surgeon is aware of the type of fluid used at all times. I limit the use of distilled water to ten to 15 minutes to avoid any problems with hemolysis or tissue irritation.

Cutting current is gradually increased until the thickened subacromial bursa underlying the coracoacromial ligament is incised. The white, closely packed, glistening fibers can be seen as the bursa is parted. The cut is placed adjacent to the acromial attachment of the ligament, and, when completed, the ends can be seen to give way as tension is released. Deltoid fibers should

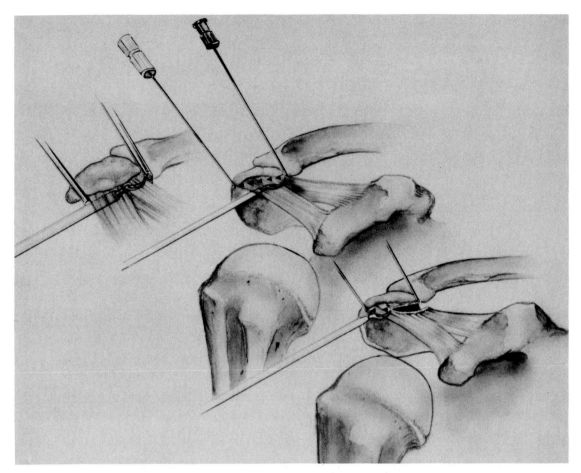

Fig. 12-4 The coracoacromial ligament is cut beginning at the medial marker pin and continuing in a straight line to the lateral pin. Cutting adjacent to the acromial attachment of the ligament minimizes the risk of injury to a branch of the coracoacromial artery. (Reproduced with permission from Ellman H: Arthroscopic subacromial decompression, in Parisien SS (ed): *Arthroscopic Surgery: Principles and Practice*. New York, McGraw-Hill, 1988.)

not be disturbed. They appear much thicker and more widely spaced than the fibers of the ligament. They also appear dull in color rather than glistening (Fig. 12–5).

Control of Bleeding

Bleeding may develop at any time during the procedure. The acromioclavicular branch of the coracoacromial artery may be encountered at this stage and produce significant hemorrhage. This can be avoided by placing the scope directly under the electrode for direct visualization of the cutting process. Caution is advised, particularly in the region of the medial pin. If this procedure is attempted without electrosurgical control, the operation may have to be terminated if significant hemorrhage develops. The electrosurgical control of hemorrhage requires additional elevation of the distilled water bags and rapid intermittent suction while the bleeding is followed to its source. External pressure may be of some value. Since most bleeding vessels are seen under direct vision, it is wise to intro-

duce the electrosurgical pencil promptly for control before visualization becomes obstructed. A change from normal saline back to distilled water improves visualization, probably as a result of local hemolysis. The appearance of a diffuse oozing generally indicates that the water bags have emptied unnoticed.

Anterior Acromioplasty

The thickened subacromial bursa attaches to the anterior undersurface of the acromion. The coracoacromial ligament also invests the undersurface of the acromion as part of its attachment. This material must be removed before the burr can work effectively. The electrosurgical pencil is used to morsellize this tissue beneath the area of acromion that will be resected. The tissue seems to melt away beneath the cauterizing current. An open curette or suction shaver can then be used to expose completely the bony undersurface.

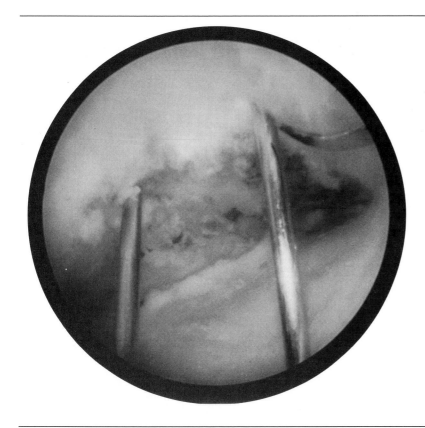

Fig. 12–5 Arthroscopic photograph taken after release of the coracoacromial ligament.

A thorough acromioplasty is essential to a successful decompression. The entire anterior acromial hook must be removed (Fig. 12–6). This involves resection of the undersurface of the acromion across its full width and extending posteriorly for at least 2.5 cm. Determining the depth and width of the removed bone is a critical part of the procedure. I use a deepening technique based on the fact that the 4.5-mm burr protrudes from its sheath approximately 3 mm (Fig. 12–7). Using this burr, a deepening hole is burrowed 3 mm into the exposed undersurface of the acromion. This hole is then extended into a trough from the anterior edge of the acromion to a point at least 2 cm posteriorly. This trough is widened successively from front to back until

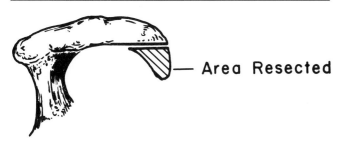

Fig. 12–6 Lateral view of the acromion shows the area that must be resected to flatten the undersurface and eliminate the anterior acromial hook.

the entire width of the acromion has been burrowed. The area is smoothed and the deepening process repeated until the desired depth of the acromial resection is achieved. The anterior edge of the acromion is tapered until it assumes the shape of the trailing edge of an airplane wing. The anterior edge of the acromion should be recessed 6 to 8 mm. During this process, the residual thickness of the acromion can be evaluated and further resection carried out, if indicated. The completed acromioplasty should extend across the full width of the acromion and both the medial and lateral borders of the acromion should be adequately resected (Fig. 12–8, *left*). An arthroscopic photograph of the completed decompression is shown in Figure 12–8, *right*. The outer end of the clavicle articulates with the medial border, and movement of the acromioclavicular joint can be detected when downward pressure is placed on the outer end of the clavicle. Spurs arising from the undersurface of the acromioclavicular joint should be removed with a burr. Peripheral leaf-like projections of bursa and periosteum can be removed with motorized trimmers or basket forceps to conclude the acromioplasty (Fig. 12–9). Prior to closure, the fluid medium is changed back to distilled water, and punctate areas of bleeding from cancellous bone are controlled with electrocautery. The joint is then flushed with normal saline and 10 ml of 0.25% bupivacaine hydrochloride is instilled into the subacromial space. The portals

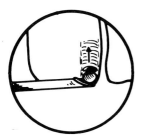 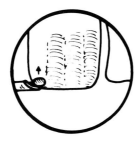 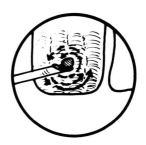 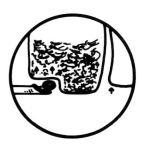

Fig. 12–7 Deepening and polishing technique. A hole 3 mm deep is made with the portion of the burr that protrudes from the sheath (**left**). Then, a furrow is created at this depth from front to back. Repeat this process across the full width of the acromion until the desired depth is achieved (**center left**). Polish in a circular fashion, smoothing and tapering the acromion toward the anterior edge (**center right**). Recess the anterior edge until it is level with the front of the clavicle (**right**).

are closed with interrupted 4-0 nylon sutures and a compression dressing is applied.

Postoperative Protocol

The arthroscopic procedure is usually performed in an outpatient setting. After surgery, patients are asked to stretch the arm overhead while they are in the supine position and also to perform external rotation and pendulum exercises every morning and evening for one minute to prevent adhesion formation. A sling is not necessary, and activities of daily living are resumed on the evening of surgery. Patients who are not required to perform strenuous overhead activities may return to work within a few days. Isometric exercises are prescribed at three weeks; at six weeks, strengthening exercises are added in the subimpingement range using surgical tubing. Most patients do not require a formal physical therapy program. The patient who occasionally demonstrates a tendency to form pericapsular adhesions is assisted in range-of-motion exercises. Patients involved in tennis, throwing activities, or occupations requiring sustained overhead work should be allowed a progressive increase in their activity after a period of two to three months.

Rotator Cuff Tears

Some method of diagnostic imaging is indicated in every patient more than 40 years old who is contemplating surgery to determine the presence or absence of a rotator cuff tear. This also applies to younger individuals in whom a full-thickness tear is suspected. Double-contrast arthrography is preferable to single-contrast, because it will permit a qualitative analysis of cuff tissue when a tear is present.[11] Double-contrast arthrography allows the thickness of the tendon to be seen, and increased uptake of dye will differentiate a frayed, degenerative margin from the edge of a sharper, more acute tear. In most cases, some estimate of the size of the tear can be made with double-contrast arthrography. The single-contrast arthrogram accurately demonstrates the presence or absence of a full-thickness tear, but the amount of dye that escapes into the subacromial space is not dependent on the size of the tear. Ultrasonography[12] by an experienced operator may demonstrate full-thickness tears and interstitial changes within a damaged rotator cuff. Magnetic resonance imaging[13] shows cuff degeneration and reactive changes within the subacromial bursa. Small tears within the tendinous portion of the cuff cannot be demonstrated accurately. However, larger tears with significant retraction may be seen. Thinning and fibrosis associated with cuff degeneration is seen best in the frontal oblique plane.

Partial-Thickness Tears

Those patients with partial-thickness cuff tears involving either the articular or bursal surface of the rotator cuff will respond favorably to light debridement of the torn cuff margins and arthroscopic subacromial decompression. The bony prominence of the anterior acromion and, at times, a bulbous enlargement arising beneath the acromioclavicular articulation will potentiate chronic impingement unless relieved. Decompression will eliminate the major contributing causes of a full-thickness rotator cuff tear.

Full-Thickness Tears

For a full-thickness rotator cuff tear, open surgical reconstruction is the optimal method of restoring near-normal function. The role of arthroscopic surgery in the treatment of full-thickness rotator cuff tears has not been established. The size of the tear may have some effect on the outcome of arthroscopic surgery. A small tear (less than 2 cm) in the nondominant arm of an older, inactive individual can be relieved of pain by debridement and decompression. The patient should

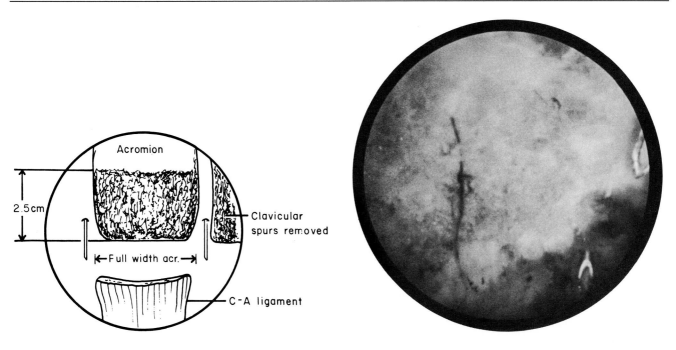

Fig. 12–8 **Left:** Diagram of arthroscopic view showing the acromioplasty extending across the full width of the acromion from the anterior aspect to a point 2.5 cm posteriorly. Clavicular spurs have also been removed. **Right:** Arthroscopic photograph of the completed decompression.

be aware that extension of the degenerative tear often occurs with trivial exertion. I recommend open reconstruction when this same small tear occurs in a patient involved in strenuous or repetitive vocational or recreational activities. The majority of rotator cuff tears treated surgically measure between 2 and 4 cm of maximum retraction. In this group, I would advise open repair.

The so-called massive tear that is greater than 4 or 5 cm may be difficult or impossible to repair. The surgeon can recognize these longstanding degenerative tears by profound weakness (classified as less than three fifths on a scale of zero to five) in abduction and external rotation, and a markedly diminished distance (3 mm or less) between the undersurface of the acromion and the superior articular surface of a high-riding humeral head.[14] The plain radiographs will show acromial concavity and sclerosis, and, in some instances, flattening and collapse of the humeral head (cuff arthropathy). Rockwood[15] has reported successful results in the treatment of massive, irreparable cuff tears using open anterior acromioplasty and debridement of the loose and floppy margins of the torn cuff. The same procedure can be performed arthroscopically and significant pain has been relieved in these cases.[16] Patients should understand that this is a procedure with limited goals, and that they are unlikely to regain any motion or strength. Neer has noted: "The rare patient with an irreparable cuff can be made more comfortable if impingement is relieved and can gain surprising function if the deltoid

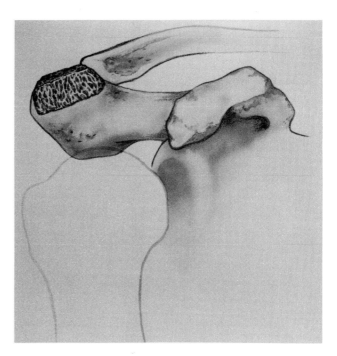

Fig. 12–9 The completed acromioplasty. Note that the anterior edge of the acromion has been recessed so that it does not protrude beyond the anterior border of the clavicle. (Reproduced with permission from Ellman H: Arthroscopic subacromial decompression, in Parisien SS (ed): *Arthroscopic Surgery: Principles and Practice*. New York, McGraw-Hill, 1988.)

is permitted to remain strong."[1] Massive cuff tears can generally be debrided through the routine subacromial space portals. The retracted tendon permits inspection of both the glenohumeral joint and subacromial space without restriction. The floppy, fibrotic edges of the torn cuff should be resected. Stubs of tendon tissue arising from the tuberosity should also be removed. Care should be taken not to resect viable tendon because this might weaken the cuff further. The long head of the biceps should be preserved. The debridement can extend into the glenohumeral joint. Synovial tags and frayed labral structures may be debrided. In some cases, I have rounded off the barren greater tuberosity to conform better with the superior articular surface of the humerus. Because the ultimate goal is to produce a ball-and-socket joint in which the humerus articulates with the undersurface of the acromion, removal of the tuberosity permits the patient a greater range of overhead elevation of the arm. This procedure is called a "tuberosity plasty." In addition to cuff debridement, an acromioplasty should be performed in each of these cases.

Treatment of Calcific Tendinitis

Patients with recurrent or symptomatic calcific deposits may benefit from arthroscopic decompression and needling with removal of the calcification.[7] This procedure is restricted to those rare patients in whom conservative treatment has failed and who would require an open procedure. Large calcific deposits are easy to locate, but smaller or multilocular calcifications can be harder to identify.

After subacromial portals are established, a needle is used to probe the rotator cuff under direct arthroscopic vision to locate the calcific deposit. In some instances, the deposit can be seen as a white, glistening substance on the surface of the cuff. When the calcium has not penetrated to the surface, the probing needle will liberate small snowflake-like pieces of calcium when a deposit is encountered. A small arthroscopic curette may be used to remove the larger deposits. Removal of calcium deposits is accompanied by arthroscopic subacromial decompression.

Problems and Complications

The arthroscopic subacromial decompression procedure is technically demanding and requires advanced arthroscopic skills. The prerequisites for successful visualization of the subacromial space are distention and hemostasis. Continuous traction is essential and accessory fluid ingress portals must be maintained throughout the procedure.

Most patients with impingement syndrome have been taking salicylates or some form of nonsteroidal anti-inflammatory medication. It is important to discontinue this medication at least two weeks before surgery. Preoperative studies include prothrombin time, partial thromboplastin time, and bleeding time. Control of intraoperative bleeding using electrosurgical techniques enhances visualization and facilitates the procedure.

Intraoperative Problems

Loosening or breaking of equipment is a potential problem in any arthroscopic procedure. I have observed that the chondroplasty burr can become detached from its revolving stem. In some models, the burr is interchangeable and held with a press fitting. I prefer the disposable burr with a solid stem. The tip of the plastic surgical cannula may chip or crack if mechanical instruments are not introduced and withdrawn gently. The rubber diaphragm can displace into the joint but can be retrieved. Improperly secured traction weights can fall to the floor, or a top-heavy fluid stand can topple across the operating field. To my knowledge, there have been no instances of skin burns related to the use of electrosurgery.

Postoperative Complications

Arthroscopic subacromial decompression has been relatively free of serious complications to date. One patient developed a localized hematoma beneath the anterior portal; this resolved spontaneously. Three patients had transient dysesthesias in the distribution of the dorsal digital nerve to the thumb; however, increased padding at the wrist level in the traction device has eliminated this difficulty. There have been no reported cases of traction neuropathy involving the brachial plexus. One patient who had a history of coronary artery bypass graft surgery developed unstable angina postoperatively and spent two days in the coronary observation unit before being released from the hospital. No infections have been reported.

Unsatisfactory Results

Persistent pain from impingement or limited range of motion are the two most common causes of an unsatisfactory result. A technically inadequate decompression is the most common cause of persistent pain from impingement. When surgery is repeated, uncut portions of ligament can be observed at both the lateral and medial margins of the ligament. Coracoacromial ligament fibers may arise from the anterior capsule of the acromioclavicular joint, and I have revised my medial pin placement somewhat more toward the lateral border of the clavicle to accommodate these fibers. It is very important to remove the full width of the acromial undersurface and avoid the tendency to dig a hole in the anterior acromion. It is possible to underestimate the size of a rotator cuff tear, even under direct visualization with the arthroscope. Tears of significant size may be laminated, and observation may be misleading from either the bursal or articular surface alone. One unsatisfactory case involved a rotator cuff tear that had escaped detection during two arthrograms and one arthroscopy. The patient recovered well after open repair of the tear. Another patient, whose open repair had failed, had a tear more than 4 cm in length and intractable pain. This patient was treated with arthroscopic debridement and decompression and did well for three years before noting a rather sudden increase of both pain and weakness. Subsequent arthroscopy documented an extension of the previous tear.

Symptoms of impingement may develop secondary to shoulder instability, and failure to recognize this diagnosis may lead to an unsatisfactory result. Surgical correction of the unstable shoulder, followed by therapy designed to strengthen and restore balance to the shoulder musculature will usually eliminate any impingement-like symptoms in these patients.

Results

The results of arthroscopic subacromial decompression are comparable to those obtained with the open technique of anterior acromioplasty.[4-10] Analysis of the first 50 consecutive operations that I performed and followed up for one to three years[7] indicated that 88% of the patients achieved a satisfactory result. When patients with full-thickness rotator cuff tears are analyzed as a group, their results are only 80% satisfactory. A subsequent study involving these and other patients suggested that the result of arthroscopic treatment of rotator cuff tears is related to the size of the tear. Patients with partial-thickness tears responded to arthroscopic shoulder decompression about as well as those patients in whom no tear was present.

My associates and I[14] reported on a series of 50 patients who had full-thickness rotator cuff tears that were treated by open reconstruction. These results were compared with our preliminary results following arthroscopic treatment of full-thickness rotator cuff tears. The results of arthroscopic treatment of small (less than 2 cm) and large (2- to 4-cm) tears are less satisfactory than the results of open surgical repair. The number of cases and length of follow-up do not permit statistically significant conclusions. It is my clinical impression that all reparable (up to 4 cm) full-thickness rotator cuff tears should be treated by open surgical reconstruction. A small tear in the nondominant arm of an older and relatively inactive individual may be treated satisfactorily by arthroscopic debridement and decompression, but the result is not likely to achieve the excellent status that may be obtained by an open repair.

Arthroscopic treatment has been effective in the management of the special category of so-called massive or irreparable tears. These patients may achieve significant pain relief following arthroscopic cuff debridement and decompression. Subsequently, when the deltoid is strengthened, function is also improved. The patient should understand that no improvement in strength will occur as a result of this operation.

Summary

Arthroscopic subacromial decompression is an alternative to open anterior acromioplasty in patients who have advanced stage II and *selected* stage III impingement syndromes. This procedure can be performed in an outpatient setting and postoperative morbidity is minimal; however, the procedure is technically demanding. Because the deltoid is not detached, immediate full range of active motion is possible, allowing an early return to activities of daily living. Substantial pain relief can be anticipated in a large majority of patients.

References

1. Neer CS II: Anterior acromioplasty for the chronic impingement syndrome in the shoulder: A preliminary report. *J Bone Joint Surg* 1972;54A:41–50.
2. Neer CS II: Impingement lesions. *Clin Orthop* 1983;173:70–77.
3. Hawkins RJ, Kennedy JC: Impingement syndrome in athletes. *Am J Sports Med* 1980;8:151–158.
4. Post M, Cohen J: Impingement syndrome: A review of late stage II and early stage III lesions. *Orthop Trans* 1985;9:48.
5. Raggio CL, Warren RF, Sculco T: Surgical treatment of impingement syndrome: 4-year follow-up. *Orthop Trans* 1985;9:48.
6. Ellman H: Arthroscopic subacromial decompression. *Orthop Trans* 1985;9:48.
7. Ellman H: Arthroscopic subacromial decompression: Analysis of 1–3 year results. *Arthroscopy* 1987;3:173–181.
8. Paulos AE, Chamberlain S, Murray S: Arthroscopic shoulder decompression: Technique and preliminary results. *Orthop Trans* 1986;10:222.
9. Gartsman GM: Arthroscopic subacromial decompression: A clinical study. Presented at the Fourth Open Meeting of the American Shoulder and Elbow Surgeons, Atlanta, Feb 7, 1988.
10. Mendoza FX, Nichols JA, Rubinstein MP: Arthroscopic treatment of stage II subacromial impingement. Presented at the Fourth Open Meeting of the American Shoulder and Elbow Surgeons, Atlanta, Feb 7, 1988.
11. Mink JH, Harris E, Rappaport M: Rotator cuff tears: Evaluation using double-contrast shoulder arthrography. *Radiology* 1985;157:621–623.
12. Mack LA, Matsen FA III, Kilcoyne RF, et al: US evaluation of the rotator cuff. *Radiology* 1985;157:205–209.
13. Seeger LL, Ruszkowski JT, Bassett LW, et al: MR imaging of the normal shoulder: Anatomic correlation. *AJR* 1987;148:83–91.
14. Ellman H, Hanker G, Bayer M: Repair of the rotator cuff. End-result study of factors influencing reconstruction. *J Bone Joint Surg* 1986;68A:1136–1144.
15. Rockwood C: Total shoulder arthroplasty. Presented at the 52nd Annual Meeting of the American Academy of Orthopaedic Surgeons, Las Vegas, Jan 24–29, 1985.
16. Ellman H: Arthroscopic subacromial decompression, in Parisien JS (ed): *Arthroscopic Surgery.* New York, McGraw-Hill, 1988, pp 243–248.

CHAPTER 13

Shoulder Arthroscopy for Shoulder Instability

David W. Altchek, MD

Michael J. Skyhar, MD

Russell F. Warren, MD

Introduction

The first arthroscopic examination of the shoulder is credited to Burman,[1] who examined several cadaver joints with a primitive arthroscope in 1931. The first clinical report of shoulder arthroscopy was by Andrén and Lundberg,[2] who in 1965 arthroscopically investigated patients with "frozen shoulders." Watanabe[3] first clearly described the anterior and posterior portals and was also the first to use the arthroscope to diagnose a variety of disorders of the shoulder. Since 1980 shoulder arthroscopy has advanced rapidly.

It is well established that the arthroscope is a valuable tool in the diagnosis of the unstable shoulder, because it provides a clear view of the intra-articular abnormality, making it possible for the surgeon to formulate a logical treatment plan. In recent years there has been increasing interest in arthroscopic stabilization procedures. The common denominator underlying all such procedures, whether performed with sutures, staples, or screws, is reestablishment of a functional inferior glenohumeral ligament both anteriorly and posteriorly. This is achieved by reattaching either the avulsed labrum with the ligament in continuity or the ligament directly to the glenoid neck.

Indications

Arthroscopy of the shoulder is indicated in patients with instability for the diagnosis and removal of loose bodies, labral debridement, stabilization (using sutures, staples, or tissue grafts), and joint debridement.

Diagnosis

The cornerstones of the diagnosis and treatment of patients with shoulder instability are an accurate history and physical examination. Although recurrent shoulder dislocation with radiologic confirmation is easy to diagnose, there is a subset of patients, particularly those with subluxation, in whom symptoms and office examination cannot prove instability to be the source of the problem. This is not uncommon in athletes involved in overhand sports, in whom instability can be the result of the high intrinsic forces generated. During throwing activities, the humeral head experiences large shear forces directed both anteriorly and posteriorly, depending on arm position. Translation of the humeral head is prevented by a competent labral ligamentous complex and by deceleration forces generated by the rotator cuff and biceps tendon. Failure or dysfunction of any part of the restraint system, whether rotator cuff, biceps tendon, or labrum-ligament complex, leads to an increased load on the other portions of the system, accounting for the coexistence of instability and impingement in the throwing athlete.

These patients often have pain as their only complaint. Accurate assessment of the amount and direction of glenohumeral translation is often difficult, and differentiating between apprehension and pain is at times impossible.

Examination with the patient under anesthesia is often not enough to confirm the instability pattern in this group of patients. Translation may be increased symmetrically both anteriorly and posteriorly. Arthroscopy of the glenohumeral joint can solve the diagnostic puzzle. A violation of the integrity of the glenoid labrum, with either frank detachment or tearing within its substance, depending on the site, can indicate the presence and direction of the instability. The location of the labral lesion is of crucial importance, as not all labral tears are indicative of instability. In general, labral lesions, whether anterior or posterior, below the equator of the glenoid are secondary to instability whereas superior lesions are not. Other findings, such as a Hill-Sachs defect, loose body, or glenohumeral ligament detachment or deficiency are important factors supporting a diagnosis of instability. In addition, the intra-articular surface of the rotator cuff and the subacromial space should be arthroscopically inspected because rotator cuff disease frequently accompanies labral damage above the equator of the glenoid.

We should emphasize that in most situations arthroscopy does not play a major role in the diagnosis of instability. We rarely rely solely on diagnostic shoulder arthroscopy to guide our final treatment plan in cases of suspected or known instability.

Technique of Diagnostic Arthroscopy and Normal Anatomy

Operating Room Setup

Necessary equipment for shoulder arthroscopy includes a 30-degree 4.5-mm arthroscope, a video camera and monitor, a suction device, motorized shaving system with various sizes of full radius resectors and arthroplasty burrs, an interchangeable cannula system with a diaphragm to allow for inflow, arthroscope, and instrument insertion, a complete set of basic hand instruments, irrigation solution suspended on poles, and an arthroscopic electrocautery.

The television monitor and video equipment are placed opposite to the shoulder being operated on. The arthroscopic irrigating solution, light source, and shaver source are placed on the same side as the monitor. For knee arthroscopy we use only normal saline as our irrigating solution. However, a nonconductive solution such as sterile water or 1.5% glycine is needed for the electrocautery. Our inflow tubing allows for four separate solution bags. For shoulder arthroscopy we use two bags each of saline and sterile water. In this way the sterile water can be used in isolation when the electrocautery is in use.

Anesthesia and Positioning

Although general anesthesia with endotracheal intubation is most widely used, we perform most of our arthroscopic shoulder procedures with the patient under scalene block. The motor block is dense enough to allow thorough examination of the shoulder. Supplementary lidocaine is occasionally needed for the posterior skin portals.

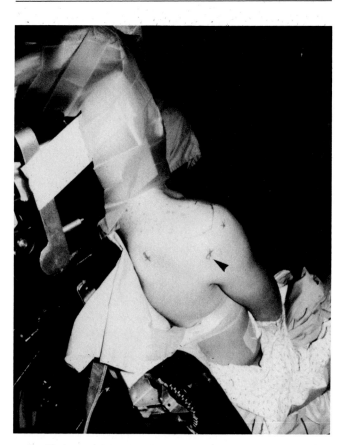

Fig. 13-1 Posterior view of the patient in the sitting position. Note the position of the posterior portal (arrowhead).

We initially performed the procedure with the patient in the lateral position with the arm suspended in a traction device. Although we have had no complications directly related to the lateral position, transient neuropraxia, presumably caused by excessive strain on the brachial plexus, has been reported by several investigators. Klein and France[4] reported a 30% incidence of transient neuropraxia following shoulder arthroscopy using traction.

Beginning in 1986 we began positioning the patient in the upright seated position with the arm free at the side. We have since used this position in more than 75 arthroscopic shoulder procedures, including diagnostic arthroscopy, subacromial decompression, and arthroscopic stabilization.

There are several advantages to this position. Patient positioning is faster and easier regardless of anesthetic technique. It is easier for the anesthesiologist to manage the airway. When scalene block anesthesia is used, the awake upright patient can observe the procedure on an overhead monitor. A patient given a scalene block tolerates the lateral position poorly but usually finds the seated position comfortable. There is no need to reprepare and redrape the patient if arthrotomy is needed after the arthroscopy.

The capsular anatomy within the joint is not placed in a nonanatomic, stretched-out attitude as occurs during arm traction. This is important in arthroscopic stabilization because an accurate assessment of glenohumeral ligament laxity must be obtained and the tissues reapproximated under minimal tension. The arm is more mobile when the beachchair position is used, allowing the assistant to manipulate the arm to afford a complete view of the intra-articular and subacromial spaces. Exact arm positioning is crucial for proper tension during arthroscopic stabilization. In addition, the anatomic vertical joint position makes triangulation and location of external anatomic landmarks easier.

We use a standard operating table that allows for hip and knee flexion, with a well-padded support placed at the foot of the table. The patient is placed supine on the table, which is adjusted to the sitting position with the torso inclined at least 70 degrees to the horizontal. A 10-lb sandbag is placed under the ipsilateral hip and a pad is placed under the medial border of the scapula to facilitate rotation of the upper torso away from the edge of the table. The shoulder should be free over the edge of the table and the entire scapula should be accessible from the posterior aspect. The arm is allowed to hang free at the side (Fig. 13-1).

Examination

After the induction of anesthesia, glenohumeral stability is assessed. The shoulder should be stressed anteriorly, posteriorly, and inferiorly. We grade instability from 1+ to 3+, with 1+ indicating that the humeral head can be translated to the glenoid rim but not over it, 2+ that the humeral head can be subluxated over the rim but will not lock in a dislocated position, and 3+ the ability to dislocate the humeral head. Inferior laxity is also judged by the presence or absence of a "sulcus sign." This means a sulcus that develops between the acromion and humeral head when traction is applied with the arm in adduction (Fig. 13–2). The examination should confirm the clinical diagnosis and dictate the treatment plan.

Occasionally a seemingly clearcut direction of instability by history can be difficult to confirm by examination. This can happen for several reasons. First, if there was erosion or fracture of the bony glenoid rim, a distinct jump may not be felt as the humeral head subluxates or dislocates. Second, in cases of anterior or posterior subluxation, the shoulder may be spontaneously subluxated while the patient is under anesthesia in the supine position; the examiner may erroneously believe that the head is subluxating anteriorly or posteriorly when in fact an already subluxated humeral head is being reduced. If equivalent translation is present in both posterior and anterior directions, the physician should rely on the preoperative impression in choosing the primary direction of instability. If this is inconclusive, however, arthroscopic evaluation may be helpful.

If an arthroscopic stabilization is being considered, significant posterior and inferior laxity must be ruled out. Inferior instability indicates that an element of multidirectional instability is present. This requires an open capsular shift for correction.[5]

Portal Placement and Portal Anatomy

The first step in accurate portal placement is identification of the external anatomic landmarks. The acromial borders, acromioclavicular joint, clavicle, and coracoid are clearly outlined. The humeral head is palpated by placing the fingers anteriorly and the thumb posteriorly. The joint can be localized by the thumb as a posterior soft spot. This point, 3 cm inferior and 2 cm medial to the posterolateral tip of the acromion, is the posterior portal site (Fig. 13–1). Anatomically this portal passes through the lower border of the infraspinatus. The final localization of the joint is performed by placing a finger on the coracoid to demonstrate the plane of the glenoid articular surface.

A spinal needle is then placed in the joint through the posterior portal site and the joint filled with 30 to 40 ml of a 1:300,000 epinephrine solution. The arthroscope is then introduced into the joint along the same path as the spinal needle, with the distended capsule providing an easier target. Inflow is initially established through the arthroscope and the joint is visualized. Using the biceps tendon as our landmark, we orient the joint in a vertical or anatomic position (Fig. 13–3).

Before examining the joint we establish an anterior portal to be used for both inflow and instrumentation. We use a disposable cannula with a side port for inflow and a diaphragm covering the main port. After localization of the biceps tendon and orientation of the joint, the triangular space of the anterior portal can be localized. The intra-articular space is bordered superiorly

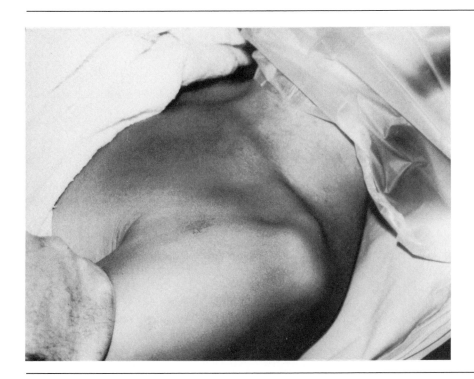

Fig. 13–2 The sulcus sign: distal traction produces a sulcus between the acromion and inferiorly subluxated humeral head. This is the most consistent physical finding in inferior laxity.

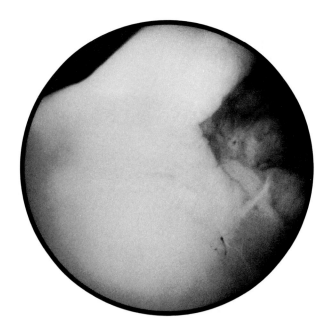

Fig. 13-3 View of the biceps tendon insertion into the glenoid with the joint oriented vertically.

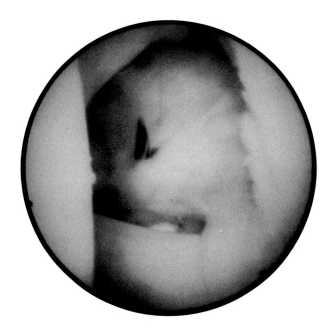

Fig. 13-4 A spinal needle piercing the triangular space for the anterior portal: the humeral head is on the left, the glenoid on the right, the biceps tendon is seen superiorly and the subscapularis tendon forms the inferior border.

by the biceps tendon, inferiorly by the subscapularis tendon, and medially by the anterosuperior portion of the glenoid (Fig. 13–4). The subscapularis tendon is a rounded, discrete, tendinous structure in the area of the anterior capsule.

Next, the exterior site of entrance is created on the anterior aspect of the shoulder. The spot chosen should be lateral and superior to the coracoid (Fig. 13–5). This avoids potential injury to the neurovascular structures in the area. Anatomic studies of the anterior portal performed by Matthews and associates[6] demonstrated that using the region medial to the coracoid places the brachial plexus and axillary vessels at risk, whereas using the inferolateral area places the musculocutaneous and subscapularis nerves at risk. The portal can then be established in either a retrograde fashion (placing the arthroscope against the anterior portal site from within and incising the skin overlying it) or an antegrade fashion (placing a spinal needle through the chosen exterior site into the intra-articular triangle under direct vision; the needle is then replaced with a cannula with removable trocar).

Primary Joint Examination and Normal Anatomy

We begin by following the biceps tendon throughout its intra-articular course from its passage out laterally into the biceps sleeve (Fig. 13–6) to the supraglenoid tubercle where it blends with the superior glenoid labrum (Fig. 13–3). The tendon should appear round and smooth with no evidence of flattening or fraying. Using the biceps tendon as our guide, we identify the glenoid

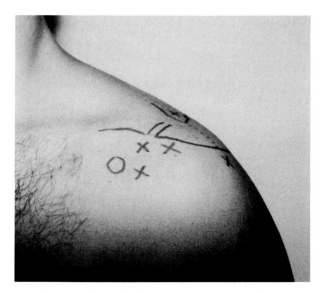

Fig. 13-5 Anterior view of the shoulder, with the coracoid represented by a circle; the three X's lateral to the coracoid demonstrate potential sites for the anterior portal.

labrum and follow it anteriorly around the glenoid face (Fig. 13–7). Moseley and Övergaard[7] demonstrated that the labrum is composed primarily of fibrous tissue, unlike the fibrocartilaginous meniscus of the knee. A small amount of fibrocartilaginous tissue is present within the

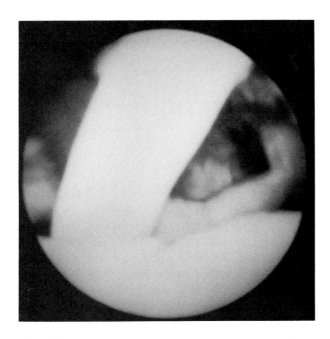

Fig. 13-6 The biceps tendon coursing laterally to exit the joint via the biceps sleeve.

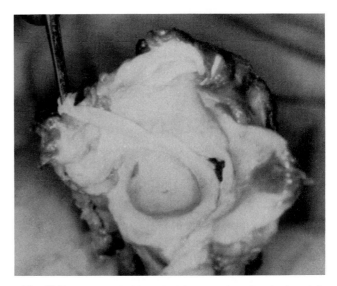

Fig. 13-7 Forceps holding the biceps tendon. Continuity of the biceps tendon with the glenoid labrum is evident.

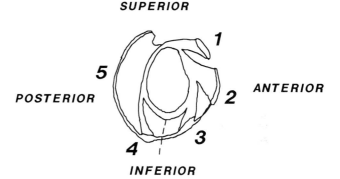

Fig. 13-8 Drawing of the capsular system: 1, biceps tendon; 2, middle glenohumeral ligament; 3, superior band of inferior glenohumeral ligament; 4, superior band of the posterior inferior glenohumeral ligament; and 5, posterior capsule.

labrum but is confined to a small transitional zone where the labrum attaches to the glenoid rim. There is great individual variation in the normal labrum. Commonly the labrum is thin superiorly and thick inferiorly. It ranges from 1 to 5 mm in width. In cross section the labrum is wedge-shaped; in the thicker portion it can be meniscoid in appearance.

The labrum can be viewed in its entirety arthroscopically from the primary posterior portal. The posterior labrum can be visualized more easily if the assistant externally rotates the humerus, relaxing the posterior capsule. The labrum should appear smooth. It should be probed to confirm that it is firmly attached at all margins of the glenoid. At the same time, the articular surface is visualized to assess the cartilage, subchondral plate, and the bony architecture of the glenoid. The normal glenoid is oval and covered by healthy articular cartilage. A central "bare area" devoid of articular cartilage occurs as a normal variant.

Returning anteriorly, the arthroscope is now focused on the anterior capsular structures. In 1883, Schlemm[8] described the capsule as having three areas of distinct thickening; he called them the superior, middle, and inferior glenohumeral ligaments (Fig. 13–8).

The superior glenohumeral ligament has been consistently described as originating, together with the biceps tendon, from the supraglenoid tubercle and adjacent labrum and inserting on the humerus in a small fovea (the fovea capitis) proximal to the lesser tuberosity. Because of its proximity to the biceps tendon, it is often obscured and is rarely visualized arthroscopi-

cally. Turkel and associates[9] found that this ligament, which becomes lax with progressive arm abduction and takes up tension only with the arm at the side, did not function in the prevention of anterior translation of the humerus on the glenoid.

Below the superior glenohumeral ligament is the most distinct structure of the anterior capsular mechanism: the subscapularis tendon. It enters the joint as a discrete, round, tendinous structure via the subscapularis bursa situated between the superior and middle glenohumeral ligaments, traveling to its insertion on the lesser tuberosity of the humerus. The tendon tightens during both external rotation and abduction of the glenohumeral joint; with internal rotation the tendon

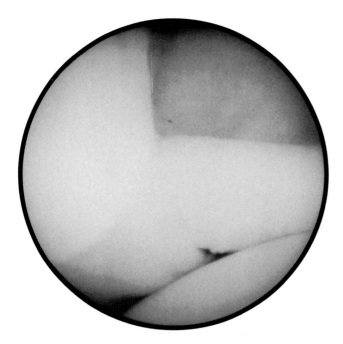

Fig. 13-9 The humeral head is at the lower right and the glenoid is at the upper left; the subscapularis tendon is seen transversely with the middle glenohumeral ligament draped over the lower border of the subscapularis.

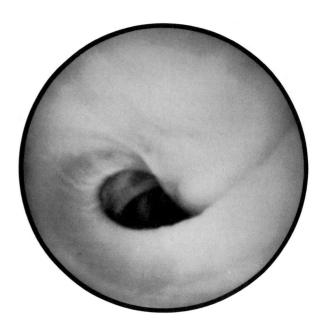

Fig. 13-10 The axillary pouch seen from a posterior view during external rotation of the humerus, demonstrating the "wind-up" of the normal axillary pouch.

becomes lax. As abduction progressively increases, the tendon of the subscapularis moves to a superior position, leaving the inferior portion of the humeral head uncovered anteriorly. Turkel and associates[9] concluded that the subscapularis is not an effective check or block to anterior dislocation at higher degrees of abduction.

Below the subscapularis tendon is the middle glenohumeral ligament. It has two alternative sites of origin. The first and most common is the supraglenoid tubercle and superior labrum just below the superior glenohumeral ligament. It sometimes arises not from the labrum but from the scapular neck. The insertion site is at the junction of the lesser tuberosity and the anatomic neck of the humerus. This variability of origin site can have important functional implications, as a scapular rather than labral origin creates a large anterior pouch that could, theoretically, contribute to anterior instability.[10] Arthroscopically it appears as a band immediately below the subscapularis tendon, between it and the thick superior edge of the inferior glenohumeral ligament (Figs. 13–8 and 13–9). Like the subscapularis, the middle glenohumeral ligament moves progressively higher relative to the humeral head with abduction of the arm. Turkel and associates[9] demonstrated that it is effective in preventing anterior dislocation only at less than 45 degrees of abduction.

When viewed from the posterior arthroscopic portal, the inferior glenohumeral ligament has three distinct parts and is the best defined of the glenohumeral ligaments. The thickened anterosuperior band (originating from the anterior margin of the glenoid labrum below the epiphyseal line of the glenoid), the axillary pouch (a diffuse thickening of the inferior portion of the capsule), and the posterosuperior band (the posterior counterpart to the anterosuperior band) insert in sequence around the anatomic neck of the humerus (Fig. 13–8). While the ligament is viewed, the arm is progressively externally rotated in adduction; the anterosuperior band becomes taut while the axillary pouch remains capacious. As the arm is progressively abducted, the axillary pouch "winds up," decreasing its volume as its fibers become taut (Fig. 13–10). At 90 degrees of abduction and maximal external rotation, the anterior and inferior aspects of the humeral head are covered by a continuous, taut ligamentous structure.

Recent work has focused on the contribution of the posterior portion of the inferior glenohumeral ligament to shoulder stability. When the arm is placed in 90 degrees of abduction and neutral rotation and the humerus is flexed 30 degrees forward in the horizontal plane, the posterior superior band of the inferior glenohumeral ligament is an important restraint to anteroposterior translation of the humeral head.[11]

After complete evaluation of the capsular mechanism, attention is directed laterally to the humeral head. By means of a sequence of internal rotation to assess the anterior aspect, external rotation to assess the posterior aspect, and abduction to examine the superior

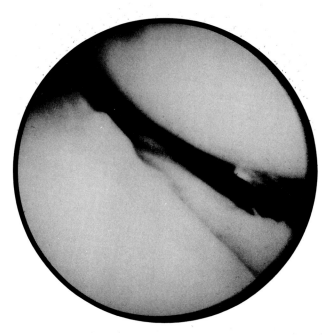

Fig. 13-11   A Bankart lesion with the glenoid below and the humeral head above. The labrum is detached from the glenoid margin.

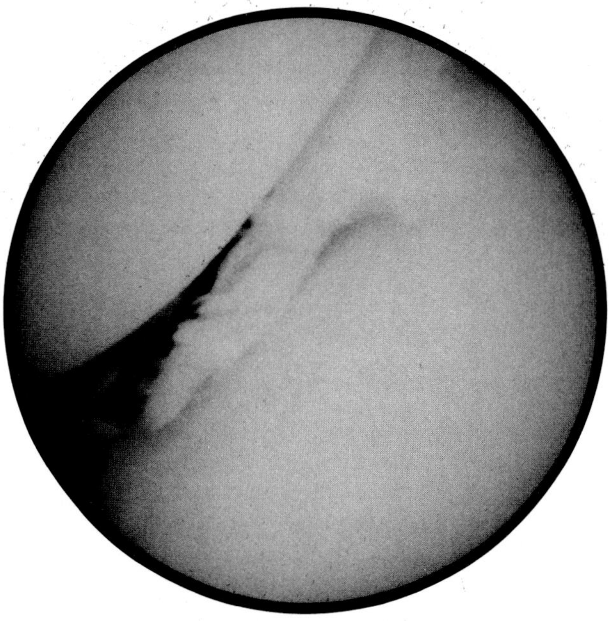

Fig. 13-12   The humeral head is at the upper left and the glenoid is at the lower right. Flap tear of the anterosuperior labrum projects into the joint.

area, the entire articular surface, including the insertion of the rotator cuff, can be visualized. A normal sulcus is present posteriorly between the insertion of the posterior capsule and overlying synovial membrane and the edge of the articular surface. DePalma and associates[12] found a variability in the size of this bare area that is directly proportional to age. In young patients no such area is seen.

Pathologic Anatomy of the Unstable Shoulder

Labrum and Glenoid The labrum plays a significant role in the prevention of shoulder instability. Through its wedge shape it increases both the depth and the conformity of the glenoid and serves as the site of attachment of the glenohumeral ligaments of the scapula. It appears that the inferior one half of the labrum, in the area of attachment of the inferior glenohumeral ligament, is relatively more important than its superior counterpart in stabilizing the glenohumeral joint.

Inferior labral lesions thought to occur secondary to increased humeral head translation take one of two forms: detachment from the scapular neck (Bankart lesion) (Fig. 13-11) or tearing of its substance (Figs. 13-12 and 13-13), similar to a knee meniscus. Associated erosion or fracture of the glenoid margin may be found in the area of labral detachment.

Superior labral lesions are frequently degenerative, resulting in tearing of the labrum. Overhand athletes, particularly throwers, often demonstrate superior labral abnormality. Andrews and Carson[13] demonstrated that tension in the biceps muscle is transmitted to the anterosuperior portion of the labrum. They hypothesized that repetitive throwing leads to tearing of the labrum in this region. Detrisac and Johnson[14] noted a labral "sulcus" at the 2 o'clock position as a normal variant in approximately 20% of individuals. This is not a detachment and can be recognized by its smooth borders (Fig. 13-14).

Glenohumeral Ligaments The inferior glenohumeral ligament is the prime stabilizer of the joint. The ligament is effective only when firmly attached to the glenoid rim. Because the labrum serves as the site of attachment, a detached inferior labrum represents a nonfunctional inferior glenohumeral ligament. Less frequently, the ligament may be avulsed from the labrum, torn within its substance, or congenitally poorly formed or absent. When a multidirectional component is present, the anterior and axillary pouch appears more capacious than usual and often the labrum appears to be intact and firmly attached. The anterosuperior band, if present, does not become taut with external rotation and the axillary portion of the inferior glenohumeral ligament does not wind up in its usual fashion.

Humeral Head In cases of recurrent anterior dislocation, more than 80% of patients have a Hill-Sachs lesion at the posterolateral margin of the humeral articular surface. The location of the Hill-Sachs lesion is just medial to the normal bare area or "sulcus" previously described. The Hill-Sachs lesion has articular cartilage lateral to it; its surface is raw and cancellous while the

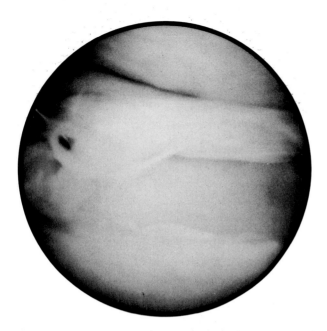

Fig. 13-13 Bucket-handle tear of the posterior labrum. The humeral head is seen above. The probe entering from the left displaces the bucket fragment into the joint. The labral rim remains on the bottom.

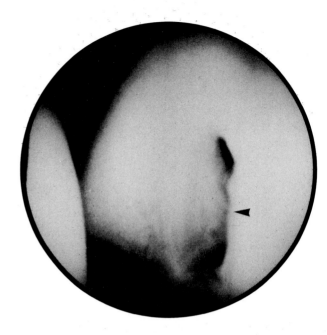

Fig. 13-14 The humeral head is at the left and the glenoid at the right. The well-rounded labral sulcus is seen in the mid-portion.

normal sulcus is smooth with vascular channels (Fig. 13-15). Patients with recurrent subluxation can demonstrate vertical ridging of the humeral subchondral surface and cartilage wear.

Loose Bodies Loose bodies secondary to the repetitive trauma of instability are present in about 10% of unstable shoulders and should be looked for, particularly in the axillary recess where they often collect (Fig. 13-16). When loose bodies are found in the shoulder of patients undergoing arthroscopy for any reason, the patient's history and physical findings should be carefully reevaluated for evidence of instability.

Treatment

Labral Debridement

Like the meniscus of the knee, the torn glenoid labrum can cause clicking or pain. Unlike the knee, locking is almost unheard of; nonetheless, a torn but attached labrum can, by interrupting the mechanics of the joint, cause a sense of instability. We have found debridement of the flaps of the labrum inferiorly or the detached or torn labrum superiorly to be successful in providing symptomatic relief in most cases. Andrews and Carson[13] pointed out that this is particularly true in throwers with an anterosuperior labral lesion. In a patient with documented or suspected instability, sim-

ple debridement of labral flaps may temporarily decrease pain but the instability will persist.

The debridement technique is similar to partial meniscectomy in the knee. Using hand or motorized shaving instruments, the surgeon resects the torn labrum back to a stable rim and contours the leading edges to achieve a smooth transition. Excessive removal of labral tissue should be avoided as this may lead to loss of ligament function.

Arthroscopic Stabilization

The common denominator underlying all arthroscopic shoulder stabilization procedures for anterior instability is reestablishment of a functional inferior glenohumeral ligament. This is achieved by reattaching the avulsed labrum with the ligament in continuity or by reattaching the ligament directly to the glenoid neck. We have performed the procedure successfully on patients with acute/recurrent, traumatic, anterior subluxation or dislocation. We have avoided cases with inferior or multidirectional components. These patients have marked redundancy of capsular tissue, making appropriate tensioning difficult to achieve arthroscopically.

Many methods of fixation have been advocated: metallic implants such as staples and screws, sutures, and, recently, biodegradable tacks. In addition, Caspari[15] developed a technique of inferior glenohumeral ligament reconstruction using a section of allograft iliotibial band. The allograft, which is fixed through a drill hole in the scapula and to the humerus by a screw with a ligament

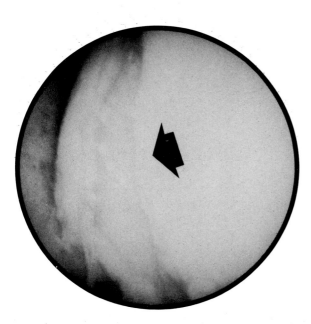

Fig. 13–15 The articular surface is at the left. There is a Hill-Sachs lesion between two areas of cartilage (arrowhead).

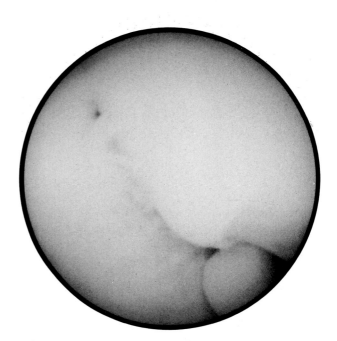

Fig. 13–16 A loose body in the axillary recess at the bottom right.

washer, functions as a sling that tightens during abduction and external rotation of the arm. Caspari has performed 100 procedures to date with no recurrent instability and excellent preservation of motion.

We are in agreement with Zuckerman and Matsen,[16] who reported an unacceptably high rate of significant complications related to the use of metal screws and staples placed in and around the shoulder. The most commonly used arthroscopic metallic device is a dual-prolonged staple. Johnson,[17] who reported on the largest series using this device, found a 15% redislocation rate in the early group. With more experience and the implementation of three weeks of immobilization and discontinuance of contact sports, the redislocation rate was reduced to 3%. In addition to redislocation, there are problems of impingement of the staple and loosening; these are thought to be related to initial positioning. The staple must be implanted with both prongs in bone and must be placed superior to the equator of the glenoid. Wiley[18] described a small series of arthroscopic stabilizations using a rivet that is removed six weeks postoperatively. Although the redislocation rate and complication rate were low, the follow-up period was too short for final judgment.

Since 1983 we have used a suture technique in which knotted sutures transfix the tissue and are passed through transglenoid drill holes. More recently, we have used a biodegradable tack placed in a predrilled hole for stabilization of anterior dislocation or subluxation.

Techniques of Arthroscopic Stabilization

Suture Technique

Besides the standard operating equipment and set-up previously described for shoulder arthroscopy, we use pins measuring 30 cm × 2 mm with two eyelets and a sharp point to drill the suture through the bone. A power drill should be available for insertion. The suture material used is absorbable 0 PDS.

After induction of anesthesia and confirmation that the instability pattern is anterior, we position the patient in the upright sitting position with the arm free at the side. The arthroscope is inserted through the posterior portal as previously described, the standard anterior portal is established with a cannula, and a complete diagnostic arthroscopy is carried out. In particular, the labrum is examined for site of detachment, continuity with ligament structures, and overall tissue quality. If a detached labrum is present, it is grasped by an instrument placed through the anterior cannula. As tension is placed on the labrum, the inferior glenohumeral ligament is viewed. A functional labrum should transmit the tension and the ligament should tighten. If the labrum is absent, nonfunctional, or of poor quality, a discrete superior band of the inferior glenohumeral ligament should be identified. This is grasped and pulled up to the 3 o'clock position on the anterior glenoid rim. As this is done, the anterior pouch should disappear and tension should be seen in the anterior ligament structures. If neither a functional labrum nor a discrete ligamentous band is present, the arthroscopic procedure should be aborted and open stabilization performed.

Next, we perform a careful but complete debridement of the anterior glenoid rim and scapular neck to achieve a raw bony surface. The drill holes are then localized. We use two drill holes: one superior at the 2 o'clock position and one inferior at the 4 o'clock position; each has two sutures. The pins should enter 2 to 3 mm medial to the edge of the glenoid rim and travel posteriorly, diverging from the articular surface of the glenoid. Excessive lateral exit of the pin posteriorly must be avoided to prevent injury to the suprascapular nerve (Fig. 13–17). If the original anterior portal is adequate for pin placement, we create a second anterior portal more superiorly to allow for grasping and tensioning of the labral or ligamentous tissue. Localization of this portal is done with a percutaneous spinal needle. The portal is established with a cannula.

The tissue is grasped through the superior portal and reduced under tension to the anterior glenoid rim. With humeral rotation at neutral, the pin is placed through the drilling portal and the sharp end is used to spear a robust section of the tissue. The point is then placed at the superior drill hole and the pin is drilled from anterior to posterior, diverging medial to the glenoid surface. The pin is drilled through the posterior cortex and to the skin posteriorly where a 5-mm skin portal is created.

The drill is then placed on the extruding pin posteriorly and the two 0 PDS sutures are threaded through the eyelets. The pin is then drilled completely through posteriorly while one end of the suture is retained anteriorly. The anterior sutures are then grasped intra-articularly through the superior portal and pulled up through this portal. This frees the suture from the drilling portal. A second set of sutures is then passed in a similar fashion at the 4 to 5 o'clock position. The posterior tails from the second set of sutures are transferred subcutaneously to the first posterior skin portal. One anterior suture from each set of two is tied to a suture from the other set with a bulky knot. The knots are then pulled through the anterior cannula by posterior tension. Under direct vision the knots should oppose the labral or ligamentous tissue to the glenoid rim under tension. Because this tightens the entire anterior recess, visualization of the anterior rim may become more difficult at this point. The tissue should be probed to be sure that the knots have not cut through. If satisfactory, the sutures are tied to themselves subcutaneously in the posterior portal over the thick fascia of the infraspinatus. The skin is closed meticulously over the sutures with no dermal pouching.

The arthroscope is then removed and the patient is placed in a shoulder immobilizer in complete internal rotation. The patient is transferred to the recovery room and may be discharged if conditions are appropriate.

Postoperative Regimen

The shoulder is maintained in internal rotation by means of an immobilizer. We use an immobilizer that

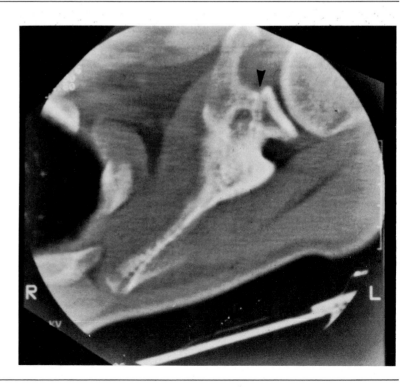

Fig. 13–17 A computed tomographic scan of the scapula of a patient who underwent arthroscopic suture stabilization. Arrowhead points to the pin tract.

allows elbow flexion and extension exercises to be performed without changing the position of the humerus. After six weeks the immobilizer is removed and range-of-motion exercises are begun. Once a complete range of motion is established through passive-and active-assisted exercises, resistance exercises for the deltoid and rotator cuff are initiated. At four months, motion is usually complete and strength sufficient to allow return to light throwing or racket sports. Contact sports and unrestricted activity begin at six months.

Technique of Stabilization Using Biodegradable Tack

The equipment for this procedure is still in an evolutionary stage. At present we use a cannulated tack made of biodegradable material. The cannula system used allows for drilling and tack insertion.

The initial setup, examination, and diagnostic arthroscopy are performed as previously described. The same criteria for tissue laxity, quality, and location are used to decide whether or not the procedure can be successfully carried out.

If conditions are appropriate, the glenoid rim is prepared and a second superior anterior portal is created. The tissue (labrum or ligament) is reduced with appropriate tension to the glenoid rim. The tissue is then speared with a pointed guidewire and positioned on the glenoid far enough superior to allow fixation of the tissue with tension. The wire is impacted into the glenoid rim 2 to 3 mm medial to the articular surface. A cannulated drill is passed over the wire and drilled to the depth of the staple. The staple is impacted under direct vision and the tissue and staple are probed to ensure that the staple has not cut through and is well fixed.

Postoperative management is identical to that for the suture procedure.

Results

We have performed 17 stabilizations with the suture technique (maximum follow-up, four years). Thus far we have had no recurrences and have had one complication. One patient developed a synovial cyst that emanated from a glenoid drill hole. The patient was aware of a posterior mass and underwent excisional biopsy with excellent results. Morgan and Bodenstab[19] reported on a series of arthroscopic stabilizations using a modification of the suture technique. During a short follow-up period, 25 patients who underwent the procedure had no episodes of recurrence and had excellent shoulder function.

The biodegradable tack has been in use since the autumn of 1987. Twenty patients have undergone the procedure and there have been no recurrences and no complications to date.

Summary

The arthroscope is a valuable adjunct in the diagnosis and treatment of shoulder instability. Throwing athletes with shoulder pain, and those with subluxation in particular, may require diagnostic arthroscopy to clarify the instability pattern. Labral debridement, if confined to the portion above the equator of the glenoid, can provide symptomatic relief. Arthroscopic stabilization of the shoulder is still in an evolutionary phase. No long-term data exist as to which technique or material provides the most secure fixation. All of these techniques are technically demanding and require a skilled arthroscopist.

References

1. Burman MS: Arthroscopy or the direct visualization of joints: An experimental cadaver study. *J Bone Joint Surg* 1931;13:669–695.
2. Andrén L, Lundberg BJ: Treatment of rigid shoulders by joint distention during arthrography. *Acta Orthop Scand* 1965;36:45–53.
3. Watanabe M: Arthroscopy: The present state. *Orthop Clin North Am* 1979;10:505–522.
4. Klein AH, France JC: Measurement of brachial plexus strain in arthroscopy of the shoulder. *Arthroscopy* 1982;3:45–52.
5. Neer CS III, Foster CR: Inferior capsular shift for involuntary inferior and multidirectional instability of the shoulder: A preliminary report. *J Bone Joint Surg* 1980;62A:897–908.
6. Matthews L, Zarins B, Michael RH, et al: Anterior portal selection for shoulder arthroscopy. *Arthroscopy* 1985;1:33–39.
7. Moseley HF, Övergaard B: The anterior capsular mechanism in recurrent anterior dislocation of the shoulder: Morphological and clinical studies with special reference to the glenoid labrum and the glenohumeral ligament. *J Bone Joint Surg* 1962;44B:913–927.
8. Schlemm F: Uber die Verstarkungsbander am Schultergelenk. *Arch Anat* 1853:45–48.
9. Turkel SJ, Panio MW, Marshall JL, et al: Stabilizing mechanisms preventing anterior dislocation of the glenohumeral joint. *J Bone Joint Surg* 1981;63A:1208–1217.
10. Uhthoff K, Piscopo M: Anterior capsular redundancy of the shoulder: Congenital or traumatic? An embryological study. *J Bone Joint Surg* 1985;67B:363–366.
11. Schwartz R, O'Brien SJ, Warren RF: Posterior shoulder. Presented at the meeting of the American Shoulder and Elbow Surgeons, Atlanta, Feb 7, 1988.
12. DePalma AF, et al: Degenerative lesions of the shoulder joint at various age groups which are compatible with good function, in Pease CN (ed): American Academy of Orthopaedic Surgeons *Instructional Course Lectures, VII.* Ann Arbor, JW Edwards, 1950, pp 168–180.
13. Andrews JR, Carson WG Jr, McLeod WD: Glenoid labrum tears related to the long head of the biceps. *Am J Sports Med* 1985;13:337–341.
14. Detrisac DA, Johnson LL: *Arthroscopic Shoulder Anatomy: Pathologic and Surgical Implications.* Thorofare, New Jersey, Slack, 1986.
15. Caspari RB: Arthroscopic evaluation and reconstruction for shoulder instability. Presented at the meeting of the Arthroscopy Association of North America, Atlanta, Feb 7, 1988.
16. Zuckerman JD, Matsen FA III: Complications about the glenohumeral joint related to the use of screws and staples. *J Bone Joint Surg* 1984;66A:175–180.

17. Johnson LL: Arthroscopic management for shoulder instability: Stapling. Presented at the meeting of the Arthroscopy Association of North America, Atlanta, Feb 7, 1988.

18. Wiley AM: Arthroscopy for shoulder instability and a technique for arthroscopic repair. *Arthroscopy* 1988;4:25–30.

19. Morgan CD, Bodenstab AB: Arthroscopic Bankart suture repair: Technique and early results. *Arthroscopy* 1987;3:111–122.

CHAPTER 14

Intra-articular Inflammatory Diseases of the Shoulder

Thomas J. Neviaser, MD

Intra-articular inflammatory diseases of the shoulder may produce acute or chronic symptoms. Among the acute conditions are acute gouty arthritis, acute bacterial infections, and acute nonspecific inflammation. Because these entities are somewhat uncommon, all extra-articular causes of acute shoulder pain must be ruled out as soon as possible. These include cervical spine disorders, acute calcific rotator cuff tendinitis, undetected fractures, acute tendinitis, and others. Aspiration of the shoulder joint fluid along with appropriate laboratory studies (crystals, Gram stain, and cultures) may help differentiate these intra-articular conditions.

Acute gouty arthritis produces a swollen, hot, and painful shoulder and severely restricted motion. After aspiration for crystal examination, and other appropriate studies, treatment will make the acute condition subside quickly.

An acute bacterial infection must be suspected in all acute intra-articular shoulder problems and must be the first diagnosis eliminated. The joint must be aspirated and aerobic and anaerobic cultures and Gram stain studies must be performed immediately. Treatment with an intravenous broad-spectrum antibiotic must be started as soon as the aspirate is taken. The antibiotic is changed as necessary. If the symptoms do not improve dramatically in 24 to 48 hours, arthroscopic irrigation and debridement should be performed in conjunction with the administration of appropriate intravenous antibiotics. If the infection fails to respond in 24 to 48 hours, open arthrotomy with anterior and posterior drainage is indicated. Intravenous antibiotic administration should continue for six weeks. After the acute infection subsides, daily physical therapy should be instituted to regain the motion lost during the acute phase.

Nonspecific inflammatory conditions of the shoulder joint are diagnosed by exclusion and are treated conservatively with rest, heat or ice, nonsteroidal anti-inflammatory medications, and, occasionally, steroids. When all conservative treatments fail and all extra-articular processes have been excluded, arthroscopic evaluation and synovectomy should be done.

Osteoarthritis

Osteoarthritis of the shoulder joint is uncommon. It can be classified as degenerative, traumatic, or postin-

fectious. Patients with intractable pain, moderate to severe restriction of motion, and radiographic evidence of severe degenerative findings are normally treated by total replacement arthroplasties. In those cases in which muscular weakness and paralysis are the primary causes, a shoulder fusion is warranted.

Patients who have pain but only mild restriction of motion and radiographic evidence of early degenerative changes, and in whom conservative management has failed, may improve after arthroscopic synovectomy and abrasion arthroplasty. This procedure removes the reactive synovitis, smooths the irregular articular surfaces of the humeral head and glenoid, and removes loose bodies. A 1-mm abrasion into the subchondral bone may promote new growth of fibrocartilage and slow the degenerative process.[1,2]

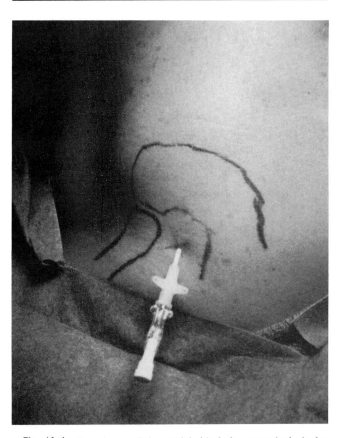

Fig. 14–1 Superior medial portal behind the acromioclavicular joint.

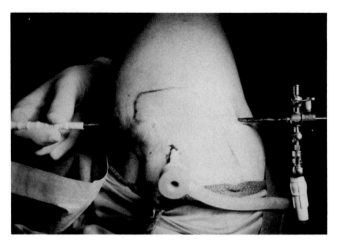

Fig. 14-2 Surgical portals in the shoulder. The anterior portal is at the left.

Rheumatoid Arthritis

After unsuccessful medical treatment in a shoulder with rheumatoid arthritis but little radiographic evidence of degeneration, a complete arthroscopic synovectomy is the treatment of choice. Almost the entire synovium of the shoulder joint can be removed; if the articular surfaces have been spared, the results can be quite good. The timing of the synovectomy is very important because rheumatoid synovitis may lead to eventual subchondral pittings, and erosions and degenerative changes develop quickly. When articular erosions exist, the principles of abrasion arthroplasty can be instituted, but the results are usually less than adequate when compared with those in osteoarthritic shoulders.

Surgical Technique

After the patient is placed in the lateral decubitus position with 10 to 15 lb of traction on the affected arm, a No. 18 spinal needle is placed within the shoulder joint from the posterior portal side. Saline is injected into the joint and the syringe removed from the needle. There should be vigorous return of fluid. If no fluid returns, the needle should be replaced and saline reinjected until fluid return occurs. Only an experienced shoulder arthroscopist should attempt to place an arthroscopic trocar into the joint blindly without distending the joint first. Once the joint is distended, the trocar can be placed gently into the joint with its stopcock opened so that the fluid again returns, proving that the arthroscopic cannula is indeed within the joint. With the arthroscope in place, it is easy to visualize the humeral head, glenoid, or the biceps tendon. Outflow can be initially established by placing a 16-gauge plastic cannulated needle through the superior medial portal behind the acromioclavicular joint (Fig. 14–1). The needle enters the joint in the vicinity of the origin of the long head of the biceps if it is angled approximately 30 to 40 degrees laterally and slightly

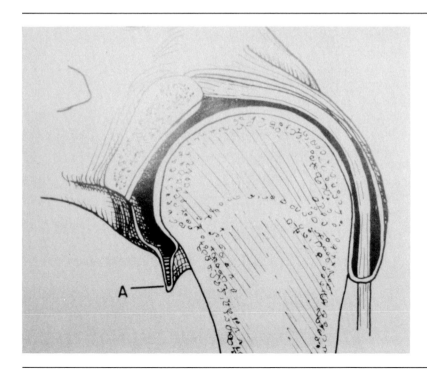

A

Fig. 14-3 Diagram of dependent fold adhesions in adhesive capsulitis.

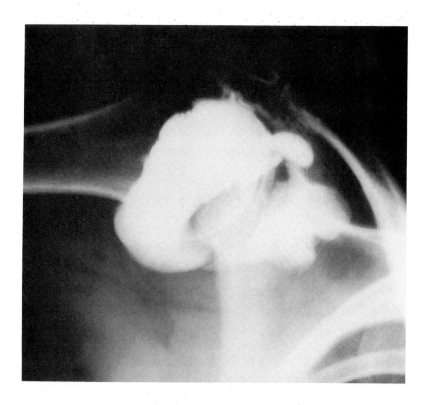

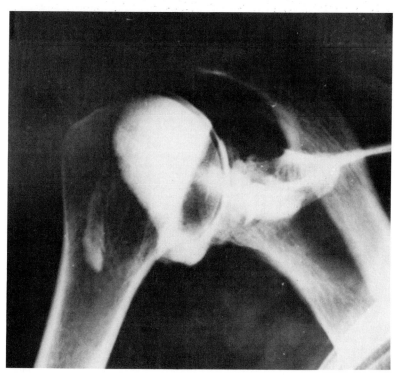

Fig. 14-4 Arthrograms of dependent fold. **Top:** Normal fold is spacious. **Bottom:** In adhesive capsulitis, the fold is very small.

anteriorly. For surgical arthroscopy, this needle can be replaced by a leak-proof instrument-compatible cannula. The saline inflow can then be attached to this cannula, allowing better distension of the joint and reducing the bleeding.

After diagnostic evaluation of the joint, the final sur-

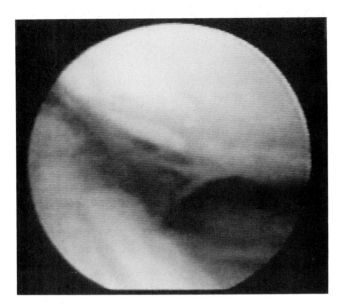

Fig. 14–5 Acute adhesion formation in stage 2 adhesive capsulitis.

gical portal is placed anteriorly through the soft spot just superior to the upper edge of the intra-articular portion of the subscapularis. This is done with a long K-wire or rod. An appropriate cannula is passed into the joint with a rod used as a guide anteriorly (Fig. 14–2). Only after all three portals have been established and saline flow is good can surgical arthroscopy be performed adequately.

In the rheumatoid shoulder, the synovectomy is usu-ally started through the anterior portal until all acces-sible areas have been shaved. The shaver is then switched to the superior medial portal and then to the posterior portal until all areas have been shaved. The posterior portal is established by means of a switching stick through the arthroscopic cannula and replacement of this cannula with an appropriate surgical cannula while the switching stick is in place. The scope can then be gently placed in the anterior or superior portal cannula for visualization while the posterior synovectomy is being done.

In the osteoarthritic shoulder, the synovectomy tech-nique is the same, but an abrasion arthroplasty is usu-ally done after the synovectomy. A full-radius resector is used to denude the diseased articular cartilage frag-ments. Next, an abrasion burr is used to smooth the bony surfaces of the humerus and glenoid that artic-ulate with one another. Pin-point bleeding is all that is necessary. Aggressive debridement and abrasion of more than 1 mm is not needed. Not all the osteophytes and degenerative changes need to be removed. The inferior humeral osteophytes are usually left alone unless they are easily resected or obviously obstruct a smooth glen-ohumeral articulation. It is important to debride and smooth at least the central half of the glenoid and the central half of the humeral head articulation. The sur-geon can get a better view of the physiologic position of the humerus and glenoid by removing the abducted arm from traction to visualize the articulation with the arm by the side. Once the bony work and synovectomy are completed, mild rotator cuff trimming and shaving

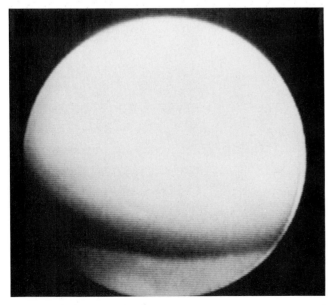 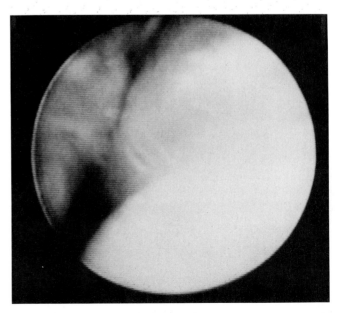

Fig. 14–6 Loss of normal spaces. **Left:** There is no space between the humeral head and glenoid. **Right:** There is no space between the biceps tendon and the humeral head.

can be accomplished. Aggressive irrigation and vacuuming are the last steps.

Adhesive Capsulitis

Adhesive capsulitis is still a poorly understood disease process of the shoulder. Its cause is unknown. The pathology of adhesive capsulitis was first described by Neviaser[3] in 1945. The adhesions found were definitely intra-articular and intracapsular. These adhesions propagate within the dependent fold of the shoulder joint, causing ever-increasing restriction of motion secondary to capsular scarring and fibrosis (Fig. 14–3). Pain usually increases as the acute process constricts the capsular structures. These adhesions were visualized during open procedures during which Neviaser cut the major capsular contracture in the dependent fold and then manipulated the shoulders. He advocated open manipulation only in those cases in which closed manipulation had failed.

Patients with adhesive capsulitis experience the insidious onset of pain and subsequent restriction of shoulder motion. Initially their pain may be somewhat similar to that of rotator cuff tendinitis in the impingement syndrome. Gradually, the pain increases and motion grossly decreases. Pure glenohumeral motion restriction and an obvious loss of external rotation are the hallmarks of adhesive capsulitis. However, these findings will appear in many stiff and painful shoulders because motion is restricted by pain and not pure capsular contracture. Arthrography is therefore necessary to prove the diagnosis. The pathognomonic arthrographic findings of adhesive capsulitis are severe restriction of the volumetric capacity of the joint (often only 5 to 8 ml of contrast medium can be introduced before the symptoms are reproduced) and obvious obliteration of the normal inferior dependent fold (Fig. 14–4).

Once the diagnosis is confirmed, physical therapy is instituted with the emphasis on passive stretching in all realms of motion, especially abduction, external rotation, and internal rotation. Wet heat and anti-inflammatory and pain medications may be needed. As well as working with the therapist, the patients must institute their own home programs and work very hard for the best and quickest outcome. The range of motion obtained with exercises may be slow to develop, but eventually most patients notice a reduction of pain as the motion improves.

For those patients whose symptoms and motion do not improve with an intensive therapy program, manipulation with the patient under general anesthesia is indicated. Arthroscopy makes possible the visualization of the disease process.[4,5] In those cases needing manipulation, adhesive capsulitis has been categorized into four separate arthroscopic stages. Stage 1 is the pread-

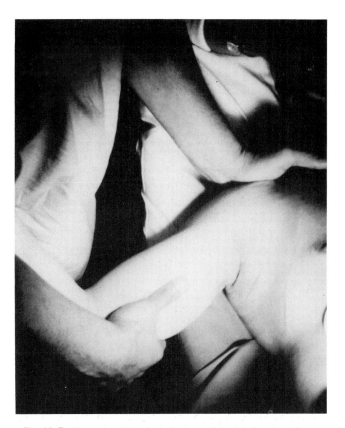

Fig. 14–7 Proper positioning of surgeon's hands for shoulder manipulation.

hesive stage in which there is a patchy low-lying fibrinous erythematous pannus of synovitis about the joint. This is particularly visible in the dependent axillary fold area. These patients have a good range of motion and their usual initial diagnosis is rotator cuff tendinitis of the impingement syndrome. Decompression produces terrible results in these cases because adhesive capsulitis progresses through all four stages. The restriction of motion caused by this disease and the pain and scar tissue from a decompression lead to a prolonged, painful postoperative course. Therefore, all surgeons are encouraged to use arthroscopy on their impingement syndrome cases before decompression. If this subtle pannus of synovitis is seen, no other surgery should be performed. These patients should begin an intensive therapy program to prevent subsequent loss of motion as adhesive capsulitis progresses.

Stage 2 of the disease is the most active and probably the most painful. Adhesions grow within the joint, accompanied by aggressive synovitis (Fig. 14–5). The restriction of the capsular structures is demonstrated by the loss of the normal space between the humeral head and the biceps tendon as well as between the humeral head and glenoid. In fact, the humeral head cannot be pulled away from the biceps tendon or glenoid even with traction (Fig. 14–6).

In stage 3, the synovitis abates and only a residual pink, fluffy synovitis is left. Again, restriction of motion and loss of the humeral head/glenoid space and humeral head/biceps space are evident.

In stage 4, synovitis is no longer evident, but it is almost impossible to visualize the dependent fold, which almost disappears once the adhesions have matured. Scarring across the dependent fold leaves very little motion.

Clinically, stage 1 of adhesive capsulitis begins with an insidious onset of pain or discomfort in the shoulder. Stage 2 is characterized by increasing pain, especially at night, and loss of motion. Most patients first note the loss of internal rotation. In stage 3, pain is usually less of a concern, and loss of motion becomes the major concern. In stage 4, the presenting complaint is usually loss of motion with the patient experiencing pain at the extremes of the range of motion. The course of the disease process lasts approximately one year to 18 months, and the time for each stage varies tremendously from patient to patient.

Manipulation of the shoulder with the patient under general anesthesia is the treatment of choice for those refractory cases of adhesive capsulitis in which pain and restriction of motion are unbearable. Once the patient is anesthetized and relaxed, the surgeon gently fixes the scapula with one hand and abducts the humerus by grasping it at its mid-point or slightly distal to the mid-point (Fig. 14–7). Forceful abduction may break the humerus, and heroic attempts at manipulation should be avoided. Gradual, gentle abduction allows the surgeon to feel and hear the adhesions tearing in the dependent fold. Once pure abduction of 90 degrees is obtained, the surgeon can then externally rotate and abduct the arm overhead as far as possible, ideally as far as the opposite, normal shoulder can be abducted. Internal rotation can then be obtained by rotating the arm inward while the humerus is abducted 90 degrees. Postoperatively, abduction and external rotation are maintained by a sling while the patient is in bed. Physical therapy is instituted on the same day and continued in the same way as the preoperative therapy.

Summary

Intra-articular disease processes of the shoulder are uncommon. Of all the processes, adhesive capsulitis is by far the most prevalent. Stage 1 of adhesive capsulitis mimics the impingement syndrome and must be ruled out by arthroscopy before decompression is performed. Other rare conditions of the shoulder joint, such as pigmented villonodular synovitis and synovial chondromatosis, can be treated with the same surgical techniques.

References

1. Johnson LL: Arthroscopic abrasion arthroplasty. Presented at the Annual Meeting of the American Academy of Orthopaedic Surgeons, Anaheim, CA, Mar 10–15, 1983.
2. Miller GK, Maylahn DJ, Drennan DB: The treatment of idiopathic osteonecrosis of the medial femoral condyle with arthroscopic debridement. *Arthroscopy* 1986;2:21–29.
3. Neviaser JS: Adhesive capsulitis of the shoulder: A study of the pathological findings in periarthritis of the shoulder. *J Bone Joint Surg* 1945;27:211–222.
4. Neviaser TJ: Adhesive capsulitis. *Orthop Clin North Am* 1987;18:439–443.
5. Neviaser TJ: Arthroscopy of the shoulder. *Orthop Clin North Am* 1987;18:361–372.

Impingement Problems in the Athlete

Frank W. Jobe, MD

Introduction

Shoulder problems in the young athlete must be viewed differently from those in the general population because of the high physical demands placed on the joint during overhand activities. The shoulder has a high degree of mobility that contributes to the function of the joint. Stability is also necessary and, when the soft tissues and supporting structures are subjected to repetitive stretches or injury during overhand activities, the delicate balance between function and stability can be upset. When the balance is upset, it is important to determine accurately whether the problem is one of impingement, instability, or, as occurs more often, a combination of both.

Once the diagnosis has been made, the decision is then whether to treat the problem with kinesiologic or anatomic repair.

Philosophy

As stated, the unique population of young (18- to 35-year-old) athletes in sports involving overhand movements requires a different perspective. For the young athlete, shoulder function and stability must be considered both anatomically and kinesiologically. The nature of the repetitive activity, whether it be throwing, swimming, or serving, and the function of the structures involved must be analyzed to understand the underlying problem.

Stabilizing Mechanisms

The shoulder joint is designed more for mobility than for stability. The stability that does exist comes from the scapular rotators, the rotator cuff, and the capsular and ligamentous structures. The scapular rotators (trapezius, rhomboids, and serratus anterior) are responsible for placing the glenoid in the optimal position for the activity being performed (Fig. 15–1). Firing of the rotator cuff muscles centers the humeral head in the most stable position in the glenoid while providing the maximal available leverage. The static stabilizers, which are the capsule and ligamentous structures, have a restraining effect at the margin of the glenoid. The structures described must work in almost perfect concert to avoid injury. There is a constant "trade-off" between stability and function at the shoulder. A gain in functional ability is achieved by a loss in stability. If the

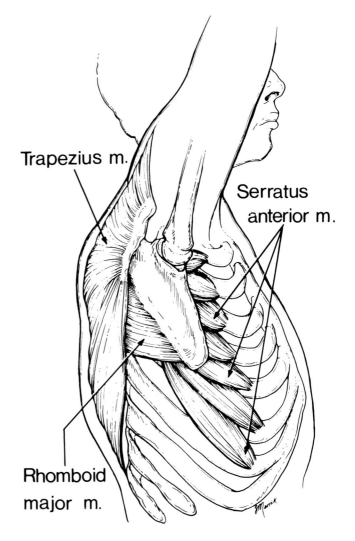

Fig. 15–1 The scapular rotators place the glenoid in the optimal position.

critical minimum for stability is exceeded, injury can occur.

Overhand Activities

Overhand activities are those activities performed at more than 90 degrees of abduction. Examples of this type of activity include, but are not limited to, pitching, swimming, racket sports, and the javelin throw. The position of maximum abduction and external rotation used in overhand sports is physiologically unstable. It stresses the stabilizing mechanisms. Overuse, common in athletic activities, stretches or injures the static stabilizers. This results in disrupting the synchronous firing of the scapular rotators and rotator cuff as these muscles attempt to provide the stability to the joint that was once provided by the static stabilizers.

Impingement and Instability

It is important to realize that impingement and instability are not two separate entities but rather are on a continuum of shoulder abnormalities. The continuum progresses from instability to subluxation to impingement to rotator cuff tear. For this reason, it is imperative that the instability problem be attacked first, before the impingement. A rotator cuff should never be surgically repaired without repairing the primary condition.

In the young athlete who participates in overhand sports, anterior instability is also most often the primary lesion. Impingement and rotator cuff tears are secondary. Anterior labrum and inferior glenohumeral ligament injuries appear to be the most common causes of instability.

Pathologic Findings

The pathologic finding associated with the impingement is a breakdown or stretching of the static stabilizers from overuse. This allows anterior subluxation of the humeral head. When the arm is abducted and externally rotated, the anterior subluxation of the humeral head causes impingement of the rotator cuff against the acromion and the coracoacromial ligament (Fig. 15–2).

Diagnostic Criteria

During the office visit, the patient will report a long history of overuse during overhand activities. Experience and sensitive fingers are the tools for the physical examination. The best test for shoulder instability is done with the patient positioned supine with the arm off the table at 90 degrees of abduction and external rotation. The examiner pushes anteriorly on the humeral head (Fig. 15–3, *left*). The test is repeated with the patient in the same position while the examiner gently pushes posteriorly (Fig. 15–3, *right*). The examiner is sometimes able to feel the sliding of the humeral head. Any subluxation noted in the anterior direction is considered pathologic. It is typically painful.

When the examiner presses posteriorly, the pain is usually relieved. Subluxation is most common in the anteroinferior quadrant. The humerus can subluxate as much as 50% in the posterior direction and still be considered normal. Impingement tests, such as the Hawkins or Neer tests, may or may not also be positive. As stated earlier, impingement is secondary to instability and, therefore, the impingement tests are not the key diagnostic tests.

If excessive subluxation is found clinically, arthroscopy will reveal damage to the anterior labrum, anterior capsule, inferior glenohumeral ligament, posterior humeral head, and/or the posterior labrum. The damage results from the humeral head coming into contact with the posterior rim of the glenoid while the shoulder is in the throwing position. This is frequently misdiagnosed as a Hill-Sachs lesion.

Kinesiologic Repair

As previously stated, the problem is both anatomic and kinesiologic. Whenever possible, it is best to correct the disturbance in kinesiology before anatomic damage occurs. In other words, kinesiologic repair is most successful as a preventive or early treatment technique. This is accomplished through a very specific exercise program.

The emphasis is on retraining the rotator cuff muscles to fire in proper synchrony to provide correct scapulohumeral rhythm and also to condition the scapular rotators. Regardless of what type of exercises are used to accomplish this, the patient should avoid hyperextension and abduction with external rotation. It is also important to strengthen the pectoralis major, coracobrachialis, and long head of the biceps brachii in patients with anterior instability as these muscles help support the anterior portion of the shoulder.

Rotator cuff strengthening can be accomplished isometrically, isotonically, or isokinetically. Internal and external rotation should be done both with the arm at the side and at 90 degrees of abduction. The supraspinatus can be isolated and strengthened with the upper extremity abducted to 90 degrees, internally rotated, and forward flexed 30 degrees.

There are three main exercises that strengthen the scapular rotators. The upper trapezius is strengthened by shoulder shrugs. The serratus anterior can be strengthened by doing push-ups. The patient can begin with wall push-ups and then progress to kneeling and full push-ups. Finally, the latissimus dorsi is strengthened by doing chin-ups. If the patient is unable to do chin-ups, then "pull-downs" can be substituted. The patient should avoid hyperextension at the shoulder while performing push-ups and pull-downs.

The remaining muscles at the shoulder should also be strengthened. The long head of the biceps, cora-

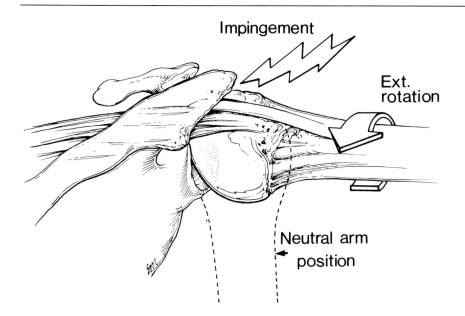

Impingement

Ext.
rotation

Neutral arm
position

Fig. 15-2 When the arm is abducted and externally rotated, the anterior subluxation of the humeral head causes impingement of the rotator cuff.

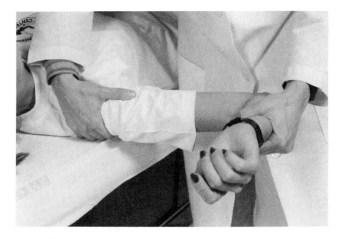
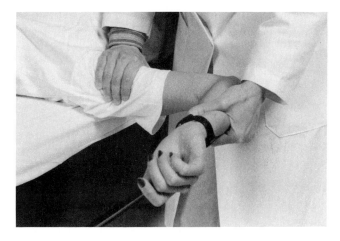

Fig. 15-3 Testing for shoulder instability. The examiner gently pushes the humeral head anteriorly (**left**) and posteriorly (**right**). (Reproduced with permission from Jobe FW, Bradley JP: Rotator cuff injuries in baseball: Prevention and rehabilitation. *Sports Med* 1988;6:377–386.)

cobrachialis, and anterior deltoid are strengthened by forward flexion. This should be limited to 90 degrees for most patients with instability. The pectoralis major and anterior deltoid muscles are strengthened by means of horizontal adduction exercises with the arm abducted to 90 degrees.

Generally, stretching exercises are contraindicated during kinesiologic repair. Some patients with anterior instability may also have tightness of the posterior deltoid, posterior capsule, and rhomboids. If the posterior deltoid is tight, it can position the head of the humerus too far forward in the fossa when it contracts. Posterior capsule tightness also causes forward displacement of the humeral head. I recommend gentle mobilization of

the posterior capsule and stretching of the posterior deltoid and rhomboids for these patients.

Anatomic Repair

Anatomic repair is done if the kinesiologic repair has failed or if there is anatomic damage.

There are four main guidelines in doing an anatomic repair: (1) The muscle attachments and proprioceptive fibers must be maintained. (2) The capsule should not be shortened too much because that would cause the shoulder to lose some of its mobility and function. (3) The anterior labrum must be built up. (4) Full range of motion must be regained quickly through abduction splinting and a rehabilitation program.

The anterior capsulolabral reconstruction technique was designed to meet these four guidelines (Fig. 15–4). Arthroscopy is done before the reconstruction to confirm the need for surgery. This, along with the history and physical examination, is a most important diagnostic tool. Special radiographs and an examination with the patient under anesthesia are not always helpful when making the diagnosis.

The patient is then placed in the supine position and a Parker armboard arranged for a modified axillary approach.

The deltopectoral groove is identified and the shoulder is approached through the deltopectoral interval. The interval is kept open by enlarged Goule retractors. The cephalic vein is dissected medially and retracted laterally; the conjoined tendon is then freed laterally and retracted with a small Richardson retractor. The subscapularis is split (two thirds of the muscle superiorly and one third inferiorly) with a coagulating Bovie cautery in the direction of its fibers.

The capsule is dissected beginning at the musculotendinous junction. A special curved Gelpi retractor is then inserted to retract, hold, and separate the two parts of the subscapularis. A three-pronged retractor is placed on the glenoid neck to expose the capsule. Then, a sharp, long blade is used to split the capsule in the same direction as the subscapularis. An additional cut is made along the rim of the glenoid. The sharp knife is then used to cut the capsule parallel to the margin of the glenoid rim from about the 6 to the 2 o'clock positions (in the right shoulder). The amount of capsule dissected from the glenoid depends on the extent of capsular shift necessary to create a stable joint. A thin humeral-head retractor is placed in the joint with its point over the posterior glenoid rim. Special care is taken not to scuff the glenohumeral cartilage. The periosteum is then elevated from the 3 to the 6 o'clock positions, providing a smooth bony surface for drill holes and aiding in the visualization for the passage of the sutures. A right-angle low-power drill (such as the Midas Rex) is used to drill three holes across the lip of the glenoid exiting into the joint near its margin. These holes are placed at approximately the 3, 4, and 6 o'clock positions.

A nonabsorbable suture is passed from outside the inferior hole to just inside the glenoid bony rim. Ten-

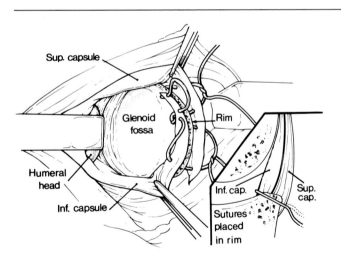

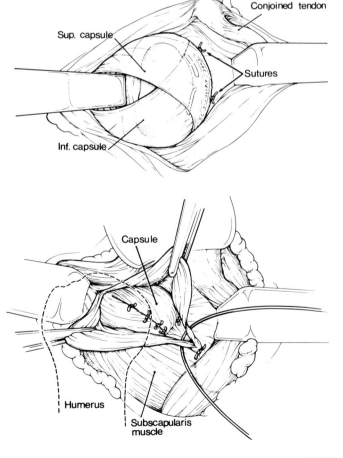

Fig. 15–4   Anterior capsulolabral reconstruction procedure. (Top right and bottom are reproduced with permission from Jobe FW, Bradley JP: Rotator cuff injuries in baseball: Prevention and rehabilitation. *Sports Med* 1988;6:377–386.)

sion is placed on the stay suture in the inferior capsular flap to approximate its final position. The suture is then inserted from outside to inside the capsule, and passed back through the capsule inside to outside, at the level of the center hole. Then, the needle is advanced through the center hole from inside the glenoid rim and tagged. Another nonabsorbable suture is inserted through the middle hole from the outside to the inside of the glenoid rim. Tension is applied as described above. The suture is then inserted from outside to inside the capsule and then passed back through the capsule at the level of the superior hole. Next, the suture is passed through the superior hole and tagged. The inferior flap should lie down inside the anterior glenoid. This recreates a reinforced labrum. The humeral-head retractor is removed and the glenoid neck sutures are tied.

The superior flap is shifted distally outside the joint and tied with the same sutures, creating an anterior bumper and tightening the inferior glenohumeral ligament. The overlapped capsule reinforces the anterior capsule at the point of previous instability. The capsule is closed with interrupted sutures (Fig. 15–4).

The range of motion is checked to ensure the correct degree of capsular tightness. The desired range is about 20 to 45 degrees of external rotation with 90 degrees of abduction and 30 degrees of horizontal adduction.

The wound is then irrigated and all bleeding is controlled with the Bovie electrocautery. The Gelpi retractor is removed, and interrupted, inverted absorbable sutures are put in the subscapularis. The remaining retractors are then removed and the skin is reapproximated with a running subcuticular stitch.

The patient is put in an airplane-type splint with approximately 20 to 45 degrees of external rotation, 90 degrees of abduction, and 30 degrees of horizontal adduction. The brace is worn for 14 days. The purpose of the brace is to allow time for the capsule to adhere to the subscapularis with as little shortening as possible, thus diminishing the rehabilitation time and allowing a quick return to full range of motion.

Rehabilitation

Immediately after surgery, the patient begins such exercises as the ball squeeze, elbow flexion-extension, and isometric abduction, horizontal adduction, and abduction. The arm can be passively ranged into abduction, flexion, and external rotation. Abduction and external rotation should be performed in 20 to 30 degrees of horizontal adduction. External rotation should not be forced.

The patient then progresses to active internal rotation with the arm at the side and active external rotation from full internal rotation to 0 degrees. Active extension can also be done, but is limited to 0 degrees or the neutral position. As the patient progresses, strengthening exercises for shoulder flexion and horizontal adduction are increased. Emphasis is on strengthening of the rotator cuff. Full range of motion will be obtained within two months of surgery.

After full range of motion is gained, muscular reeducation is begun with isokinetic devices. At first, this is done for internal and external rotation with the arm at the side. As the patient becomes stronger, and some stability has been achieved, the internal and external rotation exercises can be done with the shoulder at 90 degrees. These exercises continue for approximately one year after surgery.

The patient will be able to begin tossing a ball about four months postoperatively and throwing at six months. The patient who is a pitcher can begin pitching after approximately 12 months.

The rehabilitation process must not be overlooked or slighted. It is at least as important as the actual surgery.

Summary

In summary, there is a delicate balance between the mobility and the stability of the shoulder joint. The young athlete involved in overhand sports is at risk for injury, and must be clinically evaluated and treated differently from the rest of the population. Shoulder impingement and instability are a continuum of abnormalities, beginning with instability and progressing to subluxation, impingement, and, finally, rotator cuff tear. Thus, it is crucial to deal with the core of the problem, (that is, the instability) before dealing with the impingement. A kinesiologic repair is desirable. If that fails, or if there is anatomic damage, an anatomic repair is done. The anterior capsular labral reconstruction is a surgical procedure designed with biomechanical and kinesiologic principles in mind. A rehabilitation program is initiated immediately after surgery. The rehabilitation program is just as important as the surgery.

Posterior Instability of the Shoulder

Richard J. Hawkins, MD

Ralph M. Belle, MD

Posterior shoulder instability is rare but includes a number of subgroupings that have been classified (Outline 16–1). It may be either acute or chronic. Recurrent subluxation is encountered most frequently.

Posterior Dislocation

An acute posterior dislocation without an impression defect is extremely rare. An undiagnosed acute posterior dislocation with an impression defect can become a chronic dislocation (as described by McLaughlin[1]). Patients with this condition have several features in common. The painful shoulder of a patient who has had multiple traumas or seizures may undergo radiography. The initial radiographs are often difficult to interpret or may show an associated undisplaced fracture about the shoulder. An axillary view is seldom obtained. Physiotherapy does not improve external rotation. Such patients are often referred to an orthopaedic surgeon with the diagnosis of "frozen shoulder."

The pain improves with time and is not the primary concern. The chief complaints are stiffness and functional disability. On physical examination, the patient often finds it difficult to remove a coat or touch the head. The humeral head is prominent posteriorly and the anterior acromion squared off anteriorly. Forward elevation and abduction are limited but often functional. There is always an internal rotation deformity; this averages approximately 40 degrees.[2] This is the key physical sign. Routine anteroposterior and lateral views may be inadequate to establish the diagnosis. An axillary view confirms the diagnosis (Fig. 16–1). Associated undisplaced fractures are present in 50% of the cases.[2] The impression defect can be seen on the axillary view and an estimation of its size made; tomograms and a computed tomographic scan can delineate further the

Outline 16–1
Classification of posterior instability

I. Acute posterior dislocation
  A. Without impression defect (very rare)
  B. With impression defect (rare)
II. Chronic posterior dislocation
  A. Locked (missed) with impression defect (uncommon)
  B. Recurrent subluxation
    1. Voluntary
      a. Habitual, with personality disorder
      b. Not willful (muscular control)
    2. Involuntary
      a. Positional (demonstrable by patient)
      b. Unintentional (not demonstrable by patient)

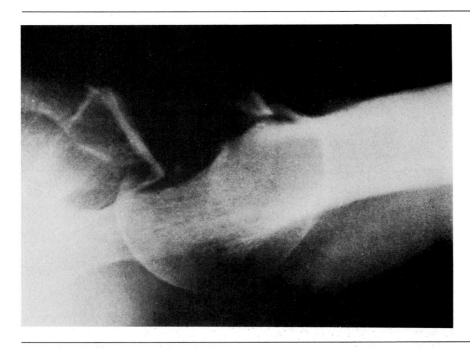

Fig. 16-1 Axillary view of locked posterior dislocation, left shoulder.

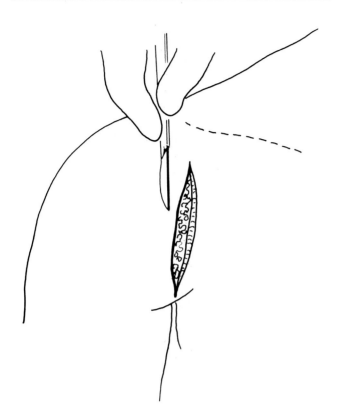

Fig. 16–2   Skin incision along posterior axillary line, left shoulder.

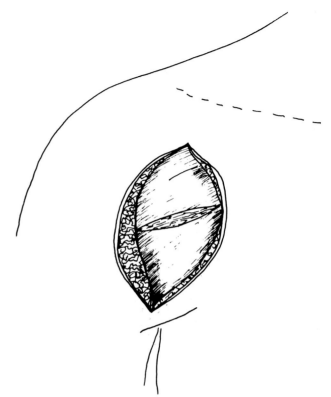

Fig. 16–3   Deltoid split.

impression defect and the remaining articular surface of the humerus.

The management of this problem depends on the size of the impression defect and the duration of the dislocation.[2] If the impression defect involves less than 20% of the head and the dislocation has lasted less than six weeks, a gentle closed reduction is attempted. If the defect involves less than 45% of the head and is less than six months in duration, a tuberosity transfer into the defect with attached subscapularis is performed. A successful transfer provides almost full range of motion and normal functional ability. If the dislocation has existed for more than six months and/or there is more than 50% head involvement, hemiarthroplasty is required. Total shoulder arthroplasty is done if the glenoid is abnormal. The prosthesis should be inserted in neutral version to the coronal plane rather than the usual 35 to 40 degrees of retroversion. This also depends on the duration of the dislocation; that is, the longer the head has been dislocated, the less retroversion. This results in less tendency to subluxate or dislocate.

Recurrent Posterior Subluxation

Recurrent posterior subluxation is the most common form of posterior instability. It is a subluxation rather than a dislocation and can usually be demonstrated by

the patient. Four subgroups have been suggested (Outline 16–1). Most cases are involuntary, although the patient is able to demonstrate the instability by arm position. Surgical results are related to this subgroup classification.

Pathoanatomy

Significant structural differences between the anterior and posterior aspects of the shoulder must be considered, particularly in reconstruction. The posterior labrum is not as structurally supportive as the anterior labrum. The anteroinferior glenohumeral ligament, which joins the inferior pouch, offers some degree of posterior stability but there is no direct posterior ligamentous reinforcement. The infraspinatus and teres minor tendons are not as strong structurally as the anterior subscapularis tendon. The pathoanatomy of recurrent posterior subluxation is not as well understood as its anterior counterpart. Reverse Bankart lesions are not usual and posterior labral defects are often only degenerative. Once recurrent posterior instability occurs, significant redundancy in the posterior capsule contributes to subsequent subluxation. Inferior redundancy may also be present and can produce multidi-

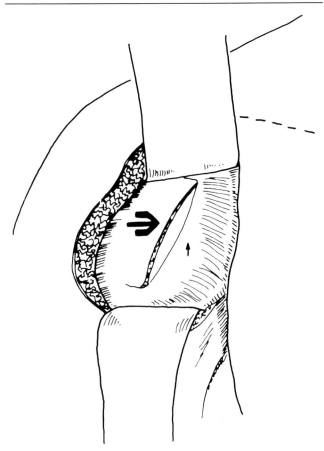

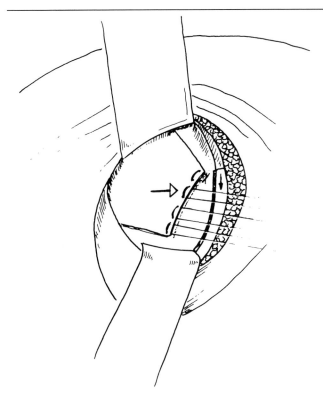

Fig. 16–5 Tendon sutured to posterior glenoid labrum (large arrow) with arm held in external rotation. Small arrow indicates remainder of infraspinatus tendon.

Fig. 16–4 Right-angle incision through infraspinatus tendon and capsule, 2 cm from its insertion. Large arrow indicates infraspinatus tendon and capsule and small arrow indicates remainder of tendon and muscle belly.

rectional instability that must be considered if surgery is contemplated.[3]

Most patients do not have histories of traumatic insults but often have some sort of overuse history. They then realize that their shoulders come out of the joints. Eventually they learn to subluxate the shoulder, usually by either arm positioning or muscular contraction. It is unusual for patients with posterior subluxation to complain of pain or functional disability sufficient to limit activities of daily living or work. Some patients, however, complain that the instability interferes with sports performance.

Only a small percentage of patients subluxate their shoulders habitually and deliberately. Such patients are psychiatrically disturbed and will not be helped by surgical reconstruction.[4] These patients must not be confused with patients who can demonstrate the instability by voluntary muscular control. Those with voluntary control usually do not have personality disorders and should not be denied reconstruction if warranted. Most patients with voluntary control also have unintentional instability associated with certain movements or activ-

ities. This may or may not be painful and functionally disabling.

The position of the arm in which the shoulder subluxates is variable. It usually involves forward flexion, internal rotation, and various degrees of abduction-adduction. The patient's fear of impending posterior subluxation is not a reliable sign of recurrent posterior subluxation. An occasional patient may be able to place the arm in an abducted externally rotated position and yet still subluxate the shoulder, not anteriorly but posteriorly.[5]

In those who cannot demonstrate the instability, the diagnosis becomes difficult. It is fortunate that this condition is rare, but we believe the diagnosis can be established by symptomatic posterior translation of the humerus in the glenoid during physical examination. This occurs when the examiner posteriorly translates the humeral head and the patient recognizes this as part of the symptom complex. In the past, the results of examination with the patient under anesthesia were confusing, but we now recognize that many patients demonstrate excessive posterior translation while under anesthesia and that this is not clinically significant. These findings must be considered in light of the presentation, history, and clinical findings.

Radiographic investigation is usually not of much help unless the shoulder is in the subluxated position. Ver-

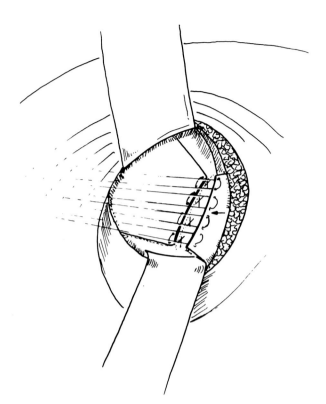

Fig. 16-6 Remainder of infraspinatus tendon and muscle belly (small arrow) imbricated and sutured down to tendon.

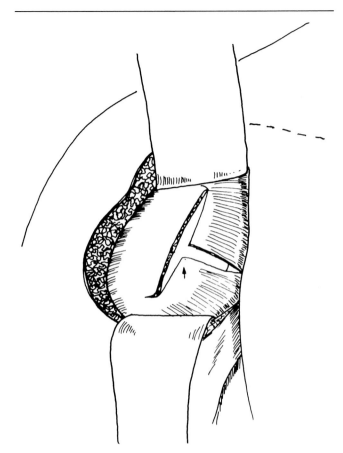

Fig. 16-7 T-shaped incision in infraspinatus tendon used when inferior capsular redundancy is present. Inferior flap (small arrow) is relocated first by pulling upward and eliminating inferior pouch.

sion is not usually abnormal. Fluoroscopy may be helpful in the diagnosis.

Treatment

Most patients with posterior subluxation do not have pain or functional disability sufficient to warrant surgical treatment. They should undergo a rotational and scapular strengthening program to diminish the instability and symptoms. Before embarking on reconstruction, it is important to ensure that there is significant pain or functional disability related to posterior subluxation. Most investigators suggest that surgical stabilization of posterior instability is indicated when recurrent unintentional posterior subluxations occur despite an adequate strengthening program. Surgical options include bony (scapular osteotomy or posterior bone block) and soft-tissue (reverse Putti-Platt, biceps tendon transfer, inferior capsular shift, or infraspinatus tendon transfer) procedures or combinations of these.

Boyd and Sisk[6] combined a posterior capsulorrhaphy with a tendon transfer of the long head of the biceps, which is rerouted around the posterior aspect of the neck of the humerus and reinserted on the posterior rim of the glenoid. Preliminary results in that series were good. There were no recurrences and the patients

were able to return to athletics. The results in other series have not been satisfactory.[5] A reverse Putti-Platt repair procedure consisting primarily of a capsular plication with infraspinatus tendon overlapping also failed to produce good results.[5]

We prefer a soft-tissue procedure using the infraspinatus tendon. The best tissue for posterior reconstruction is in the infraspinatus tendon and capsule near the insertion into the greater tuberosity. A right-angle incision is made approximately 2 cm from the insertion of the infraspinatus through the tendinous portion (Fig. 16–2). The incision is brought down through the capsule and sutured down to the posterior glenoid labrum with the arm in external rotation (Figs. 16–3 to 16–6). The substance of the posterior glenoid labrum is always good. It must be emphasized that the tendinous portion of the infraspinatus should be used for repair, because the muscle belly alone does not provide adequate tissue support for stabilization.

The arm is then immobilized in 20 degrees of external rotation for six weeks. Rehabilitation is begun slowly and is initially restricted to limited stretching. Other abnormalities (such as a malorientation of the glenoid, glenoid dysplasia, or significant architectural defects) are occasionally present. These must be considered and addressed at the time of reconstructive surgery. The posterior bone block has been used for recurrent posterior dislocation.[7] This may be of value when there is a bony deficiency posteriorly. The bone block must be extra-articular so that the humeral head does not impinge on it.

When posterior subluxation is combined with an element of inferior capsular redundancy, the inferior capsular shift should be added to the surgical procedure.[3] The soft-tissue procedure is the same, with the addition of a T-shaped incision medially through tendon and capsule (Fig. 16–7). The inferior flap is taken upward first to obliterate the inferior pouch. The superior flap is then placed in a position to overlap the inferior flap.

Many investigators have reported good results with posterior glenoid osteotomy.[8-10] The scapular osteotomy is a potentially complicated procedure that requires special attention to technique. The closer the osteotomy is to the joint, the greater is the risk of entering the joint. Entering the joint can result in devastating osteoarthritis of the glenohumeral joint.[11]

Previous reports have tended to combine subluxation and dislocation when discussing subluxation. Good results have been reported with surgical management.[1,6-10] However, the number of subjects were small and no distinction between subluxation and true dislocation was made. These dislocations may have been misnamed and the results should be considered with this in mind. Subluxation should be considered separately. The results of surgical reconstruction for posterior subluxation alone have been poor to date.[11,12]

Summary

Posterior instability is a rare entity in which subluxation is much more common than dislocation. This problem should be assessed and treated by someone particularly interested in shoulder problems. Reconstruction produces fairly high recurrence and complication rates. Accurate preoperative patient selection and improved surgical procedures and techniques are required to maximize success.

References

1. McLaughlin HL: Posterior dislocation of the shoulder. *J Bone Joint Surg* 1952;34A:584–590.
2. Hawkins RJ, Neer CS II, Pianta RM, et al: Locked posterior dislocation of the shoulder. *J Bone Joint Surg* 1987;69A:9–18.
3. Neer CS II, Foster CR: Inferior capsular shift for involuntary inferior and multidirectional instability of the shoulder: A preliminary report. *J Bone Joint Surg* 1980;62A:897–908.
4. Rowe CR, Pierce DS, Clark JG: Voluntary dislocation of the shoulder: A preliminary report on a clinical, electromyographic, and psychiatric study of twenty-six patients. *J Bone Joint Surg* 1973;55A:445–460.
5. Hawkins RJ, Koppert G, Johnston G: Recurrent posterior instability (subluxation) of the shoulder. *J Bone Joint Surg* 1984;66A:169–174.
6. Boyd HB, Sisk TD: Recurrent posterior dislocation of the shoulder. *J Bone Joint Surg* 1972;54A:779–786.
7. Jones V: Recurrent posterior dislocation of the shoulder: Report of a case treated by posterior bone block. *J Bone Joint Surg* 1958;40B:203–207.
8. English E, Macnab I: Recurrent posterior dislocation of the shoulder. *Can J Surg* 1974;17:147–151.
9. Kretzler HH Jr: Scapular osteotomy for posterior shoulder dislocation, abstract. *J Bone Joint Surg* 1974;56A:197.
10. Scott DJ Jr: Treatment of recurrent posterior dislocations of the shoulder by glenoplasty: Report of three cases. *J Bone Joint Surg* 1967;49A:471–476.
11. Johnston HH, Hawkins RJ, Haddad R, et al: A complication of posterior glenoid osteotomy for recurrent posterior shoulder instability. *Clin Orthop* 1984;187:147–149.
12. Hurley JA, Anderson TE, Dear W, et al: Posterior shoulder instability: Surgical vs. non-surgical results. *Orthop Trans* 1987;11:458.

Shoulder Instability: Management of Failed Reconstructions

Bertram Zarins, MD

Carter R. Rowe, MD

James W. Stone, MD

Introduction

The patient who develops recurrent shoulder instability after having undergone a surgical procedure to correct this problem presents a challenge. Our purposes are to identify factors associated with failure, to describe nonsurgical treatment of patients with recurrent instability, to present surgical options for stabilizing the shoulder, to discuss how previous surgery may complicate the subsequent surgical procedure, and to present the results of reoperation for recurrent shoulder instability.

We use the term "instability" to describe both glenohumeral dislocation and subluxation. These terms represent different degrees of severity of the same phenomenon. We use the term "failure" (1) if the shoulder dislocates or subluxates postoperatively for any reason, or (2) if the patient has a poor result from any cause other than recurrent instability.

Classification of Failures

Recurrent Instability: Same Direction

This category includes the shoulder that has had surgery to correct instability in one direction (such as anteriorly) that redislocates or resubluxates in the same direction. An important consideration is the severity of the traumatic episode that caused the first postoperative redislocation.

Traumatic Instability If a major injury caused the shoulder to redislocate or resubluxate, the diagnosis and initial treatment are usually straightforward. It is likely that the previous operation was successful but that the new trauma was the cause of the recurrence. If surgery is performed again, the major factor to consider is how the previous surgery altered the shoulder's anatomy. This will influence the choice of procedure and the surgical approach if reoperation is necessary (Fig. 17–1).

Atraumatic Instability If the redislocation was not the result of a significant traumatic episode, then it is important to look for other factors that could be responsible for the failure of the previous operation to correct the shoulder instability. These factors are discussed in detail later.

Recurrent Instability: Different Direction

This category includes the shoulder that has had surgery to correct instability in one direction (such as anteriorly) and that is now unstable in a different direction (such as posteriorly). The differential diagnosis includes a new injury unrelated to the previous problem, unrecognized multidirectional instability, and the possibility that the first operation was performed at the incorrect site.

Traumatic Instability It is possible to sustain a traumatic dislocation in a direction opposite to that of previous instability. This situation can present a diagnostic dilemma[1] (Fig. 17–2).

Atraumatic Instability After surgery to correct recurrent instability, a shoulder can begin to dislocate or subluxate in a different direction than it had earlier (Fig. 17–3). This complication can occur atraumatically, especially if the previous repair was too tight. For example, the surgeon may tighten the anterior capsule excessively in a patient who is at high risk for failure. Such patients include those who have multidirectional instability, Ehlers-Danlos syndrome, or some other form of generalized joint laxity and those who can voluntarily dislocate the shoulder.

If a shoulder dislocates posteriorly after surgery to correct anterior instability, one must evaluate the strength of the original evidence that led to the diagnosis of anterior instability. It is possible that the original diagnosis was incorrect. If preoperative radiographs did not document the direction of instability, it may be worthwhile to perform additional studies such as computed tomography (with or without contrast), examination with the patient under anesthesia, and/or arthroscopy.

Multidirectional Shoulder Instability If a shoulder is unstable in more than one direction and an anterior repair is performed, the operation may or may not correct a coexisting inferior or posterior instability. Patients who have excessive joint laxity (Fig. 17–4) or a connective tissue disorder, such as Ehlers-Danlos syndrome, are likely to have multidirectional instability (Fig. 17–5). Postoperative failures are common in this group of patients and alternative methods of treatment should be considered.

Other Complications

Limited Motion Several surgical procedures for anterior instability, such as the Magnuson-Stack[2,3] and the Putti-Platt procedures,[4] are designed to limit external rotation. However, excessive tightening of the anterior structures results in impaired function, especially in

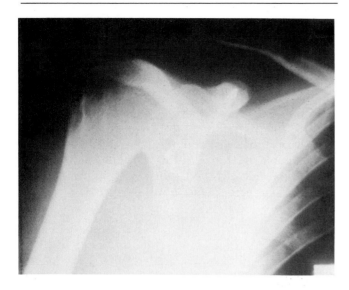

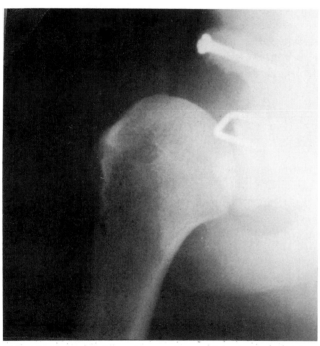

Fig. 17-1 Anteroposterior (**top**) and axillary (**bottom**) radiographs of a 25-year-old man who had undergone a right-sided Magnuson-Stack procedure four years earlier. Because of traumatic redislocation he was treated with a duToit staple capsulorrhaphy; this also failed because of minor trauma two years later. At reoperation he was found to have a Bankart lesion, an attenuated subscapularis tendon, and a defect at the superior border of the subscapularis. A Bankart repair corrected the instability.

athletes in throwing sports. Prolonged immobilization after surgery can also result in scarring of the capsule and rotator cuff, thus limiting shoulder motion.

Weakness The subscapularis muscle is an important internal rotator and stabilizer of the humeral head. If a surgical procedure weakens the subscapularis or other shoulder muscle, shoulder function will be compromised (Fig. 17–6).

Nerve Injury The axillary nerve is located approximately 1 cm caudal to the inferior shoulder capsule; it courses posteriorly over the subscapularis muscle and exits through the quadrangular space. The nerve is at risk during anterior shoulder surgery when dissection is carried out inferiorly along the capsule, such as during the inferior capsular shift operation.[5] Rockwood[6] described a method of protecting the axillary nerve during an anterior shoulder reconstruction. The inferior fourth of the subscapularis tendon is left intact and only the upper three fourths of the tendon is dissected off the anterior capsule.

The musculocutaneous nerve is a branch of the lateral cord of the brachial plexus. It courses 1 cm medial to the conjoined tendon below the coracoid process and enters the coracobrachialis approximately 6 to 8 cm below the coracoid process. This distance varies in different individuals. The nerve can usually be palpated on the undersurface of the coracobrachialis muscle. The surgeon must exercise care when retracting the conjoined tendon, especially in muscular patients. Osteotomy of the coracoid process relaxes the conjoined tendon in the direction from which the nerve arises, thus decreasing the retraction on the tendon and nerve.

Joint Injury In a long-term follow-up study, Rowe and associates[7] found no significant posttraumatic degenerative change in the glenohumeral joint after placement of holes in the anterior margin of the glenoid rim during the Bankart repair. However, the articular cartilage of the humeral head or glenoid fossa can be injured by metallic fixation devices used for repair (Fig. 17–7). A staple or bone graft placed too close to the joint margin during staple capsulorrhaphy or coracoid transplant can traumatize the humeral head.

Heterotopic Ossification Heterotopic ossification can limit motion and cause pain after shoulder surgery. We have seen a patient with heterotopic ossification after partial transection and repair of the conjoined tendon during anterior shoulder reconstruction (Fig. 17–8). The conjoined tendon should not be transected for exposure; osteotomy is safer and the healing of the bone is stronger than healing of the tendon.

Failure of Fixation Devices The glenoid cavity is relatively small compared with the humeral head. This does not allow a large margin of error when placing screws or staples into the glenoid rim. Difficulties are compounded by limited surgical exposure, narrowness of the glenoid neck, and the proximity of neurovascular structures.

Metallic fixation devices placed in the shoulder are susceptible to failure. The great mobility and the high forces generated in the shoulder girdle can result in metal fatigue or loosening (Fig. 17–9). Once loose, metallic fixation devices can cause irreversible damage to articular surfaces (Fig. 17–10) or migrate to distant

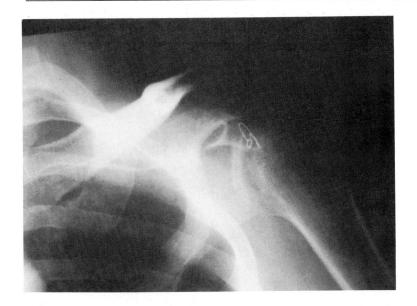

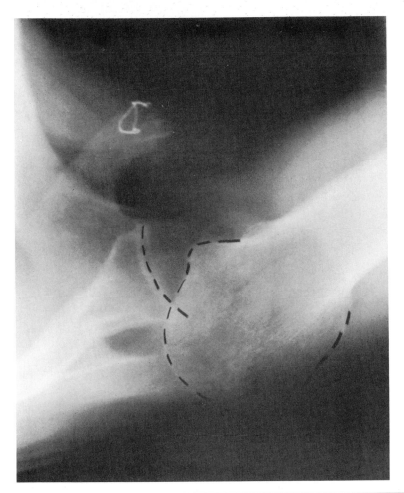

Fig. 17–2 A 33-year-old professional soccer player sustained a left shoulder injury eight years after having a successful Bankart repair. Anteroposterior radiographs were obtained **(top)** and the patient was reassured that his shoulder was not dislocated. The correct diagnosis was not made until three months later when an axillary radiograph **(bottom)** revealed an unreduced posterior glenohumeral dislocation.

sites (Fig. 17–11). We believe that arthroscopic staple capsulorrhaphy carries a significant risk for this complication (Fig. 17–12). We prefer to avoid placing metallic fixation devices into the shoulder.

Factors Associated With Failure

There are a number of factors associated with failure of surgical procedures to stabilize the shoulder. These

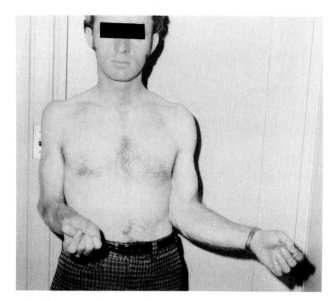

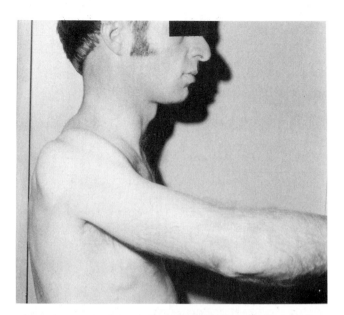

Fig. 17–3 This 28-year-old man had undergone multiple procedures on his right shoulder, including the Magnuson-Stack, Putti-Platt, and Bankart procedures. He had an internal rotation contracture **(top left)**. This picture demonstrates the maximum external rotation of his right shoulder. The lateral view demonstrates posterior glenohumeral subluxation of his right shoulder **(top right)**. The subluxation is demonstrated on axillary radiograph **(bottom)**.

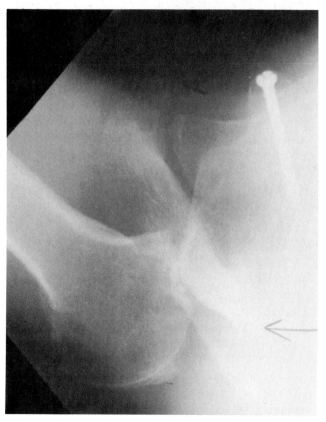

factors can be grouped into uncorrected or new pathologic lesions (Fig. 17–13), patient factors, and technical considerations.

Uncorrected or New Pathologic Lesions

The most common cause of failure is an unrepaired Bankart lesion (an avulsion of the anterior capsule and glenoid labrum from the anterior glenoid rim with or without a fragment of bone). Rowe and associates[8] found a Bankart lesion in 27 of 32 shoulders (84%) that underwent reoperation for recurrent shoulder instability. The lesions were moderately large in 11 cases and severe in 16 cases.

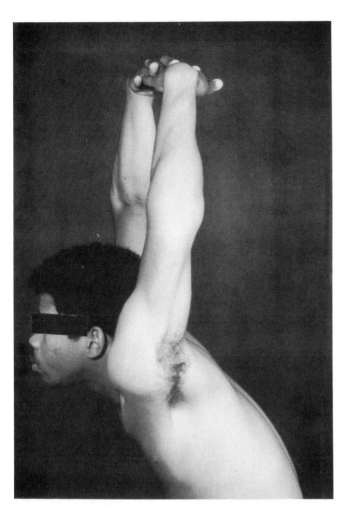

Fig. 17-4 This patient has generalized ligamentous laxity and can subluxate his shoulders.

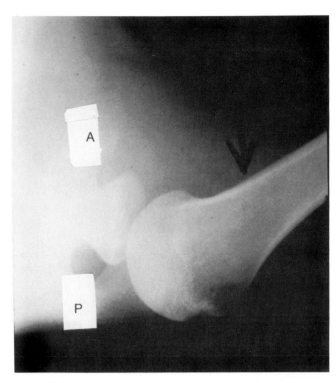

Fig. 17-5 Axillary radiograph demonstrating posterior glenohumeral subluxation in a patient who has multidirectional instability. A, anterior; P, posterior.

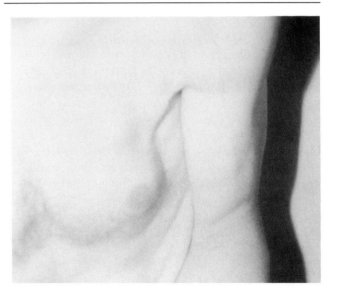

Fig. 17-6 This man had a Putti-Platt procedure performed through an axillary approach. After surgery he had shoulder weakness and a palpable defect in the anterior chest musculature. On surgical exploration he was found to have ruptured the pectoralis major insertion on the humerus.

Several surgical procedures are designed to correct the Bankart lesion: the Bankart procedure,[9] the Viek modification,[10] the duToit staple capsulorrhaphy,[11] arthroscopic staple capsulorrhaphy,[12,13] and arthroscopic transglenoid suturing.[14] On the other hand, some procedures for shoulder instability do not correct the underlying abnormality and may create an internal rotation contracture of the shoulder. These include the Putti-Platt procedure[4] and the Magnuson-Stack procedure.[2,3,15,16] The principle of the Eden-Hybinnette,[17-21] Bristow-Helfet,[22] and modified Bristow[23-26] procedures is to create a bone block along the anterior glenoid rim. Theoretically, the Bristow procedure also creates a sling formed by the conjoined tendon that holds the humeral head in place. If the failed procedure does not correct the Bankart lesion, there is a high likelihood that a patient who develops recurrent instability has an unrepaired Bankart lesion.[8]

A fracture of the anterior glenoid rim is not a contraindication to performing a Bankart procedure for

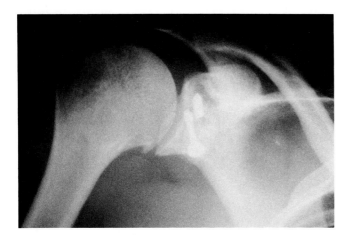

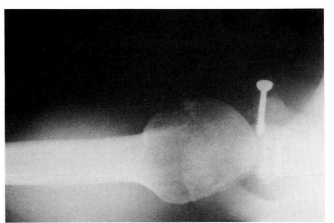

Fig. 17-7 Anteroposterior **(top left)** and axillary radiographs **(top right)** of a 32-year-old man who had undergone a Bristow procedure six years earlier. He developed shoulder pain five years after surgery; radiographs demonstrated nonunion of the coracoid process and a broken screw. Arthroscopy shows the tip of the screw in the joint, with damage to the humeral head **(bottom).**

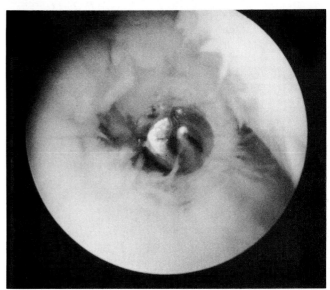

recurrent dislocation. In a long-term follow-up study, only one of 51 shoulders with fractured glenoid rims had recurrent instability after Bankart repairs.[7]

Another common finding at reoperation for shoulder instability is excessive laxity of the anterior capsule.[8] Capsular laxity can be estimated at the time of surgery after the subscapularis tendon has been dissected off the anterior capsule. With the patient's arm at the side of the body and the elbow flexed 90 degrees, the shoulder is externally rotated to 90 degrees. The anterior capsule is lifted forward with tissue forceps. If the capsule is taut and cannot be lifted up, then it is graded "tight" or "normal." If the capsule can be lifted up 1 cm, its laxity is graded as "moderate." If the capsule can be lifted up more than 1 cm, its laxity is graded as "severe."[8]

The anterior capsule was lax in 24 of 29 shoulders (83%) at reoperation for instability. The laxity was judged to be moderate in 12 and severe in 12. Excessive laxity of the capsule was considered to be the primary

cause of recurrent instability in four (14%) of these shoulders in which no other significant pathologic lesions were found at reoperation.[8] These shoulders require a reconstructive procedure that tightens the anterior capsule to restore stability.

The presence of a large Hill-Sachs lesion may increase the risk of failure after a Bankart repair[7] (Figs. 17-14 to 17-16). In a series of 145 patients followed up for an average of six years, there were five recurrences after Bankart repair (3.4%). A total of 110 shoulders (76%) had Hill-Sachs lesions. Thirty shoulders had small Hill-Sachs lesions and there were no recurrences in this group. Eighty shoulders had moderate or large Hill-Sachs lesions and there were five recurrences in this group (6%).

A Hill-Sachs lesion was found in 22 of 29 shoulders (76%) that underwent reoperation for failure of an anterior reconstruction.[8] The lesion was mild in two cases, moderately large in 17, and severe in three. This suggests that the presence of a sizable Hill-Sachs lesion is

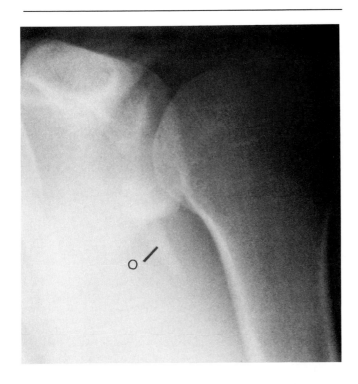

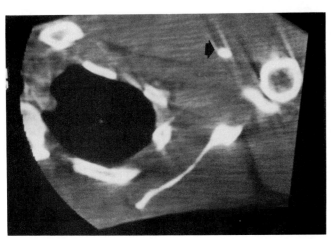

Fig. 17-8 A 26-year-old elite athlete (canoeing and white water rafting) underwent a Bankart repair. The lateral half of the conjoined tendon had been transected just below the coracoid process to enhance exposure and was then repaired. Two years after the surgery, the patient still had pain when he used the shoulder excessively. **Top:** Heterotopic ossification (O) is visible inferior to the coracoid process on the anteroposterior view. **Bottom:** A computed tomogram shows the area of ossification anteromedial to the shaft of the humerus (arrow). The heterotopic bone in the scarred conjoined tendon was excised, with a good result.

an important factor in the failure of a Bankart procedure, and that a procedure in addition to the Bankart procedure, such as the Connolly procedure,[27] may be required.

The subscapularis muscle-tendon unit is an important dynamic stabilizer of the shoulder. Along with internally rotating the shoulder, the subscapularis prevents excessive anterior translation of the humeral head.

Weakening of the subscapularis muscle can contribute to postoperative anterior shoulder instability. The subscapularis muscle can be scarred after surgery on the underlying capsule or on a transferred conjoined tendon or coracoid process. In 32 shoulders that underwent reoperation, we found the subscapularis tendon to be attenuated in five and ruptured in two.[8] Scarring was present in all other shoulders except five that had undergone a Magnuson procedure and three that had undergone a Nicola procedure.[28-30] The most severe scar formation occurred in shoulders that had Bristow-Helfet procedures. In these shoulders, the coracoid process, conjoined tendon, and subscapularis tendon were all incorporated into a mass of scar tissue.

A widening of the interval between the subscapularis and supraspinatus tendons has been implicated as a factor in anterior shoulder instability.[31] In a study of failed surgery, a large interval was found in six of 32 shoulders.[8] The widened interval can most easily be found after the coracoid process has undergone osteotomy, and should be repaired when identified.

Patient Factors and Technical Considerations

Generalized ligamentous laxity, a condition in which there is hypermobility of multiple joints, is associated with a high failure rate because of stretching of surgical repairs. An extreme example of this disorder is the Ehlers-Danlos syndrome. Generalized joint laxity can cause multidirectional shoulder instability; these patients are at high risk for failure of surgical procedures for anterior or multidirectional instability.

Patients capable of voluntary instability have a high failure rate after surgical repair.[32] If the muscles have been trained to act in synchrony to push the shoulder out of joint, the patient can use this repetitive force to loosen almost any surgical repair. A psychiatric evaluation should be considered for patients capable of voluntary recurrent instability after primary shoulder reconstruction if they exhibit emotional problems. These patients sometimes use their ability to dislocate their shoulders for secondary gains. Fortunately, only a small number have emotional problems and they generally respond successfully to conservative management.

Fractures of the glenoid rim and Hill-Sachs lesions frequently coexist, as both are caused by forceful recoil of the humeral head against the rim at the time of dislocation. We believe that a shoulder that has anterior instability and a fracture of the glenoid rim involving less than 25% of the articular surface can be treated in the same fashion as one without fracture. However, the combination of a large glenoid rim fracture and a severe Hill-Sachs lesion may be difficult to correct by means of routine soft-tissue procedures alone; a combination of procedures may be necessary. An excessively anteverted glenoid cavity may be a factor in recurrent anterior instability, just as a posteriorly inclined glenoid rim may predispose to recurrent posterior in-

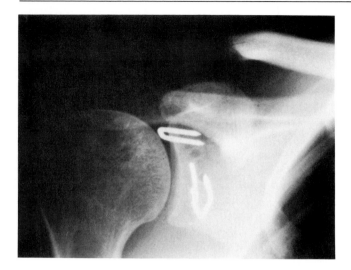
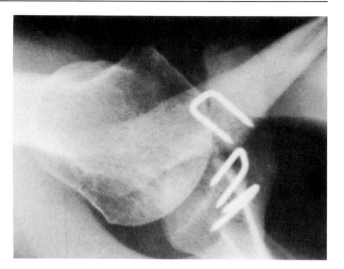

Fig. 17–9 A 30-year-old woman, who had had a duToit staple capsulorrhaphy three years earlier, experienced increasing shoulder pain. Radiographs **(top left and top right)** showed three staples, one of which appeared to be loose. The intra-articular staple was removed arthroscopically **(bottom)**.

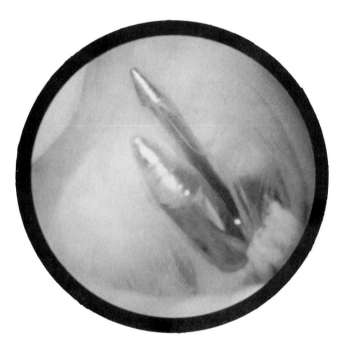

Management

The first steps in managing recurrent subluxation or dislocation after primary shoulder surgery has failed are to establish the diagnosis and to identify the factors responsible for failure. This is accomplished by a careful review of the history, physical examination, radiographic studies, examination with the patient under anesthesia, and arthroscopic examination. The next step is to institute a conservative treatment program em-

stability. In these rare instances the surgeon should consider a redirecting scapular neck osteotomy to correct the instability.

phasizing rotator cuff strengthening exercises and avoidance of activities that could cause recurrent dislocation. Surgical treatment may be required if conservative treatment fails to solve the problem. Special planning depends on the previous surgical procedures.

History

In taking the patient's history, the surgeon must determine the strength of the evidence on which the initial diagnosis of shoulder instability was made. Was anterior dislocation documented radiographically? Was there any evidence to indicate instability in more than one direction? It is important to obtain the surgical report of any procedure performed on the shoulder and to identify previous intra-articular abnormality and note if this was corrected.

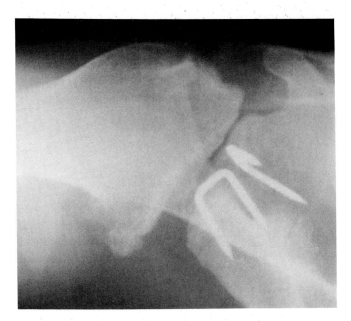

Fig. 17-10 Axillary radiograph of a patient who was treated by duToit staple capsulorrhaphy. Significant erosion of the humeral head has occurred because of the loose staple.

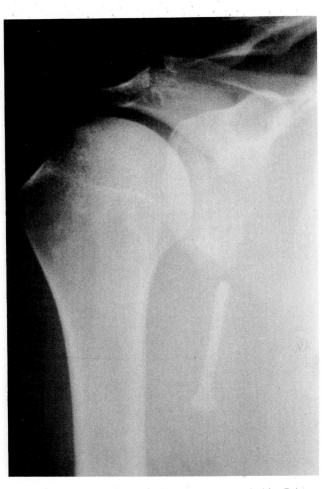

Fig. 17-11 A 22-year-old man who had been treated with a Bristow procedure nine years earlier. His shoulder was clinically stable, but the screw was palpable in the axilla.

In questioning the patient on current symptoms, one should establish the degree of trauma that was responsible for the first recurrence of instability after surgical repair. A major injury can cause new damage to the glenohumeral joint and its restraints. If the recurrent dislocation was atraumatic, it is likely that previous surgery did not correct the underlying abnormality or that other factors are involved. Aggressive physical therapy instituted too soon postoperatively, before complete healing has occurred, can stretch the surgical repair.

The surgeon should determine the position in which symptoms of instability occur. If the arm is in the overhead position (abduction, external rotation), it is likely that there is anterior instability. If the patient is symptomatic with the arm in the adducted, internally rotated position and in forward flexion, posterior instability is more likely.

Physical Examination

As with a routine shoulder examination, the range of motion and the neurovascular status of the extremity must be evaluated. Cervical spine abnormalities, brachial plexus lesions, and intrathoracic abnormalities can cause referred pain to the shoulder. These sources must be examined systematically.

The "apprehension" test is used to determine the stability of the glenohumeral joint. With complete muscle relaxation, an anteriorly directed force is applied to the arm in elevation and external rotation. A positive test occurs when the patient experiences a sudden, severe pain. Occasionally the patient may note anterior

subluxation of the shoulder and may avoid elevating and externally rotating the shoulder because of anticipated pain. Inferior instability can be detected by applying an inferiorly directed force with the shoulder at 90 degrees of abduction. To demonstrate posterior instability, the examiner internally rotates the patient's arm in front of the body at shoulder level and applies a posteriorly directed force.

Examination with the patient under anesthesia, with or without fluoroscopic control, can provide additional information, especially if the direction of instability is in question.

An assessment of general ligament laxity should be made by noting the stability of other joints, such as the fingers, the patellofemoral joint, elbow, and opposite shoulder.

Radiography

If routine radiographs, including an axillary view, do not provide sufficient information, then tomograms, computed tomograms, arthrograms, computed tomo-

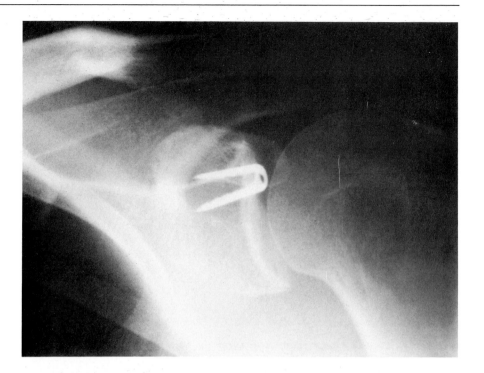

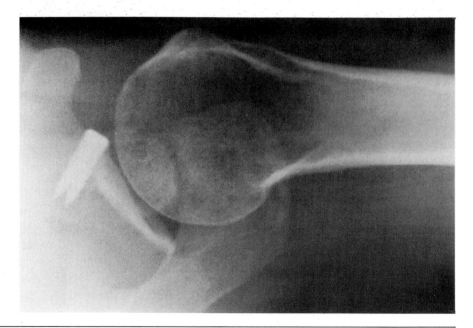

Fig. 17-12 Anteroposterior **(top)** and axillary **(bottom)** radiographs of a patient who underwent arthroscopic staple capsulorrhaphy. The humeral head was damaged by the staple.

grams with contrast, and magnetic resonance imaging studies can provide additional information on the status of the shoulder. These studies are especially useful if a bony procedure has previously been performed, or if hardware has been used.

Arthroscopy

Arthroscopy can be combined with examination under anesthesia or fluoroscopy under anesthesia to help document the direction of instability.

Arthroscopy is a useful diagnostic method for visualizing the glenohumeral joint. The surgeon can determine the presence and extent of a Bankart lesion or a Hill-Sachs lesion. The location of a glenoid labrum tear is indirect evidence that indicates the direction of instability of the humeral head.

Nonsurgical Treatment

The patient should be given rotator cuff exercises to strengthen internal rotation, external rotation, abduc-

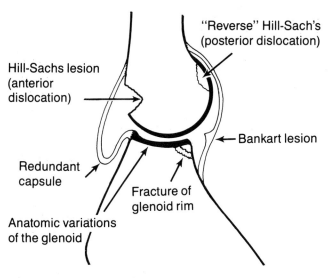

Fig. 17-13 Anatomic lesions associated with glenohumeral instability. (Reproduced with permission from Rowe CR: Dislocations of the shoulder, in Rowe CR (ed): *The Shoulder.* New York, Churchill Livingstone, 1988, p 177.)

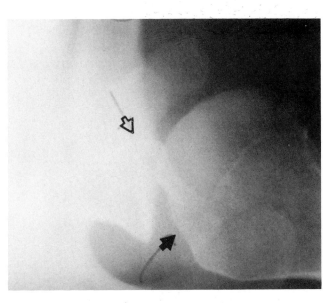

Fig. 17-15 Axillary radiograph of a patient with a large Hill-Sachs lesion (solid arrow). There is also a fracture of the anterior glenoid rim (open arrow). This combination of lesions may make it difficult to stabilize the shoulder surgically.

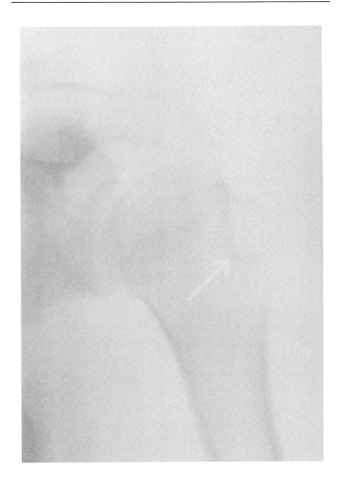

Fig. 17-14 Anteroposterior radiograph of left shoulder shows a severe Hill-Sachs lesion ("hatchet" lesion) (arrow).

tion, and adduction.[8] Exercises are performed at less than 45 degrees of elevation. The patient should not perform resistive abduction or adduction exercises at shoulder level as this produces impingement of the rotator cuff. A simple elastic resistive strap is an inexpensive method of shoulder strengthening that avoids the potential deleterious effects of exercising at more than 45 degrees of shoulder abduction, as can happen if resistive exercise machines are used.

In a review of 39 patients with recurrent glenohumeral instability after unsuccessful anterior shoulder surgery, 32 (82%) underwent reoperation.[8] Stability improved with exercises in five patients (13%); these patients did not have additional surgery. One patient continued to have functional instability but refused reoperation.

Shoulder harnesses, braces, or tape can be used to restrict glenohumeral motion and provide functional stability during athletic activities. These methods are especially useful in contact sports.

Surgical Considerations

The surgical principles to which we adhere are especially important in reoperations: (1) Carefully dissect, layer-by-layer; (2) identify the abnormality; (3) correct the lesion; and (4) return all tissues to their normal anatomic positions. It may not be possible to accomplish these goals in reoperations because the anatomy has been altered by the previous surgery or because there has been excessive scarring.

When positioning the patient for an anterior ap-

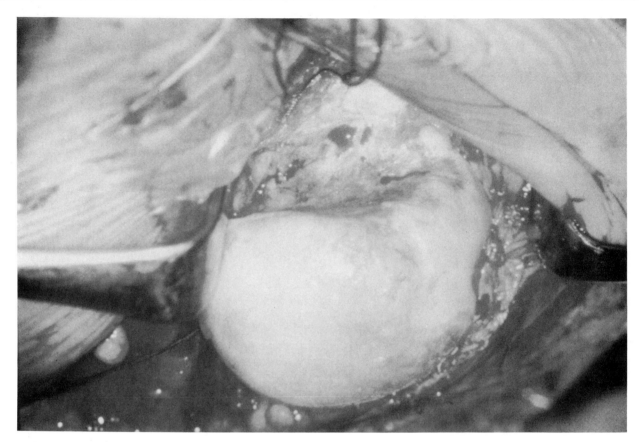

Fig. 17-16 Surgical photograph showing a large Hill-Sachs lesion.

proach, fold a towel and place it in the interscapular area to push the scapula laterally. Do not place a towel or sandbag beneath the shoulder itself, as this limits the exposure by displacing the humeral head anteriorly. Instead, elevate the elbow to displace the humeral head posteriorly. Instruments that make the procedure easier to perform include a headlight, a deep, smooth self-retaining retractor, a humeral head retractor, single- and double-pronged retractors, a scaphoid gouge, and curved spikes and awls for making the holes in the glenoid rim.

Complete muscle relaxation is needed for the duration of the operation. A long deltopectoral incision is made. A coracoid osteotomy is usually performed to enhance exposure. A meticulous dissection is carried out, identifying tissue planes and intervals that may have been distorted by previous surgery. As the surgeon approaches the shoulder joint and exposes the abnormality, it may be necessary to modify the revision procedure to be performed. This depends on the findings. The previous procedure may make the second surgery technically difficult.

Anterior Reoperations

If the patient has previously had a Bankart procedure, the surgical procedure we prefer is similar to the one performed previously. The subscapularis muscle is carefully separated from the capsule if possible. The most frequent findings are a new or previously unrepaired Bankart lesion or excessive anterior capsular laxity.[8] A Bankart repair, with or without anterior capsular reefing, should be performed if possible. However, if a severe Hill-Sachs lesion and a fracture of the anterior glenoid rim are both present, it may be difficult to stabilize the shoulder by an anterior operation alone. An anterior bone block procedure or the Connolly procedure may be necessary in addition to the Bankart repair. C.S. Neer recommends filling the Hill-Sachs defect with a bone graft (personal communication, 1988).

Patients who have previously had Bristow procedures usually have a large mass of scar tissue that incorporates the subscapularis muscle and conjoined tendon plus the anterior shoulder capsule. Our approach has been to try to restore normal anatomy. The conjoined tendon is dissected free of the subscapularis tendon if possible. The broken screw and ununited coracoid are removed. A plane is developed between the subscapularis tendon and the capsule, leaving as much tissue on the capsule as possible. A vertical or T-shaped incision is made in the capsule and the underlying abnormality is exposed. If a Bankart lesion is found, the capsule is repaired back to the glenoid rim, using sutures passed through the bony rim. The origin of the conjoined tendon is sutured locally to the capsule or subscapularis tendon. It is not reattached to the base of the coracoid process.

A previous Magnuson-Stack procedure does not scar or alter the deep shoulder structures. Therefore, reoperation is relatively simple. The subscapularis tendon should be sharply dissected from its attachment to the humerus. The underlying biceps tendon should be protected. The subscapularis tendon is removed from the anterior capsule and a routine Bankart procedure or capsulorrhaphy is performed.

A previous Putti-Platt procedure causes a moderate amount of scarring between the subscapularis tendon and the capsule, but not as much as one might expect. A plane between the two should be established with sharp dissection. An alternative method is to split the subscapularis muscle and tendon horizontally to expose the underlying capsule (F.W. Jobe, personal communication, 1987).

A previous Nicola procedure[28-30] does little to alter the normal shoulder anatomy. The transplanted biceps tendon is no obstruction to a routine Bankart procedure.

If a large Hill-Sachs lesion is present, the surgeon may have to alter the approach to recurrent anterior instability after failed surgery. This is especially true if the patient has a concurrent fracture of the anterior glenoid rim. In this situation, the shoulder may be particularly unstable and a routine anterior reconstruction may not be adequate to reestablish shoulder stability. In this situation we favor combining the anterior reconstruction with transplantation of the infraspinatus tendon into the humeral head defect. This procedure was originally described by Connolly.[27] The surgeon can expose the infraspinatus tendon insertion through a posterior approach, turning down the deltoid muscle origin from the scapular spine, or by a superior approach devised by one of us (C.R.R.).[33] The incision extends along the spine of the scapula and down the deltoid for 8 to 10 cm. The deltoid muscle is split in the direction of its fibers for a distance of 4 to 5 cm. The humerus is internally rotated, exposing the insertion of the infraspinatus into the greater tuberosity. The infraspinatus tendon insertion is divided by osteotomy, leaving a small fragment of bone attached to the tendon. The Hill-Sachs defect is curetted down to freshly bleeding bone. Drill holes are made through the greater tuberosity. The infraspinatus tendon is secured into the Hill-Sachs defect with sutures. The procedure converts an intra-articular Hill-Sachs lesion into an extra-articular one. We have not used the Connolly procedure alone to treat primary shoulder instability. We perform it only on patients in whom previous reconstructions failed and who have large Hill-Sachs lesions. We perform the Connolly procedure only in combination with surgery to correct the anterior abnormality.

There have been no failures when the procedures were used for these indications.

Inferior Instability

We have seen several patients in whom inferior glenohumeral subluxation with the arm by the side developed after anterior shoulder surgery. The inferior subluxation appeared to be new and not directly related to the anterior instability. The cause of this form of instability is not clear, but we believe that it may be secondary to disruption of the coracohumeral or superior glenohumeral ligament.

The Neer inferior capsular shift[5] has been used to treat this type of inferior glenohumeral subluxation. The axillary nerve is at risk during the inferior capsular shift. In the presence of anatomy distorted by previous surgery, it may be wise to isolate the axillary nerve before mobilizing the inferior capsule. In some cases the extent of the scarring may make this dissection very difficult. Under these circumstances, it may be prudent to perform a less complete capsular mobilization rather than risk damaging the axillary nerve.

An alternative procedure is the Thompson modification of the Nicola procedure: a core of iliac bone is driven into the hole drilled through the humeral head for passage of the long head of the biceps tendon.[34] This converts the tendon into a "ligamentum teres."

Posterior Operation After Failed Anterior Operation

If the patient has had an anterior operation in which the anterior capsule and subscapularis muscles were tightened excessively, then posterior subluxation may occur. In this instance, the anterior structures should be taken down and positioned at proper tension in addition to the posterior stabilization procedure. This requires a combined anterior and posterior approach. A posterior capsular shift or a modified Bankart procedure is carried out. If the capsular tissues are thin, we have found the Scott glenoid osteotomy to be very successful.[35]

If the anterior capsule and subscapularis tendon are not excessively tight but the shoulder is unstable posteriorly, only a posterior approach is necessary. For multidirectional instability, we try to determine in which direction the instability is most severe and operate on this side of the shoulder first.

Results

By adhering to the principles of revision surgery outlined above, Rowe and associates[8] had good results in patients with recurrent shoulder instability. More than two years of follow-up for 24 shoulders that underwent reoperation revealed excellent results in ten cases and good results in 12 (92%). Of the two failures, one shoulder continued to dislocate and the other to subluxate.

References

1. Rowe CR, Zarins B: Chronic unreduced dislocations of the shoulder. *J Bone Joint Surg* 1982;64A:494–505.
2. Magnuson PB: Treatment of recurrent dislocation of the shoulder. *Surg Clin North Am* 1945;25:14–20.
3. Magnuson PB, Stack JK: Bilateral habitual dislocation of the shoulders in twins: A familial tendency. *JAMA* 1940;114:2103.
4. Osmond-Clarke H: Habitual dislocation of the shoulder: The Putti-Platt operation. *J Bone Joint Surg* 1948;30B:19–25.
5. Neer CS II, Foster CR: Inferior capsular shift for involuntary inferior and multidirectional instability of the shoulder: A preliminary report. *J Bone Joint Surg* 1980;62A:897–908.
6. Rockwood CA Jr: Fractures and dislocations of the shoulder: Part II: Subluxations and dislocations about the shoulder, in Rockwood CA Jr, Green DP (eds): *Fractures in Adults.* Philadelphia, JB Lippincott, 1984, vol 1, pp 722–985.
7. Rowe CR, Patel D, Southmayd WW: The Bankart procedure: A long-term end-result study. *J Bone Joint Surg* 1978;60A:1–16.
8. Rowe CR, Zarins B, Ciullo JV: Recurrent anterior dislocation of the shoulder after surgical repair: Apparent causes of failure and treatment. *J Bone Joint Surg* 1984;66A:159–168.
9. Bankart ASB: Recurrent or habitual dislocation of the shoulder joint. *Br Med J* 1923;2:1132–1133.
10. Viek P, Bell BT: The Bankart shoulder reconstruction: The use of pull-out wires and other practical details. *J Bone Joint Surg* 1959;41A:236–242.
11. du Toit GT, Roux D: Recurrent dislocation of the shoulder: A twenty-four year study of the Johannesburg stapling operation. *J Bone Joint Surg* 1956;38A:1–12.
12. Henderson WD: Arthroscopic stabilization of the anterior shoulder, in Minkoff J, Sherman OH (eds): *Clinics in Sports Medicine.* Philadelphia, WB Saunders, 1987, pp 581–586.
13. Wiley AM: Arthroscopy for shoulder instability and a technique for arthroscopic repair. *Arthroscopy* 1988;4:25–30.
14. Morgan CD, Bodenstab AB: Arthroscopic Bankart suture repair: Technique and early results. *Arthroscopy* 1987;3:111–122.
15. Badgley CE, O'Conner GA: Combined procedure for the repair of recurrent anterior dislocation of the shoulder. *J Bone Joint Surg* 1965;47A:1283.
16. Bailey RW: Acute and recurrent dislocation of the shoulder, in Calandruccio RA (ed): American Academy of Orthopaedic Surgeons *Instructional Course Lectures, XVIII-J1.* St. Louis, CV Mosby, 1973, pp 70–74.
17. Eden R: Zur Operation der habituellen Schulterluxation unter Mitteilung eines neuen Verfahrens bei Abriss am inneren Pfannenrande. *Dtsch Z Chir* 1918;144:268–280.
18. Hybbinette S: De la transplantation d'un fragment osseux pour rémedier aux luxations récidivantes de l'epaule: Constatations et résultats opératoires. *Acta Chir Scand* 1932;71:411–443.
19. Lange M: Die operative behandlung der Gewohnheitsmagiben verrenkung an schulter. *Z Orthop* 1944;75:162.
20. Lavik K: Habitual shoulder luxation: Eden-Hybbinette's operation. *Acta Orthop Scand* 1961;30:251–264.
21. Palmer I, Widén A: The bone block method for recurrent dislocation of the shoulder joint. *J Bone Joint Surg* 1948;30B:53–58.
22. Helfet AJ: Coracoid transplantation for recurring dislocation of the shoulder. *J Bone Joint Surg* 1958;40B:198–202.
23. Bonnin JG: Transplantation of the tip of the coracoid process for recurrent anterior dislocation of the shoulder. *J Bone Joint Surg* 1969;51B:579.
24. Bonnin JG: Transplantation of the coracoid tip: A definitive operation for recurrent anterior dislocation of the shoulder. *Proc R Soc Med* 1973;66:755–758.
25. May V Jr: A modified Bristow operation for anterior recurrent dislocation of the shoulder. *J Bone Joint Surg* 1970;52A:1010–1016.
26. Mead NC, Sweeney HJ: Bristow procedure. *Spectator Lett*, July 9, 1964.
27. Connolly JF: Humeral head defects associated with shoulder dislocations: Their diagnostic and surgical significance, in Mac-Ausland WR Jr (ed): American Academy of Orthopaedic Surgeons *Instructional Course Lectures, XXI.* St. Louis, CV Mosby, 1972, p 42.
28. Nicola T: Recurrent anterior dislocation of the shoulder: New operation. *J Bone Joint Surg* 1929;11:128–132.
29. Nicola T: Recurrent dislocation of the shoulder: Its treatment by transplantation of the long head of the biceps. *Am J Surg* 1929;6:815.
30. Nicola T: Acute anterior dislocation of the shoulder. *J Bone Joint Surg* 1949;31A:153–159.
31. Rowe CR, Zarins B: Recurrent transient subluxation of the shoulder. *J Bone Joint Surg* 1981;63A:863–872.
32. Rowe CR, Pierce DS, Clark JG: Voluntary dislocation of the shoulder: A preliminary report on a clinical, electromyographic, and psychiatric study of twenty-six patients. *J Bone Joint Surg* 1973;55A:445–460.
33. Rowe CR: Surgical approaches to the shoulder, in Rowe CR (ed): *The Shoulder.* New York, Churchill Livingstone, 1988, pp 38–42.
34. Thompson FR, Moga JJ: *The Combined Operative Repair of Anterior and Posterior Shoulder Subluxation*, videotape. Park Ridge, American Academy of Orthopaedic Surgeons, 1965.
35. Scott DJ: Treatment of recurrent posterior dislocations of the shoulder by glenoplasty. *J Bone Joint Surg* 1967;49A:471–476.

Treatment of Two- and Three-Part Fractures of the Proximal Humerus

Louis U. Bigliani, MD

Introduction

The treatment of displaced two- and three-part fractures of the proximal humerus is a challenging and difficult problem. Accurate diagnosis, which is essential for proper treatment, depends on understanding the complex anatomy of the shoulder, obtaining adequate radiographic views, and using a classification system that allows consistent identification of fracture types. Precise radiographs in several perpendicular planes, called the trauma series, are required to identify displacement. These consist of anteroposterior and lateral views in the scapular plane as well as an axillary view. The most helpful and commonly used system is the four-part classification developed by Neer.[1] This comprehensive system integrates fracture anatomy, biomechanics, and displacement to provide the proper diagnosis, thus facilitating treatment.

Most displaced two- and three-part fractures can be treated by either closed reduction or open reduction and internal fixation (ORIF). Many methods of treatment have been proposed and I will review the preferred procedures for specific fractures.

Rehabilitation is an important aspect of the treatment of displaced fractures. Without a properly organized rehabilitation program, optimal results will not be obtained in most fractures. Management of two- and three-part fractures is difficult, and several series have reported high complication rates.[2-5] Accurate diagnosis of the type of fracture and proper selection of the appropriate treatment will reduce the incidence of complications and improve results.

Anatomy

It is important to understand the complex anatomy of the shoulder because optimal function of the glenohumeral joint depends on proper anatomic alignment. Most of the stability of the glenohumeral joint is provided by soft-tissue structures because the glenoid socket is only one third the size of the humeral head.[6] The capsule, labrum, and ligaments are the static stabilizers while the rotator cuff muscles are the dynamic stabilizers.

The proximal humerus consists of the humeral head, the lesser tuberosity, the greater tuberosity, the bicipital groove, and the proximal humeral shaft (Fig. 18–1). It is important to differentiate between the anatomic neck, which is at the junction of the head and the tuberosities, and the surgical neck, which is in the area below the greater and lesser tuberosities. Anatomic neck fractures are quite rare and have a poor prognosis since the blood supply to the head is disrupted, whereas surgical neck fractures are common and the blood supply to the head is preserved.

The subscapularis is an internal rotator that attaches to the lesser tuberosity (Fig. 18–1). The unopposed pull of this muscle pulls the lesser tuberosity medially. The supraspinatus, a head depressor, and the infraspinatus and teres minor, external rotators, attach to the greater tuberosity. When the greater tuberosity is fractured, these muscles pull this fragment superiorly and posteriorly. The pectoralis major and other internal rotators attach to the proximal shaft; when the proximal shaft is fractured, these muscles pull the shaft medially.

The biceps tendon lies in the bicipital groove and is often a useful anatomic landmark during ORIF. It identifies the rotator interval, which can be opened without injury to the cuff. Also, the biceps tendon can prevent closed reduction of unimpacted two-part surgical neck fractures because it can act as a tether between fracture fragments (Fig. 18–2, *top left* and *top right*).

The acromion, coracoacromial ligament, and coracoid form the coracoacromial arch. This is a rather rigid structure under which the proximal humerus, rotator cuff, and bursa must pass. Displaced fractures may disrupt the smooth flow of these structures below the coracoacromial arch. This can result in impingement and blockage of glenohumeral motion.

The major blood supply to the humeral head is from the ascending branch of the anterior humeral circumflex artery.[7-9] The arcuate artery is a continuation of this ascending branch as it penetrates the proximal intertubercular groove area to enter the head and tuberosities, where several branches arise.[7] An additional blood supply to the humeral head is derived from the posterior circumflex humeral artery and through anastomosis from the soft tissue of the rotator cuff. However, the contributions of these other sources are negligible compared with that of the arcuate artery.

The brachial plexus and axillary artery are anterior to the coracoid process and can be injured by anterior fracture-dislocations or by violent trauma to the proximal humerus. The axillary nerve is the most commonly injured nerve about the shoulder. It consists of fibers from the fifth and sixth cervical roots in almost all cases. It originates from the posterior cord at the level of the

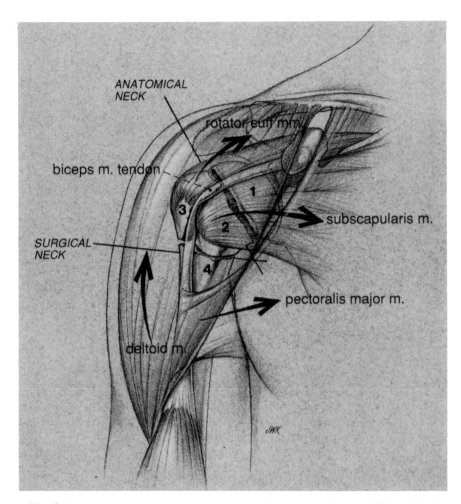

Fig. 18-1 Anatomy. The acromion, coracoacromial ligament, and coracoid form the sub-acromial arch under which the humeral head and rotator tendons must pass. The proximal humerus consists of the head, greater tuberosity, lesser tuberosity, and shaft. Displacement of bony fragments is caused by unopposed muscle pulls. The subscapularis attaches to the lesser tuberosity and pulls this fragment medially. The supraspinatus, infraspinatus, and teres minor attach to the greater tuberosity and pull this fragment superiorly and posteriorly. The pectoralis major attaches to the shaft and pulls the shaft medially. The biceps tendon is in the middle of the shoulder in the rotator interval and is a useful landmark. The anatomic neck is the area above the tuberosities at the junction of the articular surface. The surgical neck is the area below the tuberosities before the proximal shaft.

axilla. It passes along the inferior aspect of the capsule of the glenohumeral joint and then through the quadrangular space. It divides into posterior and anterior branches. The anterior branch winds along the undersurface of the deltoid, 6 to 7 cm from the edge of the acromion, giving off many small branches. It is often injured after it exits from the quadrangular space by a traction injury or near the inferior capsule during surgery. Injuries to the suprascapular and musculocutaneous nerves can occur but are much less common.

Classification

Fortunately, most fractures are minimally displaced and are easily treated by immobilization and early mo-

tion. It is important to distinguish these from the more complex displaced fractures that require more elaborate treatment. Several methods of classification have been proposed over the years, including classification by the anatomic level, the mechanism of injury, the amount of contact among fracture fragments, the degree of displacement, and the vascular status of the articular segments.[10-14] Combinations of these criteria have also been used. This has created a great deal of confusion that has resulted in inadequate treatment.

In 1934, Codman[15] made a significant contribution to the understanding of proximal humeral fractures by proposing that these fractures be separated into four distinct segmental fractures. These four segments occur along the anatomic lines of epiphyseal union and con-

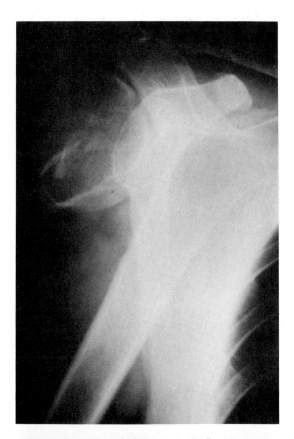

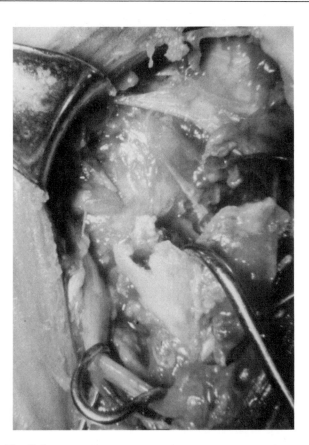

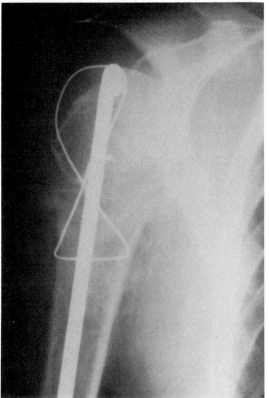

Fig. 18-2 Two-part unimpacted shaft fractures. **Top left:** Anteroposterior view of an unimpacted two-part surgical neck fracture. Closed reduction was not possible. Note the osteoporosis and fracture lines in the proximal head and greater tuberosity fragment. **Top right:** Intraoperative photograph showing the biceps tendon in the metal loop. This tendon was tethered between the shaft and the head, blocking reduction. **Bottom:** Postoperative anteroposterior view shows ORIF with figure-8 wire and Rush rod. The optional Rush rod was used for extra stability in this osteoporotic bone. It was removed after six weeks.

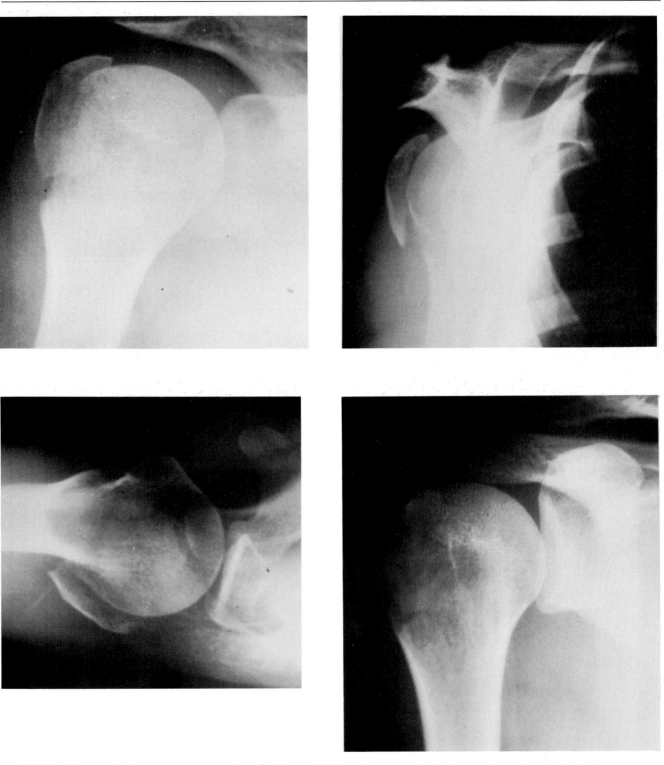

Fig. 18-3 Trauma series in two-part greater tuberosity fracture. This fracture was originally diagnosed as minimally displaced on the basis of one anteroposterior radiograph. **Top left:** Anteroposterior radiograph showing greater tuberosity fracture with minimal superior displacement. **Top right:** Lateral view in scapular plane showing posterior displacement of the fracture. **Bottom left:** Axillary view also demonstrates significant posterior displacement of the fracture. **Bottom right:** Repair of greater tuberosity fragment with nonabsorbable nylon sutures.

sist of the anatomic head, the shaft, the greater tuberosity, and the lesser tuberosity. In 1970, Neer[1] described a four-part classification that took into account these anatomic divisions. The classification is comprehensive, encompassing fracture anatomy, the biomechanics of the deforming forces, and the vascularity of

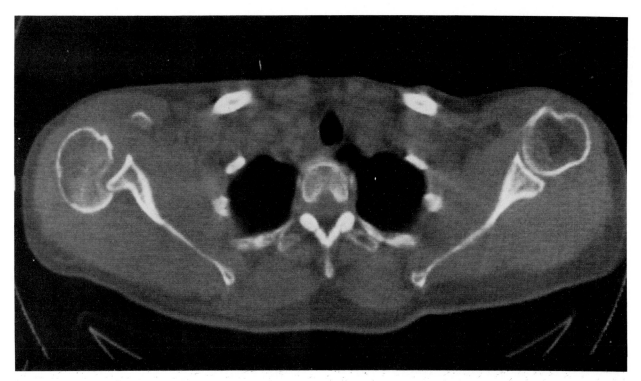

Fig. 18-4 Computed tomographic scan of posterior fracture dislocation. This scan of a posterior fracture-dislocation clearly outlines an impression defect in the humeral head of approximately 40%.

the head, and relating these factors to diagnosis and treatment. It is specific enough to allow accurate diagnosis of fractures, yet flexible enough to allow for variations. It is a consistent method on which a treatment rationale may be based.

This system is based on accurate identification of the four fragments and their relationship to one another. Therefore, a comprehensive radiographic series in several perpendicular planes, the trauma series, is essential. When any of the four major segments is displaced more than 1 cm or angulated more than 45 degrees, the fracture is considered displaced.[1,16] There can be two-part, three-part, and four-part fractures.

In a two-part fracture, one fragment is displaced in reference to the other three fragments. In a three-part fracture, two fragments are displaced in reference to each other and the two undisplaced fragments. In a four-part fracture, all four fragments are displaced. The head is out of contact with the glenoid and detached from both tuberosities, interrupting its blood supply. Fissure lines or hairline fractures are not considered displaced fragments. Therefore, a fragment may have several fissure lines in continuity. These are considered one fragment.

The normal neck shaft angle in the anteroposterior view is 143 degrees in the neutral position, but the angle can range from 134 to 166 degrees.[17] In addition, the neck shaft angle can vary as much as 30 degrees

with maximal internal and external rotation. Therefore, when radiographs are compared it is important to know the amount of rotation. The normal neck shaft angle in the lateral projection is approximately 25 degrees posteriorly. This can range from −9 degrees to 59 degrees and also can vary significantly with rotation.

A fracture-dislocation is one in which the head is displaced outside the joint space rather than subluxated or rotated. It can be a two-part, three-part, or four-part fracture and is also classified according to direction, anterior or posterior. Head-splitting and impression fractures are graded according to the percentage of the articular surface involved. The general classification guidelines adopted for these fractures are less than 20% involvement, 20% to 45% involvement, and more than 45% involvement.[16]

Radiographic Evaluation

Precise radiographs in several perpendicular planes are essential for the proper diagnosis and treatment of proximal humeral fractures. Incorrect or oblique radiographs misrepresent the fracture and create confusion. Today, this is still one of the most common errors in the treatment of displaced fractures. Often a fracture is classified on the basis of only one anteroposterior view. A trauma series, as described by Neer,[16]

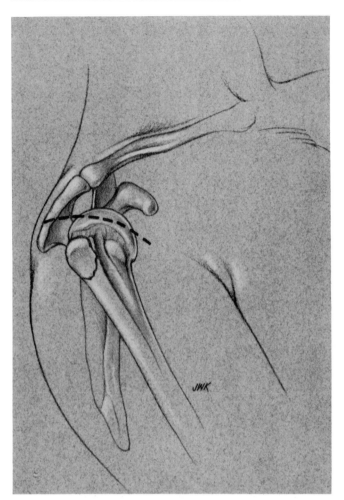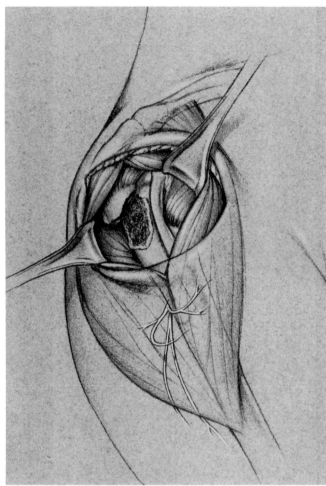

Fig. 18-5 Superior deltoid approach. **Left:** Skin incision just lateral to the anterolateral tip of the acromion extends approximately 7 to 8 cm in an oblique fashion in Langer's lines. **Right:** The deltoid is then split for approximately 5 cm from the edge of the acromion distally in the area of the junction between the anterior and middle deltoid. The split should not be longer because of possible injury to the axillary nerve.

should be performed on every patient with a proximal humeral fracture. This series consists of anteroposterior and lateral views in the scapular plane as well as an axillary view (Fig. 18–3). The glenohumeral joint does not sit in either the sagittal or the frontal plane. The scapula sits on the chest wall in an oblique fashion approximately 40 degrees posterior to the frontal plane. The axis of the glenohumeral joint is, therefore, posterior 35 to 40 degrees. To achieve a true anteroposterior view, the posterior part of the involved shoulder is placed against the plate and the other shoulder is rotated out 40 degrees. This allows clear visualization of the glenohumeral joint without bony obstruction. In the lateral view, the anterior aspect of the shoulder is placed against the radiographic plate and the other shoulder is rotated 40 degrees out. The axillary view is extremely helpful in the evaluation of anterior and posterior fracture-dislocations and the glenoid articular surface in the axial plane. It is essential for the diagnosis of a fixed posterior fracture-dislocation.

All these views can be obtained with the patient standing, sitting, or in a prone position. During the axillary view, it is helpful for the physician to hold the patient's arm in abduction to minimize any further displacement of the fracture. Also, the patient should be placed on a cushion so that the shoulder is off the table, avoiding any objects that might obscure the bony fracture. A Velpeau axillary view has been described in which the patient just leans backward 20 to 30 degrees with the tube above the shoulder and the plate below.[18] Supplemental radiographs, such as the transthoracic and various rotational views, may at times be useful in estimating the amount of displacement of specific segments. This can be especially useful in the evaluation of malunions.

Evaluation with bone imaging is not routine, but can be useful in selected displaced fractures. Magnetic resonance imaging may have potential as a useful diagnostic tool but, at present, the computed tomographic scan is the most accurate test. Further, it produces a

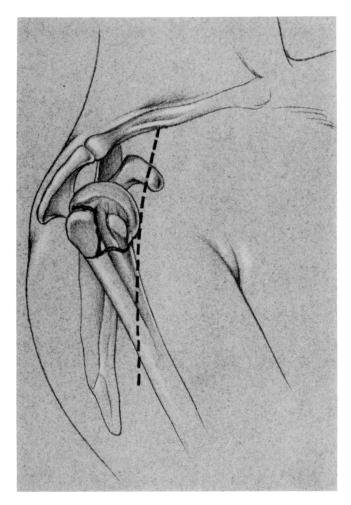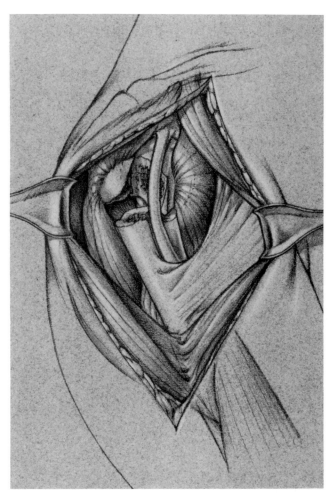

Fig. 18-6 Deltopectoral approach. **Left:** Skin incision showing the long deltopectoral approach starting at approximately the clavicle and extending distally along the coracoid to the shaft of the humerus. **Right:** The deltoid is split in a longitudinal fashion. The deltoid's origin is not removed. If more exposure is needed, the insertion may be elevated, as may the insertion of the pectoralis major.

relatively low radiation exposure. It has replaced tomography as the procedure of choice in most situations. Computed tomography is extremely useful in evaluating the articular surfaces of both the glenoid and the humeral head (Fig. 18–4). Morris and associates[19] reported that it is also useful in evaluating the amount of greater tuberosity displacement. If the radiographs are not optimum and do not show the fracture clearly, it is important to repeat these tests.

Surgical Approaches

The deltoid muscle is not injured or disrupted in most proximal humeral fractures, whereas the rotator cuff muscles are usually involved. Therefore, it is important to preserve the integrity of the deltoid muscle and not detach its origin or injure the axillary nerve. Two basic approaches are sufficient to expose most dis-

placed two- and three-part proximal humeral fractures adequately.

The first is the superior deltoid split. A 7- to 8-cm incision is made in the Langer's lines just lateral to the anterolateral tip of the acromion (Fig. 18–5, *left*). The deltoid is then split from the lateral tip of the acromion distally for approximately 5 cm (Fig. 18–5, *right*). The lower part of the split is sutured to avoid further dissection and injury to the axillary nerve during retraction. This procedure is extremely useful in the treatment of greater tuberosity fractures because the fragment and rotator cuff can be easily mobilized. It is also useful for the insertion of an intramedullary rod through the greater tuberosity.

All other fractures can be adequately treated with the long deltopectoral approach (Fig. 18–6, *left*). This approach does not remove the deltoid's origin. If more exposure is needed, the insertion may be partially elevated. In most instances, however, exposure adequate for ORIF, as well as for prosthetic replacement, can be

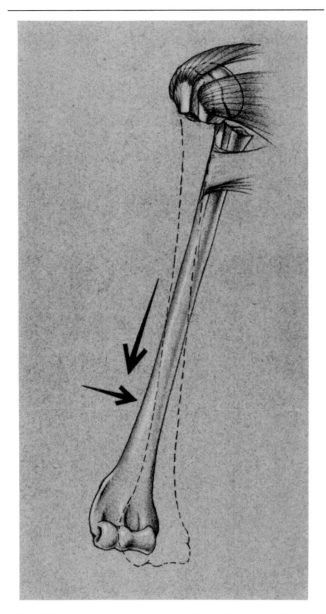

Fig. 18-7 Reduction maneuver for a displaced unimpacted surgical neck fracture. The deforming force in an unimpacted two-part surgical neck fracture is the pectoralis major. The head remains in neutral position in the glenoid since both tuberosities are attached. Longitudinal traction is placed on the arm as it is gently flexed and adducted. The head is then brought beneath the humerus and impacted and the arm is placed in the Velpeau position. The reduction is checked by image-intensifier control.

obtained (Fig. 18–6, *right*). It is important to identify the biceps tendon quickly as this is an important landmark. It leads to the glenoid by splitting the rotator interval and also helps identify displaced fragments. The surgeon should avoid making a longitudinal cut in the muscle of the deltoid more than 5 cm from the edge of the acromion because this may injure the axillary nerve. Compromised function of the anterior deltoid produces a poor result, despite adequate fracture fixation and healing.

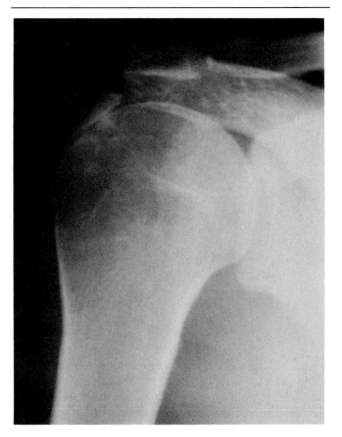

Fig. 18-8 Greater tuberosity malunion. Anteroposterior view of a greater tuberosity malunion in a fracture treated by closed reduction. The patient had significant impingement secondary to a superiorly and posteriorly retracted greater tuberosity.

Treatment of Displaced Two-Part Fractures

Closed Reduction

Several types of displaced two-part fractures are amenable to closed reduction. These include the rare lesser tuberosity fracture, shaft fractures (angulated, unimpacted, and comminuted), anterior and posterior fracture-dislocations, and head impression fractures with less than 20% articular involvement.

Isolated lesser tuberosity fractures are extremely rare and generally can be treated with closed reduction. If the fragment is large and prevents medial rotation, ORIF may be necessary. These fractures are usually associated with a posterior fracture-dislocation, and in acute injuries a closed reduction can be attempted. Longitudinal traction is placed on the arm as it is gently flexed and brought out of adduction to unhook the head from the glenoid. Continued traction and a slight degree of abduction and external rotation will achieve reduction. Digital pressure on the posterior aspect of the head can be helpful. Repeated, forcible attempts at reduction and sudden rotation should be avoided because they may lead to a fracture or a nerve injury. The arm is immobilized at the side in a cast or brace that maintains neutral or slight external rotation. If the lesser tuberosity fragment is large and involves a significant part of the articular surface, ORIF is necessary.

Two-part greater tuberosity fracture-dislocations can also be treated by closed reduction, but the greater tuberosity fragment is more apt to displace after reduction, and serial radiographs are needed to check for subsequent displacement. Closed reduction is achieved with longitudinal traction, flexion, and adduction of the arm to the neutral position. Digital pressure on the head anteriorly can also be helpful.

Impacted surgical neck fractures with more than 45 degrees of angulation should be disimpacted and reduced to decrease the amount of anterior angulation. A malunion with excessive anterior angulation will compromise forward elevation of the arm.

In an unimpacted two-part surgical neck fracture, the shaft is usually pulled medially by the pull of the pectoralis major and other internal rotators. The head is generally situated in a neutral position in the glenoid. A closed reduction is achieved by longitudinal traction, flexion, and adduction (Fig. 18–7). The shaft is gently impacted beneath the head and the reduction is checked with an image intensifier. At times, soft-tissue interposition from the biceps tendon, muscle, or capsule prevents closed reduction (Fig. 18–2, *top left* and *top right*). Furthermore, the proximal fragment may be osteoporotic and repeated attempts at closed reduction will further comminute the fracture. If reduction can be achieved but remains unstable, percutaneous pinning may be required. Under image-intensifier control, two distal pins are directed proximally from just above the level of the deltoid's insertion into the head. A power drill is necessary as it may be difficult to penetrate the cortex of the shaft. Threaded-tip 2.5-mm AO pins are preferred. A third pin directed proximally through the greater tuberosity into the shaft improves fixation. The pin should be cut subcutaneously and removed after six weeks when there is adequate fracture healing. Jakob and associates[14] reported good results with this technique in 35 of 40 patients, but emphasized that it is a very demanding procedure.

Comminuted proximal shaft fractures can be treated by closed reduction and a spica cast, but this may not provide adequate alignment for the displaced fracture fragments. Traction is an option but it is difficult to maintain as well as contraindicated in the patient with multiple injuries since it significantly curtails mobilization. However, it may be useful until ORIF is possible.

ORIF

ORIF is generally indicated for displaced greater tuberosity fractures, anatomic neck fractures, unreduced shaft and lesser tuberosity fractures, and fracture-dislocations. In most instances, the greater tuberosity is

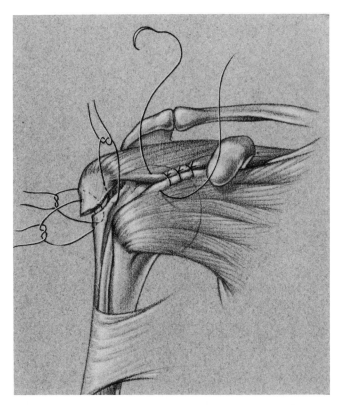

Fig. 18–9 Repair of greater tuberosity fracture. Greater tuberosity fractures are exposed by the superior deltoid approach. The fragment is mobilized with several nylon sutures. It is important to repair the rent in the rotator cuff first, as this relieves tension on the bony fragment. The arm should be rotated for optimum exposure. Nylon sutures are then placed in the bony fragment and it is reattached to its humeral bed.

displaced superiorly and posteriorly by the unopposed pull of the supraspinatus, infraspinatus, and teres minor. If left to heal in this displaced position, it will block forward elevation and external rotation, especially with the arm in 90 degrees of abduction (Fig. 18–8). The surgical technique for this fracture is a superior deltoid approach in which the deltoid is split for 5 cm distal to the acromion and not detached from its origin (Fig. 18–5). The greater tuberosity fragment is attached back to its bed with several nylon sutures. The tear in the rotator cuff interval should be repaired first as this takes tension off the bone-to-bone repair (Fig. 18–9). Nonabsorbable nylon sutures provide firm fixation and decrease the irritation in the subacromial space (Fig. 18–3, *bottom right*). A second procedure is not needed to remove the fixation.

Anatomic neck fractures are exceedingly rare but do occur. ORIF should be attempted, especially if the patient is young. If the patient is older and the bone is quite osteoporotic, a primary prosthesis is probably the best choice. Unimpacted two-part shaft fractures may require ORIF because of interposition of the biceps ten-

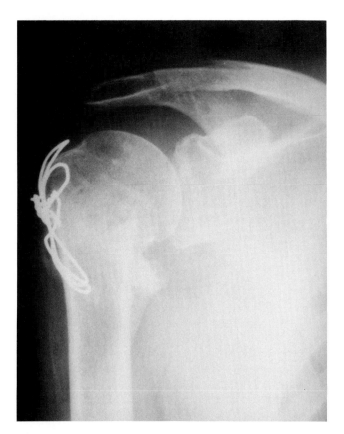 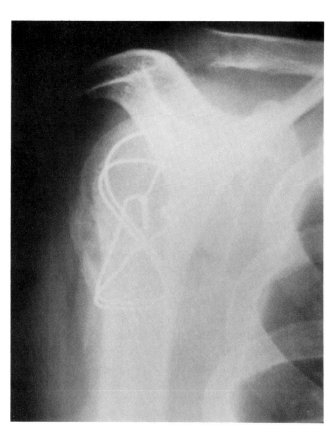

Fig. 18–10 Two-part unimpacted shaft fractures. **Left:** Anteroposterior view three months after ORIF with two figure-8 tension band wires that gave excellent internal fixation. **Right:** Lateral view in the scapular plane at three months reveals excellent alignment of the fracture.

don, capsule, or muscle that prevents closed reduction (Fig. 18–2, *top left* and *top right*). A long deltopectoral approach is usually the preferred method. Internal fixation may be achieved by a figure-8 wire or several nylon sutures (Fig. 18–10). If there is significant comminution, a Rush rod or other form of intramedullary fixation may occasionally be required for extra stability (Fig. 18–2, *bottom*). Excellent fixation that permits early motion can be achieved with this technique. The fixation should be tested at surgery and the arm put through a limited range of motion. A buttress T-plate can also be used, but this requires more soft-tissue exposure and good bone stock for adequate screw fixation. Severely comminuted fractures may require ORIF. The fixation may not be rigid but it at least aligns the fracture fragments so that plaster fixation will be successful. The goal in these fractures is not early motion but fracture healing. A second procedure may be needed to lyse adhesions and to remove hardware so that adequate motion can be achieved.

Treatment of Displaced Three-Part Fractures

Closed reduction is generally less successful in the treatment of displaced three-part fractures. These frac-

tures are unstable because there is shaft displacement as well as the displaced tuberosity fragment. Repeated attempts at closed reduction should be avoided because the fractures are often in osteoporotic bone and further fragmentation and displacement of the fragments can occur. Leyshon[20] and Young and Wallace[21] reported satisfactory results with closed reduction of displaced three-part fractures. However, it should be noted that the patients in these series were elderly and that their expectations in regard to treatment and use of the extremities were limited. Pain relief was adequate. In younger, active individuals, open reduction is the treatment of choice.

Many methods of ORIF have been described, but the preferred technique is one that uses minimal, but secure, internal fixation with limited soft-tissue dissection. In the past, T-plate fixation was a popular technique, but several recent studies have reported high failure rates.[2-4] The bone in these fractures is usually osteoporotic and unable to hold screw fixation. The excessive soft-tissue dissection needed for plate fixation may also be a factor leading to avascular necrosis.[2] This technique seems better suited for young individuals with bone of good quality. Multiple compression screws and intramedullary rods are inadequate to control the deforming forces in these complex fractures.

Nonabsorbable nylon or wire is the preferred method of fixation.[16] Several No. 2 or 5 nylon sutures or 18-gauge figure-8 wires provide adequate fixation in most cases (Fig. 18–11). The sutures should be passed through the rotator cuff as well as the bone because the rotator cuff may be stronger and provide better fixation than the osteoporotic bone. A large 14- or 16-gauge spinal needle or plastic catheter is helpful in passing sutures or wire through the cuff. The displaced tuberosity should be attached to the head and the remaining tuberosity fragment as well as to the shaft below. Hawkins and associates[22] obtained satisfactory results in 14 patients with a figure-8 tension band technique. I have had satisfactory results with nonabsorbable sutures as well as with the wire technique (Fig. 18–12). Fixation is surprisingly secure and early range-of-motion exercises can be started.

In selected older patients with comminuted fractures in osteoporotic bone, a primary prosthesis may be a better alternative. Because of the soft bone, secure internal fixation may not be possible; a prosthesis permits a more stable repair so that early mobilization of the fracture can be started. Tanner and Cofield[23] reported good results with this technique. In anterior three-part fracture-dislocations, the head is situated below the coracoid and lies against the neurovascular bundle. It is extremely important to dissect out the head with caution to avoid injuring the neurovascular bundle.

Rehabilitation

Rehabilitation of proximal humeral fractures is essential because adequate motion is needed for optimum shoulder function. Once a fracture or a fracture repair is stable, therapy should be started. The most useful system presently available is the three-phase one devised by Neer.[16] The first phase consists of passive assisted exercises. The second phase consists of active and resistance exercises as well as stretching. The third phase is a maintenance program designed to further stretch and strengthen the tissues. Application of this system is variable and depends on the type of fracture, the stability of the fracture, and the ability of the patient to comprehend the exercise program. In most instances it is advisable to involve a physical therapist.

If a fracture is stable, passive exercises are begun once the acute pain from the trauma has subsided. This is generally between seven and ten days. At that time, pendulum exercises and supine external rotation with a stick can be started. During the next few weeks, pulley exercises and assisted supine forward elevation can be added. Active and resistance exercises are not started until six to eight weeks after the injury or when there is adequate fracture healing. There is a tendency for displacement of fracture fragments during rehabilita-

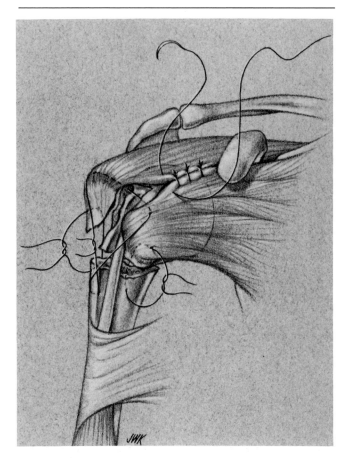

Fig. 18–11 Technique of three-part repair. Several nonabsorbable nylon sutures or wire can be used to repair displaced three-part fractures. It is important to attach the displaced tuberosity to the head and remaining tuberosity fragment as well as to the shaft fragment. It is important to preserve the biceps tendon.

tion and it is important to check the reduction by serial radiographs. Greater tuberosity fractures are particularly likely to displace after reduction.

Once ORIF has produced a stable repair, exercises are begun within 48 to 72 hours. These are conducted by the physician and involve assisted forward elevation and external rotation. By the fourth or fifth postoperative day, a formal physiotherapy program with a physical therapist can be started. This includes pendulum exercises, supine external rotation with a stick, supine assisted forward elevation, and pulley exercises. These exercises should be done at least three times a day, and preferably four times. An analgesic administered 20 to 30 minutes before the exercise period often facilitates range of motion. This program is maintained for approximately six weeks, at which time the active and resistance exercise phase of the program is begun. It is essential that fracture healing be adequate before active exercises are started. Initially these consist of isometrics and Theraband. Light weights (1 to 3 lb) are used much later in the program, usually after three months. An advanced stretching and strengthening program is gen-

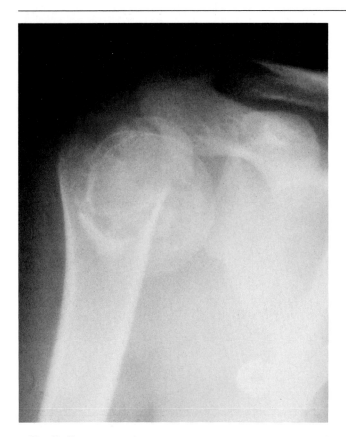

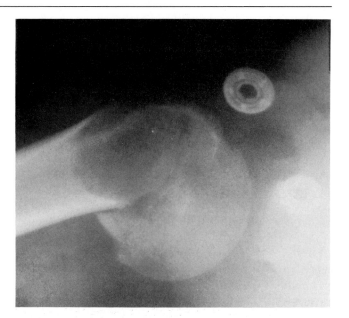

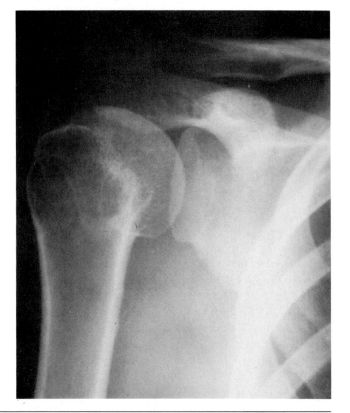

Fig. 18-12 Three-part greater tuberosity displacement. **Top left:** Anteroposterior view of a three-part greater tuberosity displacement. **Top right:** Axillary view of the three-part greater tuberosity displacement. **Bottom right:** Postoperative anteroposterior view after ORIF with nonabsorbable nylon sutures. Six months after the injury, patient had a full, normal range of motion with excellent bony union.

erally started after three months, during the third phase of the program. It is important to emphasize that the final result may not be achieved for at least a year after injury and the physician must encourage the patient to continue the exercise regimen throughout this period.

Complications

Many complications have been reported after both closed and open treatment. The more common com-

plications include malunion, nonunion, hardware failure, frozen shoulder, infection, and neurovascular injury. Avascular necrosis is generally considered to be a complication of four-part fractures, but it is not uncommon after three-part fractures and can occur after some two-part fractures.[1-5,24] Hägg and Lundberg[5] reported a high incidence of avascular necrosis in three-part fractures in their review of several large series. The rate of avascular necrosis in three-part fractures after closed treatment was between 3% and 14% and the rate after ORIF was between 12% and 25%. Sturzenegger and associates[2] also reported a high incidence of avascular necrosis after T-plate fixation of displaced fractures. They believed that the extensive soft-tissue dissection and exposure needed for the T-plate contributed to the high incidence. Others have also reported problems with T-plate fixation, including loosening of plate and screw fixation and plate malposition.[3-5,22]

Malunion can significantly limit range of motion, thereby compromising shoulder function. The space beneath the subacromial arch is limited and malunion will cause impingement. Reconstruction of a malunion is especially difficult since displacement of the fragments distorts the anatomy and scarring can compromise the surrounding soft tissues. Nonunion usually occurs after two-part unimpacted shaft fractures and three-part fractures, but can also occur after undisplaced proximal humeral fractures.[16] The factors associated with nonunion include interposition of soft tissue, overly aggressive physiotherapy before adequate fracture healing has taken place, infection, loss of internal fixation, metabolic bone disease, and poor patient compliance. Treatment includes ORIF, autogenous iliac crest bone graft, and a shoulder spica cast for at least six weeks postoperatively. Figure-8 wires and a Rush rod for longitudinal support, if needed, are the preferred methods of internal fixation. A second procedure is generally necessary to remove the hardware and lyse adhesions so that adequate motion can be achieved.

Stableforth[24] reported injury to the axillary artery in four of 81 fractures (roughly 4.9%). This injury is usually associated with penetrating or violent blunt trauma that causes multiple fractures, but it can also occur after ORIF.[25] The most common site of injury is at the junction of the anterior circumflex and axillary arteries. Early diagnosis and repair are essential. It is important to check the radial pulse in the injured extremity. However, peripheral pulses may be caused by the collateral circulation. This does not, therefore, guarantee that no significant arterial injury has occurred. Paresthesias are probably the most reliable sign of inadequate distal circulation and a vascular injury should be suspected if they are present. Doppler ultrasonography can be helpful in detecting a pulse but can also be misleading because the collateral circulation can create a pulse detectable by Doppler examination. If arterial injury is suspected, angiography should be performed without delay to confirm the diagnosis.

Brachial plexus injuries were reported in five of the 81 fractures in Stableforth's series (6.2%).[24] The axillary nerve is the nerve most commonly injured after shoulder fractures. The deltoid patch area should be tested for sensation because pain can make testing deltoid muscle function difficult. If a nerve injury is suspected, an electromyogram should be obtained within four to six weeks. If a complete axillary nerve injury does not improve

within three months, surgical exploration may be indicated.

Injuries to the suprascapular and musculocutaneous nerves are uncommon in proximal humeral fractures. They are more likely in scapular fractures. Injury to the thorax can also occur after fractures of the proximal humerus. Intrathoracic dislocation of the head has been reported in surgical neck fractures.[26,27] In addition, a pneumothorax or hemopneumothorax can occur. A complete chest examination is essential in all fractures and if pneumothorax is suspected, a chest radiograph is indicated. Myositis ossificans is a rare complication, but may occur after fracture-dislocations.

References

1. Neer CS II: Displaced proximal humeral fractures: I. Classification and evaluation. *J Bone Joint Surg* 1970;52A:1077–1089.
2. Sturzenegger M, Fornaro E, Jakob RP: Results of surgical treatment of multifragmented fractures of the humeral head. *Arch Orthop Trauma Surg* 1982;100:249–259.
3. Kristiansen B, Christensen SW: Plate fixation of proximal humeral fractures. *Acta Orthop Scand* 1986;57:320–323.
4. Paavolainen P, Björkenheim J-M, Slätis P, et al: Operative treatment of severe proximal humeral fractures. *Acta Orthop Scand* 1983;54:374–379.
5. Hägg O, Lundberg B: Aspects of prognostic factors in comminuted and dislocated proximal humeral fractures, in Bateman JE, Welsh RP (eds): *Surgery of the Shoulder*. Philadelphia, Decker, 1984, pp 51–59.
6. Saha AK: Dynamic stability of the glenohumeral joint. *Acta Orthop Scand* 1971;42:491–505.
7. Laing PG: The arterial supply of the adult humerus. *J Bone Joint Surg* 1956;38A:1105–1116.
8. Moseley HF, Goldie I: The arterial pattern of the rotator cuff on the shoulder. *J Bone Joint Surg* 1963;45B:780–789.
9. Rothman RH, Parke WW: The vascular anatomy of the rotator cuff. *Clin Orthop* 1965;41:176–186.
10. Kocher T: *Beiträge zur Kenntniss einiger praktisch wichtiger Fracturformen*. Basel, Carl Söllmann, 1896.
11. Watson-Jones R: *Fractures and Joint Injuries*, ed 5. Baltimore, Williams & Wilkins, 1955.
12. Drapanas T, McDonald J, Hale HW Jr: A rational approach to classification and treatment of fractures of the surgical neck of the humerus. *Am J Surg* 1960;99:617–624.
13. Knight RA, Mayne JA: Comminuted fractures and fracture-dislocations involving the articular surface of the humeral head. *J Bone Joint Surg* 1957;39A:1343–1355.
14. Jakob RP, Kristiansen T, Mayo K, et al: Classification and aspects of treatment of fractures of the proximal humerus, in Bateman JE, Welsh RP (eds): *Surgery of the Shoulder*. Philadelphia, Decker, 1984, pp 330–343.
15. Codman EA: *The Shoulder: Rupture of the Supraspinatus Tendon and Other Lesions in or About the Subacromial Bursa*. Boston, Thomas Todd, 1934.
16. Neer CS II: Fractures and dislocations of the shoulder: Part I. Fractures about the shoulder, in Rockwood CA Jr, Green DP (eds): *Fractures in Adults*, ed 2. Philadelphia, JB Lippincott, 1984, vol 1, pp 675–721.
17. Keene JS, Huizenga RE, Engber WD, et al: Proximal humeral fractures: A correlation of residual deformity with long-term function. *Orthopedics* 1983;6173–6178.
18. Bloom MH, Obata WG: Diagnosis of posterior dislocation of the

shoulder with use of Velpeau axillary and angle-up roentgenographic views. *J Bone Joint Surg* 1967;49A:943–949.

19. Morris ME, Kilcoyne RF, Shuman W, et al: Humeral tuberosity fractures: Evaluation by CT scan and management of malunion. *Orthop Trans* 1987;11:242.

20. Leyshon RL: Closed treatment of fractures of the proximal humerus. *Acta Orthop Scand* 1984;55:48–51.

21. Young TB, Wallace WA: Conservative treatment of fractures and fracture-dislocations of the upper end of the humerus. *J Bone Joint Surg* 1985;67B:373–377.

22. Hawkins RJ, Bell RH, Gurr K: The three-part fracture of the proximal part of the humerus: Operative treatment. *J Bone Joint Surg* 1986;68A:1410–1414.

23. Tanner MW, Cofield RH: Prosthetic arthroplasty for fractures and fracture-dislocations of the proximal humerus. *Clin Orthop* 1983;179:116–128.

24. Stableforth PG: Four-part fractures of the neck of the humerus. *J Bone Joint Surg* 1984;66B:104–108.

25. Zuckerman JD, Flugstad DL, Teitz CC, et al: Axillary artery injury as a complication of proximal humeral fractures: Two case reports and a review of the literature. *Clin Orthop* 1984;189:234–237.

26. Hardcastle PH, Fisher TR: Intrathoracic displacement of the humeral head with fracture of the surgical neck. *Injury* 1981;12:313–315.

27. Glessner JR Jr: Intrathoracic dislocation of the humeral head. *J Bone Joint Surg* 1961;43A:428–430.

CHAPTER 19

Lesions of the Brachial Plexus Revisited

Robert D. Leffert, MD

In this chapter, I will examine the current status of brachial plexus lesions, emphasizing the treatment advances made since my previous discussion of this topic in 1977.[1] I have chosen not to repeat material that is, in my opinion, still current but rather to provide updated information in areas where the previous material is no longer timely.

Clinical and Anatomic Correlations

The anatomy of the brachial plexus has been the subject of many investigations.[2-5] Although the correlations between diagnosis and prognosis are well known and clearly useful in the treatment of patients, it was not until recently that intraneural topography was applied to surgery of the brachial plexus. Sunderland,[6] Mansat,[7] Alnot and associates,[8] Bonnel,[9,10] and Narakas[11] have shown that knowledge of intraneural topography is essential for selective grafting within the plexus (Fig. 19–1). Slingluff and associates[12] have published a significant work on the quantitative microanatomy of the brachial plexus (Fig. 19–2). Although all this work represents a significant advance in our knowledge and ability to design surgery more intelligently, no universal approach can be applied to all patients. Additional methods of investigation are needed in the areas of electrical stimulation in vivo, discussed later, and the definition of different varieties of nerve fiber by histochemical methods that can be applied intraoperatively.[13]

Methods of Evaluation and Examination

The examination of a patient with a brachial plexus injury must be carried out in a standardized and minutely detailed manner with the objective of establishing the location of the nerve lesions and their degree of abnormality. It must be determined whether the loss of motor and sensory function in the distribution of a particular nerve root represents avulsion of that root from the spinal cord (supraganglionic lesion) or a lesion distal to the dorsal root ganglion (infraganglionic). The latter can range from a lesion in continuity that will recover spontaneously to a distal rupture that will require surgical repair for functional recovery to occur. Presently, the prognosis for spontaneous recovery of the avulsed root is poor, and there is no proven surgical

technique for reestablishing continuity with the spinal cord to allow reinnervation. Because most clinically observed complete brachial plexus injuries represent combinations of root avulsions and distal ruptures, all diagnostic maneuvers are intended to establish the presence or absence of root avulsion. The variations in individual patterns of innervation make absolute accuracy in diagnosis problematical. Nevertheless, once this differentiation has been made, the more treatable infraganglionic lesions can be further identified and a therapeutic plan formulated.

The history of the injury is significant because the mode and the mechanism determine the neuropathologic abnormality. High-velocity injuries, such as those received in a fall from a speeding motorcycle onto a helmet and the shoulder, are likely to result in major supraclavicular traction injuries. Paralysis of the entire limb accompanied by severe burning pain is a sign of avulsion of one or more nerve roots. A fracture of the clavicle with lateral dislocation of the scapula on the thorax indicates greater traction on the nerves than would have occurred if the clavicle had remained intact.[14] In contrast, a stretch injury of the plexus received by an anesthetized patient on an operating table is almost always of lesser severity and usually has a good prognosis for spontaneous recovery.[15] Intermediate situations, such as falls on stairs or when a worker's sleeve is pulled by a machine, can result in a variety of nerve injuries that are correspondingly less severe in nature.

In all cases of brachial plexus injury, it is important to establish the previous state of the patient's upper extremity. Then, after the detailed history of the injury is obtained and recorded, a physical examination, which begins with the head and neck, is conducted. The eyes are examined for Horner's syndrome, which is a useful indicator of root avulsion at the level of the first thoracic vertebra. It may be partially present and expressed as myosis or a slight droop of the upper eyelid. The supraclavicular fossa is examined for Tinel's sign, and if the patient can feel the paresthesia in the limb without sensation when the plexus is percussed in the neck, then at least one nerve root has not been avulsed and is potentially available as a source of axons for surgical reconstruction. The passive range of motion of the joints of the upper limb is documented and then manual muscle testing is done. It must include the periscapular muscles such as the trapezius and serratus anterior, because these are significant in reconstruction, particularly in shoulder fusion. In addition, since the serratus

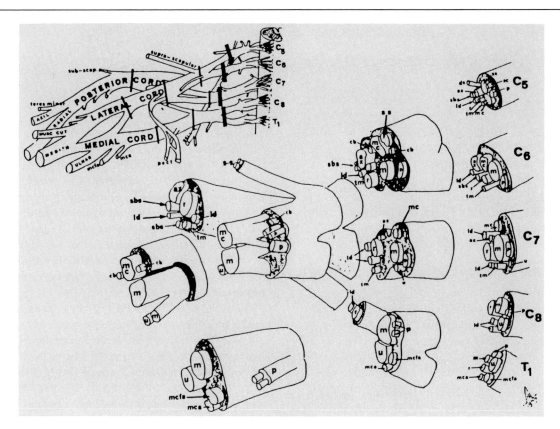

Fig. 19-1   Intraneural topography of the brachial plexus. (Reproduced with permission from Narakas AO: Surgical treatment of traction injuries of the brachial plexus. *Clin Orthop* 1978;133:71.)

and rhomboids are supplied by nerves that are root collaterals, finding them denervated is strong evidence that the damage to the fifth cervical vertebra (rhomboids) or the fifth through seventh vertebrae (serratus) is intraspinal and represents root avulsion.

Plain radiographs of the cervical spine and shoulder are taken in all cases. Significant cervical scoliosis is compatible with a diagnosis of multiple root avulsions,[16] and an avulsion of a cervical transverse process or the first rib indicates that the nerve root at that level has been avulsed. Although the fracture fragments from a broken clavicle usually do not themselves account for the acute nerve injury, they may occasionally transect the nerves and injure the vessels. In the presence of a nonunion with a slowly enlarging callus, the resulting mass may cause subclavicular compression of the nerves. This situation is best evaluated by means of a computed tomographic scan, and it may well require surgical correction.

Since the initial report by Murphey and associates[17] that contrast myelography was a useful method of detecting root avulsion, many others have studied this technique.[18-20] Clearly, this application is not without controversy and has changed with the evolution of imaging techniques during the past four decades.[21,22] Both false-positive and false-negative results can be obtained

and the test must be evaluated in this context. Millesi,[23,24] for example, stated that the test is not reliable because only the presence of a meningocele is significant. Gilbert and associates,[25,26] in a study of infants with obstetric brachial plexus injuries, found three false-negative results among 495 roots studied. In these cases, the myelographic findings were normal although the roots were avulsed. There were 14 false-positive results. Alnot and associates[8] stated that most of their patients with normal myelograms who were treated surgically had either distal lesions in continuity, leading to progressive recovery, or ruptures in the scalene region or more distally, in which repair was possible.

In addition, whereas oil-based contrast material was formerly injected via lumbar puncture, our present technique employs a puncture at the first and second cervical vertebrae with the aid of a C-arm and the instillation of metrizamide, a water-soluble contrast material. The test is usually well tolerated and, although we formerly preferred polytomes as the method of imaging, we have found that computed tomography significantly improves the yield of the test (Fig. 19–3). Marshall and DeSilva[27] confirmed this impression, particularly with reference to the fifth and sixth cervical root levels. In addition to pseudomeningoceles, the findings in root avulsion may include absence of the

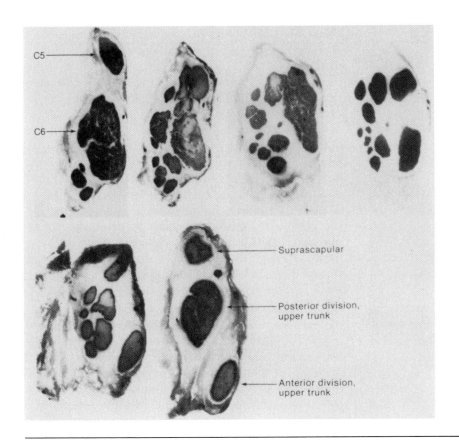

C5

C6

Suprascapular

Posterior division,
upper trunk

Anterior division,
upper trunk

Fig. 19-2 This sequence of six sections samples a 3-cm span of the upper trunk from the initial merging of C5 and C6 spinal nerves, through the gross mixing of fascicles, to the rearrangement into three monofascicular components, the anterior and posterior divisions of the upper trunk, and the suprascapular nerve. (Reproduced with permission from Slingluff CL, Terzis JK, Edgerton MT: The quantitative microanatomy of the brachial plexus in man: Reconstructive relevance, in Terzis JK (ed): *Microreconstruction of Nerve Injuries*. Philadelphia, WB Saunders, 1987.)

root shadows, as well as obliterated root pouches. These are well demonstrated in the multiple views possible with a computed tomographic scan. Although we have made some use of magnetic resonance imaging in this situation, the present technique's inadequate resolution offers no advantage over computed tomography.

Surgical exploration of traction injuries of the brachial plexus has been done progressively sooner during the past ten years. Some investigators now advocate exploration in the first week after injury if there is clinical evidence of either a complete lesion of the brachial plexus or of a reparable lesion.[27] The timing of myelography has followed the same pattern. I presently believe that neither should be done before one month after injury to allow any hemorrhage in the spinal fluid to clear and pseudomeningoceles to form if meningeal tears are present.

Axon responses to intradermal histamine have been used to differentiate root avulsions from distal ruptures in flail arms without sensation as a result of traction injury to the brachial plexus.[18,28] The findings are difficult to interpret, particularly with reference to the seventh cervical vertebra root, and have the additional problem of potentially serious systemic reaction to the histamine in some patients. For these reasons, and the availability of other contemporary means of evaluation, I no longer use it as described previously.[1]

Electromyography of the posterior cervical region, as described by Bufalini and Pescatori,[29] continues to be of value in differentiating supraganglionic from infraganglionic lesions. In addition to this test, the determination of the velocity of conduction of the peripheral nerves of the affected limb can provide additional information regarding the state of the nerves at the level of the spinal cord.[30,31] If, for example, sensory conduction velocity is normal in a patient whose anesthetic limb is without sensation, wallerian degeneration has not taken place in these fibers; this indicates root avulsion. The explanation lies in the fact that the axon and cell body are not separated, and the lack of sensation is caused by loss of central connection proximal to the dorsal root ganglion. Loss of motor conduction in this same paralyzed limb can reflect either root avulsion or distal rupture since, in either case, the cell body (the anterior horn cell) is intraspinal and is separated from its axon.

The use of somatosensory-evoked potential determinations, in both preoperative and intraoperative situations but particularly in the latter, has proved to be indispensable diagnostically.[30] It is the only physiologic measure of continuity with the spinal cord available to the surgeon who must determine the suitability of a damaged root as a source of axons for a nerve graft.

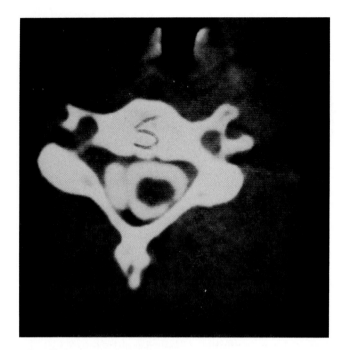

Fig. 19-3 A pseudomeningocele at C5 as seen on a computed tomographic scan in a patient who has root avulsion due to a traction injury incurred in a motorcycle accident.

Surgical Treatment

Surgical Reconstruction of the Brachial Plexus

Since the first published report of successful surgery on the brachial plexus by Thoburn[32] in 1903, there has been continuing controversy over the efficacy of surgical repair of these nerves. In 1903, Kennedy[33] described three patients in whom he had resected and sutured the upper trunk. In the next 15 years, increasing numbers of operations were performed, particularly for obstetric palsies, and by 1920 Taylor and associates[34-36] had a series of 70 surgically treated cases. However, after further evaluation and follow-up of the results of these operations, a more conservative therapy was generally accepted.[37] It was not until the resurgence of interest in the mechanical techniques of peripheral nerve repair and the generalized use of the operating microscope that documentation of the benefits of repair of the brachial plexus emerged. Millesi[24] of Vienna reported his results with autografting and neurolysis in plexus injuries in adults, as did Samii and Kahl,[38] Narakas,[11,39] and Lusskin and associates[40] in New York and Mansat,[7] Alnot and associates,[8] Allieu,[41] Dolenc,[42] and Sedel[43] in France. Detailed analyses of the results and comparisons of these series are not possible, but preliminary studies are available.[44,45]

On the basis of these published reports and my own observations of patients over the past 25 years, my approach to surgical treatment of the nerves has evolved in the following four conditions:

Flail Arm In the adult patient with a flail arm without sensation as a result of supraclavicular traction injury to the brachial plexus, the prognosis for spontaneous recovery is poor, so that every attempt to restore even minimal function must be made. Thus, surgery is necessary. Because most plexus injuries are combinations of root avulsions and distal ruptures (usually of the upper three roots and outflow), exploration and attempted grafting are indicated. Direct repair of the nerves, which usually requires bridging gaps by means of autografting, is the only means by which restoration of even imperfect sensibility can be accomplished. In cases in which root avulsion has occurred, neurotization of the plexus should be considered. Although there have been some encouraging reports,[46,47] they must be viewed from the perspective of whether the patient will really use the limb so reconstructed.

Partial Preservation of Function In a patient who has partial preservation of function in the limb, a combined approach, using all available techniques of nerve repair and peripheral reconstruction, must be formulated.[48] Although peripheral reconstruction using conventional tendon transfers and arthrodeses can provide extremely useful function, it cannot restore sensibility. I have observed in my own patients that the results of the best tendon transfer are inferior to those of the best nerve repair in terms of strength and function of the reconstructed limb (Fig. 19–4). The surgeon must realize, however, that just as using a functioning muscle as the motor unit in a tendon transfer risks loss of the

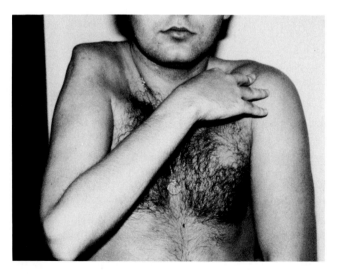

Fig. 19-4 A patient with a C5, C6, and C7 traction lesion of the brachial plexus who had his elbow flexors reinnervated by a graft of the sural nerve from the upper trunk to the lateral cord. Note the excellent bulk of his biceps compared with the atrophy of the deltoid, which was not reinnervated. His shoulder was fused.

original function, operations on the nerves have the same potential. The best example of this is in the upper trunk lesion. If even a modicum of sensibility is preserved in the thumb and index finger, as is often the case, then transecting the nerves to provide a source of axons for a graft will, at the same time, deprive the patient of any feeling in the hand. This deficit may be permanent.

Obstetric Palsies The treatment of obstetric palsies has paralleled that in adults, and remains a problem that must be addressed. In 1983 Tassin[49] described 110 infants who underwent brachial plexus surgery by Gilbert in Paris. This series was compared with a control group of 44 infants who were followed up long enough to document spontaneous recovery or lack thereof. It was found that Gilbert's reconstructions improved the functional results significantly for the shoulder and elbow. Reports by Gilbert[25] and Solonen and associates[50] showed similar results. I believe that the evidence is sufficient to advocate early surgery in these infants. If there has been no evidence of neurologic recovery, particularly in the biceps, by the age of 3 months, infants should undergo myelography and electromyographic examination under general anesthesia to determine whether there are available roots. Surgery should then be done to salvage whatever can be reconstructed.

Progressive Dysfunction After Irradiation The problem of the patient with progressive neurologic dysfunction of the hand and upper extremity occurring at variable times after irradiation of the breast and axilla for malignant disease remains difficult. The first question that must be addressed is whether this represents a recurrence of tumor or whether it is a late effect of the radiation.[51] Since the latency period for both is about the same, and there are no absolute diagnostic criteria for differentiation, the surgeon and oncologist may have difficulty planning therapy in terms of the diagnosis. In general, patients with recurrence of malignant disease have significantly more pain than those with radiation neuropathy of the plexus, but this is by no means universal. Although there should be additional evidence of spread of disease in terms of systemic symptoms, laboratory abnormalities, or positive bone scans, these are often unhelpful. The malignant disease can remain localized to the plexus for a considerable period, and it may not be detectable by means of computed tomographic scanning, although magnetic resonance imaging offers some additional diagnostic aid. For those patients in whom none of the indicators of malignant disease are positive and who have severe, intractable pain, the question is whether the pain can be relieved surgically. Neurolysis of the plexus for this problem is not generally recommended because of the high risks and serious complications reported in such patients.[52] Nevertheless, there have been attempts to revascularize the plexus by free transfer of omentum.

This has produced a positive response to pain in a small series of patients.[53] My experience with the treatment of irradiation neuropathy of the brachial plexus by neurolysis without revascularization has been confined to three patients and the results were disappointing.

The diagnostic maneuvers and general indications for surgery have been described. As to the timing of the technique, the sooner the diagnostic evaluation can be completed and the status of the nerve injury clarified, particularly in those patients who have flail arms without sensation, the easier the surgery, because scarring has less time to develop and there will be less atrophy of the end-organs. Ultimately, the results will be best if surgery is done in the first six months after injury. Surgery is probably not worthwhile after 18 months. However, the interval to surgical intervention is becoming progressively shorter. In my opinion, surgery can be done any time after one month in patients with complete lesions but should be delayed for three months in those with partial lesions.

Surgical Technique

The patient is placed in a semisitting, supine position and given general anesthesia with a Foley catheter in place. Surgery may take from eight to ten hours, and sterile draping must allow access to both lower limbs, because graft material may be required from them. The incision begins at the mid-point of the posterior border of the sternomastoid; although a direct perpendicular limb to the clavicle is the shortest route to the plexus, it tends to result in a hypertrophic scar. This can be minimized by making the incision oblique to the medial end of the clavicle, from which it then proceeds parallel, and about 1.5 cm caudad, to the bone to the level of the coracoid process (Fig. 19–5). The deltopectoral groove is then opened, and the incision can be extended into the arm as necessary. Depending on the degree of scarring and difficulty of identifying the pertinent anatomy and planes of dissection, the surgeon may start at the supraclavicular part of the incision or that below the clavicle. The objective is to establish a position in relatively normal tissues and then proceed to the scarred areas after having identified intact neural elements. The surgeon may choose to detach the pectoralis minor initially so that the nerves at the level of the cords of the plexus and the terminal branches can be dissected. They can then be followed cephalad, and as much of the pectoralis major detached from the clavicle as is necessary for adequate exposure. The bone itself is usually not osteotomized unless it is necessary to expose the subclavian artery and the eighth cervical root completely, which is difficult with the clavicle in place. If it is done, provision should be made for later reconstitution with a compression plate.

The external jugular vein, as well as the suprascapular and transverse cervical vessels, must be divided along with the omohyoid muscle in the supraclavicular

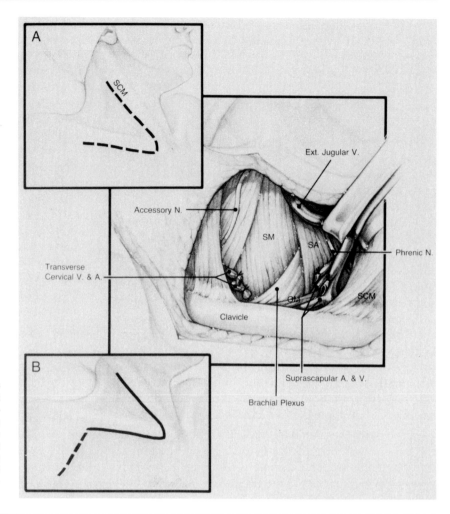

Fig. 19-5 The surgical approach to the brachial plexus. The external jugular vein has been retracted rather than excised to show its relationship to other structures. Part B shows the extension of the skin incision into the deltopectoral groove. (Reproduced with permission from Elizabeth Roselius and previously published in Leffert RD: Brachial plexus, in Green DP (ed): *Operative Hand Surgery.* New York, Churchill Livingstone, 1988, vol 2, chap 41.)

fossa. If the scarring between the nerves and the scalene muscles is dense, as it often is in traction lesions, it may be difficult to identify individual nerve elements. The use of electrical stimulation in the area where the phrenic nerve should be on the anterior surface of the anterior scalene may help. If the nerve is intact and the anesthesiologist has not paralyzed the patient completely, the diaphragm will contract when the phrenic nerve is stimulated. It can then be followed proximally to locate the foramen of the fifth cervical nerve root. Additional exposure can be gained from partial reflection of the lateral border of the sternomastoid and detachment of the anterior scalene from the first rib. The neural elements can then be defined and inspected to determine whether they are intact, avulsed, ruptured distally, or injured in continuity. Although the magnification afforded by the operating microscope or high-power loupes is essential to any surgical manipulation of the nerves, it cannot provide physiologic evidence of continuity with the spinal cord. A clear gap or actual absence of the nerve elements can, however, provide evidence of discontinuity. For this determination, it is necessary to have prepared the patient preoperatively

with electrodes placed so that somatosensory-evoked potentials can be determined. These have proved to be extremely useful in determining the suitability of nerve roots as donors of axons for nerve reconstruction.[30] In general, if the nerve elements can be stimulated and muscles in the limbs can be made to contract, these elements must not be disturbed. More often, however, the scarring in a traction lesion will have abolished these responses, and the surgeon must determine which nerves can be reconstituted. In general, traction lesions involve large gaps that must be closed by means of grafts. The intraneural topography of the plexus has, therefore, assumed great importance in the placement of these grafts.

The upper and intermediate trunks are the most often grafted because they are least often avulsed, and the results of surgery on them have been shown to be the most favorable.[8,11,23,24,39,43] Specifically, the ability to restore the power of elbow flexion has been most often noted, with shoulder function less likely, particularly in adults. Not only must the innervation to the deltoid be restored, but that to the suprascapular nerve as well, or there will be no control of the shoulder when the patient attempts abduction or forward flexion. The most commonly used donor nerve is the sural, which can be obtained through multiple, small transverse incisions in the leg. The nerve is used in 10- to 15-cm segments if placed between the upper trunk and the lateral cord or musculocutaneous nerve; these are sutured in place with 8-0 to 10-0 nylon sutures. Nerve gaps in the other parts of the plexus below the level of the roots may be similarly reconstructed. Whenever possible, attention should be paid to the local intraneural topography so that the integrity of the fascicular pathway can be maintained. The presence of root avulsion produces a shortage or absence of donor axons for reinnervation. These situations may require the use of axons from intercostal, spinal accessary, or cervical plexus nerves in the process of neurotization. Some surgeons have found the plasma clot technique helpful.[54]

The indications for neurolysis are limited. A patient whose recovery has ceased or regressed is a candidate for neurolysis. The same approach and safeguards are used. In patients with partial lesions, there is a definite risk of making an existing deficit greater. In general, if neurolysis is performed, it should be external and done with a microscope and physiologic monitoring.

The postoperative care of the patient with a grafted brachial plexus is relatively simple. The patient uses a sling for two weeks until the wound is healed or uses additional support as dictated by the treatment of the clavicle.

Published results of surgery of the brachial plexus should be reviewed for comparisons between series and with the results of peripheral reconstructions for motor function.[8,11,23,24,39,43,55]

Reconstruction for Partial Impairment

The general principles described previously[1] are still applicable, but it is possible to combine neurologic repair with reconstruction of the periphery. While arthrodesis remains the most frequently performed operation for the completely paralyzed shoulder, patients who have some shoulder function should be considered for tendon transfer if there is adequate musculature. For those patients who do have a fusion, I routinely use the compression plate technique so that the long period of immobilization in a shoulder spica can be eliminated (Fig. 19–6). This has resulted in considerably less stiffness of other joints and a significant improvement in the quality of the patient's life during the postoperative period. Immobilization is achieved with a light plastic brace, used for six weeks, that can be removed for dressing and bathing.

Rehabilitation of the Patient With a Brachial Plexus Injury

Although the general principles have not changed since 1977,[1] some alterations in emphasis and technique should be noted.

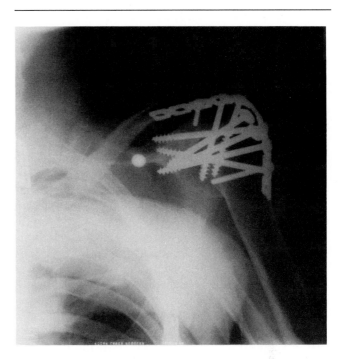

Fig. 19–6 Postoperative radiograph of a shoulder fusion using ankle orthosis screws and a pelvic reconstruction plate.

Intractable pain in the patient with a brachial plexus injury remains problematic, and conservative management is difficult. Severe pain is a common complaint in patients who have sustained multiple root avulsions, and its presence may indicate a poor prognosis. Fortunately, most patients who initially complain of severe pain tend to have less pain with the passage of time or simply learn to live with it. The problem for the clinician is providing treatment during this period, which may last as long as a year or more. Then, it is important to provide guidance and assistance in the management of pain, along with prescribing nonnarcotic analgesics. I make it a practice not to prescribe narcotics after the immediate postoperative period. Aspirin remains the benchmark against which all of the nonnarcotics can be measured for analgesic power. The necessary high doses of aspirin and its tendency to irritate the stomach or cause tinnitus have led to the general use of the nonsteroidal anti-inflammatory agents as substitutes, and they are generally better tolerated, although considerably more expensive. Propoxyphene in combination rather than alone is preferred by some patients but is really no more effective than aspirin as an analgesic and may be habit-forming. The anticonvulsants, phenytoin and carbamazepine, have been used to treat a variety of neuralgias. By analogy, they have been suggested for the pain of brachial plexus injury. In my experience, phenytoin is rarely effective. Carbamazepine is sometimes effective, but the patient must be carefully observed for side effects, including a feeling of weakness. Patients must also be screened before administration of the drug for hematopoietic, renal, and hepatic dysfunction, and these tests must be periodically repeated during treatment. The dosage is gradually increased to between 400 and 800 mg/day and should not exceed 1,200 mg/day.

The use of the transcutaneous nerve stimulator for the treatment of brachial plexus pain is theoretically attractive. In actuality, it has almost no side effects other than dermatitis under the electrode pads but its effectiveness has been questionable in my patients.

The surgical treatment of intractable pain in brachial plexus injury continues to be a significant problem. The dorsal column stimulator has not retained its popularity. The most promising procedure available today is the radiofrequency lesion of the substantia gelatinosa (DREZ—dorsal root entry zone) procedure described by Nashold,[56,57] who reported encouraging long-term results. Several of my patients have derived substantial benefit from this operation.

Some patients do not want to live with a flail arm without sensation, but requests for amputation have become considerably fewer. Because of the possibility of neurologic reconstruction, even with minimal function, most patients do choose to retain the arm. The option of a forearm amputation remains for the patient who regains elbow control in the absence of a useful hand function,[58] but some of these patients will elect to be fitted with a functional splint rather than undergo ablation. I have not offered myoelectric prostheses to these patients because I do not believe that the level of function to be gained in this situation is worth the expense and need for maintenance.

References

1. Leffert RD: Lesions of the brachial plexus, including thoracic outlet syndrome, in American Academy of Orthopaedic Surgeons *Instructional Course Lectures, XXVI.* St. Louis, CV Mosby, 1977, pp 77–102.
2. Harris W: The true form of the brachial plexus and its motor distribution. *J Anat Physiol* 1903–1904;38:399–422.
3. Hovelacque A: *Anatomie des nerfs craniens et rachidiens et du systeme grand sympathique.* Paris, Doin, 1927.
4. Kerr AT: The brachial plexus of nerves in man, the variations in its formation and branches. *Am J Anat* 1918;23:285–395.
5. Stevens JH: Brachial plexus paralysis, in Codman EA (ed): *The Shoulder.* Brooklyn, G Miller, 1934, pp 332–381.
6. Sunderland S: *Nerves and Nerve Injuries,* ed 2. Edinburgh, Churchill Livingstone, 1978.
7. Mansat M: Anatomie topographique chirurgicale du plexus brachial. *Rev Chir Orthop* 1977;63:20–26.
8. Alnot JY, Jolly A, Frot B: Traitement direct des lésions nerveuses dans les paralysies traumatiques du plex brachial chez l'adulte: A propos d'une série de 100 cas opérés. *Int Orthop* 1981; 5:151–168.
9. Bonnel F: Microscopic anatomy of the adult human brachial plexus: An anatomical and histological basis for microsurgery. *Microsurgery* 1984;5:107–118.
10. Bonnel F: Paralysie traumatique du plexus brachial chez l'adulte: III. Configuration interne histo-physiologique. *Rev Chir Orthop* 1977;63:35–38.
11. Narakas A: Surgical treatment of traction injuries of the brachial plexus. *Clin Orthop* 1978;133:71–90.
12. Slingluff CL, Terzis JK, Edgerton MT: The quantitative microanatomy of the brachial plexus in man: Reconstructive relevance, in Terzis JK (ed): *Microreconstruction of Nerve Injuries.* Philadelphia, WB Saunders, 1987.
13. Engel J, Ganel A, Melamed R, et al: Choline acetyltransferase for differentiation between human motor and sensory nerve fibers. *Ann Plast Surg* 1980;4:376–380.
14. Seddon HJ: *Surgical Disorders of the Peripheral Nerves.* Baltimore, Williams & Wilkins, 1972.
15. Jackson L, Keats AS: Mechanism of brachial plexus palsy following anesthesia. *Anesthesiology* 1965;26:190–194.
16. Roaf R: Lateral flexion injuries of the cervical spine. *J Bone Joint Surg* 1963;45B:36–38.
17. Murphey F, Hartung W, Kirklin JW: Myelographic demonstration of avulsing injury of the brachial plexus. *AJR* 1947;58:102–105.
18. Yeoman PM: Cervical myelography in traction injuries of the brachial plexus. *J Bone Joint Surg* 1968;50B:253–260.
19. Jaeger R, Whiteley WH: Avulsion of the brachial plexus: Report of 6 cases. *JAMA* 1953;153:633–635.
20. Mendelsohn RA, Weiner IH, Keegan JM: Myelographic demonstration of brachial plexus root avulsion. *Arch Surg* 1957;75:102–107.
21. Héon M: Myelogram: A questionable aid in diagnosis and prognosis in avulsion of brachial plexus components by traction injuries. *Conn Med* 1965;29:260–262.
22. Jelasic F, Piepgras U: Functional restitution after cervical avulsion injury with "typical" myelographic findings. *Folia Haematol* 1974;101:158–163.
23. Millesi H: Brachial plexus injuries: Management and results. *Clin Plast Surg* 1984;11:115–120.
24. Millesi H: Surgical management of brachial plexus injuries. *J Hand Surg* 1977;2:367–378.
25. Gilbert A: Obstetrical palsy: A clinical, pathologic and surgical review, in Terzis JK (ed): *Microreconstruction of Nerve Injuries.* Philadelphia, WB Saunders, 1987.
26. Gilbert A, Khouri N, Carlioz H: Exploration chirurgicale du plexus brachial dans la paralysie obstetricale: Constatations anatomiques chez 21 malades opérés. *Rev Chir Orthop* 1980;66:33–42.
27. Marshall RW, De Silva RD: Computerised axial tomography in traction injuries of the brachial plexus. *J Bone Joint Surg* 1986;68B:734–738.
28. Bonney G: The value of axon responses in determining the site of the lesion in traction injuries of the brachial plexus. *Brain* 1954;77:588–609.
29. Bufalini C, Pescatori G: Posterior cervical electromyography in the diagnosis and prognosis of brachial plexus injuries. *J Bone Joint Surg* 1969;51B:627–631.
30. Landi A, Copeland SA, Parry CB, et al: The role of somatosensory evoked potentials and nerve conduction studies in the surgical management of brachial plexus injuries. *J Bone Joint Surg* 1980;62B:492–496.
31. Bonney G, Gilliatt RW: Sensory nerve conduction after traction lesion of the brachial plexus. *Proc R Soc Med* 1958;51:365–367.
32. Thoburn W: Obstetrical paralysis. *J Obstet Gynecol Br Emp* 1903; 3:454–458.
33. Kennedy R: Suture of the brachial plexus in birth paralysis of the upper extremity. *Br Med J* 1903;1:298–301.
34. Taylor AS: Conclusions derived from further experience in the surgical treatment of brachial birth palsy (Erb's type). *Am J Med Sci* 1913;146:836–856.
35. Taylor AS: Brachial birth palsy and injuries of similar type in adults. *Surg Gynecol Obstet* 1920;30:495–502.
36. Clark LP, Taylor AS, Prout FP: A study on brachial birth palsy. *Am J Med Sci* 1905;130:670–707.

37. Jepson PN: Obstetrical paralysis. *Ann Surg* 1930;91:724.

38. Samii M, Kahl RI: Clinische Resultate der autologen nerven Transplantation. *Melssunger Med Mitteil* 1972;46:197.

39. Narakas A: Surgical treatment of traction injuries of the brachial plexus. *Clin Orthop* 1978;133:71–90.

40. Lusskin R, Campbell JB, Thompson WAL: Post-traumatic lesions of the brachial plexus: Treatment by transclavicular exploration and neurolysis or autograft reconstruction. *J Bone Joint Surg* 1973;55A:1159–1176.

41. Allieu Y: Exploration et traitement direct des lesions nerveuses dans les paralysies traumatiques par elongation du plexus brachial chez l'adulte. *Rev Chir Orthop* 1975;63:107.

42. Dolenc V: Diagnostic et traitement des lésions du plexus brachial: A propos de 100 cas. *Neurochirurgie* 1982;28:101–105.

43. Sedel L: The results of surgical repair of brachial plexus injuries. *J Bone Joint Surg* 1982;64B:54–66.

44. Solonen KA, Vastäma M, Ström B: Surgery of the brachial plexus. *Acta Orthop Scand* 1984;55:436–440.

45. Simesen K, Haase J: Microsurgery in brachial plexus lesions. *Acta Orthop Scand* 1985;56:238–241.

46. Allieu Y, Privat JM, Bonnel F: Les neurotisations par le nerf spinal (nerf accessoriua) dans les avulsions radiculaires du plexus brachial. *Neurochirurgie* 1982;28:115–120.

47. Kotani T, Toshima Y, Matsuda H, et al: Postoperative results of nerve transposition in brachial plexus injury. *Orthop Surg* [*Tokyo*] 1971;22:963–966.

48. Leffert RD: *Brachial Plexus Injuries.* New York, Churchill Livingstone, 1985.

49. Tassin JL: *Paralysies obstetricales du plexus brachial: Evolution spontanee, resultats des interventions reparatrices precoces,* thesis. Paris, 1983.

50. Solonen KA, Telaranta T, Ryöppy S: Early reconstruction of birth injuries of the brachial plexus. *J Pediatr Orthop* 1981;1:367–370.

51. Thomas JE, Colby MY Jr: Radiation-induced or metastatic brachial plexopathy? A diagnostic dilemma. *JAMA* 1972;222:1392–1395.

52. Match RM: Radiation-induced brachial plexus paralysis. *Arch Surg* 1975;110:384–386.

53. Clodius L, Uhlschmid G, Hess K: Irradiation plexitis of the brachial plexus, in Terzis J (ed): *Microreconstruction of Nerve Injuries.* Philadelphia, WB Saunders, 1987.

54. Tarlov IM: *Plasma Clot Suture of Peripheral Nerves and Nerve Roots: Rationale and Technique.* Springfield, Charles C Thomas, 1950.

55. Leffert RD, Pess G: Tendon transfers for paralysis following brachial plexus injury. *J Hand Surg,* in press.

56. Nashold BS Jr, Ostdahl RH: Dorsal root entry zone lesions for pain relief. *J Neurosurg* 1979;51:59–69.

57. Nashold BS Jr: Modification of DREZ lesion technique, letter. *J Neurosurg* 1981;55:1012.

58. Yeoman PM, Seddon HJ: Brachial plexus injuries: Treatment of the flail arm. *J Bone Joint Surg* 1961;43B:493–500.

Lower Extremity Disorders in the Child

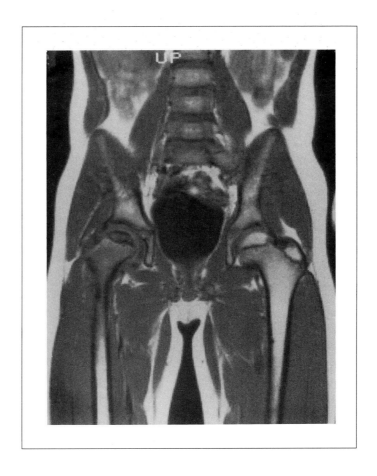

Principles of in Situ Fixation in Chronic Slipped Capital Femoral Epiphysis

Raymond T. Morrissy, MD

Slipped capital femoral epiphysis (SCFE) presents a paradox to the treating surgeon. On the one hand, it is easy to put a pin in the hip to treat the disorder; on the other hand, the postoperative course often includes significant complications. The resolution of this paradox is found in an understanding of the natural history of the disease.

In any disease it is most important to understand the natural history, for treatment is our effort to alter the natural history.[1] Howorth[2] demonstrated a keen insight into this reality when he wrote:

> It should be recognized that the disease always heals, regardless of treatment, and that the results of untreated hips often are good, sometimes better than some of the results of treatment. Treatment is of no value unless the result is better than if the hip were not treated. Further, it should be recognized that aseptic necrosis does not occur in the untreated hip and that untreated hips rarely cause serious trouble before middle or late adult life.

The observation that it is the complications that lead to a bad result is now widely accepted. The complications are primarily two: avascular necrosis and chondrolysis. Howorth's statement that aseptic necrosis does not occur in the untreated hip does not seem to have received wide acceptance in the orthopaedic community. This may be because no direct link between in situ pinning and avascular necrosis is immediately apparent.

In 1960 Brodetti[3] reported on experiments designed to show how aseptic necrosis could occur in the femoral head of an adult as a result of the placement of the nail. In his injection studies, he outlined the course of the interosseous blood vessels, and in particular pointed out the importance of the lateral ascending cervical vessels. He noted that these vessels were in the superior and posterior part of the femoral neck. This pattern can be seen in published reports of injected specimens in children and adolescents as well as adults[4,5] (Fig. 20-1). Next, Brodetti placed nails in the femoral heads in various positions, noting that the valgus position in which the nail reached the superior part of the head had the greatest chance of interrupting the blood supply. His recommendation was to keep the nail in the "central zone" of the femoral head where it would interfere less with the blood supply.

This somewhat obscure article presents a plausible connection between in situ pinning and avascular necrosis. A recent study of the relationship between pin placement within the femoral head and complications showed that the lowest complication rate occurred when

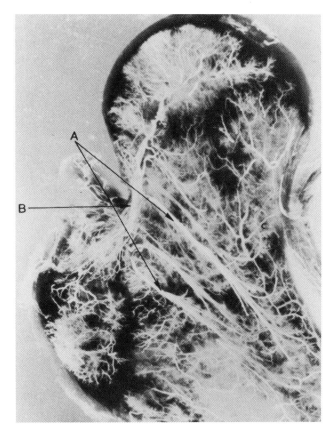

Fig. 20-1 The blood supply to the proximal femoral epiphysis of a 14-year-old girl (A, descending metaphyseal arteries). The segmental blood supply to the weightbearing portion is from the lateral ascending cervical artery (B) with little cross connection. Interruption of this artery could result in avascular necrosis. (Reproduced with permission from Chung SM: The arterial supply of the developing proximal end of the femur. *J Bone Joint Surg* 1976;58A:961–970.)

the pins were in the varus position and avoided the superior quadrant of the femoral head.[6]

Chondrolysis is a peculiar disease that seems to affect only the hip. It rarely occurs in the absence of SCFE, providing support for the commonly held view that it is a complication somehow related to the slipping and not the treatment. However, in 1980 Walters and Simon[7] presented evidence that chondrolysis was related to persistent pin penetration, and that this penetration could remain unrecognized on the radiographs. This report was also greeted with skepticism for it was, and still is, not clear what links the presence of a pin in the hip joint to the biologic process of chondrolysis. A partial explanation might be found in the fact that patients with a SCFE have synovitis that differs from synovitis in other joints by the presence of immune complex in the synovial fluid.[8] This milieu might be different enough in some way to result in chondrolysis when the pin abrades the joint cartilage.

Perhaps of equal significance in Walters and Simon's report was the demonstration of unrecognized pin penetration. A radiograph is a shadow of the outline of the femoral head. Thus, a pin that projects out of the femoral head but does not project beyond the periphery of the head casting the shadow on the radiographic plate is not seen as penetrating the femoral head (Fig. 20–2). Walters and Simon went on to demonstrate what they called a "blind spot." If two radiographs are taken at right angles to each other, there will always be an area where a projecting pin is not seen. If the pin is in the central axis of the femoral head, this area is very small; by keeping the pin 5 mm within the head, the surgeon can be sure it is not penetrating. However, the farther the pin is from the central axis, the larger is the "blind spot" where the pin can penetrate without being seen. In some positions the pin may appear to be 1 cm within the femoral head while it is actually penetrating.

With all this information, the paradox becomes easier to resolve. It is easy to put a pin in the femoral head.

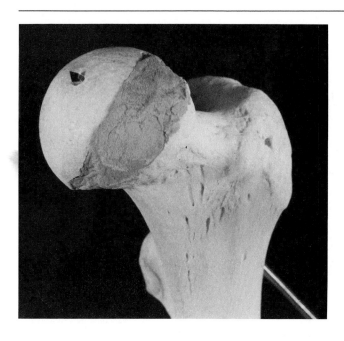

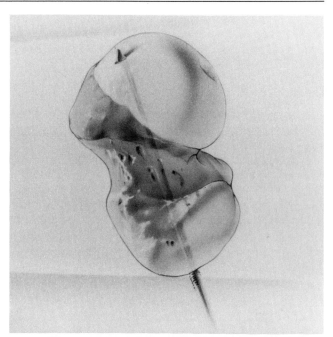

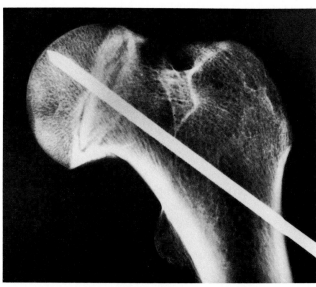

Fig. 20–2 A pin penetrating the femoral head may not be seen on a routine or lateral radiograph. This is because the shadow of the femoral head that appears on the radiograph is made by the beam passing at a tangent to the edge of the femoral head. **Top left:** The penetration of the pin is clear in the gross specimen. **Top right:** The X-ray beam passes at a tangent to the outline of the femoral head. **Bottom:** The X-ray beam casts a shadow of the outline of the femoral head. Note that the pin appears to be within the femoral head on the two-dimensional radiograph.

However, without understanding the natural history of SCFE and the etiology of the complications, the surgeon does not know that the pin must be in a certain place within the femoral head. Thus, it is important to know where the femoral head is so that the pin can be properly placed.

To place the pin in the central axis of the femoral head, it is necessary for the pin to enter the physeal plate in its center as well as be perpendicular to it so that the pin remains in the central axis (Fig. 20–3). In addition, the pin must pass through the femoral neck to secure fixation. Lastly, all of this must be accomplished without the ability to visualize any of the structures directly. This emphasizes a very important point: in situ pinning is a radiographic technique.

Although the surgeon may eventually achieve correct pin placement by trial and error using good radiographs, it is better to have a conceptual understanding of the relationship between the femoral neck and head before starting. The direction in which the displacement of the femoral head occurs is determined by muscular forces, gravity, and anatomy. In chronic slips this process of displacement takes place slowly, as if the epiphyseal plate had become putty. First, the femoral neck rotates externally. The femoral head slides posteriorly around the axis of the femoral neck, remaining in the acetabulum and tilting posteriorly. Inferior displacement of the head is prevented by the shape of the femoral neck. In most chronic slips this is the only direction the slip takes (Fig. 20–4).

On radiographs the femoral head appears to have slipped inferiorly. In the usual chronic SCFE, however, this is not the case. This can be verified by computed axial tomography. The appearance is the result of parallax.[9] However, in late and neglected cases or in an acute slip, the femoral neck may begin to move cephalad in relation to the femoral head, so that the metaphysis comes to approximate the lateral edge of the acetabulum. This is the radiographic appearance typical of a complete acute slip (Fig. 20–4).

The degree of external rotation of the femoral neck or posterior slipping of the femoral head is often dif-

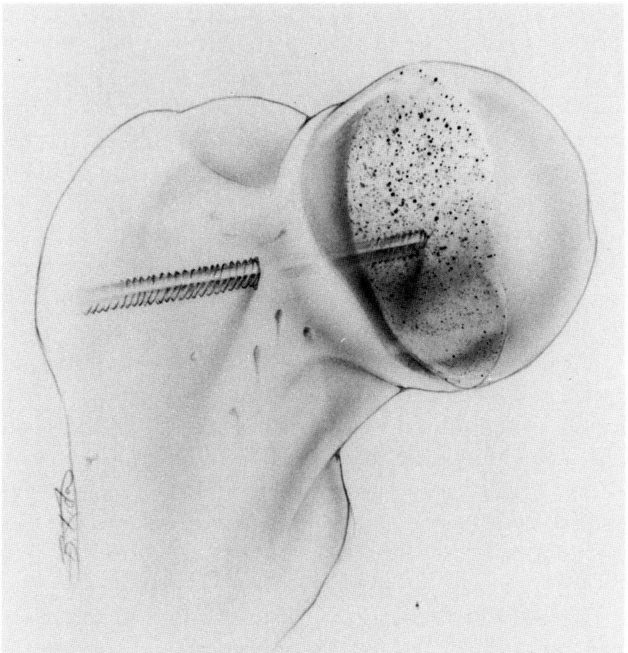

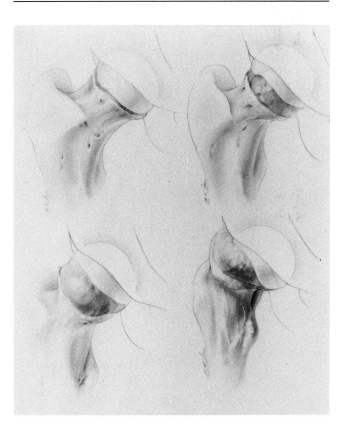

Fig. 20–4 In the earliest phases of a slipped capital femoral epiphysis, no displacement may be seen **(top left)**. The muscles producing external rotation on the femur will cause the shaft to rotate externally, leaving the femoral head in the acetabulum. At this stage, the femoral head will have migrated posteriorly around the axis of the femoral neck **(top right)**. Because of the shape and contour of the femoral neck and the epiphyseal surface, however, it will not have slipped inferiorly. As this continues, the posterior displacement becomes more severe **(bottom left)**. In the late stages, as the slip is neglected, or in cases of acute slip, the femoral shaft or metaphysis may begin to migrate superiorly in relationship to the femoral epiphysis. However, this can only occur when the femoral neck has first rotated externally **(bottom right)**.

Fig. 20–3 The important landmarks in the pinning of a slipped capital femoral epiphysis are the location and plane of the surface of the epiphysis. The pin must enter its center and be perpendicular to its surface. This differs from the traditional point of view that the pin starts on the lateral femoral cortex and then seeks the head. The further the femoral head slips posteriorly, the more anterior the starting position on the femur must be.

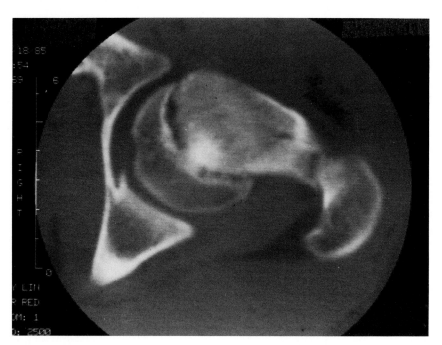

Fig. 20-5 Computed tomographic scan of a slipped capital femoral epiphysis more clearly illustrates the pathology. Notice the position that the femoral head has assumed on the femoral neck as it is rotated posteriorly. It remains in intimate contact with the femoral neck. Notice the amount of resorption and rounding that has occurred in the posterior femoral neck region.

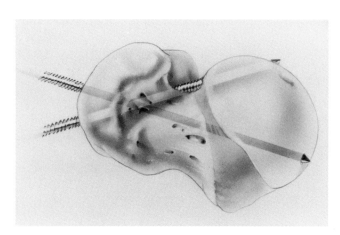

Fig. 20-6 A pin that enters the lateral femoral cortex and passes directly down the center of the femoral neck will, by necessity, enter the slipped epiphysis at an acute angle passing toward its periphery. Penetration may not be seen in this location on a radiograph. If the pin in angled posteriorly, it still does not enter the femoral epiphysis in a perpendicular direction but instead passes posteriorly toward the periphery, again being hidden from radiographic view. The only proper starting point for the pin in a slip such as the one illustrated is on the anterior femoral cortex.

ficult to appreciate on routine anteroposterior, frog-leg lateral, or even true lateral views with the leg in external rotation. However, the amount of posterior slip along with the tremendous amount of remodeling of both the anterior and posterior femoral neck can readily be appreciated by computed tomography (Fig. 20-5).

Appreciating the relationship of the femoral head and neck makes it easier to analyze the two common errors made in in situ pinning and their origin. In the classical description, illustration, and teaching of the method of in situ pinning, the surgeon begins with an incision on the lateral side of the femur. The fixation device is then passed down the femoral neck and into the head, as in fixation for a fractured femoral neck. However, the femoral head is no longer in its normal relationship to the femoral neck. Thus, in cases of SCFE the device does not enter the center of the femoral head but rather passes obliquely toward the anterior surface—the very position in which radiographs are inaccurate in regard to the actual position of the pin (Fig. 20-6).

The second common error is to pass the fixation device out the posterior neck and into the head. This results in the pin being out of the central axis and can lead to the pin penetrating the femoral head posteriorly where it will not be recognized in subsequent radiographs. In addition, it results in less secure fixation of the device in the metaphysis as well as the head (Fig. 20-6).

The correct solution to this problem is to select the starting point of the fixation device on the basis of the position of the femoral head. The device should be started on the femoral neck so that when the device leaves the neck it enters the femoral head perpendicular to the physeal surface and in its center. This starting point, of necessity, is on the anterior neck. There is often concern that this device may be intra-articular. This would probably cause no difficulty, but in reality

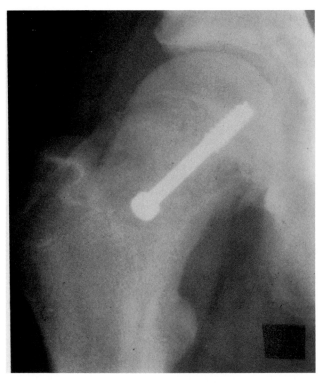
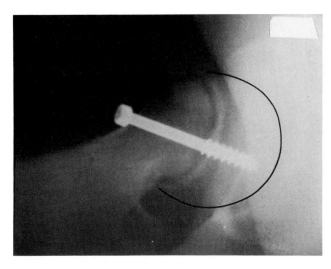

Fig. 20-7 Anteroposterior **(left)** and lateral **(right)** radiographs of a properly pinned slipped epiphysis. Notice that on both views the screw is in the central axis of the femoral head. On the anteroposterior view, the starting point for such correct placement is not the lateral femoral cortex but well anterior on the femoral neck.

the posterior displacement of the head has drawn the capsule tight across the anterior femoral neck, obliterating what would ordinarily be joint space in this region of the femoral neck.

The ideal fixation device should possess several characteristics. It should be strong enough so that only one is needed. Since there is only one correct place for the device—the central axis of the head—additional pins only increase the risk of complications. The device should be easy to remove. For this it should have reverse cutting threads, and be strong enough not to break as reverse cutting begins. It should be cannulated to facilitate easy percutaneous placement and removal.

Technique of Percutaneous in Situ Fixation

The patient is secured to the fracture table. The affected leg is abducted about 20 degrees to facilitate placement of the image intensifier. Before anything else is done, anteroposterior and lateral views are obtained. It is essential that the subchondral outline of the femoral head be seen on both views. If the image intensifier is not strong enough to obtain a good lateral view, a portable radiographic unit should be used.

Positioning of the machine for the lateral view is crit-

ical. Abduction or adduction of the leg has little to do with obtaining a good image since the hip remains in the same location. However, the angle of the tube in relation to the femoral head will determine the image obtained.

The patient's skin is then prepared and the field draped. With the image intensifier taking anteroposterior images, a guide wire can be inserted percutaneously through the anterolateral area of the thigh down to the femoral neck. This can be adjusted on the anteroposterior projection to ascertain the axis of the femoral neck. At this time a lateral view can also be obtained to determine the amount of posterior inclination the device should take.

When the starting point on the femoral neck and the amount of posterior inclination have been estimated, the guide assembly can be inserted through a small puncture wound and advanced. When it has reached the epiphyseal plate, both anterior and posterior views should be obtained to ensure that the guide assembly enters the femoral head in its central axis. Drilling the guide assembly across the plate without doing this may result in either penetration of the femoral head or passage of the pin into the superior quadrant of the femoral head, disrupting the lateral epiphyseal artery. If the position is correct, the guide assembly is advanced across the plate. It should not be advanced any farther than to within 0.5 cm of the subchondral bone and should only be advanced this far if the pin is in the center of the femoral head on both views. When it is properly positioned, the cannula is removed, with the guide wire left in the bone. A screw of proper length is then advanced over the guide pin (Fig. 20–7).

Postoperative Care

How quickly the patient recovers from a percutaneous epiphysiodesis depends largely on the irritability of the hip before surgery since there will be little pain from the surgery itself.

The patient begins range-of-motion exercises the morning after surgery. In most cases motion will be good, and the patient has less pain than preoperatively. Most patients can begin ambulation with a three-point partial weightbearing crutch gait on the first postoperative day, and can leave the hospital the same day.

Patients continue to use crutches until all signs of synovitis are gone and motion is free and painless. This usually takes one week. All rigorous sports and activities are forbidden until the epiphyses have closed. This protects the affected hip and lessens the possibility of an acute slip on the opposite side. The prodromal symptoms of thigh pain or groin pain are emphasized, and the patient is instructed to obtain immediate attention if such symptoms occur in the opposite hip. The patients are also instructed to return immediately if any symptoms of pain or stiffness develop in the affected hip. Anteroposterior and frog-leg lateral radiographs are taken every three months until the epiphyses are closed. The fixation device is then removed.

References

1. Morrissy RT: Slipped capital femoral epiphysis: Part II. Natural history and etiology in treatment, in American Academy of Orthopaedic Surgeons *Instructional Course Lectures, XXIX*. St. Louis, CV Mosby, 1980, pp 81–86.
2. Howorth B: Slipping of the upper femoral epiphysis. *Clin Orthop* 1957;48:148–173.
3. Brodetti A: The blood supply of the femoral neck and head in relation to the damaging effects of nails and screws. *J Bone Joint Surg* 1960;42B:794–801.
4. Chung SM: The arterial supply of the developing proximal end of the human femur. *J Bone Joint Surg* 1976;58A:961–970.
5. Crock HV: *The Blood Supply of the Lower Limb Bones in Man*. London, E & S Livingstone Ltd, 1967.
6. Stambough JL, Davidson RS, Ellis RD, et al: Slipped capital femoral epiphysis: An analysis of 80 patients as to pin placement and number. *J Pediatr Orthop* 1986;6:265–273.
7. Walters R, Simon SR: Joint destruction: A sequel of unrecognized pin penetration on patients with slipped capital femoral epiphysis, in *The Hip: Proceedings of the Eighth Open Scientific Meeting of the Hip Society*. St. Louis, CV Mosby, 1980, pp 145–164.
8. Morrissy RT, Steele RW, Gerdes MH: Localised immune complexes and slipped upper femoral epiphysis. *J Bone Joint Surg* 1983;65B:574–579.
9. Griffith MJ: Slipping of the capital femoral epiphysis. *Ann R Coll Surg Eng* 1976;58:34–42.

Bone Graft Epiphysiodesis in the Treatment of Slipped Capital Femoral Epiphysis

Dennis S. Weiner, MD

Introduction

As a direct result of a virtual cascade of scientific reports documenting an alarming incidence of inferior results secondary to the use of metallic internal fixation in the treatment of both chronic and acute slipped capital femoral epiphysis (SCFE),[1-49] there has been a resurgence of interest in the use of bone-graft epiphysiodesis. The array of complications associated with metallic fixation includes pin penetration, avascular necrosis, chondrolysis, metal failure, and failure to cross the growth plate. Less common complications include distraction of the head from the neck during insertion,[41] fracture at the lateral entry site on the upper femur,[41,43] and even pseudoaneurysm.[22]

Most of the more serious complications clearly stem from a direct failure to appreciate the distorted architectural anatomy of the slipping process at the site of head-neck displacement (Fig. 21–1). This local geometric disturbance at the slip site demands that the surgeon inserting metallic pins or screws be aware of the exact direction the metal must traverse to avoid penetrating the neck of the femur or piercing the articular cartilage of the head. Numerous reports have shown pin penetration to be a direct proximate cause of chondrolysis. Furthermore, inexact placement induces a stress riser at the site of exit of the metal from the neck or at the site of entry into the lateral proximal femur. Using an anterolateral entry on the neck to accommodate the more posteroinferior location of the head has been associated with pseudoaneurysm and also commonly necessitates penetration of the hip capsule (intra-articular entry), one of the common objections to intra-articular bone-graft epiphysiodesis.

Current awareness of this disturbed geometric architecture[47] has been accompanied by a more careful scrutiny of techniques, a more precise definition of pin placement, and recognition that this procedure requires an experienced surgical team. Dismay at the disturbing incidence of penetration has also led to a reevaluation of the role of bone-graft epiphysiodesis, particularly in more severe degrees of slipping. More than 30 reported series have highlighted complications of metallic internal fixation.[1-49] My colleagues and I, in a review of cases treated at Toronto's Sick Children's Hospital and the Akron Children's Hospital Medical Center, identified a startlingly high incidence of complications.[41] This series included 308 hips in 202 patients with SCFE treated by metallic internal fixation (pins and screws). We found an alarming 26% overall complication rate with an additional 18% of the entire series undergoing a second operation to deal with the complications of the primary treatment.

Since Ferguson and Howorth's[50] initial report in 1931, there have been more than 600 reported cases in which bone-graft epiphysiodesis was used in the treatment of SCFE.[51-66] My colleagues and I described a series of 185 hips in 159 patients in 1984.[66] The remarkably low incidence of complications with this procedure has influenced its increased use in many centers treating SCFE.

Surgical Procedure

Between 1950 and 1985, my colleagues and I used the anterior iliofemoral (Smith-Peterson) incision as our standard approach (Fig. 21–2). After 1985 we shifted to an anterolateral approach similar to that used in some total hip surgery[67] (Fig. 21–3). The ease of entering the hip with this approach, the reduced operating time, the reduced blood loss, and the ease with which the hollow mill can be inserted led us to replace the older incision with this improved version. Our experiences with this approach will be reported elsewhere.[67] Regardless of the approach, the hip joint capsule is exposed, an H-shaped incision is made into the capsule, and the joint is opened. Large Cobra retractors are placed around the femoral neck, further exposing the anterior aspect of the neck, the area of slipping, and usually a portion of the femoral head. The Cobra retractors do not place excessive leverage against the critical posterosuperior epiphyseal blood supply. If a bony prominence ("hump") on the anterolateral metaphyseal region resulting from the slipping is severe enough to act as an impediment to motion, it is removed with an osteotome. The remaining area is fashioned so as to remove any obstacle to flexion, abduction, and internal rotation.

The physis is identified by visual inspection or, if necessary, by probing with a straight needle. A small osteotome is used to cut a metaphyseal cortical window in the femoral neck immediately lateral and distal to the physis. A 1-cm hollow mill drill is then passed through this window, across the growth plate, and into the epiphysis and a core biopsy specimen is extracted (Fig. 21–4). The hollow mill is carefully advanced under image intensification control and placed as close as pos-

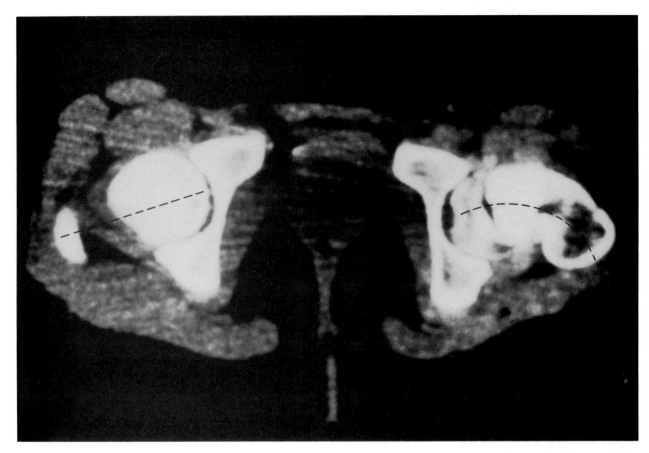

Fig. 21-1 Computed tomographic image of femoral neck and displaced left femoral head (lateral view). Remodeling of the head and neck lead to marked posterior curvature.

sible to the center of the growth plate and the epiphysis (Fig. 21-5). The biopsy specimen includes bone from the metaphysis, cartilage of the physis, and bone from the epiphysis. The growth plate is then extensively drilled and curetted adjacent to the track of the core biopsy, under direct vision and, if necessary, image intensification (Fig. 21-6). The cylindrical tunnel is enlarged to accommodate at least three cortical cancellous grafts taken from the adjacent ilium. These are roughly 1 cm wide and long enough to bridge the physis. The grafts are then placed "sandwich" fashion across the physis and tamped into place (Fig. 21-7). The cortical window removed from the femoral neck initially is replaced after the cylindrical tunnel is packed with pieces of cancellous bone from the outer table of the ilium. The hip joint capsule is then closed.

We generally obtain roentgenographic evidence that the graft crosses the physis. This is facilitated by the dense appearance of the cortical portion of the bone graft. This technique differs only slightly from that initially described by Ferguson and Howorth,[50] Howorth,[55,64] and Heyman and associates.[52-54] Our procedure includes more extensive curettage of the growth plate and the routine extraction of the core biopsy specimen guarantees identification of the physis by direct vision.

The same procedure is performed in both acute and chronic slipping with the exception that a patient with an acute slip is placed on a fracture table and, after the displacement is reduced under direct vision, the limb is affixed to the fracture table to maintain reduction before the epiphysiodesis is done. A bilateral hip spica cast is applied after surgical epiphysiodesis in the acute cases.

Chronic SCFE

Chronic slipping of the capital femoral epiphysis implies that the proximal femoral epiphysis is firmly anchored to the neck (that is, healing is sufficient to prevent displacement during manipulation of the hip). Fortunately, this constitutes a large majority of cases. That such healing probably occurs in two weeks or less is suggested by experimental studies of Salter-Harris

procedure easy to accomplish without the use of a hip spica cast. There is indeed inherent stability in the chronic slip but the exact amount of force necessary to distract a chronic slip further is as yet unknown. My colleagues and I do not believe that temporal factors should be used to distinguish chronic from acute slips because many supposedly acute cases are firmly stable despite only one to three weeks of symptoms.

Data and Results

Between 1950 and 1980, 134 patients, (159 hips) were treated by bone-graft epiphysiodesis and followed up for a minimum of one year.[66] There was one case of avascular necrosis. In four cases in which reslipping occurred, all were salvaged by closed reduction and casting or pinning. Not a single case of acute cartilage necrosis was encountered. In an updated study of chronic SCFE treated between 1980 and 1987, 34 patients (43 hips) underwent bone-graft epiphysiodesis. There were two cases of graft resorption salvaged by regrafting in one case and pinning in the other. In two additional cases reslips were salvaged by closed reduction and hip spica casting for six weeks without sequelae (Figs. 21–8 to 21–10). In two cases deep infection led to residual stiffness and inferior results; the infections probably resulted from the intra-articular surgical exposure rather than from the type of operation employed. Not a single case of avascular necrosis or acute cartilage necrosis was found in this group of recent cases.

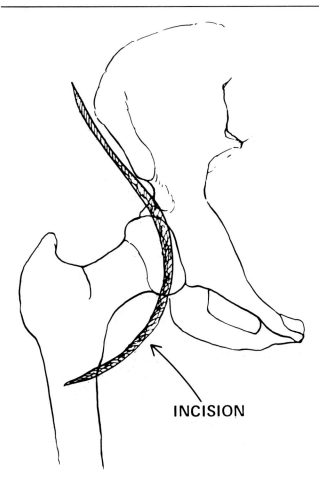

Fig. 21-2 Anterior iliofemoral approach.

type I and type II fractures in animals, providing there is no further head-on-neck movement (slipping).

In chronic SCFE head and neck stability is directly observed during bone-graft epiphysiodesis, making the

Acute SCFE

Acute SCFE is characterized by all the prodromal symptoms and findings of chronic SCFE, plus the acute onset of pain on any attempt to mobilize the limb and a sudden inability to bear weight. Commonly, but not

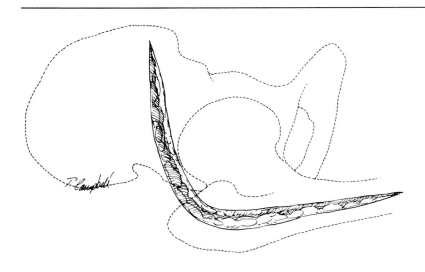

Fig. 21-3 Anterolateral approach.

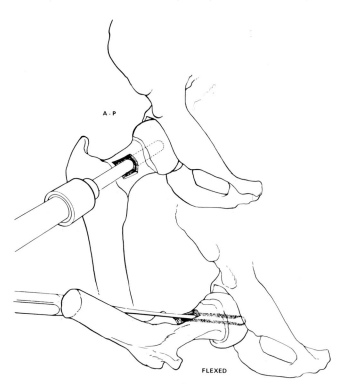

Fig. 21-4 Drawing shows insertion of hollow mill and further curettage of the growth plate.

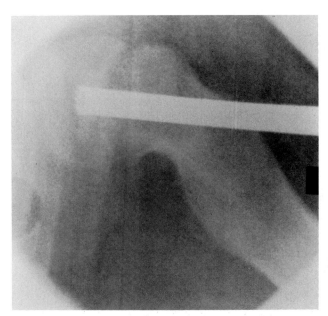

Fig. 21-5 Image intensifier shows hollow mill crossing growth plate.

always, the slippage is radiographically greater (second- or third-degree) in the acute form. Clearly, the risk of complications, particularly avascular necrosis, is greater. I believe this results from tension on the vascular pedicle (sleeve of periosteum with the lateral epiphyseal artery) supplying the femoral head. In the presence of the posteroinferior rotated head and an anterolateral rotated neck, the pedicle is "kinked" (Fig. 21–11). There is a tear in the periosteal sleeve along the anterosuperior portion of the metaphysis of the femoral neck, exposing the bare reddened bony metaphysis anteriorly. The periosteal sleeve remains at least partially intact posteriorly and attached to the epiphysis.[68]

I also believe that quick reduction (within 24 hours) is likely to decompress this tenuous vascular compromise. My colleagues and I, in our small series of 14 such cases, have so far avoided avascular changes. Similarly, we do not consider the synovial fluid to be a potential source of tamponade of the superolateral epiphyseal arterial blood supply. Clearly, all treatment methods employed to date have produced cases of avascular necrosis associated with acute slipping. It is, therefore, highly likely that avascular necrosis is a function of the acute displacement and perhaps of our technique and timing of reduction of that displacement, rather than a function of the type of treatment employed.

The bone-graft epiphysiodesis has been used in the

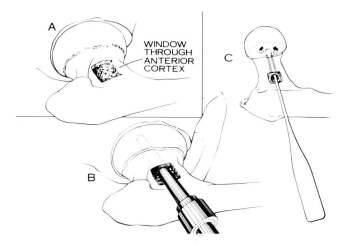

Fig. 21-6 Drawing shows cortical window, insertion of hollow mill, and curettage of the growth plate.

treatment of acute slips since the mid 1950s at Akron Children's Hospital Medical Center.[53,66] The "slip site" is directly visualized and the slip reduced by manipulation (flexion, internal rotation, traction, and abduction) (Fig. 21–12). Undoubtedly, bone-graft epiphysiodesis temporarily further weakens the link between the femoral head and neck until union across the growth plate occurs. This lack of inherent stability is counteracted by application of a bilateral hip spica cast in the operating room.

The hip spica cast is removed after six weeks and a

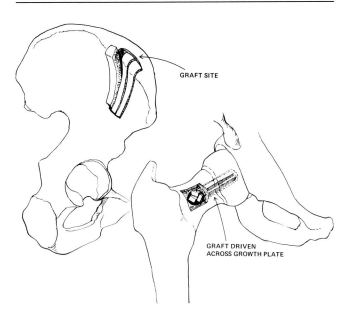

Fig. 21-7   Drawing shows cortical cancellous grafts inserted across femoral neck.

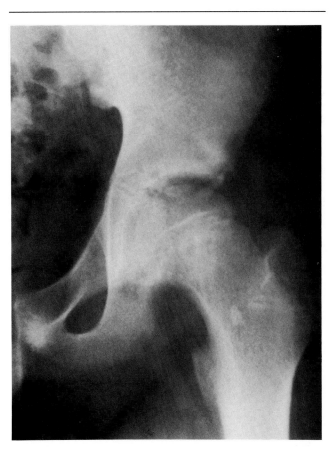

remarkably high percentage of acute slips show advanced growth plate closure at that time (Fig. 21–13). Theoretically at least, the cylindrical channel across the growth plate through which the bone-graft material passes, allows for an additional potential source of vascularization. Aadalen and associates[68] reported that bone-graft epiphysiodesis markedly reduced the incidence of avascular necrosis compared with multiple pin fixation.

Data and Results

Between 1950 and 1980, my colleagues and I treated 25 patients (26 hips) for acute SCFE.[66] We found two cases of avascular necrosis and one case of acute cartilage necrosis. Between 1980 and 1987, an additional four hips were treated by bone-graft epiphysiodesis (making a total of 29 patients and 30 hips). All recent cases healed uneventfully without evidence of avascular necrosis or acute cartilage necrosis.

Current Experience

Our statistics to date are derived from experience with 197 patients (232 hips). Of these, 168 patients (202 hips) had chronic SCFE and 29 patients (30 hips) had acute slips. Overall, there were six reslips, all of which were salvaged by either remanipulation and cast application (four cases) or pinning (two cases). Two cases of graft resorption occurred without reslipping, each salvaged by regrafting and pinning. There were three cases of avascular necrosis but only a single case of

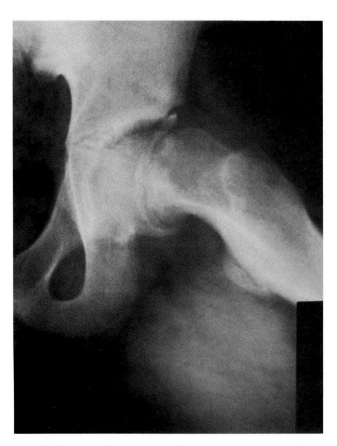

Fig. 21-8   Chronic SCFE. **Top:** Anteroposterior view. **Bottom:** Lateral view.

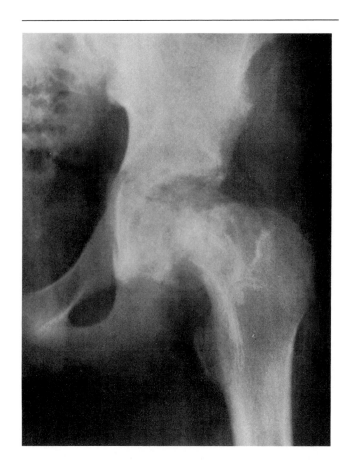

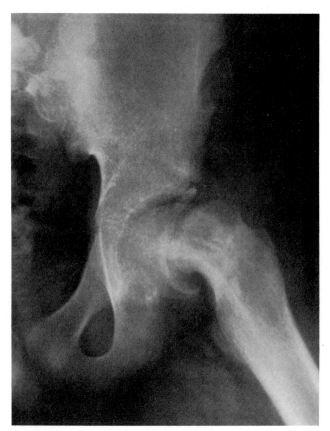

Fig. 21-9 SCFE was treated with bone-graft epiphysiodesis. Three weeks later, the patient tried to walk and fell, sustaining an acute-on-chronic slip. **Top:** Anteroposterior view. **Bottom:** Lateral view.

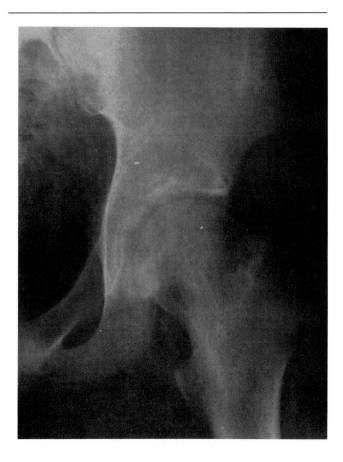

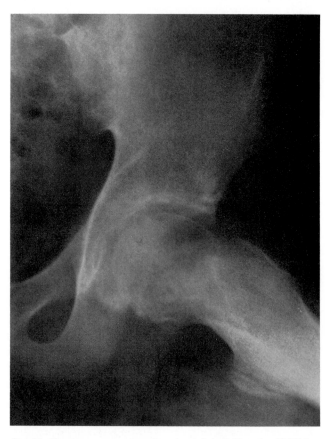

Fig. 21-10 Sixteen months after the original slip, the SCFE has healed without sequelae. Acute slip was treated by closed reduction and spica cast. **Top:** Anteroposterior view. **Bottom:** Lateral view.

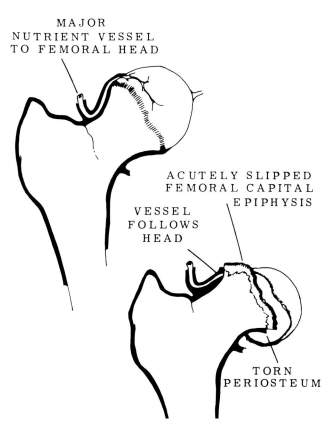

Fig. 21-11   Drawing shows vascular kinking in acute SCFE.

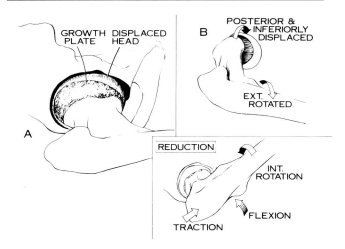

Fig. 21-12   Drawing shows mechanics of reduction of acute SCFE: flexion, internal rotation, traction, and abduction.

acute cartilage necrosis in the entire series. All three were in acute slips.

Discussion

There is little question that all slips will eventually "stop" slipping and that the head will become anchored to the neck. Further, although Oram[69] reported progressive slipping in untreated cases, most cases are chronic and likely to heal with little deformity and no significant additional slipping. Because it is difficult to determine which slips will progress, which will become stable, and which will become acute-on-chronic slips with a much poorer overall prognosis, surgical treatment is now universally accepted as the standard of care.

The goals of treatment are simple: to arrest any further progression and induce closure of the growth plate as rapidly as possible, thereby allowing the patient to return to regular activities with minimal difficulty. Thus, any surgical procedure should prevent further slipping, induce rapid and reliable growth plate closure with a minimum of hardship to the patient, be technically achievable by the surgeon, carry the least possible risk

of all complications, and avoid the necessity of additional surgery at a later time.

Before 1930, SCFE treatment included bedrest, proximal femoral osteotomy of the upper femoral shaft, osteotomy of the femoral neck, osteoplasty of the neck of the femur, crutches, and casting. In 1931, Ferguson and Howorth[50] reported the use of bone-graft epiphysiodesis in the treatment of SCFE. In the late 1920s and 1930s, multiple drilling across the growth plate (inforation) became popular.[70,71] The successes and failures of this technique probably influenced the development of bone grafting to enhance the opportunity for growth plate closure. In 1933 Phemister[72] clearly demonstrated the efficacy of bone grafting in inducing growth plate closure in long bones.

After the development of the Smith-Peterson nail, many surgeons began bridging the growth plate with durable metal to provide stable fixation and to allow for growth plate closure while avoiding further slipping. Disastrous results with the triflanged nailings[19,25] led to the use of multiple threaded pins; by the 1950s, internal fixation by multiple threaded pins had become the most common method of treatment in SCFE.

No scientific study has provided the exact criteria needed for assessing the extent of growth plate closure correlated with time. Inferences have been drawn,[24] but it is not known exactly when and how growth plate closure occurs after metallic internal fixation. Most investigators report that growth plate closure occurs six to 18 months after pinning, but information about the extent of plate closure and, thus, what activities may be allowed can be difficult to ascertain. Growth plate closure after threaded pinning seems to occur by new bone growth directly adjacent to the threads that cross and bridge the growth plate in response to the trauma and local damage induced by inserting the threaded portion of the metal.

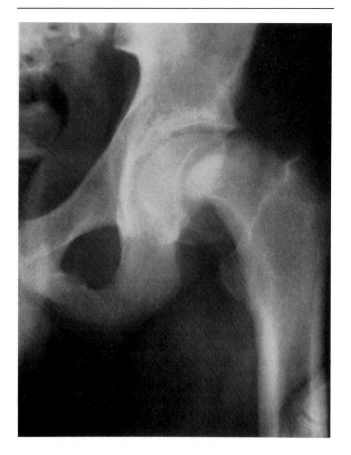

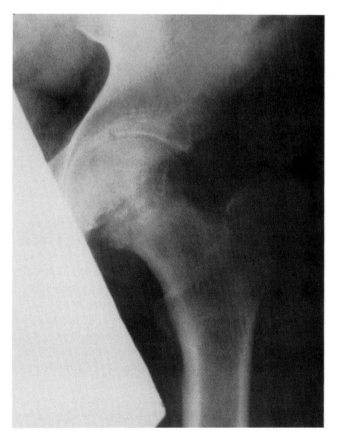

Fig. 21-13   Acute SCFE. **Top:** Anteroposterior view before bone-graft epiphysiodesis. **Bottom:** Anteroposterior view six weeks after bone-graft epiphysiodesis shows advanced closure of growth plate.

Although growth plate closure after bone-graft epiphysiodesis has been reported to occur after an average of ten weeks,[53,59,65,66] strict criteria for assessing the manner and extent of closure were not provided. Therefore, a study was done to obtain such data (P. Fleissner and D. Weiner, unpublished data). We demonstrated in 79 carefully scrutinized cases that one third of the growth plate is closed after an average of ten weeks, one half after 15 weeks, and three fourths after six months. Return to full unprotected activities would probably have been safe after an average of 15 weeks (50% closure). A study using similar criteria to assess a large group of hips treated by multiple pins is now underway.

Campbell and associates[73] demonstrated in dogs that the incidence and rapidity of growth plate closure were directly proportional to the size of the bone graft employed. It is presently unclear whether the location of the graft (central or eccentric) has a similar effect. It is likely that roughly 20% to 30% of the growth plate is removed by our present technique of bone-grafting epiphysiodesis.

The use of a single-threaded screw has recently become popular in some centers. Although it will be some time before there are enough cases for statistical analysis, there are some obvious concerns. The procedure still necessitates a second operation for removal; extraction may ultimately prove to be difficult (like Hagie pins)[48] because of bone growth behind the screw threads adjacent to the screw shaft; and the ability of the metal to resist shear forces across the growth plate in an acute slip with a mobile femoral head is unknown.[74] Distraction of the femoral head during insertion of threaded pins or screws occasionally occurs, probably increasing the risk of avascular necrosis. Despite these concerns, this technique, augmented by image intensification control at the time of surgery, may well replace or decrease the use of multiple pins.

Conclusion

In cases of minimal slipping (first-degree), metallic fixation and bone-graft epiphysiodesis (which has the fewest overall complications) both seem to be justified on the basis of studies of complications, provided that extreme care is used in the insertion of metallic fixation. In cases of moderate or severe slipping (second- or third-degree), bone-graft epiphysiodesis is strongly recommended to avoid the obvious problems caused by the disturbed architectural geometry at the site of slipping. It is hoped that using the anterolateral approach in bone-graft epiphysiodesis will allow more surgeons to familiarize themselves with this technique, one that has been shown to be safer in a large number of cases.

References

1. Badgley CE, Isaacson AS, Wolgamot JC, et al: Operative therapy for slipped upper femoral epiphysis: An end-result study. *J Bone Joint Surg* 1948;30A:19–30.

2. Baker G, Louis H: Treatment of slipped capital femoral epiphysis with pinning. Presented at the meeting of the Western Orthopaedic Association, 1982.

3. Barrett J, Imrie D, Derian P: Chondrolysis: A severe complication of slipped capital femoral epiphysis. Presented at the meeting of the Orthopaedic Research Society, 1976.

4. Bennet GC, Koreska J, Rang M: Pin placement in slipped capital femoral epiphysis. *J Bone Joint Surg* 1981;63B:637.

5. Bishop JO, Oley TJ, Stephenson CT, et al: Slipped capital femoral epiphysis: A study of 50 cases in black children. *Clin Orthop* 1978;135:93–96.

6. Borofsky E, LaMont R: Result of multiple pinning in slipped capital femoral epiphysis. Presented at the American Orthopaedic Association Resident's Conference, 1982.

7. Boyd HB, Ingram AJ, Bourkard HO: The treatment of slipped femoral epiphysis. *South Med J* 1949;42:551–560.

8. Boyer DW, Mickelson MR, Ponseti IV: Slipped capital femoral epiphysis: Long-term follow-up study of one hundred and twenty-one patients. *J Bone Joint Surg* 1981;63A:85–95.

9. Brodetti A: The blood supply of the femoral neck and head in relation to the damaging effects of nails and screws. *J Bone Joint Surg* 1960;42B:794–801.

10. Brodsky JW, Barnes DA, Tullos HS: Unrecognized pin penetration of the hip joint. *Contemp Orthop* 1984;9:13–19.

11. Cameron HU, Wang M, Koreska J: Internal fixation of slipped femoral capital epiphyses. *Clin Orthop* 1978;137:148–153.

12. Durbin FC: Treatment of slipped upper femoral epiphysis. *J Bone Joint Surg* 1960;42B:289–302.

13. Eisenstein A, Rothschild S: Biochemical abnormalities in patients with slipped capital femoral epiphysis and chondrolysis. *J Bone Joint Surg* 1976;58A:459–467.

14. El-Khoury GY, Mickelson MR: Chondrolysis following slipped capital femoral epiphysis. *Radiology* 1977;123:327–330.

15. Frymoyer JW: Chondrolysis of the hip following Southwick osteotomy for severe slipped capital femoral epiphysis. *Clin Orthop* 1974;99:120–124.

16. Goldman AB, Schneider R, Martel W: Acute chondrolysis complicating slipped capital femoral epiphysis. *AJR* 1978;130:945–950.

17. Greenough CG, Bromage JD, Jackson AM: Pinning of the slipped upper femoral epiphysis: A trouble-free procedure? *J Pediatr Orthop* 1985;5:657–660.

18. Griffith MJ: Slipping of the capital femoral epiphysis. *Ann R Coll Surg Engl* 1976;58:34–42.

19. Hall JE: The results of treatment of slipped femoral epiphysis. *J Bone Joint Surg* 1957;39B:659–673.

20. Hartman T, Gates D: Recovery from cartilage necrosis following slipped capital femoral epiphysis. *Orthop Rev* 1972;1:33–37.

21. Heppenstall RB, Marvel JP Jr, Chung SM, et al: Chondrolysis of the hip. *Clin Orthop* 1974;103:136–142.

22. Herndon WA, Yngve DA, Janssen TP: Iatrogenic false aneurysm in slipped capital femoral epiphysis. *J Pediatr Orthop* 1984;4:754–755.

23. Ingram A, Clarke M, Clark C: The effect of treatment on the incidence of chondrolysis complicating slipped capital femoral epiphysis. Presented at the meeting of the Pediatric Orthopaedic Society, Palm Springs, Nov 10–14, 1976.

24. Rosenzweig AH, Irani RN: Epiphysiodesis in slipped capital femoral epiphysis: Comparison of various surgical modalities. Presented at the 47th Annual Meeting of the American Academy of Orthopaedic Surgeons, Atlanta, Feb 7–12, 1980.

25. Jerre T: Early complications after osteosynthesis with a three flanged nail in situ for slipped epiphysis. *Acta Orthop Scand* 1957;27:126–134.

26. Korn MW, States JD: Slipping capital femoral epiphysis: A long-term follow-up and review of cases in Rochester, New York. *Clin Orthop* 1966;48:119–128.

27. Kulick RG, Denton JR: A retrospective study of 125 cases of slipped capital femoral epiphysis. *Clin Orthop* 1982;162:87–90.

28. Lehman WB, Menche D, Norman A, et al: The problem of in situ pinning of slipped capital femoral epiphysis. Presented at the 49th Annual Meeting of the American Academy of Orthopaedic Surgeons, New Orleans, Jan 21–26, 1982.

29. Lehman WB, Menche D, Grant A, et al: The problem of evaluating in situ pinning of slipped capital femoral epiphysis: An experimental model and a review of 63 consecutive cases. *J Pediatr Orthop* 1984;4:297–303.

30. Lowe HG: Necrosis of articular cartilage after slipping of the capital femoral epiphysis: Report of six cases with recovery. *J Bone Joint Surg* 1970;52B:108–118.

31. MacEwen GD: Advantages and disadvantages of pin fixation in slipped capital femoral epiphysis, in American Academy of Orthopaedic Surgeons *Instructional Course Lectures, XXIX.* St. Louis, CV Mosby, 1980, pp 86–90.

32. Mankin H, Sledge C, Rothschild S, et al: Chondrolysis of the hip. *Hip* 1975:127–135.

33. Maurer RC, Larsen IJ: Acute necrosis of cartilage in slipped capital femoral epiphysis. *J Bone Joint Surg* 1970;52A:39–50.

34. Menche D, Lehman WB: In situ pinning of slipped capital femoral epiphysis, abstract. *Orthop Rev* 1982;11(2):129–130.

35. Morrissy R: In-situ fixation of chronic slipped capital femoral epiphysis, in American Academy of Orthopaedic Surgeons *Instructional Courses Lectures, XXXIII.* St. Louis, CV Mosby, 1984, pp 319–327.

36. Ninomiya S, Nagasaka Y, Tagawa H: Slipped capital femoral epiphysis: A study of 68 cases in the eastern half area of Japan. *Clin Orthop* 1976;119:172–176.

37. Ogden JA, Simon TR, Southwick WO: Cartilage space width in slipped capital femoral epiphysis: The relationship to cartilage necrosis. *Yale J Biol Med* 1977;50:17–30.

38. Orofino C, Innis J, Lowrey CW: Slipped capital femoral epiphysis in Negroes: A study of ninety-five cases. *J Bone Joint Surg* 1960;42A:1079–1083.

39. Pierce R, Mott W: Observations on slipped capital femoral epiphysis. *Orthop Trans* 1980;4:335.

40. Ponseti I, Barta CK: Evaluation of treatment of slipping of the capital femoral epiphysis. *Surg Gynecol Obstet* 1948;86:87–97.

41. Riley P, Weiner DS, Weiner S, et al: Perils of pin fixation in slipped capital femoral epiphysis. *J Pediatr Orthop*, in press.

42. Ross PM, Lyne ED, Morawa LG: Slipped capital femoral epiphysis long-term results after 10–38 years. *Clin Orthop* 1979;141:176–180.

43. Schmidt R, Gregg J: Subtrochanteric fractures complicating pin fixation of slipped capital femoral epiphysis. Presented at the meeting of the Pediatric Orthopaedic Society, San Antonio, 1985.

44. Southwick WO: Osteotomy through the lesser trochanter for slipped capital femoral epiphysis. *J Bone Joint Surg* 1967;49A:807–835.

45. Swiontkowski M: Slipped capital femoral epiphysis: Complications related to internal fixation. *Orthopedics* 1983;6:705–712.

46. Tillema DA, Golding JSR: Chondrolysis following slipped capital femoral epiphysis in Jamaica. *J Bone Joint Surg* 1971;53A:1528–1540.

47. Walters R, Simon S: Joint destruction: A sequel of unrecognized pin penetration in patients with slipped capital femoral epiphysis. *Hip* 1980;8:145–164.

48. Weiner D: Letter to the editor. *J Bone Joint Surg* 1975;57A:433.

49. Wilson PD, Jacobs B, Schecter L: Slipped capital femoral epiphysis: An end-result study. *J Bone Joint Surg* 1965;47A:1128–1145.

50. Ferguson AB, Howorth MB: Slipping of the upper femoral epiphysis: Study of 70 cases. *JAMA* 1931;97:1867–1872.

51. Herndon CH, Heyman CH, Bell DM: Treatment of slipped capital femoral epiphysis by epiphyseodesis and osteoplasty of the femoral neck: A report of further experience. *J Bone Joint Surg* 1963;45A:999–1012.

52. Heyman CH: Treatment of slipping of the upper femoral epiphysis: A study of results of forty-two cases. *Surg Gynecol Obstet* 1949;89:559–565.

53. Heyman CH, Herndon CH: Epiphyseodesis for early slipping of the upper femoral epiphysis. *J Bone Joint Surg* 1954;36A:539–555.

54. Heyman CH, Herndon CH, Strong JM: Slipped femoral epiphysis with severe displacement: A conservative operative treatment. *J Bone Joint Surg* 1957;39A:293–303.

55. Howorth MB: Slipping of the upper femoral epiphysis. *Surg Gynecol Obstet* 1941;73:723–732.

56. Howorth MB: Slipping of the upper femoral epiphysis. *J Bone Joint Surg* 1949;31A:734–747.

57. Howorth B: Slipping of the upper femoral epiphysis, in Pease CN (ed): American Academy of Orthopaedic Surgeons *Instructional Course Lectures, VIII.* Ann Arbor, JW Edwards, 1951, pp 306–317.

58. Howorth MB: *A Textbook of Orthopedics.* Philadelphia, WB Saunders, 1952, pp 689–711.

59. Howorth B: The treatment of slipping of the upper femoral epiphysis. *J Int Coll Surg* 1953;20:716–735.

60. Howorth B: Slipping of the upper femoral epiphysis. *Clin Orthop* 1957;10:148–173.

61. Howorth B: Slipping of the capital femoral epiphysis. *J Bone Joint Surg* 1963;45A:1776.

62. Howorth B: Slipping of the capital femoral epiphysis. *Am J Orthop* 1965;7:10–17.

63. Howorth B: The bone-pegging operation for slipping of the capital femoral epiphysis. *Clin Orthop* 1966;48:79–87.

64. Howorth B: Slipping of the capital femoral epiphysis: Treatment. *Clin Orthop* 1966;48:53–70.

65. Melby A, Hoyt WA Jr, Weiner DS: Treatment of chronic slipped capital femoral epiphysis by bone-grafted epiphyseodesis. *J Bone Joint Surg* 1980;62A:119–125.

66. Weiner DS, Weiner S, Melby A, et al: A 30-year experience with bone graft epiphysiodesis in the treatment of slipped capital femoral epiphysis. *J Pediatr Orthop* 1984;4:145–152.

67. Weiner DS, Weiner SD, Melby A: Anterolateral approach to the hip for bone graft epiphysiodesis in the treatment of slipped capital femoral epiphysis. *J Pediatr Orthop* 1988;8:349–352.

68. Aadalen RJ, Weiner DS, Hoyt W, et al: Acute slipped capital femoral epiphysis. *J Bone Joint Surg* 1974;56A:1473–1487.

69. Oram V: Epiphysiolysis of the head of the femur: A follow-up examination with special reference to end results and the social prognosis. *Acta Orthop Scand* 1954;23:100–120.

70. Kiaer S: Epiphyseolysis capitis femoris treated with inforation. *Acta Orthop Scand* 1948;17:81–92.

71. Mathiesen FR: Slipping of the proximal femoral epiphysis: Thirty-six cases treated by drilling. *Acta Orthop Scand* 1957;27:115–125.

72. Phemister DB: Operative arrestment of longitudinal growth of bones in the treatment of deformities. *J Bone Joint Surg* 1933;15:1–15.

73. Campbell CJ, Grisolia A, Zanconato G: The effects produced in the cartilaginous epiphyseal plate of immature dogs by experimental surgical traumata. *J Bone Joint Surg* 1959;41A:1221–1242.

74. Herring JA: Slipped capital femoral epiphysis: Case 2 (clinical conference). *J Pediatr Orthop* 1984;4:764–767.

The Role of Osteotomy in the Treatment of Slipped Capital Femoral Epiphysis

Alvin H. Crawford, MD

The treatment of advanced slipping of the upper femoral epiphysis remains an unsolved problem despite the fact that it was first described by Pare[1] some 400 years ago. The primary goal of osteotomy in the treatment of slipped capital femoral epiphysis (SCFE) is to restore the anatomy to the best position possible with the least amount of compromise to the femoral-acetabular components. Howorth[2] stated that the lesion always heals spontaneously and that treatment is of no value unless it produces a better result than would have been accomplished by nature. He further stated that nature, even in the presence of considerable slipping, did a better job in many cases than he had been able to do surgically.

O'Brien and Fahey[3] reported remodeling of the femoral neck in patients in whom the triradiate cartilage was open. However, they believed that this treatment would not be satisfactory for a slip of more than 60 degrees. Wilson[4] stated that a slip of up to one third of the metaphyseal diameter is "acceptable" and that fixation in situ is all that is needed, a view supported by Newman[5] and Boyer and associates.[6] Although most authorities believe that without restoration of normal alignment of the head and neck arthritis will eventually develop, debate still surrounds the degree or amount of restoration of normal alignment needed to prevent osteoarthritis. Almost all reports indicate that severe slipping and malunion have a poor long-term prognosis.[3,7-9] There are only two well-documented studies on the long-term follow-up of unrealigned severe slips. Herndon and associates[10] described patients treated by bone grafting and osteoplasty with no attempt at alignment. Twenty-five of 32 hips had good or excellent results. Boyer and associates[6] described seven patients with severe uncorrected slips, six of whom had good clinical results. Although motion was quite restricted, their overall function was good and painless. There is general agreement that malunion of less than 60 degrees in the skeletally immature patient and of less than 30 to 40 degrees in the skeletally mature patient is consistent with adequate function for several decades. Thus, the indications for realignment osteotomy have become more stringent during the last decade.[11,12]

Objectives

The objectives of treatment are (1) stabilization of the epiphysis and prevention of further slippage, (2) stimulation of early closure, (3) prevention of avascular necrosis, (4) prevention of chondrolysis, and (5) improvement of joint function. These objectives are important in the management of all cases of SCFE whether they are treated with in situ stabilization or realignment. Because of the potential complications of osteotomy, the risk-reward ratio must be assessed carefully before this treatment is initiated.

The Goals of Osteotomy

The goals of osteotomy in this condition are straightforward: realignment of the slip, improved kinematics of the acetabular and femoral components, and delaying the onset of degenerative joint disease. The first two goals are mechanical and relatively easy to achieve. The third is more difficult and depends on the avoidance of chondrolysis and avascular necrosis. Unfortunately, long-term personal follow-up is beyond the scope of the average orthopaedic surgeon because long-term follow-up requires at least 30 years of observation and the original treating physician would probably no longer be in practice. Since we know that stabilization of minimal and moderate slippage is consistent with good long-term results, it appears that realignment procedures should be used only in cases of severe slippage.

The Rationale for Osteotomy

The rationale for osteotomy assumes that the forces resulting from a slip of more than 30 to 45 degrees produce a varus posterior tilting deformity of the head of the femur with respect to the neck, leading to a deformity of external rotation and shortening with varus angulation.

Realignment can be approached directly or by compensatory procedures. Theoretically, an open surgical correction by transcervical osteotomy (involving removal of the callus and anatomic alignment of the head on the neck followed by internal fixation) gives the best chance of good recovery of function.[13,14] Unfortunately, this technique has produced many of the significant problems associated with the treatment of SCFE.[5,15-17]

Levels of Osteotomy

My purpose is to review the levels of osteotomy performed historically in regard to their advantages and disadvantages. The techniques have been described elsewhere.[8,9,13,15,16,18-33] The levels include the subcapital, the base of the neck, the transtrochanteric rotational, and the trochanteric.

Subcapital

Through the Callus An osteotomy at this level has the distinct advantage of anatomic reduction. None of the procedures performed at a lower level achieves the anatomic correction that this procedure achieves. One can excise the callus, remove whatever bony posterior beak has formed, replace the head on the neck, and maintain it there with rigid internal fixation, thus producing essentially full correction of the deformity.[34,35] I consider this procedure "orthopaedic roulette" because the alarming incidence of avascular necrosis (the average incidence was 21% in a comprehensive American study[24] and 34% in a similar British study[16]) far outweighs its advantages.[2,5,16,36-40] Chondrolysis has also been reported with this procedure; however, the incidence has not been as high nor the consequences as devastating.

Cuneiform Osteotomy The cuneiform osteotomy described by Fish[41] has the fewest complications. In his discussion of the procedure, Fish cited two points: (1) In the pre-adolescent hip, the cartilaginous physis acts as a barrier to the vessels of the metaphysis, so the blood supply from the lateral epiphyseal vessels must pass through the posterolateral part of the periosteum of the neck to reach the epiphysis.[38] Therefore, one should avoid an osteotomy through this area and manipulation that produces tension on the posterior part of the periosteum and damages the blood vessels. (2) Fish credits DePalma and associates[42] with the speculation that an osteotomy through the physis, followed by removal of the physeal cartilage and meticulous osteotomy of the metaphysis, would obtain a bony apposition allowing some of the blood supply to the epiphysis to come directly from the metaphysis. For these reasons, Fish's procedure includes thorough and careful removal of the physeal cartilage with a curette at the same time that the deformity is corrected. This careful handling of the periosteal vessels of the posterior neck and complete removal of the physeal cartilage may account for his low incidence of avascular necrosis.

Subcapital osteotomy and realignment for SCFE remains one of the most dangerous procedures performed on a child for acquired deformities of the musculoskeletal system.[43]

Base of Neck

More frequently performed procedures include Hungria's osteotomy,[24] the compensating osteotomy of Kramer and associates,[27] and extracapsular osteotomy.[18] These are safer than subcapital procedures and they often achieve satisfactory anatomic restoration. The

extracapsular procedure attempts to avoid the problem of circulatory compromise.

The disadvantage of base-of-neck osteotomies is that they are limited in their ability to achieve correction. The maximum correction is limited to slips of 35 to 55 degrees. In patients with marked varus deformity in whom realignment causes shortening of the femoral neck and decreased articulotrochanteric distance, a trochanteric osteotomy (or a trochanteric apophysiodesis if the child is under 11 years of age) may be necessary.[27] The wedge required for correction may leave the leg so short that epiphysiodesis of the opposite side must be considered to achieve equalization of limb length at skeletal maturity. There is also the possibility of avascular necrosis associated with the procedure, most often as a result of failure to maintain stability of the proximal and distal fragments during the surgical procedure.[24] This problem is lessened by not placing retractors behind the femoral neck, something that may disrupt the cortex or—worse—strip the blood supply from the posterior femoral neck. Combining this osteotomy with manipulation of an acute slip is strongly condemned.

Transtrochanteric Rotational Osteotomy

The theoretical advantages of the Sugioka transtrochanteric rotational osteotomy far outweigh its actual advantages. In theory, it corrects severe deformities of more than 60 degrees and permits direct observation of the amount of correction and relocation of the alignment of the head or neck with the shaft. This, in turn, allows preservation of the abductor mechanism of the trochanter and avoids any shortening or subtrochanteric deformity.[30] A review of SCFE treated by this method showed significant complications in two of five cases (40%), an unacceptable rate.[44]

The disadvantage of the Sugioka osteotomy is a tendency to produce avascular necrosis and chondrolysis. In one study of 250 hips treated by this procedure,[30] one of nine hips with SCFE developed avascular necrosis. It is a technically demanding procedure and the general orthopaedist probably does not perform the procedure often enough to refine the technique.

Trochanteric Osteotomy

Trochanteric osteotomies can be biplanar or multiplanar and compensatory. They have advantages that far outweigh their disadvantages. Trochanteric osteotomy is one of the safest methods because it does not cause avascular necrosis, is extracapsular, stimulates epiphyseal closure, improves hip function, and, in most cases, does not adversely affect future surgery.[6] The procedure is less rewarding when used for severe slips because of the possible shortening. Southwick[9] believes that severe deformity does not require absolute technical compensation and correction. A lesser correction (which minimizes shortening) produces a realignment (20 to 30 degrees) adequate to improve function. The

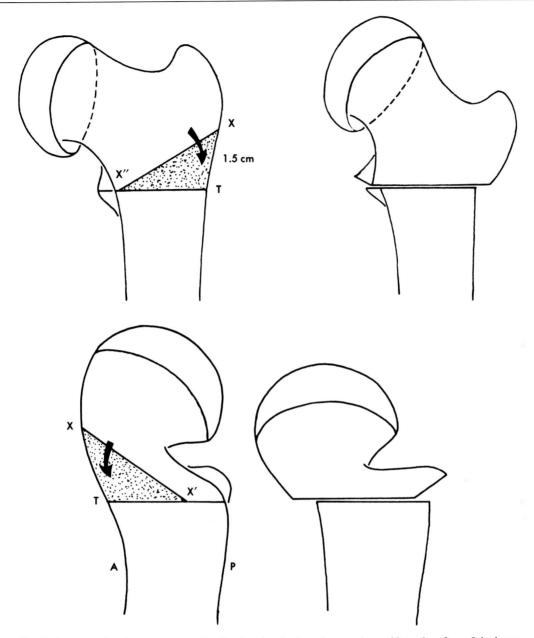

Fig. 22-1   Top left: After a transverse line has been scribed on the anterior and lateral surface of the bone at the level of the lesser trochanter, the junction of the lateral and anterior surface is identified and also marked as an orientation mark (X-T). The usual size of the wedge to be removed is indicated as 1.5 cm along the anterolateral orientation mark. **Top right:** Postoperative position as it would be seen on an anteroposterior radiograph. **Bottom left and right:** Lateral aspect of the osteotomy before and after removal of bone. (Reproduced with permission from Clark CR, Southwick WO, Ogden JA: Anatomic aspects of slipped capital femoral epiphysis and correction by biplane osteotomy, in American Academy of Orthopaedic Surgeons *Instructional Course Lectures, XXIX.* St. Louis, CV Mosby, 1980, pp 90–100.)

operation does not restore the normal anatomy of the proximal end of the femur because the osteotomy is distal to the muscle insertions on the greater trochanter. The recent modification of Southwick's technique by Clark and associates[22] (fixed dimensioned rather than constructed templates) decreases the calculations required and should improve the technical results. They recommend that the anterior osteotomy include an area

two-thirds the distance across the anterior surface at the level of the lesser trochanter, directed from a height of 1.5 cm proximally. The posterior angle extends one-half the distance across the femur from an anterolateral orientation line (Fig. 22–1).

The 20 to 30 degrees of latitude in the position of the osteotomy makes this operation fairly successful. Undercorrection of the severe slip not only prevents ex-

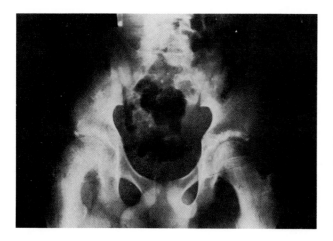

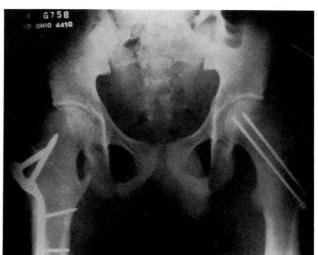

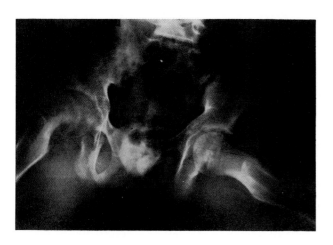

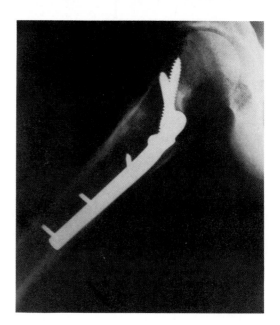

Fig. 22-2 **Top left and bottom left:** Anteroposterior radiographs of a skeletally immature child showing obvious slipped capital femoral epiphysis of the right hip and minimal preslip on the left side. **Top right:** Eighteen months after Southwick osteotomy on the right side and in situ pin fixation on the left. **Bottom right:** True lateral view of right hip. (Reproduced with permission from Crawford AH: Osteotomies in the treatment of slipped capital femoral epiphysis, in American Academy of Orthopaedic Surgeons *Instructional Course Lectures, XXXIII*. St. Louis, CV Mosby, 1984, pp 327–349; original Figures 22–2, *top left and bottom left* were provided by Timothy L. Stephens, MD, Cleveland.)

cessive shortening but makes the correction consistent with in situ fixation of mild to moderate slips (Fig. 22–2).

The less experienced surgeon can use the techniques of Gruber and Laskin[25] and MacEwen and Shands[28] to perform a biplane osteotomy with maximum efficiency and minimal difficulty.

None of the results obtained with trochanteric osteotomy are as good as the best results obtained by neck osteotomies, but none are as bad as the worst results obtained by neck osteotomies. The advantages and disadvantages of each procedure are summarized in Figure 22–3.

Complications

Avascular Necrosis

Avascular necrosis is the most unsettling of all the complications associated with the treatment of SCFE. It is rare in the untreated slip but has been reported after almost all forms of treatment. The incidence appears to be higher in series reporting on neck osteotomy and lower in those reporting on trochanteric osteotomies. It is rarely, if ever, seen with bone-graft epiphysiodesis. The management of this complication must be individualized because of the lack of consis-

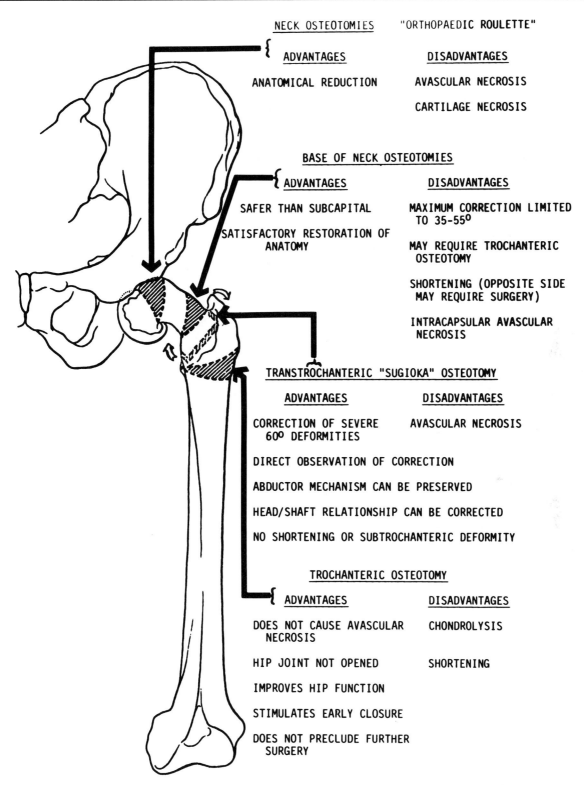

NECK OSTEOTOMIES   "ORTHOPAEDIC **ROULETTE**"

ADVANTAGES	DISADVANTAGES
ANATOMICAL REDUCTION	AVASCULAR NECROSIS
	CARTILAGE NECROSIS

BASE OF NECK OSTEOTOMIES

ADVANTAGES	DISADVANTAGES
SAFER THAN SUBCAPITAL	MAXIMUM CORRECTION LIMITED TO 35-55°
SATISFACTORY RESTORATION OF ANATOMY	MAY REQUIRE TROCHANTERIC OSTEOTOMY
	SHORTENING (OPPOSITE SIDE MAY REQUIRE SURGERY)
	INTRACAPSULAR AVASCULAR NECROSIS

TRANSTROCHANTERIC "SUGIOKA" OSTEOTOMY

ADVANTAGES	DISADVANTAGES
CORRECTION OF SEVERE 60° DEFORMITIES	AVASCULAR NECROSIS
DIRECT OBSERVATION OF CORRECTION	
ABDUCTOR MECHANISM CAN BE PRESERVED	
HEAD/SHAFT RELATIONSHIP CAN BE CORRECTED	
NO SHORTENING OR SUBTROCHANTERIC DEFORMITY	

TROCHANTERIC OSTEOTOMY

ADVANTAGES	DISADVANTAGES
DOES NOT CAUSE AVASCULAR NECROSIS	CHONDROLYSIS
HIP JOINT NOT OPENED	SHORTENING
IMPROVES HIP FUNCTION	
STIMULATES EARLY CLOSURE	
DOES NOT PRECLUDE FURTHER SURGERY	

Fig. 22-3 Advantages and disadvantages of osteotomies for slipped capital femoral epiphysis. (Reproduced with permission from Crawford AH: Osteotomies in the treatment of slipped capital femoral epiphysis, in American Academy of Orthopaedic Surgeons *Instructional Course Lectures, XXXIII.* St. Louis, CV Mosby, 1984, pp 327–349.)

tently good results with any method short of arthrodesis.

Chondrolysis

Narrowing of the joint space may occur in treated as well as untreated patients. Its association with the biplane osteotomy has caused enthusiasm for that procedure to wane in recent years.[45] To decrease, if not prevent, the occurrence of chondrolysis in the chronic slip undergoing osteotomy, I recommend (1) preoperative traction to relieve muscular spasms, (2) complete detachment of the iliopsoas muscle to decrease intra-articular pressure, and (3) rigid internal fixation of the osteotomy fragments to avoid external immobilization. Motion is important in prevention as well as in treatment of chondrolysis.

If chondrolysis does occur after osteotomy, prolonged traction and physical therapy should be instituted. Recovery of the joint space has been noted one to two years after the onset of chondrolysis and one should wait at least a year before considering surgical treatment. If the problem is unresponsive to traction and physiotherapy, I recommend subtotal circumferential capsulectomy, intraoperative manipulation, and postoperative continued passive motion with bupivacaine analgesia. If there is still no improvement in joint space narrowing or joint motion, a hip fusion or replacement arthroplasty should be considered.

Shortening

All the compensating osteotomies require removal of a bony wedge and, as a result, shortening is a potential complication. The problem is more likely to occur in patients with severe slippage, especially if the attempted correction is overzealous. The problem occurs more frequently with intracapsular and base-of-neck osteotomies. Trochanteric transfer and trochanteric apophyseal arrest of the ipsilateral limb can be carried out if there is excessive neck shortening; however, the resulting limb-length inequality may necessitate a contralateral epiphyseal arrest at the appropriate time to achieve equalization of the limbs at skeletal maturity.

Peritrochanteric Deformity

Although the primary indication for osteotomy about the head and neck of the femur for SCFE is to prevent degenerative arthritis, this does, nevertheless, occur. A significant number of children treated for SCFE will later have degenerative arthritis requiring arthroplasty.[46,47] Most of the compensating osteotomies result in deformities of the proximal femur. This should be kept in mind when performing the initial procedure. If rigid internal fixation is used in a young child, it should be removed after complete epiphyseal closure has occurred to permit as much remodeling as possible. The removal also makes the task of the reconstructive surgeon much easier. Crutch-assisted ambulation after

removal of hardware is strongly recommended for at least four to six weeks because stress fractures through the screw holes are more likely to occur if motion of the hip joint is decreased.

Current Management of SCFE

Most patients admitted to my institution with SCFE have been symptomatic for some time. The hips are usually somewhat sensitive and the range of motion is limited. If the femoral epiphysis is stable, we place the patient in split Russell's traction until the pain has been relieved. If the epiphysis is unstable, as in an acute slippage, a distal femoral skeletal pin is placed on the ipsilateral femur along with a derotation sling. Weights are increased and radiographs taken every other day until head-neck alignment improves. Once the pain has abated, in situ fixation by open epiphysiodesis is performed. If the procedure is unilateral, the child is placed on crutches and undergoes rehabilitation. If bilateral fixation is required, the child is placed in traction at home or in a spica cast (depending on the home environment) for approximately four to six weeks and rehabilitation with crutch-assisted ambulation is initiated.

Once the child has completed rehabilitation and there is evidence of a bony fusion across the epiphyseal plate, the child is allowed to resume normal activities. If after one year there is persistent limitation of motion with external rotation deformity and the slip is more than 60 degrees after remodeling, a peritrochanteric biplane osteotomy using rigid internal fixation is performed.

References

1. Pare A: Fractures of the neck of the femur, in *Cinq livres de chirurgie.* Paris, Andre Wechel, 1572, vol 2, p 95.
2. Howorth B: The bone-pegging operation for slipping of the capital femoral epiphysis. *Clin Orthop* 1966;48:79–87.
3. O'Brien ET, Fahey JJ: Remodeling of the femoral neck after in situ pinning for slipped capital femoral epiphysis. *J Bone Joint Surg* 1977;59A:62–68.
4. Wilson PD: The treatment of slipping of the upper femoral epiphysis with minimal displacement. *J Bone Joint Surg* 1938;20:379–399.
5. Newman PH: The surgical treatment of slipping of the upper femoral epiphysis. *J Bone Joint Surg* 1960;42B:280–288.
6. Boyer DW, Mickelson MR, Ponseti IV: Slipped capital femoral epiphysis: Long-term follow-up study of one hundred and twenty-one patients. *J Bone Joint Surg* 1981;63A:85–95.
7. Howorth B: Slipping of the capital femoral epiphysis. *Am J Orthop* 1965;7:10–17.
8. Jerre T: Early complications after osteosynthesis with a three flanged nail in situ for slipped epiphysis. *Acta Orthop Scand* 1957;27:126–134.
9. Southwick WO: Osteotomy through the lesser trochanter for slipped capital femoral epiphysis. *J Bone Joint Surg* 1967;49A:807–835.
10. Herndon CH, Heyman CH, Bell DM: Treatment of slipped cap-

ital femoral epiphysis by epiphyseodesis and osteoplasty of the femoral neck: A report of further experiences. *J Bone Joint Surg* 1963;45A:999–1012.

11. Cordell LD: Slipped capital femoral epiphysis: Long-term results. *Postgrad Med* 1976;60:135–141.

12. Ross PM, Lyne ED, Morawa LG: Slipped capital femoral epiphysis long-term results after 10–38 years. *Clin Orthop* 1979;141:176–180.

13. Klein A, Joplin RJ, Reidy JA: Treatment of slipped capital femoral epiphysis. *JAMA* 1948;136:445–451.

14. Klein A, Joplin RJ, Reidy JA, et al: Roentgenographic changes in nailed slipped capital femoral epiphysis. *J Bone Joint Surg* 1949;31A:1–22.

15. Badgley CE, Isaacson AS, Wolgamot JC, et al: Operative therapy for slipped upper femoral epiphysis: An end-result study. *J Bone Joint Surg* 1948;30A:19–30.

16. Hall JE: The results of treatment of slipped femoral epiphysis. *J Bone Joint Surg* 1957;39B:659–673.

17. Lowe HG: Avascular necrosis complicating slipped upper femoral epiphysis. *J Bone Joint Surg* 1959;41B:618.

18. Barmada R, Bruch RF, Gimbel JS, et al: Base of the neck extracapsular osteotomy for correction of deformity in slipped capital femoral epiphysis. *Clin Orthop* 1978;132:98–101.

19. Barton JR: On the treatment of ankylosis by the formation of artificial joints. *North Am Med Surg J* 1887;3:279.

20. Blount WP: Proximal osteotomies of the femur, in Pease CN (ed): American Academy of Orthopaedic Surgeons *Instructional Course Lectures, IX.* Ann Arbor, JW Edwards, 1952, pp 1–29.

21. Dunn DM, Angel JC: Replacement of the femoral head by open operation in severe adolescent slipping of the upper femoral epiphysis. *J Bone Joint Surg* 1978;60B:394–403.

22. Clark CR, Southwick WO, Ogden JA: Anatomic aspects of slipped capital femoral epiphysis and correction by biplane osteotomy, in American Academy of Orthopaedic Surgeons *Instructional Course Lectures, XXIX.* St. Louis, CV Mosby, 1980, pp 90–100.

23. Compere CL: Correction of deformity and prevention of aseptic necrosis in late cases of slipped femoral epiphyses. *J Bone Joint Surg* 1950;32A:351–362.

24. Gage JR, Sundberg AB, Nolan DR, et al: Complications after cuneiform osteotomy for moderately or severely slipped capital femoral epiphysis. *J Bone Joint Surg* 1978;60A:157–165.

25. Gruber MA, Laskin RS: A single stage osteotomy and epiphysiodesis for treatment of moderately displaced femoral capital epiphyses. *Clin Orthop* 1975;107:159–167.

26. Ireland J, Newman PH: Triplane osteotomy for severely slipped upper femoral epiphysis. *J Bone Joint Surg* 1978;60B:390–393.

27. Kramer WG, Craig WA, Noel S: Compensating osteotomy at the base of the femoral neck for slipped capital femoral epiphysis. *J Bone Joint Surg* 1976;58A:796–800.

28. MacEwen GD, Shands AR Jr: Oblique trochanteric osteotomy. *J Bone Joint Surg* 1967;49A:345–354.

29. Salvati EA, Robinson JH Jr, O'Down TJ: Southwick osteotomy for severe chronic slipped capital femoral epiphysis: Results and complications. *J Bone Joint Surg* 1980;62A:561–570.

30. Sugioka Y: Transtrochanteric rotational osteotomy of the femoral head. *Hip* 1980.

31. Thompson VP: The telescoping V osteotomy: A general method for correcting angular and rotational disalinements. *Arch Surg* 1943;46:772–779.

32. Whiteside LA, Schoenecker PL: Combined valgus derotation osteotomy and cervical osteoplasty for severely slipped capital femoral epiphysis: Mechanical analysis and report preliminary results using compression screw fixation and early weight bearing. *Clin Orthop* 1978;132:88–97.

33. Wiberg G: Wedge osteotomy in serious slipping of the upper femoral epiphysis. *Acta Orthop Scand* 1956;25:63–68.

34. Green WT: Slipping of the upper femoral epiphysis: Diagnostic and therapeutic considerations. *Arch Surg* 1945;50:19–33.

35. Martin PH: Slipped epiphysis in the adolescent hip: A reconsideration of open reduction. *J Bone Joint Surg* 1948;30A:9–19.

36. Crowe HE, in discussion, Badgley CE, Isaacson AS, Wolgamot JC, et al: Operative therapy for slipped upper femoral epiphysis: An end-result study. *J Bone Joint Surg* 1948;30A:19–30.

37. Joplin RJ: Slipped capital femoral epiphysis: The still unsolved adolescent hip lesion. *JAMA* 1964;188:379–381.

38. Trueta J, in discussion, Lowe HG: Avascular necrosis complicating slipped upper femoral epiphysis. *J Bone Joint Surg* 1959;41B:618.

39. Wilson PD, in discussion, Klein A, Joplin RJ, Reidy JA, et al: Roentgenographic changes in nailed slipped capital femoral epiphysis. *J Bone Joint Surg* 1949;31A:1–22.

40. Southwick WO: Slipped capital femoral epiphysis, editorial. *J Bone Joint Surg* 1984;66A:1151–1152.

41. Fish JB: Cuneiform osteotomy of the femoral neck in the treatment of slipped capital femoral epiphysis. *J Bone Joint Surg* 1984;66A:1153–1168.

42. DePalma AF, Danyo JJ, Stose WG: Slipping of the upper femoral epiphysis. *Clin Orthop* 1964;37:167–183.

43. Crawford AH: Osteotomies in the treatment of slipped capital femoral epiphysis, in American Academy of Orthopaedic Surgeons *Instructional Course Lectures, XXXIII.* St. Louis, CV Mosby, 1984, pp 327–349.

44. Masuda T, Matsuno TS, Hasegawa I, et al: Transtrochanteric anterior rotational osteotomy for slipped capital femoral epiphysis: A report of five cases. *J Pediatr Orthop* 1986;6:18–23.

45. Frymoyer JW: Chondrolysis of the hip following Southwick osteotomy for severe slipped capital femoral epiphysis. *Clin Orthop* 1974;99:120–124.

46. Wilson PD, Jacobs B, Schecter L: Slipped capital femoral epiphysis: An end-result study. *J Bone Joint Surg* 1965;47A:1128–1145.

47. Chandler HP, Reineck FT, Wixson RL, et al: Total hip replacement in patients younger than thirty years old: A five-year follow-up study. *J Bone Joint Surg* 1981;63A:1426–1434.

Problems and Complications of Slipped Capital Femoral Epiphysis

S. Terry Canale, MD

According to *Webster's Dictionary*, a problem is "an unsettled matter demanding a solution or decision requiring considerable thought or skill," whereas a complication is a "difficult factor or issue often appearing suddenly and unexpectedly and changing existing plans, methods or attitudes." In the treatment of slipped capital femoral epiphysis (SCFE), certain problems can be anticipated and thus avoided or circumvented. Complications, however, arise unexpectedly and cannot be avoided. Such complications may necessitate a change in treatment and may even alter the result of treatment. This review of the problems and complications in SCFE is based on 329 patients treated at the Campbell Clinic between 1935 and 1973.[1,2]

Problems

The problems associated with SCFE are related to (1) classification, (2) indications, and (3) surgical procedures and techniques.

Classification

Problems related to classification include differentiating between acute and chronic SCFE. In acute SCFE the symptoms and radiographic changes are less than two weeks old, whereas in chronic SCFE they are more than two weeks old. Two weeks is an arbitrarily chosen dividing line (some investigators use three weeks) selected because a slipped epiphysis usually can be reduced within the first two weeks. After this period, the slip is considered chronic and not reducible. Whether reduction should be undertaken is a matter of controversy, but it is important to know the treatment options and whether the slip can be reduced. Another point of confusion is the definition of a third temporal stage, "acute-on-chronic" SCFE, in which chronic symptoms or radiographic changes more than two weeks old are exacerbated by new acute symptoms and radiographic changes less than two weeks old. It is important to know the sequence of change and to be able to compare old radiographs with recent ones. In an acute-on-chronic slip the entire capital femoral epiphysis must be "loose" if it is to slip further. Finally, the confusing term "pre-slip" needs to be defined. This entity consists of mild hip symptoms (whether acute or chronic) and radiographic evidence of minor widening of the epiphyseal line compared with the contralateral hip, along with small areas of peripheral callus formation but without any evidence of actual "slipping" or displacement on anteroposterior and lateral views (Fig. 23–1).

Another problem concerning classification is meas-

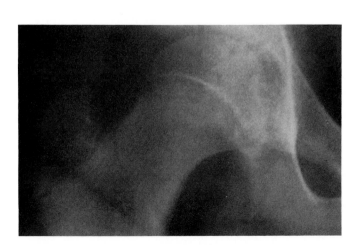
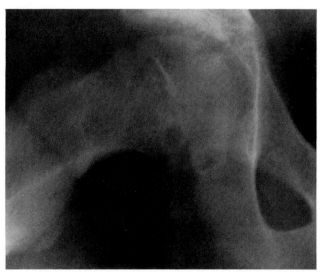

Fig. 23–1 Anteroposterior (**left**) and lateral (**right**) views reveal slight widening of the epiphyseal line. The lateral view shows minimal but definite SCFE.

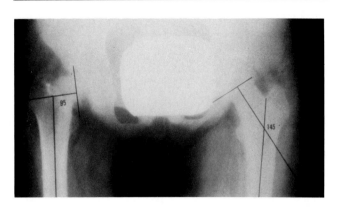

Fig. 23-2   Comparison of SCFE angle of 95 degrees with normal contralateral hip angle of 145 degrees.

uring the amount of slip. Some investigators have used the "percent" of the slip of the capital femoral epiphysis in relationship to the femoral neck. However, this relationship can be influenced by rotation and by "chronic bending" (remodeling) of the neck in chronic SCFE. My colleagues and I, like Southwick,[3] use the "epiphyseal line-femoral shaft angle" on both the anteroposterior and lateral radiographs. This angle should be measured in degrees and compared with that of the contralateral hip (Fig. 23–2). A mild slip is less than 30 degrees, a moderate slip is 30 to 60 degrees, and a severe slip is more than 60 degrees.

Indications

Problems also exist concerning the exact indications for surgery. It must be determined whether surgery will be of any benefit. In the Campbell Clinic series, 22 of the 329 hips did not undergo surgery. Eleven patients refused surgery; of these 11, seven had increased displacement. In three patients who had no treatment at all, chondrolysis developed. In the remaining 11, surgery was not recommended. Four of these ultimately had good results and two had poor results (one case of arthritis and one case of chondrolysis). Five patients were treated with spica casts; in these five there were six complications (two cases of increased displacement, two of chondrolysis, and two of avascular necrosis).

Thus, it seems that surgery is indicated to prevent all the sequelae of further slipping, and that complications occur even when surgery is not performed.

For simplicity, Table 23–1 outlines treatment recommendations (guidelines) related to time and severity. For example, pre-slips and mild acute slips should be pinned in situ. Whether a more severe acute slip should be reduced or not depends on the surgeon's beliefs about the relationship of closed reduction and avascular necrosis. It should be noted that some investigators do not believe that osteotomy is ever indicated in chronic SCFE.[4] Others believe that the epiphyseal plate should be stabilized with pins or an epiphysiodesis before a compensatory osteotomy is done.[4]

Prophylactic pinning of the contralateral hip is also a problem area. In the past, it was common to pin the contralateral hip in patients who were statistically likely to develop bilateral disease, especially blacks (Figs. 23–3 and 23–4). In our series, the bilateral incidence was 32%, with blacks having a higher incidence of bilateral disease (37%) than whites (27%). When the incidence of bilateral slipping is 32%, contralateral prophylactic pinning should be considered; however, both hips had already slipped at the time of initial presentation in one half of the 32%. Because only 16% had later slipping of the opposite hip, my colleagues and I do not believe that prophylactic pinning is indicated. This was recently substantiated by Greenough and associates.[5]

Surgical Procedures and Techniques

There are also problems with the types and techniques of surgical procedures. One basic problem is whether a reduction should be attempted or not. There appears to be a direct relationship among the severity of the slip, the reduction, and avascular necrosis.[6] Boyer and associates[7] noted that slips pinned in situ, even moderate and severe slips, did better because of lower avascular necrosis and chondrolysis rates than those that were reduced and pinned. We noted a 20% rate of avascular necrosis after closed reduction and pinning, compared with a 2% rate after in situ pinning. It appears that leaving the slip unreduced is preferable to performing a manual reduction. If reduction is deemed necessary, then skeletal or skin traction over

Table 23-1
Treatment guidelines based on time and severity of slip

Time	Slip (degrees)		
	Mild (<30)	Moderate (30 to 60)	Severe (>60)
Pre-slip	Pin or peg in situ	—	—
Acute (<2 weeks)	Pin in situ	Reduce/pin in situ	Reduce/pin in situ
Acute-on-chronic	Pin in situ	Reduce/pin in situ	Reduce/pin in situ/osteotomy
Chronic (>2 weeks)	Pin in situ	Pin in situ/osteotomy	Pin in situ/osteotomy

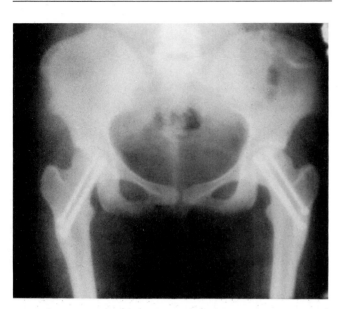

Fig. 23-3 SCFE was reduced and fixed with multiple pins in 1954. The contralateral hip "slipped" one year later and was reduced and held with multiple pins. Good long-term results are evident in both hips almost 20 years after pinning.

three to four days in the hospital should be used and should include longitudinal traction and medial internal rotation traction. Forceful traction at surgery, manually or with the aid of the fracture table, should be avoided. If the slip is severe ("all the way off") and the surgeon believes it cannot be pinned in situ, a gentle,

closed reduction may be necessary. In this case, the surgeon should be prepared to deal later with avascular necrosis. Open reduction of slips should be avoided because of the high incidences of chondrolysis and avascular necrosis. The 33% incidence of avascular necrosis and the 37% incidence of chondrolysis after open reduction and pin fixation in our series indicate that this procedure is very unlikely to be successful.

On rare occasions, the surgeon, thinking the slip is acute, plans to reduce and pin the hip. At surgery, however, the slip cannot be reduced. The surgeon erroneously attributes this to an interposition of material when, in fact, the slip is probably chronic and the history inaccurate. The surgeon proceeds with open reduction only to find that it is indeed a chronic slip necessitating a "cuneiform" osteotomy for reduction, a procedure associated with a high incidence of avascular necrosis and chondrolysis. This scenario, obviously, should be avoided. If the femoral head cannot be reduced (which may be fortunate), the hip should be pinned in situ; a compensatory osteotomy can be performed later if it is needed.

The final problem with surgery is the technique of pinning. Because of the relationship between pin penetration into the hip joint and the incidence of chondrolysis, an image intensifier should be used with the fracture table. "Penetration and withdrawal" techniques, as described by Moseley,[6] and rotation of the image intensifier as the leg and hip are rotated are helpful in determining the placement of the pins and whether there is any penetration into the joint. It should

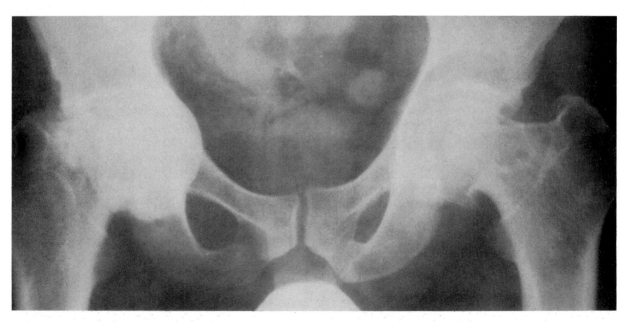

Fig. 23-4 This patient had unilateral SCFE on the right side. Prophylactic pinning was done on the left hip. Twenty-two years after bilateral pinning, the patient has painful traumatic arthritis in both hips.

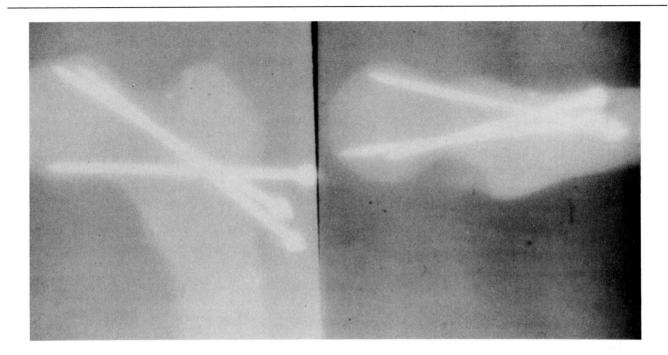

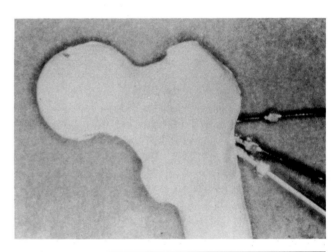

Fig. 23–5 **Top:** In anteroposterior and lateral views of bone model all three pins appear to be in the femoral head. **Bottom:** Actual model, however, shows that at least two, and maybe all three, pins are outside the femoral head. A two-plane roentgenogram may not reveal pin penetration because the femoral head is a three-dimensional sphere. (Reproduced with permission from Canale ST: Fractures and dislocations in children, in Crenshaw AH (ed): *Campbell's Operative Orthopaedics*, ed 7. St. Louis, CV Mosby, 1987, vol 3, pp 1833–2013.)

be remembered, however, that when an image intensifier is rotated from the anteroposterior to the lateral plane the rotation is only through 180 degrees; flexing, abducting, and externally rotating the hip adds only 90 more degrees, resulting in a total of 270 degrees. One cannot be completely certain that the pins have not protruded out of the sphere of the head in the last 90-degree quadrant, regardless of how they look on a two-plane radiograph or the image intensifier (Fig. 23–5). At present, a cannulated pin or cannulated pediatric hip screw, which allows more exact placement of the final pin, probably should be used. Occasionally, the limits of the femoral head are difficult to determine, especially in an overweight patient. Dye can be injected before surgery (arthrogram) and dye techniques[8] can be used during surgery to determine if pin penetration

has occurred (Fig. 23–6). Recently, percutaneous pinning has been advocated by Morrissy.[9]

The threads of the pins should be placed across the epiphyseal plate, resulting in the cartilage columnar cells "piling-up" on themselves and causing epiphyseal growth arrest and plate closure. The Campbell Clinic rule on Knowles pins is that two are too few and five are too many. The subchondral bone area should be avoided, especially in the superolateral quadrant where avascular necrosis is more prevalent.[10] Pin penetration should be avoided at all costs because this may lead to chondrolysis; using fewer pins and placing them centrally in the head, 7 mm distal to the subchondral joint line (Fig. 23–7), helps avoid pin penetration. The larger cannulated pediatric hip screw causes the fewest problems simply because fewer pins are necessary. One screw

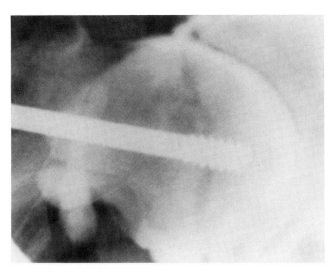

Fig. 23-6 Arthrogram outlines the hip joint and confirms that cannulated pediatric hip screws do not penetrate the joint.

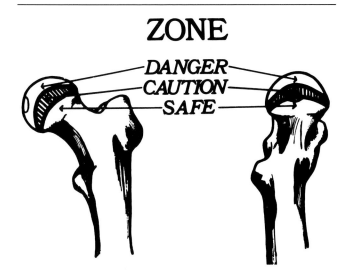

Fig. 23-7 Three zones of pin placement in the femoral head. To avoid the "danger" zone, pins should be placed in the center of the femoral head. (Reproduced with permission from Canale ST: Fractures and dislocations in children, in Crenshaw AH (ed): *Campbell's Operative Orthopaedics*, ed 7. St. Louis, CV Mosby, 1987, pp 1833–2013.)

defies orthopaedic tradition, but appears to work with the fewest complications.

Complications

Complications include increased displacement (further slipping), pathologic fracture, avascular necrosis, and chondrolysis.

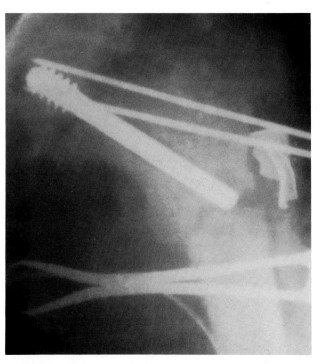

Fig. 23-8 This hip with acute SCFE was reduced and the slip held with multiple pins. Three weeks after reduction and pinning, the patient sustained a subchondral fracture through an "unfilled" drill hole. The original pins were removed and smooth pins were inserted to avoid displacing the capital femoral epiphysis; the fracture was treated with open reduction and fixation with an adult compression hip screw.

Increased Displacement

Increased displacement or further slipping can be avoided by not delaying pinning or pegging. Pins, screws, or bone pegs of sufficient length across the epiphyseal plate, left in place until the epiphyseal plate closes (a minimum of 12 to 18 months), usually prevent further slipping. Pegging avoids the complication of pin penetration into the joint but further displacement has been reported in most series.[10] If bone pegging is used in an acute slip, it should probably be supplemented with immobilization for six to 12 weeks in a spica cast to avoid this complication. In a chronic slip, sufficient bone across the epiphyseal plate should be used to prevent further chronic slipping.

Because there is a short "lag time" before closure during which the epiphyses can still grow, causing further displacement when the pins are "outgrown," the pins should extend beyond the epiphyseal growth plate.

Pathologic Fracture

The second complication, pathologic fracture, may occur from the placement of unnecessary drill holes. This is an iatrogenic problem usually compounded by a noncompliant patient. Attention to detail and the use of an image intensifier and cannulated hip screws can lessen the incidence of this complication. If an unnec-

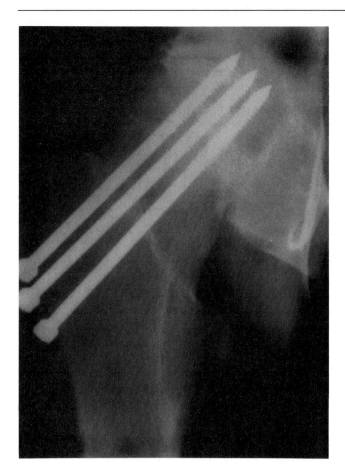

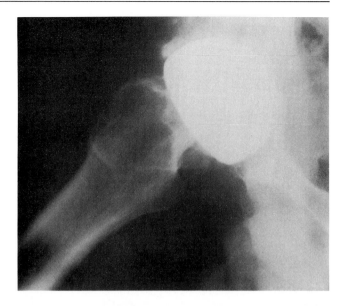

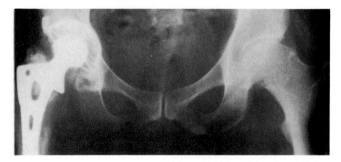

Fig. 23–9 Moderate, chronic SCFE. **Left:** Five years after cuneiform osteotomy there is evidence of avascular necrosis, pin penetration, and progressive traumatic arthritis. **Top right:** Cup arthroplasty was performed six years after osteotomy. **Bottom right:** Twenty-six years after osteotomy, the cup arthroplasty was converted to a total hip arthroplasty; the patient was 43 years old at this time.

essary drill hole is made, it should be "filled" or the patient warned; a noncompliant patient should be placed in a spica cast (Fig. 23–8). A stress fracture of the femoral neck following the use of a cannulated hip screw was recently reported by Cummings and associates.[11] They postulated that this complication occurred because of overzealous reaming of the femoral neck and cortex, or because the reamers were not of sufficient quality and actually burned or "weakened" the femoral neck, causing a stress fracture distal to the capital femoral epiphysis in the neck without breakage of the cannulated pediatric hip screw. This can be avoided by using sharp reamers and, if necessary, by predrilling the cannulated area.

Avascular Necrosis

Avascular necrosis occurred in 13% of the Campbell Clinic series and was related to the severity of the slip. The incidence in mild slips was 4%, in moderate slips 25%, and in severe slips 20%. The incidence was also related to the surgical procedure. Patients who did not undergo surgery had an 18% incidence of avascular

necrosis. Those treated with in situ pinning had an avascular necrosis rate of 2%. Those with closed reduction (20%) and open reduction (27%) had higher rates than those with in situ pinning. Avascular necrosis has been reported with spica cast treatment, in situ pinning, and bone-pegging epiphysiodesis. The avascular necrosis rate of approximately 2% for these three procedures is much less than for closed or open reduction, subtrochanteric osteotomy (10%), and cuneiform neck osteotomy (33%) (Fig. 23–9). The cuneiform or neck osteotomy has been advocated by Fish,[12] who reported only one case of avascular necrosis in 42 hips. His neck osteotomy, which is a "relaxing" osteotomy and a closing wedge osteotomy, probably relieves tension on the blood vessels that supply the capital femoral epiphysis (Fig. 23–10). This is similar to the procedure reported by Dunn and Angel.[13] The avascular necrosis rate after cuneiform osteotomy in the Campbell Clinic series was 33% and the chondrolysis rate was 37%—totally unacceptable results. Even though these complications were related to the severity of the slip, the difference between the Fish series and the Campbell Clinic series is difficult to ex-

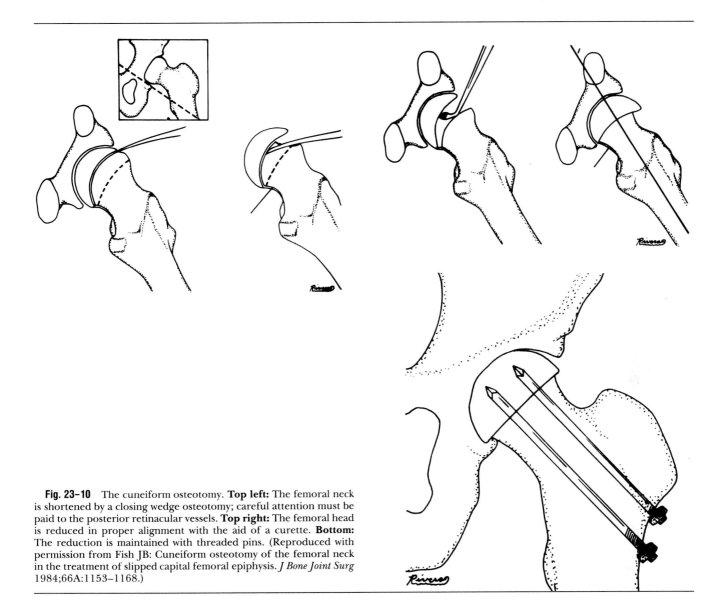

Fig. 23-10 The cuneiform osteotomy. **Top left:** The femoral neck is shortened by a closing wedge osteotomy; careful attention must be paid to the posterior retinacular vessels. **Top right:** The femoral head is reduced in proper alignment with the aid of a curette. **Bottom:** The reduction is maintained with threaded pins. (Reproduced with permission from Fish JB: Cuneiform osteotomy of the femoral neck in the treatment of slipped capital femoral epiphysis. *J Bone Joint Surg* 1984;66A:1153–1168.)

Table 23-2
Chondrolysis rate and type of treatment

Treatment	Chondrolysis Rate (%)
No operation	5
In situ pinning	9
Closed reduction/pinning	15
Open reduction/pinning	55
Neck osteotomy (cuneiform)	37
Trochanteric osteotomy	59

plain. Possibly, Fish used a more generous osteotomy that permitted more relaxation of the femoral vessels and thus produced less avascular necrosis.

The adolescent patient in whom avascular necrosis of the entire femoral head develops is too young for a total hip replacement because of future wear and tear on the prosthesis. If only a segment of the head is involved, a varus flexion osteotomy should be considered, as well as a graft, either vascularized or not, into the area of the avascular subchondral bone. However, the most definitive operation, although a salvage procedure at best, is an arthrodesis of the hip joint, especially when there is severe pain and total head involvement.

Chondrolysis

The final complication is chondrolysis. The exact cause of chondrolysis is unknown. Decreased joint motion, especially hip flexion, abduction, and internal rotation, and flexion contracture are almost always present. Radiographs reveal a joint space measurement of less than 3 mm. The overall chondrolysis rate in the Campbell Clinic series was 24%. Chondrolysis after SCFE is more common in blacks and females, and the incidence is especially high in black females. In the

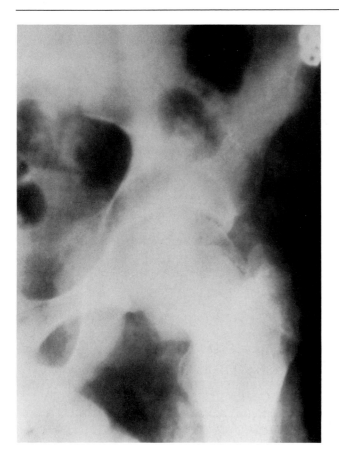

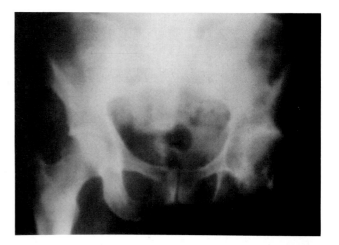

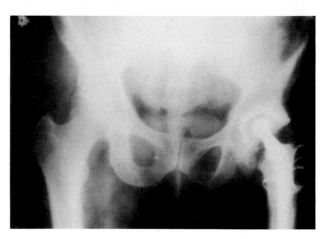

Fig. 23-11 Acute SCFE. **Left:** Six months after reduction and spica cast immobilization, there is narrowing of the joint space and evidence of chondrolysis. **Top right:** Ten years after reduction the patient has severe traumatic arthritis secondary to chondrolysis. **Bottom right:** Total hip arthroplasty was required 20 years after reduction because of severe pain and stiffness of the hip joint.

Campbell Clinic series, 51% of black females with SCFE developed chondrolysis. The incidence was also directly related to the severity of the slips. Those with mild slips had a 10% incidence of chondrolysis, those with moderate slips had a 35% incidence, and those with severe slips had a 45% incidence. In our series, acute-on-chronic and chronic slips produced the highest incidences of chondrolysis.

Various surgical procedures have been implicated in the development of chondrolysis, but chondrolysis also occurs in patients who have had no treatment for SCFE. As Table 23–2 shows, chondrolysis developed in 5% of patients who had no surgery (Fig. 23–11). In patients treated surgically, in situ pinning caused the lowest incidence of chondrolysis, whereas open reduction and pinning, neck osteotomy (cuneiform osteotomy), and subtrochanteric osteotomy (compensatory osteotomy) all had high incidences of chondrolysis (Fig. 23–12).

Finally, pin penetration has been strongly implicated as a cause of chondrolysis. Walters and Simon[14] noted the correlation between pin penetration and chondrol-

ysis and the difficulty in determining whether pin penetration has occurred. In an effort to avoid chondrolysis, my colleagues and I use the cannulated pediatric hip screw system because it allows for more exact placement and fewer screws. Recently, bone-pegging epiphysiodesis has been advocated to decrease the complication of chondrolysis. It should be emphasized that chondrolysis occurred in 5% of the Campbell Clinic patients who had no surgery and in three children who had no treatment. This implies that chondrolysis can occur for reasons other than pin penetration and that not all chondrolysis is iatrogenic.

Chondrolysis, like avascular necrosis, is devastating. Historically, treatment for chondrolysis has consisted of range-of-motion exercises and nonweightbearing for a two-year period. This protocol reportedly restores approximately 50% of joint motion, and increases the joint space 50% on radiographic assessment. We have tried many methods of treatment, including bedrest, nonweightbearing on crutches, range-of-motion exercise programs, and anti-inflammatory drugs and sali-

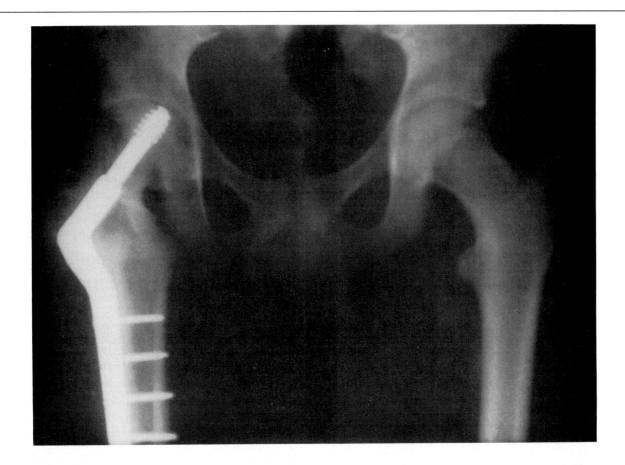

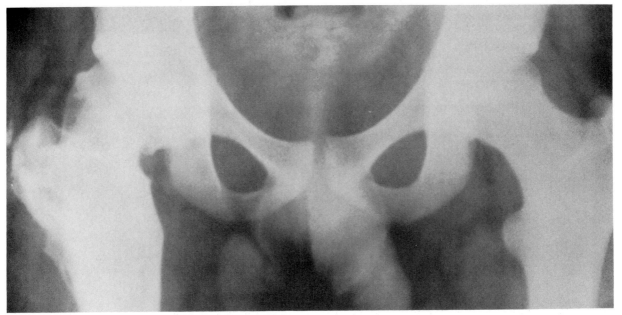

Fig. 23-12   Chronic SCFE was pinned in situ with multiple threaded pins. **Top:** After subtrochanteric biplane osteotomy, there is joint narrowing and stiffness and evidence of chondrolysis. Four years later there was evidence of some widening of the joint space. **Bottom:** Three years after osteotomy the joint space is almost normal, but there is still some restriction of motion of the hip joint. (Reproduced with permission from Canale ST: Fractures and dislocations in children, in Crenshaw AH (ed): *Campbell's Operative Orthopaedics*, ed 7. St. Louis, CV Mosby, 1987, pp 1833–2013.)

cylates. We have limited experience with the "hanging hip" operation[15] to relieve tension about the hip joint. We have had some limited success with intra-articular injection of cortisone into the hip joint with the patient under general anesthesia; after injection, the hip is gently manipulated through an acceptable range of motion. This is followed by skeletal traction and an extensive range-of-motion exercise program in the hospital.

Summary

In summary, epiphysiodesis, by either "pinning" or "pegging," seems to be necessary to further prevent displacement of the SCFE. To minimize complications, aggressive closed reduction, open reduction, pin penetration, and unnecessary drill holes should be avoided. Avascular necrosis and chondrolysis, the most frequent and devastating complications, appear to be related to the severity of the slip and the type of treatment.

References

1. Ingram AJ, Clarke MS, Clarke CS Jr, et al: Chondrolysis complicating slipped capital femoral epiphysis. *Clin Orthop* 1982;165:99–109.
2. Canale ST: Fractures and dislocations in children, in Crenshaw AH (ed): *Campbell's Operative Orthopaedics*, ed 7. St. Louis, CV Mosby, 1987, vol 3, pp 1913–2013.
3. Southwick WO: Osteotomy through the lesser trochanter for slipped capital femoral epiphysis. *J Bone Joint Surg* 1967;49A:807–835.
4. Roberts JM, Canale ST, Crawford AH, et al: Symposium: Slipped capital femoral epiphysis. *Contemp Orthop* 1986;13(5):71–119.
5. Greenough CG, Bromage JD, Jackson AM: Pinning of the slipped upper femoral epiphysis: A trouble-free procedure? *J Pediatr Orthop* 1985;5:657–660.
6. Moseley CF: The biomechanics of the pediatric hip. *Orthop Clin North Am* 1980;11:3–16.
7. Boyer DW, Mickelson MR, Ponseti IV: Slipped capital femoral epiphysis: Long-term follow-up study of one hundred and twenty-one patients. *J Bone Joint Surg* 1981;63A:85–95.
8. Lehman WB, Grant A, Rose D, et al: A method of evaluating possible pin penetration in slipped capital femoral epiphysis using a cannulated internal fixation device. *Clin Orthop* 1984;186:65–70.
9. Morrissy RT: Percutaneous in situ screw fixation of SCFE: Rationale for the technique. Presented at the annual meeting of the Pediatric Orthopaedic Society of North America, Colorado Springs, CO, May 8, 1988.
10. Irani RN, Rosenzweig AH, Cotler HB, et al: Epiphysiodesis in slipped capital femoral epiphysis: A comparison of various surgical modalities. *J Pediatr Orthop* 1985;5:661–664.
11. Cummings RJ, Baynham GC, Lucie RS: Femoral neck fracture complicating in situ pinning of slipped capital femoral epiphysis. Presented at the annual meeting of the Pediatric Orthopaedic Society of North America, March 1988.
12. Fish JB: Cuneiform osteotomy of the femoral neck in the treatment of slipped capital femoral epiphysis. *J Bone Joint Surg* 1984;66A:1153–1168.
13. Dunn DM, Angel JC: Replacement of the femoral head by open operation in severe adolescent slipping of the upper femoral epiphysis. *J Bone Joint Surg* 1978;60B:394–403.
14. Walters R, Simon SR: Joint destruction: A sequel of unrecognized pin penetration in patients with slipped capital femoral epiphysis. *Hip* 1980;145–164.
15. Mensor MC, Scheck M: Review of six years' experience with the hanging-hip operation (follow-up note). *J Bone Joint Surg* 1968;50A:1250–1254.

Legg-Calvé-Perthes Disease: Diagnostic and Prognostic Techniques

James H. Beaty, MD

During the initial history-taking and physical examination of children with Legg-Calvé-Perthes disease, it is important to remember that this is a "dynamic" disease. The history and physical findings can vary markedly depending on the particular stage of the disease process. During the early stages, the history is most often that of a limp or increasing groin, thigh, or knee pain. The physical findings at this time are similar to those in a child with an "irritable" hip. The initial synovitis may cause a small decrease in range of motion at the extremes of internal and external rotation and there may be mild muscle atrophy in the thigh or calf consistent with an antalgic gait. In later, more severe stages of Perthes' disease there may be contractures of the adductor and hip flexor musculature in addition to the decreased range of internal and external rotation of the hip.

Techniques for diagnosing Perthes' disease and determining its prognosis include radiography, technetium scanning, magnetic resonance imaging (MRI), arthrography, and computed tomographic (CT) scan. They are all equally useful and each has its advantages and disadvantages.

To determine the best imaging technique for a particular patient some questions must be answered. Which technique can make the diagnosis of Perthes' disease earliest? Which gives the best estimate of the percentage of the femoral head involved? Which can best assess the mechanical shape of the femoral head and acetabulum? Which best determines the revascularization stage so that decisions about discontinuing bracing can be made? Which is the best prognosticator of long-term results when the disease process is completed? No one technique is the answer to all of these questions, but each has its special merits.

Radiography

Radiography has been the standard technique for the diagnosis and evaluation of treatment of Perthes' dis-

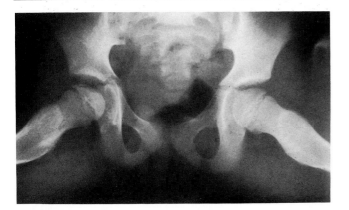

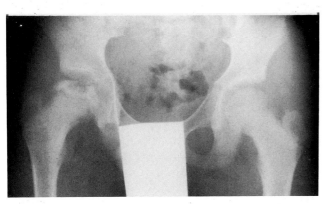

Fig. 24-1 A 7-year-old boy had a two-month history of pain in his right hip. **Top:** The subchondral fracture is through 75% of the femoral head. **Bottom:** Anteroposterior radiograph made nine months later confirms Catterall group III classification.

Fig. 24-2 Epiphyseal extrusion (E), which is the percentage of diseased femoral head lateral to Perkins' line (line EF), is computed by dividing the amount of involved head that is uncovered (line AB) by the width of the opposite normal femoral head measured at the epiphyseal plate (line CD). Thus, E = (AB divided by CD) × 100. (Reproduced with permission from Green NE, Beauchamp RD, Griffin PP: Epiphyseal extrusion as a prognostic index in Legg-Calvé-Perthes disease. *J Bone Joint Surg* 1981;63A:900–905.)

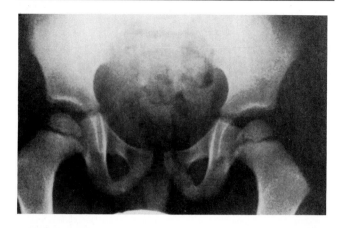

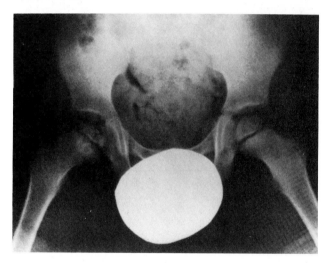

Fig. 24-3   A 3-year-old boy had a one-week history of a painful limp related to his right hip. **Top:** Anteroposterior radiograph was considered normal, but bone scan taken four days later showed Legg-Calvé-Perthes disease. **Bottom:** Radiograph taken 13 months later confirms the accuracy of the bone scan diagnosis. (Reproduced with permission from Paterson D, Savage JP: The nuclide bone scan in the diagnosis of Perthes' disease. *Clin Orthop* 1986;209:23–29.)

the radiographic findings can change, necessitating reclassification from one Catterall group to another. The ultimate Catterall classification may not be determined for six to nine months after the initial onset.[2,3]

After radiographic investigation of 1,057 children with Perthes' disease, Salter and Thompson[4] described the prognostic value of the subchondral fracture of the femoral head (Fig. 24–1). They concluded that in the early stage of Perthes' disease the extent of the subchondral fracture was useful in predicting the eventual extent of involvement of the femoral head. They proposed a two-group classification: Group A, in which less than one half of the head is involved, and Group B, in which more than one half of the head is involved. This classification is applied in the early stages of the disease if a subchondral fracture is detectable and is useful if decisions concerning treatment are based on the percentage of head involvement. Not all children, however, have a subchondral fracture when the decision concerning treatment must be made. Other investigators have questioned whether the extent of the subchondral fracture correlates absolutely with the ultimate extent of femoral head involvement.[5]

Green and associates,[6] in their review of 200 children, described epiphyseal extrusion as a long-term prognostic index (Fig. 24–2). When the epiphyseal extrusion was greater than 20%, the prognosis was poor, and when it was less than 20% the prognosis was good. The number of poor results also increased as femoral head involvement increased, so that when epiphyseal extrusion was greater than 20% and femoral head involvement was greater than 50%, only 8% of hips had good results.

Technetium Scanning

A technetium scan can be used to diagnose Perthes' disease when initial radiographs are normal, and certainly this is its main advantage (Figs. 24–3 and 24–4). Paterson and Savage[7] found the sensitivity of technetium bone scan for Perthes' disease to be 0.98 in their review of 131 consecutive referrals of children with suspected abnormality of the hip. They recommended using ^{99m}Tc medronate methylene diphosphonate in an intravenous dose of approximately 215 μCi/m^2 of body surface area. Ninety minutes after injection, the patient is scanned in the anterior supine position by means of pin-hole collimation. Delaying the bone scan for 90 minutes to three hours after injection eliminates the soft-tissue uptake that occurs in the flow and blood-pool stages of bone scans. Pin-hole collimation magnifies the hip being studied and appears to provide a better delayed image of the femoral head.

One disadvantage of technetium scanning is that it is a relatively invasive procedure. There may be some false-negative results in children with synovitis super-

ease for many decades. It is the simplest form of imaging to obtain and the one with which physicians have the most experience. It can help differentiate Perthes' disease from other skeletal disorders. Radiography, however, may not be diagnostic of Perthes' disease in its early stages, during the first three to six weeks of the disease process.[1] The femoral head at any one time may contain both necrotic and living bony tissue, making a radiographic assessment of this dynamic disease difficult. That radiographic findings may be normal in early Perthes' disease has led to interest in other imaging techniques.

Many investigators have attempted to use radiographic findings to predict the ultimate outcome in Perthes' disease. The Catterall classification is useful in classifying the percentage of femoral head involvement and the "head-at-risk" signs that predict children at risk for a poor result. However, many have noted that

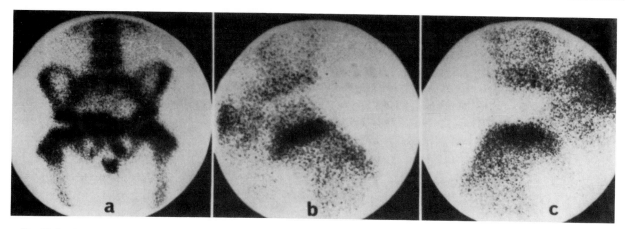

Fig. 24–4   Bone scans of early Legg-Calvé-Perthes disease. **Left:** Parallel-hole collimator view of both hips. **Center:** Pinhole view of normal left hip. **Right:** Pinhole view of right hip, showing the void in the epiphysis. (Reproduced with permission from Paterson D, Savage JP: The nuclide bone scan in the diagnosis of Perthes' disease. *Clin Orthop* 1986;209:23–29.)

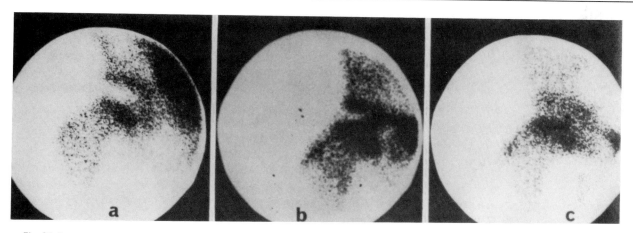

Fig. 24–5   Legg-Calvé-Perthes disease. **Left:** Early stage. **Center:** Advanced revascularization. **Right:** Complete revascularization. (Reproduced with permission from Paterson D, Savage JP: The nuclide bone scan in the diagnosis of Perthes' disease. *Clin Orthop* 1986;209:23–29.)

imposed on the ischemic necrosis of the femoral head. Technetium scanning is not quantitative and cannot be used to measure the exact degree of nuclide uptake in each femoral head. Paterson and Savage described some promising results in the evaluation of revascularization of the femoral head, but these are not conclusive at present (Fig. 24–5). The final drawback of technetium bone scanning is the difficulty of making assessments in children with bilateral disease.

MRI

MRI is the most recent advance in imaging for children with Perthes' disease (Fig. 24–6). MRI uses a powerful magnet and radiofrequency waves to produce de-

tails of anatomic structures. Imaging techniques using the T_1 relaxation time provide the most valuable information in orthopaedic patients.[8] The signal strength is determined by the water content of the structure. The tissues, in order from highest to lowest signal strength, are fat, blood, marrow, cancellous bone, brain and spinal cord, viscera, muscle, ligaments and tendons, cortical bone, and air. Cortical bone, therefore, emits little or no signal and is erased from the image as if it did not exist. Ischemic necrosis in the femoral head emits a weaker signal than does the normal portion of the femoral head so these can be differentiated on the scan.

The advantages of this technique are that it provides early diagnosis of Perthes' disease when radiography gives normal results, the children are not exposed to

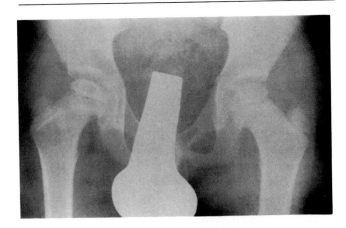

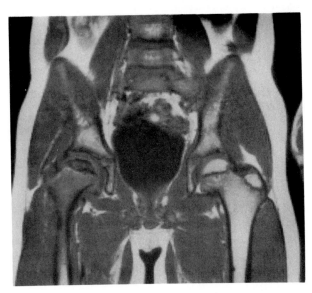

Fig. 24-6 A 9-year-old boy with a four-month history of pain in his right hip. **Top:** Radiograph. **Bottom:** Magnetic resonance imaging shows ischemic necrosis of the entire femoral head on the right in contrast to the normal left hip.

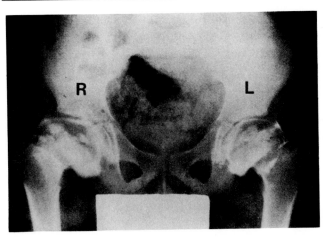

Fig. 24-7 Arthrogram of patient with bilateral Legg-Calvé-Perthes disease. Right side already shows advanced deformity of femoral head and acetabulum. (Reproduced with permission from MacEwen GD: Treatment of Legg-Calvé-Perthes disease, in Murray DG (ed): American Academy of Orthopaedic Surgeons *Instructional Course Lectures, XXX.* St. Louis, CV Mosby, 1981, pp 75–84.)

radioactivity, and the information obtained is probably the most sophisticated available at the present time.

The disadvantages include the cost, which may be approximately $800 against $250 for a technetium scan. In addition, the test may require 30 to 45 minutes in an enclosed unit, something difficult for very young children to endure. MRI may assess the percentage of head involvement and revascularization, but there are currently no data to support MRI correlation with percentage of femoral head involvement nor have enough children undergone sequential MRI to correlate staging of Perthes' disease.

Arthrography

Arthrography has no significant diagnostic value because the diagnosis of Perthes' disease is usually made before arthrographic examination is undertaken. The purpose of arthrography is to obtain information that may help determine the shape of the femoral head and acetabulum and assist in decision-making concerning treatment.

One advantage of arthrography is that it allows a more thorough assessment of the mechanical shape of the femoral head and acetabulum, including the cartilaginous portion not seen by radiography (Fig. 24–7). In the early stages of Perthes' disease, arthrography may reveal progressive deformation of the femoral head, indicating that institution of treatment is appropriate to prevent further deformity. When surgical treatment is considered in the older child, arthrography may show the femoral head to be aspherical and significantly misshapen, a possible contraindication for surgery. In addition, the phenomenon of hinged abduction, seen as a late sequel of Perthes' disease, is best viewed with dynamic arthrography[9] (Fig. 24–8).

The disadvantages of arthrography are that it is an invasive procedure and that, in general, it is performed during the mid or late stages of Perthes' disease. If the physician is biased toward nonsurgical treatment of Perthes' disease, any information obtained regarding the sphericity of the femoral head may be of academic or prognostic interest, but is of no use in decision-making.

CT Scanning

CT scanning is of limited value from either a diagnostic or a prognostic standpoint. The information gained from a CT scan primarily concerns the intra-

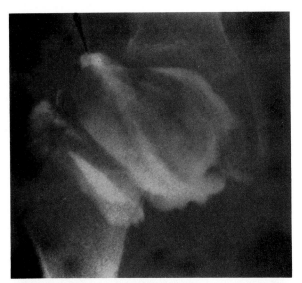

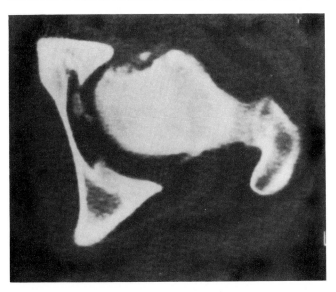

Fig. 24–9 Computed tomographic scan shows marked fragmentation and flattening of anterior aspect of left femoral head; bony fragment can be seen inside joint space. (Reproduced with permission from Hernandez RJ, Poznanski AK: CT evaluation of pediatric hip disorders. *Orthop Clin North Am* 1985;16:513–541.)

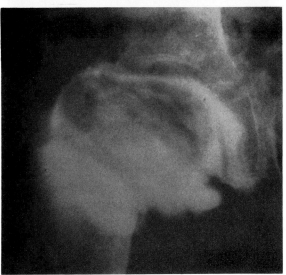

Fig. 24–8 Arthrogram in neutral (**top**) and stressed (**bottom**) abduction shows hinging of deformed femoral head on corner of acetabulum with pooling of dye medially (hinged abduction). (Reproduced with permission from MacEwen GD: Treatment of Legg-Calvé-Perthes disease, in Murray DG (ed): American Academy of Orthopaedic Surgeons *Instructional Course Lectures, XXX.* St. Louis, CV Mosby, 1981, pp 75–84.)

articular abnormality, especially in children with the rare late complication of osteochondritis dissecans or a loose body after Perthes' disease[10] (Fig. 24–9). The disadvantages are the cost involved and the fact that no other useful clinical information is gained from CT scanning.

Discussion

The answers to our original questions, then, may help determine which imaging modality is appropriate for a particular patient or purpose. Which makes the earliest diagnosis of Perthes' disease? Both technetium scanning and MRI are diagnostic earlier than radiography. Which gives the best estimate of head involvement so that treatment decisions can be made? At present, radiography still gives the best information concerning percentage of femoral head involvement, although technetium scanning and MRI have shown promising results. Which best assesses the mechanical shape of the femoral head and acetabulum? Arthrography gives the clearest information on which to base treatment decision-making. Which best indicates the stage of revascularization? Information gained from radiography lags behind the actual process; technetium scanning and MRI have shown promising results. Which gives the best long-term prognosis? Radiography is still the best indicator of the ultimate result of Perthes' disease.

At present, no one of these techniques is best for all patients at all stages of the disease process. Each can be useful for obtaining specific information. Radiography remains the simplest and least expensive tool for diagnosis and prognosis, but the newer modalities offer great promise. The ultimate usefulness of technetium scanning and MRI as prognostic tools depends on their ability to assess accurately the percentage of femoral head involvement and revascularization, two findings that as yet have not been documented in a significant number of cases.

References

1. Gershuni DH: Preliminary evaluation and prognosis in Legg-Calvé-Perthes disease. *Clin Orthop* 1980;150:16–22.

2. Van Dam BE, Crider RJ, Noyes JD, et al: Determination of the Catterall classification in Legg-Calvé-Perthes disease. *J Bone Joint Surg* 1981;63A:906–914.

3. Kelly FB Jr, Canale ST, Jones RR: Legg-Calvé-Perthes disease: Long-term evaluation of non-containment treatment. *J Bone Joint Surg* 1980;62A:400–407.

4. Salter RB, Thompson GH: Legg-Calvé-Perthes disease: The prognostic significance of the subchondral fracture and a two-group classification of the femoral head involvement. *J Bone Joint Surg* 1984;66A:479–489.

5. Weinstein SL: Legg-Calvé-Perthes disease, in Evarts CM (ed): American Academy of Orthopaedic Surgeons *Instructional Course Lectures, XXXII.* St. Louis, CV Mosby, 1983, pp 272–291.

6. Green NE, Beauchamp RD, Griffin PP: Epiphyseal extrusion as a prognostic index in Legg-Calvé-Perthes disease. *J Bone Joint Surg* 1981;63A:900–905.

7. Paterson D, Savage JP: The nuclide bone scan in the diagnosis of Perthes' disease. *Clin Orthop* 1986;209:23–29.

8. Powers JA: Magnetic resonance imaging in marrow diseases. *Clin Orthop* 1986;206:79–85.

9. MacEwen GD: Treatment of Legg-Calvé-Perthes disease, in Murray DG (ed): American Academy of Orthopaedic Surgeons *Instructional Course Lectures, XXX.* St. Louis, CV Mosby, 1981, pp 75–84.

10. Hernandez RJ, Poznanski AK: CT evaluation of pediatric hip disorders. *Orthop Clin North Am* 1985;16:513–541.

Legg-Calvé-Perthes Disease

Morbid Anatomy and Natural History

Anthony Catterall, M Chir, FRCS

Despite an increasing volume of studies, the cause of Legg-Calvé-Perthes disease remains obscure, and management, therefore, is empirical. In many instances treatment is based on radiologic images with little thought given to the changes in morbid anatomy within the femoral head and neck represented by these radiologic images. This paper reviews these morphologic changes and their natural history.

Morbid Anatomy

The scarcity of pathologic material has permitted few accounts of the pathology of this disease[1-4] and fewer still in which the sequential changes observed radiologically were correlated with the morphologic findings.[2,5,6]

The evidence in these few reports suggests that there is thickening of the articular cartilage with infarction of the bony epiphysis. In some cases involvement is partial whereas in others the whole epiphysis is involved.[2,5,6] In most cases there is reason to believe there is more than one episode of infarction.[3,7]

Early Stages

In the early stages (Table 25A–1), there is major overgrowth of the articular cartilage on the medial and lateral aspects of the femoral head. This results in enlargement of the femoral head. Infarction is present within the bony epiphysis, and there is an early loss of epiphyseal height because of trabecular fracture. The density noted on fine-detail radiography results in part from this trabecular fracture and appositional new bone formation but primarily from calcification of the necrotic marrow. The growth plate is also abnormal, with distortion of the cellular columns and an increase in the quantity of calcified cartilage in the primary spongiosa.

Intermediate Stages

Once the infarction has occurred, a process of repair revascularizes the intact avascular trabeculae by the process of creeping substitution and removes the loose necrotic bone in the apex of the femoral head, replacing it with fibrocartilage (Table 25A–1). This repair process produces the radiologic appearance of fragmentation. In the thickened articular cartilage this repair is by endochondral ossification, occurring as a natural growth process from the subchondral bone plate of the viable portion of the epiphysis and as islands of new bone formation in the thickened anterior and lateral articular cartilage. These areas gradually enlarge and then fuse with the bony epiphysis. Initially these small islands appear radiologically as areas of calcification lateral to the epiphysis. In the growth plate, areas of unossified cartilage stream down from the growth plate into the metaphyseal region, producing a metaphyseal cyst. When these areas are large, the normal architecture of the growth plate is lost and no further growth forms from this part of the femoral neck. Because these lesions are usually anterior and lateral, this results in a growth disturbance in the femoral neck that produces a tilt deformity of the femoral head on the neck.

Healing and Late Phases

In the healing phases of this disease (Table 25A–1), most of the loose necrotic trabeculae have been removed, and the fibrocartilage is progressively reossified with the establishment of a new subchondral bone plate and, thus, the reestablishment of normal epiphyseal growth. The last portions to re-form are in the anterosuperior portion of the epiphysis. The pathologic process, therefore, converts an initially round head to one that is oval, particularly in its anterior and lateral aspects.

The Process of Femoral Head Deformity

These findings suggest that, in the early phases of this disease, overgrowth of the articular cartilage and loss of epiphyseal height from trabecular fracture produce a change in head shape from round to oval. This does not, however, account for the severe deformity seen to occur in some cases. In the long term it is important to realize that there are two possible results: When the femoral head is round or oval, a ball-and-socket joint occurs. When the femoral head is progressively flattened, a roller-bearing shape evolves. Stulberg and associates[8] referred to this as aspherical incongruity. Clinical examination reveals that the roller-bearing joint moves in a flexion-extension range only and is adducted in extension and abducted and exter-

Table 25A–1
Clinical findings in Legg-Calvé-Perthes disease

Stage	Articular Cartilage	Epiphysis
Onset	Thickened	Variable degree of infarction
Sclerosis	Thickened, especially laterally	Variable infarction; trabecular fracture; calcification of necrotic marrow
Fragmentation	Overgrowth laterally; islands of ossification in thickened cartilage laterally; calcification lateral to epiphysis	Repair proportional to trabecular structure; loose necrotic bone replaced by fibrocartilage; intact necrotic trabeculae revascularized by creeping substitution
Healing	Resumption of normal growth	Progressive removal of necrotic bone with ossification of fibrocartilage, reestablishing normal subchondral bony plate and growth

nally rotated in flexion because a varus deformity in the femoral neck makes the leg lie short. Clinical examination also shows that in cases of severe femoral head deformity this position of adduction begins in the early phases and that flexion with abduction is also an early sign. It is radiologically and arthrographically apparent that abduction is progressively lost in the early phases of the disease and that the movement changes from one of pure rotation to one of rotation with hinging on the lateral aspect of the acetabulum. As overgrowth of the femoral head continues, the moment of this hinging comes to lie outside the confines of the bony acetabulum; at this stage the subluxation becomes fixed and the roller-bearing joint is the inevitable long-term result. This process is called hinge abduction.

Clinical Recognition of Progressive Deformity of the Femoral Head

Clinical recognition of the early stages of progressive deformity of the femoral head is obviously important. If treatment is to be effective it must be started as early as possible. I[9] introduced the concept of the "head at risk" to identify these cases. Numerous clinical and radiologic signs identify cases in which serious deformity may occur. The clinical signs include progressive loss of movement, flexion with abduction, adduction contracture, and obesity. The radiologic signs are associated with epiphyseal and metaphyseal changes. Epiphyseal signs include Gage's sign, in which there is a lytic area on the lateral aspect of the epiphysis and adjacent metaphysis, and calcification lateral to the epiphysis. Both suggest overgrowth of the articular cartilage laterally. The metaphyseal signs (a diffuse reaction and a horizonal growth plate) reflect the growth disturbance within the femoral neck and the tilt of the femoral head on the neck that occurs with time. The horizontal growth plate reflects the position of abduction and external rotation and is another early sign of the hip's being adducted and externally rotated and, therefore, of the

roller-bearing joint. It has been shown that two or more of these signs adversely affect the prognosis.[6,10] A poor result does not occur in untreated cases unless two or more of the radiologic signs were present during the active stages of the disease.

Factors Influencing Natural History

In a disease in which 57% of cases do well without treatment, it is obviously important to discover factors that help to identify the 43% of cases in which treatment is required. A number of factors may be useful in assessing individual cases. The clinician may be able to influence some of them. These factors can be subdivided into short- and long-term factors.

Short-Term Factors

Age and Sex The prognosis is better for the younger child than for the older one; boys have a more favorable outlook than girls. This is not true in every case, particularly in some of the younger Catterall group IV patients, who may have a poor result even with adequate treatment. Girls have an unfavorable prognosis because they have a more serious form of the disease.[6,11]

Stage of the Disease at Diagnosis The earlier in the disease process that treatment is started, the better the prognosis will be because deformity will be less. Also, once healing has been established radiologically, the shape of the femoral head will not deteriorate further.[12] The signs of healing are increases in the height and size of viable bone on the medial side of the epiphysis and the height and quality of new bone formed laterally. Treatment is indicated at this stage of the disease only if it will improve congruity of the femoral head. Arthrography is essential to prove this point.

Group The prognosis for an individual case depends on the degree of radiologic involvement of the epiphysis (Table 25A–2). I[9] have defined four radiologic groups. These correspond to the extent of infarction

Table 25A-1 (*continued*)

Growth Plate	Radiograph
Distortion of cell columns with abnormal ossification of primary spongiosa	Normal
Continued growth disturbance, more marked anteriorly than posteriorly	Dense, slightly flatter epiphysis; subchondral fracture line; widening of growth plate
Gross disorganization in metaphyseal lesions with local cessation of growth; in anterior lesions this tilts femoral head on neck; in central lesions this shortens neck	Fragmentation
Ossification of metaphyseal lesion, possibly resulting in local growth plate closure	Healing

Table 25A-2
Results in untreated cases

Group	Results*		
	Good	Fair	Poor
I	27	1	0
II	25	6	2
III	4	7	11
IV	0	4	10
Total No.	56	18	23
%	57	19	24

*Good results were obtained in 92% of those in groups I and II, whereas results were poor in 91% of those in groups III and IV.

within the epiphysis[2,5] (Table 25A–3). Good-quality radiographs are essential.[6,9,13,14]

Signs of the Head at Risk These have already been discussed with reference to progressive deformity in the femoral head. The presence of two or more radiologic signs and the clinical sign of flexion with abduction should be regarded as absolute indications for treatment.

Long-Term Factors

There are still relatively few long-term studies of the consequences of this disease but the conclusions are clear. Although 86% of patients will develop osteoarthritis by the age of 65 years, most will not have a problem until the fifth or sixth decade.[15,16] One third of cases will improve after the disease heals but a small proportion will deteriorate. About 9% of patients will require reconstructive surgery by the age of 35 years.[17] Children who will develop early osteoarthritis have late-onset disease, usually after the age of 9 years, that produces an irregular, uncovered femoral head (aspherical incongruity) with partial arrest of the growth plate and a reduced range of movement with flexion with abduction.[15,16] These signs are a continuation of the earlier signs of the head at risk and, therefore, provide the long-term justification for treatment in these children. In some cases, however, an oval head with some deformity shows congruity with the acetabulum when the leg is in the neutral position of weightbearing. Curtis[18] called this congruous incongruity and Stulberg and associates[8] called it aspherical congruity. Thus, if femoral head deformity is present the object of treatment should be to realign the leg so that there is max-

Table 25A-3
Radiologic signs in Legg-Calvé-Perthes disease

Radiologic Signs	Group I	Group II	Group III	Group IV
Epiphyseal signs				
Sclerosis	No	Yes	Yes	Yes
Subchondral fracture line	No	Anterior	Posterior	Complete
Junction of involved and uninvolved segments	Clear	Clear, often V-shaped	Sclerotic	No
Viable bone on growth plate	Anterior margin	Anterior half	Posterior half	No
Medial/lateral aspects appear triangular	No	No	Occasionally	Yes
Metaphyseal signs				
Localized	No	Anterior	Anterior	Anterior or central
Diffuse	No	No	Yes	Yes
Posterior remodeling	No	No	No	Yes

imum contact between the femoral head and acetabulum when the leg is in the neutral position of weightbearing.

Obviously, there are only a few factors that the clinician is in a position to control. Age, sex, and radiologic group are already determined by the time the patient is initially examined. Public education and awareness of symptoms can encourage early examination, allowing needed treatment to be begun sooner. Early clinical recognition of children with poor prognoses through the concept of the "head at risk" will also provide a better opportunity for effective treatment. Treatment is intended to control the growth disturbance and restore the normal growth mechanism within the femoral head and neck.

Indications for and Principles of Treatment

Because of the usually benign natural course of the condition, it is important to identify indications for treatment so that unnecessary therapy can be avoided. Treatment is contraindicated during the early stages for all cases in group I and for all cases in groups II and III without "at-risk" signs. In the late stages, contraindications are (1) established healing and (2) serious femoral head deformity without hinge abduction. Those who should be treated in the early stages are all patients with "at-risk" signs, all those in groups II and III who are more than 7 years old, and all those in group IV who have no serious deformity. The indication for late-stage treatment is hinge abduction. Conservative treatment is indicated in cases in which the growth disturbance is mild or has already occurred (late-stage cases). Definitive treatment is required in cases in which the growth disturbance is likely to be severe (all "at-risk" cases and older children) or deformity in the late stages is associated with pain and hinge abduction.

The principles of treatment should be redefined as the restoration of movement, the reduction of forces through the hip joint, revascularization of necrotic bone, and the prevention of further ischemia. Normal movement is required to prevent progressive deformity of the femoral head and to encourage remodeling. Abduction of the leg has two effects on the hip: to reduce the forces through the joint[19] and to reposition the uncovered anterolateral aspect of the femoral head within the remodeling influence of the acetabulum. This reduction of forces through the joint should promote revascularization of the infarcted bone and the reestablishment of normal growth. In addition, removing the abnormal forces from the lateral cartilaginous aspect of the acetabulum allows it to assume a more normal appearance and resume growth. When the volume of necrotic bone is large, as in the older child, a period of immobilization may be needed for revascularization

in order to prevent further trabecular fracture and, therefore, collapse of the femoral head.

Applying these principles in the early and late stages of the disease leads to different methods of treatment. In the early stages, when the predominant abnormality is cartilage overgrowth, restoration of movement with the femoral head repositioned or contained within the acetabulum is the method of choice. In the later stages, when serious deformity of the femoral head has already occurred or healing is established, restoration of movement with the joint congruous in the neutral position of weightbearing allows the best long-term remodeling and prevents the long-term effects of hinge abduction.

Conclusions

It is unfortunate most clinicians manage the problems of Legg-Calvé-Perthes disease by studying radiologic images rather than understanding what these images imply in terms of morbid anatomy. Careful thought on this point will permit a better understanding of the natural history of the process and, thus, a better application of the principles of treatment.

References

1. Jensen OM, Lauritzen J: Legg-Calvé-Perthes' disease. Morphological studies in two cases examined at necropsy. *J Bone Joint Surg* 1976; 58B:332–338.
2. Catterall A, Pringle J, Byers PD, et al: A review of the morphology of Perthes' disease. *J Bone Joint Surg* 1982;64B:269–275.
3. McKibbin B, Ralis Z: Changes found in a case of Perthes' disease at necropsy: A case report. *J Bone Joint Surg* 1974;56B:438–447.
4. Dolman CL, Bell HM: The pathology of Legg-Calvé-Perthes' disease. *J Bone Joint Surg* 1973;55A:184–188.
5. Catterall A, Pringle J, Byers PD, et al: Perthes' disease: Is the epiphysial infarction complete? *J Bone Joint Surg* 1982;64B:276–281.
6. Catterall A: *Perthes' Disease.* London, Churchill Livingstone, 1982.
7. Inoue A, Freeman MA, Vernon-Roberts B, et al: The pathogenesis of Perthes' disease. *J Bone Joint Surg* 1976;58B:453–461.
8. Stulburg SD, Cooperman DR, Wallensten R: The natural history of Legg-Calvé-Perthes' disease. *J Bone Joint Surg* 1981;63A:1095–1108.
9. Catterall A: The natural history of Perthes' disease. *J Bone Joint Surg* 1971;53B:37–53.
10. Murphy RP, Marsh HO: Incidence and natural history of head-at-risk factor in Perthes' disease. *Clin Orthop* 1978;132:102–107.
11. Lovell WW, MacEwen GD, Stewart WR, et al: Legg-Perthes' disease in girls. *J Bone Joint Surg* 1982;64B:637.
12. Westin G, Thompson GH: Legg-Calvé-Perthes' disease: The results of discontinuing treatment in reformative phase. First International Symposium on Legg-Calvé-Perthes' Syndrome, Los Angeles, November 1977.
13. Catterall A: *Recent Advances in Orthopaedics,* ed 5. London, Churchill Livingstone, 1987.
14. Catterall A: Perthes' disease, in *Hip and Its Disorders.* Philadelphia, WB Saunders, in press.
15. Mose K, Hjorth L, Ulfeldt M, et al: Legg-Calvé-Perthes' disease: The late occurrence of coxarthrosis. *Acta Orthop Scand* 1977;169:1–39.

16. Weinstein SL: Legg-Calvé-Perthes' disease: Results of long-term follow-up. *Hip* 1985;28–37.
17. Catterall A: Adolescent hip pain after Perthes' disease. *Clin Orthop* 1986;209:65–69.
18. Curtis BH: A method for assessing outcome in Legg-Calvé-Perthes' syndrome. Presented at the First International Symposium on Legg-Calvé-Pethes' Syndrome, Los Angeles, November, 1977.
19. Heikkinen E, Puranen J: Evaluation of femoral osteotomy in the treatment of Legg-Calvé-Perthes' disease. *Clin Orthop* 1980;150:60–68.

P A R T B

Surgical Treatment

Anthony Catterall, M Chir, FRCS

Introduction

Surgical treatment of Legg-Calvé-Perthes disease is relatively recent. Both soft-tissue and bony procedures have been developed, although the indications for soft-tissue procedures are rare. Because surgery is associated with possible complications such as infection, the indications for treatment must be selective.[1] There are two other important aspects to surgical management that must be emphasized: (1) Surgical treatment should not be considered in cases in which conservative treatment has failed because this failure implies a serious deformity of the femoral head. Surgery has no more chance of improving the condition than the conservative treatment that failed. In the early stages, therefore, the conservative and surgical treatments are parallel and not sequential. (2) There are indications for surgical treatment in the late stages if the patient has pain, leg shortening, and hinge abduction. The goals here are to produce congruity of the femoral head within the acetabulum in the neutral position of weightbearing and to encourage long-term remodeling. However, these must be regarded as salvage procedures. One must also consider the problem of the child who is more than 9 years old and for whom conservative treatment is unsatisfactory.

The Soft-Tissue Releases

Children with Perthes' disease classically have loss of movement of the hip joint and, often, fixed flexion and fixed adduction that shorten the involved leg. A recent trend in treatment is a soft-tissue release followed by traction and physiotherapy to restore movement to the joints. However, when these children are examined under anesthesia, there is often no fixed deformity. These hips have a good range of abduction and no fixed flexion. In those with femoral head deformity, moreover, hinge abduction may be observed. If there is no fixed deformity, using an adjustable broomstick plaster to restore abduction and rotation frequently results in a rapid improvement in the range of movement without soft-tissue release. When fixed deformity is associated with hinge abduction, soft-tissue release is contraindicated as encouraging the process of hinging, thus exacerbating the condition. It is my conclusion, therefore, that soft-tissue releases are seldom indicated, except in the older child who has a marked degree of fixed flexion or adduction without serious deformation of the femoral head. This is rare.

The Realignment Osteotomies

Movement must be restored to the hip joint and the femoral head centered within the acetabulum before a splint can be used or realignment achieved by surgery. Whether splinting or surgery is the more effective procedure is a matter of controversy. In essence, both the containment braces and the surgical treatment achieve the same objectives and have similar results in children under the age of 7 years[2] compared with untreated children in groups II, III, and IV who have "at-risk" factors. The main advantages of surgery are that the treatment is short, effectively maintains the concentric position, and allows better long-term remodeling while the varus of the femoral neck is remodeling.[3–6] A disadvantage, however, is that the varus will not remodel with time in children more than 10 years old; this leads to persistent shortening that may require further reconstructive surgery such as trochanteric advancement or lower femoral epiphysiodesis (M.O. Tachdjian, personal communication, 1986). The containment splints, of which there are many kinds, have the immediate advantage of not requiring surgery, but treatment is long and there is no precise end point. All splints present psychological problems and there is no long-term varus to permit good remodeling. In addition, if full movement is not maintained, pelvic obliquity may result in a flexion abduction contracture that can prejudice the long-term results. This is often the case in the older child for whom treatment is most necessary. Most authorities agree that bracing is an unsatisfactory method for children more than 7 years old and that a weight-relieving caliper, although maintaining good movement, does not seriously alter the natural history of the untreated disease.

Both the innominate osteotomy described by Salter[7] and femoral osteotomy have been advised as realignment procedures in the management of this condition.

Innominate Osteotomy

The reported results of treatment by innominate osteotomy are variable. Salter[7] reported good results when the femoral head was round and no serious subluxation was present at the time of surgery. A deformity of the pelvis must, by definition, restrict movement by altering the arcs of movement and this is a possible long-term disadvantage. Many cases, however, are not first examined at the stage of the subchondral fracture and the problem that confronts the surgeon is how much deformity of the femoral head is acceptable if the result is to be considered "successful." There is no definite evidence on this point.

Femoral Osteotomy

Femoral osteotomy was introduced by Soeur and DeRacker[8] for the treatment of Perthes' disease. There are, however, few reports that consider the results of femoral osteotomy in the overall global management of this condition; they usually concentrate simply on the results obtained in a number of cases treated surgically. Muirhead-Allwood and I[6] addressed this problem. Given the selective indications for treatment already identified,[1] it is important to show that no more than 40% of patients require surgery. Muirhead-Allwood and I[6] reported overall results similar to those of Lloyd-Roberts and associates[3] and Canario and associates,[5] but only 45% of their cases required surgery. Those treated with femoral osteotomy had fewer poor results than those in groups II, III, and IV who had "at-risk" factors and who were untreated (Table 25B–1). When the disease process was in an early stage and prospective management was possible, 79% achieved good results, substantially better results than for untreated controls (Table 25B–2). For the most part, poor results occurred in late cases in which femoral head deformity was already established and for which containment treatment was not indicated. Results were also poor in early-stage cases in children who were first seen when they were more than 9 years old.

The Problem of the Older Child

Management is always difficult in children over 9 years of age. In these older children the ratio of epiphysis to cartilage within the femoral head is high by comparison with younger children, who have a greater proportion of cartilage. Initial examination is often at the stage of the subchondral fracture when there is marked loss of movement and an adduction contracture. Collapse of the epiphysis is commonly rapid because of the fixed deformity that compresses the fragile infarcted bone. Early subluxation of the femoral head exacerbates this process. To overcome this subluxation, innominate osteotomy has been recommended[7,9] for the same reason as in congenital dislocation of the hip.

In these older children the principles of treatment must be redefined as the restoration of movement, reduction of the forces through the hip joint, and revascularization of the infarcted bone with union of the subchondral fracture. There must be no further ischemia. Because of the marked muscle spasm, the position of abduction, which is of value in the younger child, is difficult to achieve and an alternative method of reduction of forces through the hip joint must be considered.

Enlargement of the acetabulum, by either a Chiari procedure or a lateral shelf acetabuloplasty, reduces the forces through the hip joint and also prevents lateral subluxation. This protection reduces the irritability of the hip joint and allows better movement, producing good long-term remodeling. In theory, the Chiari procedure has the same effect as the lateral shelf acetabuloplasty, but in practice it is commonly associated with stiffness and the medial displacement weakens the abductor lever arm and induces shortening, both of which encourage a persisting limp. Lateral shelf acetabuloplasty causes no weakening of the abductor lever arm and the positioning of the graft prevents the forces that induce subluxation.

Table 25B–1
Results of femoral osteotomy in patients in groups II, III, and IV who have "at-risk" factors

Results	Femoral Osteotomy (No. = 40)	Control Group (No. = 54)
Good (%)	67	31
Fair (%)	25	27
Poor (%)	8	42

Table 25B–2
Overall results

Management*	No. of Cases	Results (%)		
		Good	Fair	Poor
Prospective (early untreated and femoral osteotomy cases)	70	79	14	7
Late presentation (no surgery)	19	11	47	42
Overall	89	64	21	15

*There were 95 untreated controls not included in the overall results. Of these, 57% had good results, 19% had fair results, and 24% had poor results.

Van der Heyden and Van Tongeroloo[10] have reported good results for this procedure, and I have had an encouraging experience in this older group of children.

Late Presentation

Children in the healing phases of the disease may or may not have serious deformity of the femoral head. In the series Muirhead-Allwood and I[6] reported, 21% were in this stage and only 11% achieved good results. When leg lengths are equal and there is only slight restriction of movement, any serious deformity of the femoral head is unlikely. The hip is congruous in the neutral position of weightbearing.[2,11] Persistent pain during the healing phase is always a worrying symptom, particularly if there is shortening from a fixed deformity. An arthrogram in these circumstances commonly demonstrates hinge abduction.

The object of treatment in children with late femoral head deformity is to restore movement with the femoral head congruous in the neutral position of weightbearing. There should also be relief of pain and improvement in leg length. The procedures advocated for this are abduction-extension osteotomy of the femur, chielectomy, and the Chiari operation. Chielectomy,[12] or removal of the lateral obstructing lip of the femoral head, seems to be indicated only after healing of the disease when hinging cannot be eliminated except in the extreme position of flexion and abduction. In practice, this clinical situation is seldom encountered. The Chiari operation[13,14] undoubtedly covers the lateral aspect of the femoral head but does not reverse the process of hinging or improve leg length. The effect of the medial displacement is to exaggerate the limp. Abduction-extension osteotomy[15] fulfills the requirements of treatment. It reverses the process of hinging and allows remodeling of the femoral head and the lateral acetabulum. This seems to be the most logical procedure for cases late in the disease process.

Summary

The place of surgical treatment in the management of Perthes' disease has yet to be defined. There is no doubt that in children who have late-stage disease or who are more than 9 years old conservative treatment or the use of splints is unlikely to be effective or to produce great improvement. In such cases surgery seems to be the best method of management. In the younger child, the results obtained with braces and with surgery are similar. It must be emphasized, however, that failed conservative treatment is not a good indication for surgery because once the femoral head is deformed containment treatment is no more likely to be effective than the splint.

References

1. Catterall A: Legg-Calvé-Perthes' disease: Part A. Morbid anatomy and natural history, in Barr JS Jr (ed): American Academy of Orthopaedic Surgeons *Instructional Course Lectures, XXXVIII.* Park Ridge, American Academy of Orthopaedic Surgeons, 1989, pp 297–301.
2. Cooperman, DR, Stulberg SD: Ambulatory containment treatment in Legg-Calvé-Perthes disease. *Hip* 1985, pp 38–62.
3. Lloyd-Roberts GC, Catterall A, Salamon PB: A controlled study of the indications for and the results of femoral osteotomy in Perthes' disease. *J Bone Joint Surg* 1976;58B:31–36.
4. Axer A, Gershuni DH, Hendel D, et al: Indications for femoral osteotomy in Legg-Calvé-Perthes disease. *Clin Orthop* 1980;150:78–87.
5. Canario, AT, Williams L, Wientroub S, et al: A controlled study of the results of femoral osteotomy in severe Perthes' disease. *J Bone Joint Surg* 1980;62B:438–440.
6. Muirhead-Allwood W, Catterall A: The treatment of Perthes' disease: The results of a trial of management. *J Bone Joint Surg* 1982;64B:282–285.
7. Salter RB: Legg-Perthes disease: Part V. Treatment by innominate osteotomy, in American Academy of Orthopaedic Surgeons *Instructional Course Lectures, XXII.* St. Louis, CV Mosby, 1973, pp 309–316.
8. Soeur R, DeRacker C: L'aspect anatomo-pathologique de l'osteochondrite e les theories pathogeniques qui s'y rapportent. *Acta Orthop Belge* 1952;18:57.
9. Klisic PJ: Treatment of Perthes' disease in older children. *J Bone Joint Surg* 1983;65B:419–427.
10. Van der Heyden AM, Van Tongeroloo RG: Shelf operation in Perthes' disease. Presented at the Continental Meeting of Dutch, Nordic and British Orthopaedic Associations, October 1980.
11. Stulberg SD, Cooperman DR, Wallensten R: The natural history of Legg-Calvé-Perthes' disease. *J Bone Joint Surg* 1981;63A:1095–1108.
12. McKay DW: Chielectomy of the hip. *Orthop Clin North Am* 1980;11:141–160.
13. Handelsman JE: The Chiari pelvic sliding osteotomy. *Orthop Clin North Am* 1980;11:105–125.
14. Schepers A, Von Bormann PFB, Craig JJG: Coxa magna in Perthes' disease: Treatment by Chiari's pelvic osteotomy. *J Bone Joint Surg* 1978;60B:297.
15. Quain S, Catterall A: Hinge abduction of the hip: Diagnosis and treatment. *J Bone Joint Surg* 1986;68B:61–64.

Nonsurgical Treatment of Legg-Calvé-Perthes Disease

Carl D. Fackler, MD

An understanding of the natural history of Legg-Calvé-Perthes disease is essential in managing its treatment. The clinician must apply this knowledge to each patient individually in order to recommend appropriate treatment because there is no one method that applies to all patients. The purpose of treatment is to minimize the forces that cause deformity of the femoral head during the active or "plastic phase." The long-term goal of treatment is to prevent arthritis later in life.

Methods

Nonweightbearing

This method was the first to be employed. It was believed that prevention of weightbearing through the hip meant there would be no force on the soft femoral head to cause deformity. This can be accomplished either by prolonged bedrest or by mobilizing the patient while protecting the leg by means of crutches, the Snyder sling, the Forte harness, or the ischial weightbearing brace. This method used alone provides results no better than those in untreated patients[1,2] and has been abandoned except for occasional, short-term symptomatic use.[3]

Containment

Containment is achieved by abduction to contain the involved femoral head within the acetabular "mold" and by maintaining motion. Any collapse that might occur is controlled and congruous with the acetabulum during the plastic or active phase. The concept of containment was proposed by Parker[4] and Eyre-Brook[5] and has been developed by many others.[6-8] It forms the basis of most current methods of treatment.

Nonweightbearing Containment Containment was originally used in combination with nonweightbearing. Patients were confined to bed for months with abduction maintained by spica casts, broomstick plasters, or traction.[6,8-11] This method is still proposed by some[12] but social and economic forces in most areas make it impractical. Some orthoses have been developed that abduct the hip and prevent weightbearing through it, but these have not gained wide acceptance and there are few reports on their effectiveness.

Ambulatory Containment Petrie and Bitenc[7] described ambulatory or weightbearing containment with plasters in 1971. A variety of orthotic devices have followed, including the Toronto, Craig, Newington, and Scottish Rite orthoses. These devices allow weightbearing through the involved hip and allow the patient to be more mobile.

Initial Management

The goal of initial care is to regain and maintain motion and protect the femoral head until the full extent of its involvement can be determined. Frequently, this takes several months.

The patient who has a stiff and painful hip is required to rest and is given salicylates. Traction (or slings and springs) is begun. This is usually done in the hospital but can be done at home if equipment is available and parents are able to cooperate. Abduction is slowly increased as comfort permits. Once adequate abduction is achieved, ambulatory containment is started with either Petrie casts or an orthosis. Coverage is considered adequate when the abduction is at least 45 degrees and when the lateral aspect of the epiphyseal plate is covered by the lateral margin of the acetabulum.[3] If adequate abduction is not achieved after seven to ten days of rest in traction, adductor tenotomy is done with the patient under anesthesia and Petrie casts are applied. Alternatively, traction is continued.

When the patient is mobilized with an abduction device, a radiograph of the pelvis should be taken with the patient standing to be sure that adequate lateral coverage (as defined above) is being maintained. This should be repeated every two to three months, along with a test of the range of motion, until it can be determined that treatment is no longer needed. If hip irritability or loss of motion occurs, the patient is placed back in traction at home or in the hospital until the symptoms subside and adequate abduction is regained.

If the patient is less than 5 years of age, is asymptomatic, and has no limitation of motion, close follow-up and mild limitation of activities are all that is needed. If symptoms of hip irritability develop along with some limitation of motion, temporary bedrest in slings and springs or traction is indicated.

Petrie Casts

Petrie casts are simply long leg casts with an abduction bar placed in 0 to 10 degrees of internal rotation and adequate abduction. They enforce compliance and are less expensive than an orthosis but can be cumbersome to apply. Their main use is as a temporary device until staging can be determined or until an orthosis can be fabricated, although there is

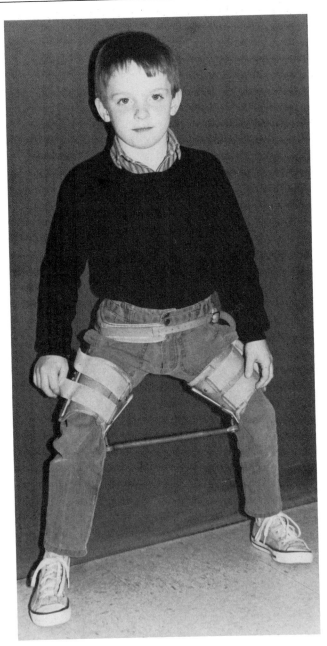

Fig. 26–1 A 5-year-old patient wearing the Scottish Rite orthosis for Legg-Calvé-Perthes disease.

renewed interest in their long-term use. They are applied after adequate abduction and motion have been achieved and are changed every six to eight weeks. When the casts are changed, the patient is generally hospitalized, is restricted to bedrest, and spends two or three days out of the casts to regain knee and ankle motion with the help of a physical therapist. No late problems with knee or ankle stress have been reported with their use.

Orthotic Treatment

Of the many orthoses available, I prefer the Scottish Rite orthosis (Fig. 26–1). It allows free and full knee

and ankle motion. Although this orthosis does not control internal rotation, anterior coverage is gained by mild hip flexion. It is fitted once the patient has achieved a full and comfortable range of motion with adequate abduction. It is worn at all times except when bathing or swimming with a life preserver. The patient is encouraged to be fully active and frequently masters many activities, including bike riding, running, and roller skating. The child is examined every three months to test range of motion out of the brace. At each examination a standing anteroposterior radiograph of the pelvis is taken while the brace is on (Fig. 26–2). If motion or adequate lateral coverage is lost, the child is placed back in traction or Petrie casts.

Definitive Management

Patients in Catterall group I do not require ambulatory containment because they do well with no treatment as long as range of motion is maintained. The same is true for group II patients under 7 years of age. For group II patients who are 7 years of age and older, ambulatory containment is continued six months from onset[3] because of the risk of progression to group 3.

Patients with group III or group IV involvement should continue ambulatory containment until the sclerotic areas in the femoral epiphysis are gone and new bone formation is evident in the lateral column.[3] This usually occurs by 12 to 18 months after onset. Because this is often difficult to determine, the patient is weaned from the orthosis gradually over six weeks and is monitored closely. If pain or decreased motion occurs during weaning, the orthosis is resumed (after motion is regained) for three more months.

Discussion

The studies reporting the results of treatment use the radiologic appearance of sphericity of the femoral head and joint congruence as criteria for grading. There are no long-term studies showing the effect of treatment on the onset of arthritis. However, on the basis of radiologic criteria, containment methods have shown improvement over no treatment and over the non-weightbearing methods.[1,5–8,13,14] All ambulatory containment methods appear to be equally effective but the study groups have not been large enough to compare statistically.

Recent long-term, natural history studies[15,16] suggest a decrease in severity and delay in onset of arthritic symptoms in patients with radiologic sphericity and joint congruity. It seems logical that the improvement in sphericity as a result of ambulatory containment will delay or prevent degenerative arthritis at a later age.

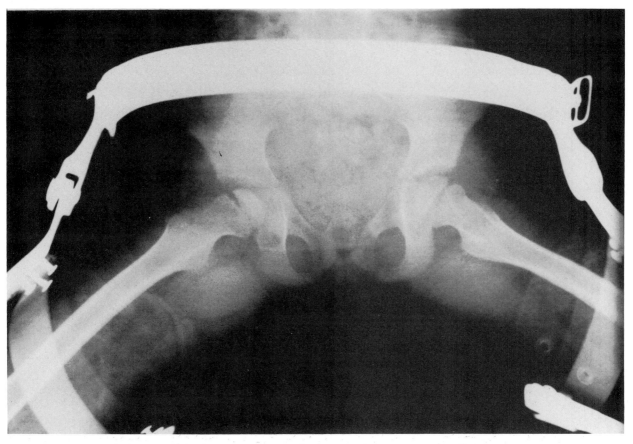

Fig. 26–2 Anteroposterior radiograph of the pelvis taken during a follow-up visit with patient standing in the Scottish Rite orthosis. Abduction of the involved right hip is adequate.

Personal Observations

Patients and their families seem to cope better with the treatment of this condition if they understand that it will last for several months or years and that the goal is to manage the problem and minimize its effects since it cannot be cured. This should be explained when the diagnosis is made and reinforced at follow-up visits.

Nonsurgical treatment of Legg-Calvé-Perthes disease is the preferred method of most clinicians, with surgery reserved for those patients who are at risk for femoral head deformity but who cannot, or will not, accept orthotic devices. In some cases, surgery may be a better method of treatment and the patient and the family should be informed of this option.

A long-term, multicenter prospective study should be encouraged and supported. We need to know more about the natural history and the results of treatment to be more certain that this treatment is effective and that we are not overtreating or undertreating these young patients.

References

1. Cooperman DR, Stulberg SD: Ambulatory containment treatment in Perthes' disease. *Clin Orthop* 1986;203:289–300.
2. O'Hara JP, Davis ND, Gage JR, et al: Long-term follow-up of Perthes' disease treated nonoperatively. *Clin Orthop* 1977; 125:49–56.
3. MacEwen GD, Bunnell WP, Ramsey PL: The hip, in Lovell WW, Winter (eds): *Pediatric Orthopedics*, ed 2. Philadelphia, JB Lippincott, 1986, vol 2, pp 750–770.
4. Parker AO, cited by Harrison MHM, Menon MPA: Legg-Calvé-Perthes disease: The value of roentgenographic measurement in clinical practice with special reference to the broomstick plaster method. *J Bone Joint Surg* 1966;48A:1301–1318.
5. Eyre-Brook AL: Osteochondritis deformans coxae juvenilis or Perthes' disease: The results of treatment by traction in recumbency. *Brit J Surg* 1936;24:166–182.
6. Harrison MHM, Menon MPA: Legg-Calvé-Perthes disease: The value of roentgenographic measurement in clinical practice with special reference to the broomstick plaster method. *J Bone Joint Surg* 1966;48A:1301–1318.
7. Petrie JG, Bitenc I: The abduction weight-bearing treatment in Legg-Perthes' disease. *J Bone Joint Surg* 1971:53B:54–62.
8. Salter RB: Legg-Perthes disease: The scientific basis for the methods of treatment and their indications. *Clin Orthop* 1980;150:8–11.
9. Eaton GO: Long-term results of treatment in coxa plana: A follow-up study of eighty-eight patients. *J Bone Joint Surg* 1967;49A:1031–1042.

10. Katz JF: Conservative treatment of Legg-Calvé-Perthes disease. *J Bone Joint Surg* 1967;49A:1043–1051.

11. Perpich M, McBeath A, Kruse D: Long-term follow-up of Perthes disease treated with spica casts. *J Pediatr Orthop* 1983;3:160–165.

12. Brotherton BJ, McKibbin B: Perthes' disease treated by prolonged recumbency and femoral head containment: A long-term appraisal. *J Bone Joint Surg* 1977;59B:8–14.

13. Richards BS, Coleman SS: Subluxation of the femoral head in coxa plana. *J Bone Joint Surg* 1987;69A:1312–1318.

14. Purvis JM, Dimon JH III, Meehan PL, et al: Preliminary experience with the Scottish Rite Hospital abduction orthosis for Legg-Perthes disease. *Clin Orthop* 1980;150:49–53.

15. Stulberg SD, Cooperman DR, Wallensten R: The natural history of Legg-Calvé-Perthes disease. *J Bone Joint Surg* 1981;63A:1095–1108.

16. McAndrew MP, Weinstein SL: A long-term follow-up of Legg-Calvé-Perthes disease. *J Bone Joint Surg* 1984;66A:860–869.

Legg-Calvé-Perthes Disease:
A Review of Current Knowledge

John A. Herring, MD

Introduction

The disorder known as Legg-Calvé-Perthes disease was recognized early in this century and is a relatively common affliction of children today. In dealing with this disorder we tend to assume that we have extensive knowledge about the problem and that most of this knowledge has been discovered recently. As we shall see, this is not always the case. Many of the established facts about this disorder were discovered within a few years of the identification of the process. Treatment programs began empirically before the natural history was known, and have yet to be carefully analyzed against untreated controls. No true experimental model exists and major assumptions have been made from dissimilar models of the disease. The cause is probably a combination of vascular and constitutional factors, but little is known about what initiates the disease. We have a fair understanding of the natural history but are still hampered by the lack of accurate prognostic indicators for a given patient.

History

Q: Who first described Perthes' disease?

A: The usual answer is Waldenström,[1] who published radiographs of this condition in 1909, considering it a mild form of tuberculosis. However, the first radiograph was published in 1905 by Köhler, who also described an osteochondrosis that is still known as Köhler's disease.[2]

Q: Who first described it as a disease entity?

A: Although Legg's paper was actually published first, the record probably should go to Calvé. Sourdat, who worked with Calvé at the marine hospital at Berck, France, included several of Calvé's newly described cases in his doctoral thesis, published in 1909.[2] Although Calvé's paper was still in the publication process when Sourdat published his thesis, this established Calvé as the first to describe the disease. Legg[3] of Boston was second, describing five cases in 1910, and Perthes,[4] who also published a description in 1910, was third.

Q: Why did all this happen almost simultaneously?

A: The X-ray machine, invented in 1895, was the catalyst for a myriad of discoveries.[2] In fact, someone has located a radiograph of a hip with Perthes' disease taken in 1898, only three years after the machine was invented![2] When Calvé, for example, obtained an X-ray

machine, he proceeded to do radiographs on 500 patients with hip disease at his tuberculosis hospital. There were ten children who did not have the usual signs of tuberculosis but who limped. These ten were found to have the new disease, which he called "old rickets."[2]

Q: Did scientific investigators first elucidate the natural history of the disease, then observe in controlled trials the effect of treatment compared with untreated controls, and finally formulate appropriate treatment protocols?

A: The answer is no on all counts. For example, Legg's initial paper not only described the disease but also the treatment of all five cases.[3] The first patient was treated with traction followed by a splint (presumably a patten bottom brace). The second, third, and fourth patients were treated with spica casts, and the fifth patient underwent curettage of the femoral neck.

Q: Did subsequent studies go back and compare untreated controls with treated cases?

A: Yes and no. A number of articles described controls—patients who were not treated with containment methods. However, these patients all had some treatment that may or may not have affected the outcome of the disease. Most of these methods involved years of treatment, including traction, bedrest, bracing, and cast immobilization. A review of the early articles shows rather convincingly that these "control" patients were treated vigorously. Thus, all along we have been hampered by the historic fact that the disease was treated as soon as it was recognized.

It is interesting to note that Legg in later years may have seen a new light. In 1927 in a discussion of an article in the *Journal of Bone and Joint Surgery*, he is quoted as stating, "It must be admitted that while any process which suggests a weakening in bone structure is going on in the hip joint, it would seem theoretically sound treatment to allow no weight-bearing. It has been my experience, however, that relief from weight bearing has in no way affected the end result." The other discussants disagreed and Legg replied, "In my cases relief from weight bearing did not stop the process from going on, and it was kept up for five years."[5]

Q: When did the idea of a vascular cause for Perthes' disease originate?

A: The concept of vascular infarction of the femoral head in Perthes' disease was first postulated by Schwarz[6] in 1913. He stated, "If the disease, whose cause I would like to consider to be a disturbance of blood supply, involves the whole epiphysis, then all of the vascular channels which provide blood must be blocked" (Fig. 27–1).

Subsequent investigators discovered two other significant facts. Pathologic specimens have shown evidence of a double infarction. There are two types of infarcted bone in these specimens. The existing lamellar bone is infarcted and, in addition, there is often a layer of new woven bone that is also necrotic. Similar double-infarction patterns were seen in an experimental canine model in which a single infarction did not produce changes like those in Perthes' disease but in which a double infarction did cause typical avascular necrosis patterns.[7]

The second interesting finding is that there are vascular abnormalities in the femoral neck. This information comes from studies in which needles were inserted into the femoral neck at the time of femoral osteotomy. Venograms were performed and metaphyseal pressures were measured. These studies showed a distortion of the pattern of venous drainage of the femoral neck with abnormal filling of the femoral diaphysis. There was also apparent blockage of the veins of the femoral neck. In addition, the pressures in the neck were increased. This suggests a possible venous infarction pattern rather than the usually presumed arterial occlusion.[8,9]

Q: Why do some children develop this unusual avascular necrosis?

A: The best answer we have at this point is that there are constitutional factors that are somehow related to the development of the disorder. Although the exact pathophysiologic mechanisms have not been identified, these associated factors may provide the clues that will lead to a complete understanding in the future.

Children with Perthes' disease have significant abnormalities of growth and maturation that are evident in a systemic way. The skeletal age of these children, determined by wrist radiographs, is significantly delayed. Skeletal age is usually about two years or more behind the chronologic age. In addition, the bone fails to mature during the two years after disease onset after which there is a "catch-up" period of growth.[10] Perhaps related to this is the finding that somatomedin (growth hormone) levels do not increase with age in patients with Perthes' disease as they do in control subjects.[11] In addition, patients show a decreased serum growth hormone response to insulin-induced hypoglycemia.[12]

Other constitutional factors have been documented but as yet defy explanation. For one, the incidence of Perthes' disease is 0.45 per 100,000 in black children and 10.8 per 100,000 in white children. Why this is so is unknown, but this may be an important etiologic clue that merits further study.[13] Lower socioeconomic status is associated with an increase in the incidence of the disease, and in some studies a weak familial tendency has been identified.[14,15]

These observations have led to various theories. One concept is that these skeletally immature children overload their immature, mostly cartilaginous femoral heads with normal or hyperactive activity levels. The resulting injury to the femoral head initiates several ischemic episodes that produce all the manifestations of avascular necrosis.[16]

Q: What happens when the head infarcts?

A: As with much of our knowledge of this syndrome, the early observations provided us with as good an answer as any we have now. Note, for example, that the first pathologic specimen was described by Frangenheim in 1909.[2]

Waldenström[17] described five radiographic stages of the progression of the disease. In the first, or synovitic stage, the patient limps and has pain and/or a decreased range of motion. The radiographs are either normal or show a decrease in the size of the ossific nucleus with widening of the medial cartilage space. The pathologic correlate of this is continued growth of articular cartilage based on nutrition by means of diffusion while the avascular osseous head fails to grow.

In the second, or avascular, stage, there is increased radiodensity of the femoral head. This is now known to represent a combination of new bone laid down on dead bone, crushing together of avascular trabeculae, and deposition of dead granulation tissue in marrow spaces.

In the third, or fragmentation, stage, the femoral head has areas of decreased density, often interspersed with areas of continuing increased density. The lucent areas represent areas of nonossified granulation tissue.

In the fourth, or reossification, stage, the areas of previous lucency reossify. The process is very gradual and residual areas of lucency may persist until skeletal maturity.

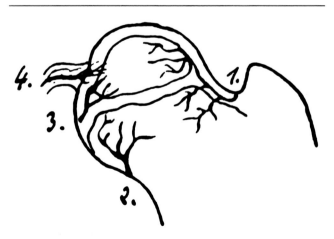

Fig. 27-1 Drawing of the blood supply of the femoral head, originally published in 1913. (Reproduced with permission from Schwarz E: A typical disease of the upper femoral epiphysis. *Clin Orthop* 1986;209:5–12 [reprint].)

In the fifth, or residual, stage, the femoral head is fully reossified with residual changes of shape.

Q: What is known of the disease's natural history?

A: Three things are known: (1) Most patients do well. (2) Older patients do less well. (3) The disease is quite variable.

Q: What percentage of patients do well?

A: Several long-term studies have addressed this question. Whitman[18] commented on the usual benign nature of the disease in 1928. He stated, "In the majority of cases, particularly those of childhood, the disability is slight, and practically full functional recovery may be predicted within a comparatively short period."

Ratliff,[19] who evaluated 34 hips after an average follow-up of 30 years, found that 80% of the patients were active and had no complaints of pain but that 60% of the hips showed significant degenerative changes on radiographic examination. Gower and Johnston[20] found that only 8% of the patients they studied had significant pain or loss of function at follow-up. Lloyd-Roberts[21] stated, "59% or so of untreated patients are known to evolve satisfactorily without the benefit of our attentions." These studies were further confirmed by Englehardt[22] in 1985. Of 55 patients monitored for 42 years, 46% had excellent functional results, 33% good results, and only 16% were disabled.

As patients with Perthes' disease reach their fifth and sixth decades, there may be significant functional deterioration. McAndrew and Weinstein[23] found that 40% of patients in these age groups had undergone total hip replacement and another 10% had enough pain and disability to qualify for the procedure.

Q: What is the prognostic significance of age at onset?

A: Age at onset is probably the most significant and reliable prognostic factor we have. One of the first to note the effect of age was Møller[24] in 1926. A multitude of subsequent publications verified the observation.

Brotherton and McKibbin[25] reported the results of ambulatory containment treatment. They noted that the average age at onset for all patients was 5.4 years whereas the average age at onset for those with poor results was 8.7 years. Evans[26] described a series of patients treated with traction and spica casts and made the following observation: "The age of onset of the disease is important. Except in one case, a good result did not occur with an age at onset of over six, and with one exception the result was always poor if the age at onset was over eight years."

The effect of age at onset is readily apparent in reports of modern treatment modes. Hoikka and associates[27] in a series of 112 varus osteotomies found that the result worsened as age at onset increased and was seldom good if the age at onset was more than 9 years. Ingman and associates[28] compared innominate osteotomy with spica cast treatment and found that:

The most significant factor determining the clinical and radiological results, whether treated by innominate osteotomy or hip spica, was

the age of the patient. There were 8 patients over the age of 8 years treated in plaster, with only one good result. There were only three radiographic good results out of 14 such patients treated by osteotomy.

Almost all other studies comparing outcome to age at onset have shown the same relationship.

Q: Are there other ways to predict the severity of the disease?

A: From the early days the variability of the disease was noted and a number of radiographic risk factors have been identified. Waldenström[17] found ". . . three groups, the first two mentioned are somewhat more normal, so to speak. Of my 22 cases, 14 belong to this type. It is then the more usual. The third type embraces the most severe deformities." In this paper Waldenström also introduced the idea of risk factors. He found that the prognosis was poor

if decalcinated areas have appeared in the collum (neck). . . . and if the epiphysis in the fragmentation phase is separated into small granules and severely flattened, and if further a part of the epiphysis lies outside the articular cavity at the top of the collum.

Thus, he rather clearly described the risk factors of metaphyseal lucency, early flattening, and lateral extrusion (Fig. 27–2). In 1927, Legg[5] identified two types of disease, a "mushroom type which remains spherical, and a cap type which becomes flat and is less common." Goff[2] in 1954 proposed a three-part classification consisting of a spherical type, a cylindrical or mushroom type, and an irregular type. The first usually occurred in those less than 7 years old at onset, the second in those 7 to 10 years old, and the third in those aged 11 years or more.

The classification commonly used today was proposed by Catterall[29] in a classic article in 1971. He defined four groups on the basis of percentage of head involvement. Toward the end of the article he explained the further variability of outcome within the groups by the presence of five "head at risk" signs. These were lateral extrusion, lateral calcification, lucency of the lateral portion of the head, diffuse metaphyseal reaction, and horizontal growth plate. (The last factor has since been dropped from the list of useful predictors.)

Salter and Thompson[30] simplified the classification of head involvement by using the extent of the subchondral fracture, a finding usually seen on the frog-position lateral radiograph of a patient in the early phase of the disease. If the fracture extends over less than half of the head, it is group A, corresponding to Catterall groups I and II. If the fracture involves more than half the head, it is group B, resembling Catterall groups III and IV.

Stulberg and associates[31] proposed a five-part classification applied after healing of the femoral head. Type 1 is almost normal. In type 2 the femoral head and acetabulum are spherical. In type 3 the femoral head and acetabulum are not spherical but are not truly

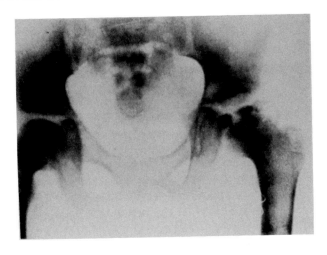

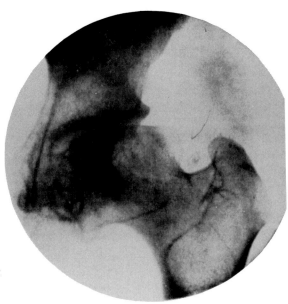

Fig. 27-2 Radiographic findings predictive of a poor outcome. (Reproduced with permission from Waldenström H: The definitive forms of coxa plana. *Acta Radiol* 1922;1;384–394.)

flat. In type 4 there is flattening of the femoral head and concomitant flattening of the acetabulum. Type 5 has flattening of the femoral head but the acetabulum remains spherical, producing severe incongruity. Type 5 is usually seen only in children more than 9 years of age at onset. In a long-term follow-up study, Stulberg and associates[31] found that radiographic osteoarthritic changes were present in no patients with type 1 disease, in 16% with type 2, 58% with type 3, 75% with type 4, and 78% with type 5. Only patients with type 5 disease had symptomatic degenerative disease.

Q: What is the history of treatment of Perthes' disease?

A: Treatment of the disorder has largely evolved on an empiric basis. By and large, this means that an assumption about the problem was made and a logical means to affect the outcome was tried. While this approach has been associated with many medical advances, it is always necessary to verify the outcome relative to some control or standard. This has rarely, if ever, been done with Perthes' disease.

Let's start at the beginning. As was mentioned earlier, Legg treated his first five patients with traction, bracing, spica casts, and femoral neck curettage.[3] (The last was probably done to rule out infection.) Subsequently, the usual treatment was bedrest with or without splinting. Some patients in this era were treated with a patten bottom brace. This device suspended the affected leg from an ischial weightbearing caliper and required an elevated shoe on the other foot. The principle was to relieve weightbearing forces across the hip joint. Modern biomechanical studies have revealed, however, that the compressive muscular forces acting across the hip joint produce as much or more intra-articular pressure when this device is worn as is produced by normal activities. Nonetheless, this was a widely used mode of treatment and many of the early "control" patients were treated in this manner.

Snyder, in a most candid 1947 article, described the birth of a new form of treatment.[32]

F. H., an 8-year-old boy with unilateral LCP had an initial period of bed rest, after which he was allowed up with crutches; he continued however to bear weight on the involved leg, either walking or standing on it at times. His father asked for some sort of sling to help the child hold his leg off the ground and the one shown in the figure was the result.

The article resulted in widespread use of the Snyder sling (Fig. 27–3) and it is interesting to note its "scientific" basis:

Several children are now wearing this type of sling, and are able to walk with crutches and attend orthopedic school. The muscle spasm disappears after a few weeks, and quite normal rounding of the head of the femur results in due time without much atrophy and in most cases with very little shortening of the limb.

No data, no radiographic evaluation, and no follow-up were presented. This report was the basis of a treatment program used widely throughout the world for many years. (An occasional patient still appears with a sling around the waist.)

These modes of management have been termed non-containment treatment. There are a few studies of the results of such treatment. The most complete was that of Kelly and associates.[33] They had 64 good results (80%), nine fair results (11%), and seven poor results (9%). Of the hips classified in Catterall groups III and IV, 72% had good results. Few subsequent studies of patients treated with containment methods reported overall results as good as these.

The next major empiric idea for treatment was containment. The theory starts with the observation that the femoral head in the early stages of the disease becomes softer than normal and tends to flatten out and extrude laterally from the acetabulum. The basis of the theory is the concept that maintaining the softened head within the confines of the acetabulum may cause it to respond to the concentric pressure of the joint and maintain its shape. The earliest reports of containment dealt with bedrest and abduction splinting. Pike[34] had 36% good and excellent results in patients kept in bed only, and 83% good and excellent results when abduction splinting was also used. Katz[35] had 12% poor results in patients treated in bed with abduction splints when the age at onset was under 7 years and 50% poor results when it was more than 7 years. (This obviously raises the question of whether we are seeing the effects of treatment or of age at onset.) Many patients in this era were hospitalized for long periods of time, often for as long as three or four years. Brotherton and McKibbin[25] used a nonambulatory program of abduction braces and plasters and prolonged recumbency in the hospital. They had 88% good results, 10% fair results, and 2% poor results. In patients with hips classified as Catterall group III, results were 44% good, 38% fair, and 18% poor; results in hips in Catterall group IV were 50% good and 50% fair. The average time of treatment was 26 months with some patients hospitalized as long as 44 months.

The next logical step in containment theory was to begin allowing the children to ambulate in an abduction orthosis or cast. Petrie and Bitenc's[36] results were 60% good, 31% fair, and 8% poor in patients allowed to ambulate in "broomstick" plasters held in abduction and internal rotation. Harrison and associates[37] used the Birmingham brace—which abducted and internally rotated the hip, had a kneeling bar, and was padlocked on to ensure compliance—with "good" results. Kamhi and MacEwen[38] compared the results of treatment with and without containment. Without containment the results were 13% good, 30% fair, and 57% poor. With containment the results were 13% good, 53% fair, and 33% poor, a marginal reduction in the number of poor results. The effect of age appeared in their series too: for the total group of patients, the age at onset averaged 5.4 years and for those with poor results, 8.7 years. Purvis and associates[39] reported their results with the Atlanta Scottish Rite brace, a relatively uncomplicated device that allows a greater degree of freedom than the previous designs. It consists of a pelvic band connected to thigh cuffs. The hips are held in abduction

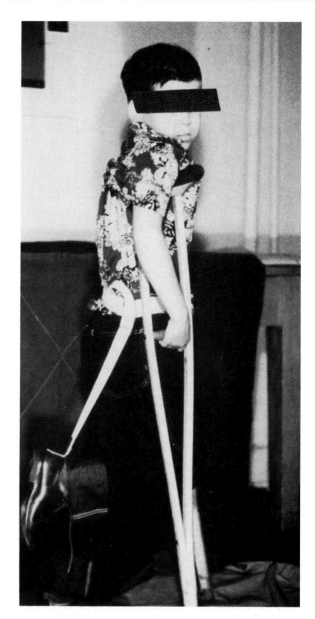

Fig. 27-3 The Synder sling.

by an extensile center bar connected to the cuffs with ball joints. They had 32% good results, 42% fair results, and 26% poor results. In patients in Catterall groups III and IV, results were 24% good, 52% fair, and 24% poor.

The most recent step in containment management is surgical repositioning of either the femoral head or the acetabulum to redirect the hip geometry. The two common methods are the femoral varus osteotomy and the innominate osteotomy of Salter. The concept is that the osteotomies place the femoral head deeper within the confines of the acetabulum, thereby preventing flattening. As with other forms of containment, the prerequisite to definitive containment is the regaining of an adequate range of motion and relief of muscle spasm and irritability. Lloyd-Roberts and associates'[40] results were 44% good, 22% fair, and 34% poor in patients who were older than 6 years at disease onset, had risk factors, and were treated with femoral varus osteotomy. In the "control" group (who had noncontainment treatment) results were 17% good, 33% fair, and 50% poor. Lloyd-Roberts and Catterall[41] later reported the results of selective surgical treatment and again showed improvement of outcome relative to controls (osteotomy: 51% good, 25% fair, and 24% poor; control: 14% good, 38% fair, and 48% poor). Hoikka and associates[27] reported a series of 112 osteotomies; in hips in Catterall groups III and IV at risk, they had 51% good results, 26% fair results, and 23% poor results. They too noted the disturbing effect of age at onset. "The result worsened with the increasing age of the patient at operation. It was seldom good if the patient's age was over nine years. No correlation was found between the result and the femoral neck-shaft angle."

There also have been a number of articles dealing with innominate osteotomy. It is important to note that the actual effect of the surgery is difficult to ascertain in these reports because of the variability of the disease. For example, when Ingman and associates[28] compared innominate osteotomy with spica cast treatment, they noted that age was more significant than treatment in determining outcome.

A similar conclusion comes from a large, multicenter study reported by the Perthes' Study Group.[42] They saw differences in treatment groups (crutches, Scottish Rite brace, Newington orthosis, and femoral osteotomy) that favored containment treatment. They cautioned, however, "It is difficult to draw firm conclusions about the relative merits of the three ambulatory treatment methods because of the differences in prognosis of the patients in the treatment groups."

At first it may seem that the reported results of treatment so strongly support the concept of containment treatment that the only real choice is not whether to use containment treatment, but rather what type. To the contrary, it must be noted that no report regarding treatment of Perthes' disease includes a truly untreated control group. Furthermore, no investigator has reported statistically significant differences among the treated groups. Many of the evident differences may be nothing more than selection biases. A major shortcoming affecting everyone trying to study Perthes' disease is that our ability to determine the probable severity of disease in an individual patient before treatment is quite poor. In a 1980 study, experienced observers showed little ability to apply the Catterall classification to hip radiographs taken within the first three months after diagnosis.[43] Thus, it is likely that the apparent effects of treatment in many series were really just differences in selection of patients. While the noncontainment series of Kelly and associates[33] had results equal

to or better than those of the current containment series, the same selection biases may have been responsible for their good results.

The other vital factor, sometimes not delineated in studies, is the age factor. If one examines the reported results relative to age at onset, the outcome is more consistently related to the age factor than to treatment. In fact, the extreme variability of disease severity makes meaningful interpretation of any uncontrolled series difficult, if not impossible. Early "control" patients were all treated by many different methods, and thus were not controls at all. Our current dilemma may be best summed up by a distinctly skeptical statement from an editorial by Burwell and Harrison[44]:

Perthes' disease, managed largely by orthopedic surgeons, has stood relatively isolated from knowledge and theory of contemporary bone biology as the latter has evolved during this century. . . . The concept of "matched controls" is, in our opinion, a sterile self-delusion. . . . We must submit to the discipline of the independent prospective trial. . . . It may be that Perthes' disease is now moving out of the stage of being a kitchen art.

How far we have progressed! Listen to Waldenström[45] in 1922.

As early as 1909 or 1910 I had the idea that no intervention should be undertaken. No improvement is to be expected from it. The prognosis is so good without any treatment whatever and with an operation of the joint we may of course do great harm, even if no effect therefrom is noticed until some long time afterwards. Operative therapy is tried by some few; the indications are based on the incorrect interpretation of the bad functional results of coxa plana. In my own opinion, the functional results are remarkably good, and a surgical intervention only injures the sufferer.

His method of treatment was as follows: "During the first three to five years [of the disease] it should not take part in gymnastics, neither should it jump on one leg, nor jump too much at all, nor take very long walks, etc."

References

1. Waldenström H: Der obere tuberkulöse Collumherd. *Z Orthop Chir* 1909;24:487–512.
2. Goff CW: *Legg-Calvé-Perthes' Syndrome and Related Osteochondroses of Youth.* Springfield, Charles C Thomas, 1954.
3. Legg AT: An obscure affection of the hip-joint. *Boston Med Surg J* 1910;162:202–204.
4. Perthes G: Über Arthritis deformans juvenilis. *Dtsch Z Chir* 1910;107:111–159.
5. Legg AT: The end results of coxa plana. *J Bone Joint Surg* 1927;9:26–36.
6. Schwarz E: A typical disease of the upper femoral epiphysis [1913]. Reprinted in *Clin Orthop* 1986;209:5–12.
7. Inoue A, Freeman MA, Vernon-Roberts B, et al: The pathogenesis of Perthes' disease. *J Bone Joint Surg* 1976;58B:453–461.
8. Green NE, Griffin PP: Intra-osseous venous pressure in Legg-Perthes disease. *J Bone Joint Surg* 1982;64A:666–671.
9. Iwasaki K: The change of venous circulation of the proximal part of the femur after varus osteotomy. *Nippon Seikeigeka Gakkai Zasshi* 1986;60:237–249.
10. Kristmundsdottir F, Burwell RG, Hall DJ, et al: A longitudinal

study of carpal bone development in Perthes' disease: Its significance for both radiologic standstill and bilateral disease. *Clin Orthop* 1986;209:115–123.

11. Burwell RG, Vernon CL, Dangerfield PH, et al: Raised somatomedin activity in the serum of young boys with Perthes' disease revealed by bioassay: A disease of growth transition? *Clin Orthop* 1986;209:129–138.

12. Rayner PH, Schwalbe SL, Hall DJ: An assessment of endocrine function in boys with Perthes' disease. *Clin Orthop* 1986;209:124–128.

13. Purry NA: The incidence of Perthes' disease in three population groups in the Eastern Cape region of South Africa. *J Bone Joint Surg* 1982;64B:286–288.

14. Barker DJ, Hall AJ: The epidemiology of Perthes' disease. *Clin Orthop* 1986;209:89–94.

15. Hall DJ: Genetic aspects of Perthes' disease: A critical review. *Clin Orthop* 1986;209:100–114.

16. Douglas G, Rang M: The role of trauma in the pathogenesis of the osteochondroses. *Clin Orthop* 1981;158:28–32.

17. Waldenström H: The definitive forms of coxa plana. *Acta Radiol* 1922;1:384–394.

18. Whitman R: Observations on Legg-Perthes' disease with particular reference to operative treatment. *Am J Surg* 1928;4:185–187.

19. Ratliff AHC: Perthes' disease: A study of thirty-four hips observed for thirty years. *J Bone Joint Surg* 1967;49B:102–107.

20. Gower WE, Johnston RC: Legg-Perthes disease: Long-term follow-up of thirty-six patients. *J Bone Joint Surg* 1971;53A:759–768.

21. Lloyd-Roberts GC: The management of Perthes' disease, editorial. *J Bone Joint Surg* 1982;64B:1–2.

22. Englehardt P: Die Spatprognose des Morbus Perthes: Welche Factoren bestimmen desarthroserisiko? *Z Orthop* 1985;123:168–181.

23. McAndrew MP, Weinstein SL: A long-term follow-up of Legg-Calvé-Perthes disease. *J Bone Joint Surg* 1984;66A:860–869.

24. Møller PF: The clinical observations after healing of Calvé-Perthes disease compared with the final deformities left by that disease, and the bearing of those final deformities on ultimate prognosis. *Acta Radiol* 1926;5:1–36.

25. Brotherton BJ, McKibbin B: Perthes' disease treated by prolonged recumbency and femoral head containment: A long-term appraisal. *J Bone Joint Surg* 1977;59B:8–14.

26. Evans DL: Legg-Calvé-Perthes' disease: A study of late results. *J Bone Joint Surg* 1958;40B:168–181.

27. Hoikka V, Lindholm TS, Poussa M: Intertrochanteric varus osteotomy in Legg-Calvé-Perthes disease: A report of 112 hips. *J Pediatr Orthop* 1986;6:600–604.

28. Ingman AM, Paterson DC, Sutherland AD: A comparison between innominate osteotomy and hip spica in the treatment of Legg-Perthes' disease. *Clin Orthop* 1982;163:141–147.

29. Catterall A: The natural history of Perthes' disease. *J Bone Joint Surg* 1971;53B:37–53.

30. Salter RB, Thompson GH: Legg-Calvé-Perthes' disease: The prognostic significance of the subchondral fracture and a two-group classification of the femoral head involvement. *J Bone Joint Surg* 1984;66A:479–489.

31. Stulberg SD, Cooperman DR, Wallensten R: The natural history of Legg-Calvé-Perthes disease. *J Bone Joint Surg* 1981;63A:1095–1108.

32. Snyder CF: A sling for use in Legg-Perthes disease. *J Bone Joint Surg* 1947;29:524–526.

33. Kelly FB Jr, Canale ST, Jones RR: Legg-Calvé-Perthes disease: Long-term evaluation of non-containment treatment. *J Bone Joint Surg* 1980;62A:400–407.

34. Pike MM: Legg-Perthes' disease: A method of conservative treatment. *J Bone Joint Surg* 1950;32A:663–670.

35. Katz JF: Conservative treatment of Legg-Calvé-Perthes disease. *J Bone Joint Surg* 1967;49A:1043–1051.

36. Petrie JG, Bitenc I: The abduction weight-bearing treatment in Legg-Perthes' disease. *J Bone Joint Surg* 1971;53B:54–62.

37. Harrison MH, Turner MH, Smith DN: Perthes' disease: Treatment with the Birmingham splint. *J Bone Joint Surg* 1982;64B:3–11.

38. Kamhi E, MacEwen GD: Treatment of Legg-Calvé-Perthes disease: Prognostic value of Catterall classification. *J Bone Joint Surg* 1975;57A:651–654.

39. Purvis JM, Dimon JH III, Meehan PL, et al: Preliminary experience with the Scottish Rite Hospital abduction orthosis for Legg-Perthes disease. *Clin Orthop* 1980;150:49–53.

40. Lloyd-Roberts GC, Catterall A, Salamon PB: A controlled study of the indications for and the results of femoral osteotomy in Perthes' disease. *J Bone Joint Surg* 1976;58B:31–36.

41. Lloyd-Roberts GC, Catterall A: A controlled study of the results of femoral osteotomy in severe Perthes' disease. *J Bone Joint Surg* 1980;62B:438–440.

42. Cooperman DR, Stulberg SD: Ambulatory containment treatment in Perthes' disease. *Clin Orthop* 1986;203:289–300.

43. Hardcastle PH, Ross R, Hamalainen M, et al: Catterall grouping of Perthes' disease: An assessment of observer error and prognosis using the Catterall classification. *J Bone Joint Surg* 1980;62B:428–431.

44. Burwell RG, Harrison MHM: Editorial comment. *Clin Orthop* 1986;209:2–4.

45. Waldenström H: On coxa plana. *Acta Chir Scand* 1923;55:577–590.

Equalization of Lower-Limb Inequality by Lengthening

Sherman S. Coleman, MD

Mechanical lengthening of a shortened lower limb is a well-accepted and widely employed surgical procedure. Previous techniques that stimulated growth have been abandoned because of their unpredictable results and the frequency of unattractive side effects. Thus, procedures such as sympathectomy[1] (designed to increase blood supply), creation of arteriovenous fistulas,[2] insertion of subepiphyseal foreign bodies,[3] and multiple osteotomies or other repeated surgical trauma[4] have been relegated to history.

Because of technical advances and our greater understanding of the problems and complications in limb lengthening, nearly all modern techniques use some form of osteotomy and gradual distraction to achieve the lengthening desired. This can be done safely, but there are still many unavoidable problems. In many instances, especially those having to do with congenital or developmental shortening, efforts to elongate the limb are basically nonphysiologic.

Several different technical and therapeutic programs have evolved. Some of these have clearly established track records,[5] whereas others require further study. Because too few patients have been operated on for statistically significant conclusions to be drawn, innovations must be regarded with caution. Nonetheless, it is important that these newer techniques be considered, because early reports suggest that they will assume a place in our surgical treatment.

It is essential that our enthusiasm for surgical techniques does not overshadow the all-important issues of indications and prerequisites for lengthening a lower limb. Thus, we must weigh all the various factors carefully before embarking on a procedure that is ambitious, lengthy, and oftentimes worrisome, regardless of the technique chosen. The most important considerations include both objective and subjective issues. The former are rather straightforward, because they can be measured and assessed rather accurately. The latter are much more difficult to put into perspective because of the many philosophic and individual concerns involved.

Criteria for Surgery

The objective determinants include the degree of discrepancy, the anticipated adult height of the patient, the cause of the shortening, the sex of the patient, the radiographic and clinical configuration and function of the foot, ankle, knee, and hip, and any general or ex-

tenuating health circumstances. Of these, the most critical are the degree of the discrepancy and the configuration of the hip joint (in femoral lengthening) and whether or not the foot and ankle are or can be made plantigrade with acceptable function (in tibial lengthening). If the discrepancy, for example, exceeds 18 cm, then lengthening is rarely a realistic goal, even lengthening of both major lower limb bones simultaneously with later appropriate shortening of the contralateral side. On the other hand, if the ultimate discrepancy is likely to be less than 3 to 4 cm, limb lengthening is probably not justified.

Further, if the foot is not plantigrade or cannot be made plantigrade, or if the ankle is grossly unstable, limb lengthening is probably inadvisable. I believe that the first question that must be settled is whether or not the patient and the patient's parents are willing to accept the status of the foot and ankle for the remainder of the patient's life. If so, then serious consideration of limb lengthening is appropriate. If not, then such a procedure is probably contraindicated. The other objective data that must be considered in this decision-making process have been discussed in considerable detail elsewhere.[6]

The subjective criteria that must be assessed include the patient's and parents' desires, especially as they relate to ultimate adult height, and the prolonged nature of the lengthening process. These are highly personalized issues and can only be decided by the patient and the parents. This does not mean, however, that the physician's advice and knowledge are not important ingredients in defining the problem and outlining the options.

Surgery

The lower limb can be lengthened through the femur, the tibia, or both. Furthermore, in some unusual and highly specialized instances, it is possible to lengthen the femur and tibia simultaneously.[7] This requires substantial experience with both tibial and femoral lengthening and should be done only when extensive discrepancies exist. The problems and complications inherent in performing simultaneous tibial and femoral elongations are substantial, and this ambitious and extensive program should not be undertaken by a surgeon who performs these procedures only occasionally.

Tibial Lengthening

Tibial lengthening has been the most commonly used method. Although several attempts to lengthen the lower limb were reported after Codivilla[8] performed a femoral elongation in 1905, Abbott and Crego[9] and Anderson[10] (a student of Abbott) were the ones who established the practicability of tibial lengthening in modest discrepancies of more than 4 to 5 cm. The popularity of femoral lengthening lagged behind that of tibial lengthening, presumably because of the technical problems created by the unique anatomy of the thigh, until Bost and Larsen[11] and Westin[12] developed a technique to lengthen the femur.

The most popular tibial lengthening technique in the United States is the one described and popularized by Wagner.[5] The procedure is based upon three basic concepts. It is an open diaphyseal lengthening in which the osteotomy is made transversely, precisely midway between two sets of pins (6.5-mm Schanz-type pins) placed into both proximal and distal metaphyses of the tibia (Fig. 28–1). These pins are placed through the medial aspect of the tibia and traverse both cortices. Before this is done, the distal fibula is transfixed to the tibia by means of a 3.5- or 4.5-mm hexagon-head screw to stabilize the ankle mortice. The fibula is then transected just proximal to the screw. After radiographic verification of the placement of the Schanz screws with respect to both location and depth, the distraction device is applied and the transverse tibial osteotomy is done. In all cases I routinely perform an anterior compartment fasciotomy. In all instances of congenital or developmental shortening I decompress the common peroneal nerve at the level of the neck of the fibula and proximally under the shelving edge of the biceps tendon, because Wagner[5] showed that peroneal palsies are more apt to result from compression of the deep fascia over the peroneal nerve than from neuropraxia caused by traction. After a few turns of the distraction knob, the wound is closed. Radiographic verification of alignment of the fragments completes the operation (Fig. 28–2).

Postoperatively, the foot and ankle go through daily or twice-daily range-of-motion exercises. At least 20 degrees of motion in each range should be maintained. This usually requires the assistance of a qualified physical therapist. If this range of motion cannot be accomplished, then the lengthening process must be interrupted temporarily. Ankle motion is necessary for proper articular cartilage joint nutrition and to avoid permanent ankle stiffness. One or two days after the osteotomy and application of the distraction device, the formal lengthening process is begun. One full turn of the knob on the Wagner device equals 1.6 mm. In most cases, the full turn is accomplished on a once-daily basis; twice-daily half turns are sometimes used when the distraction produces unusual discomfort.

The neurovascular status of the foot and ankle must be carefully monitored during the lengthening process. Also, the patient's blood pressure and ankle joint range of motion must be measured and recorded. Both systolic and diastolic blood pressures tend to rise in some patients during the elongation process. If the diastolic pressure exceeds 100 mm Hg, further lengthening must cease until the diastolic pressure has returned to an acceptable level (90 to 100 mm Hg). Correspondingly, if the range of ankle joint motion is less than 20 degrees, lengthening should be interrupted until the range increases. These appear to be minor issues, but they often make the difference between success and major compromise or failure.

In most instances, 4 to 5 cm of distraction can be achieved in three to four weeks without much difficulty. However, some degree of ankle equinus often develops during the elongation process. It is rare to see any evidence of osseous union within this period, and I have followed Wagner's program of stabilizing the distracted fragments by insertion of a specially constructed lengthening plate and screws. I have also accompanied it by implantation of an autogenous iliac bone graft (Fig. 28–3). If ankle equinus is excessive, I may also perform a heel cord lengthening at the same time. In such cases, however, a below-knee cast must be applied to hold the ankle in its corrected position. This cast is removed in four to six weeks.

Bony consolidation of the distracted area usually occurs within three to six months after plating and bone grafting (Fig. 28–4). Weightbearing is then begun gradually, depending on the radiographic appearance of the grafted area of the bone. Physical activities are restricted until the marrow cavity has re-formed and the cortical bone of the lengthened area has been restored to normal. This often requires one to two years in children and skeletally immature adolescents.

It has been my policy to remove the plate and screws in two separate sessions. At about 18 months, depending on the radiographic appearance of healing, I remove every other screw and loosen the remaining screws at least one or two full turns (Fig. 28–5). Any excess bone about the plate is also removed to permit some longitudinal weightbearing forces to be transmitted through the tibia. The patient is then permitted protected weightbearing (with one crutch) for four to six weeks. Thereafter, full weightbearing is allowed, but contact or high-velocity sports are not recommended.

Six months later, when further osseous consolidation has usually taken place, the entire plate and the remainder of the screws are removed (Fig. 28–6). The same postoperative restrictions on activities are imposed as for the first screw removal. By doing it in this manner, I have had no late fractures either through the area of lengthening or through the screw holes. Before this program was instituted, the incidence of fractures after one-step plate and screw removal was substantial (Fig. 28–7).

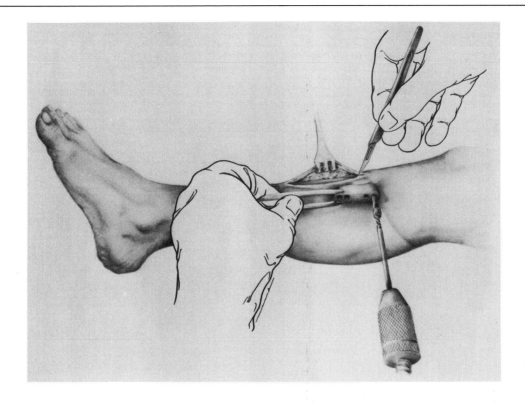

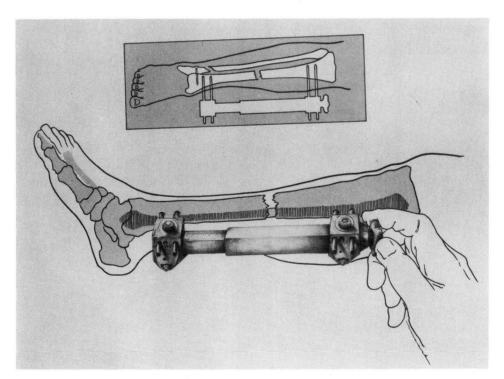

Fig. 28-1 The Wagner technique. **Top:** The holes for insertion of the Schanz pins are predrilled with a 3.5-mm drill. A drill guide and template are used. **Bottom:** A diaphyseal osteotomy is done after placement of the distraction device. The fragments are then separated about 1 cm.

Throughout the entire postoperative period, continuous efforts must be made to regain the preoperative range of ankle motion and muscle strength. An occasional patient may require heel cord lengthening; in some instances lengthening of the posterior tibial tendon was necessary. Such cases are, however, uncom-

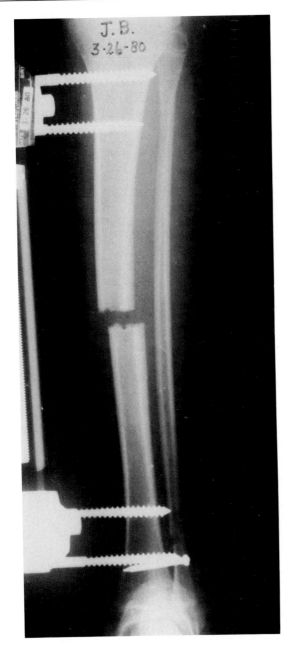

Fig. 28-2 Radiograph shows the Schanz pins properly positioned in the proximal and distal fibula and the osteotomy in mid shaft.

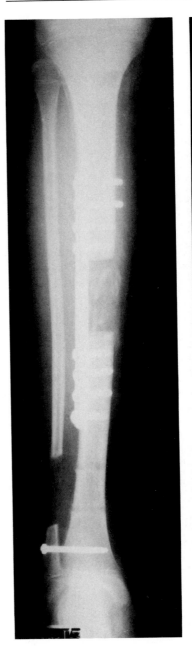
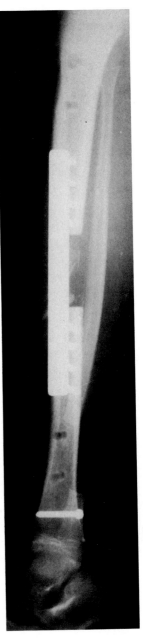

Fig. 28-3 Once the desired lengthening is achieved, the gap between the distracted fragments is grafted and a lengthening plate is applied.

mon, and almost always occur in patients with congenital or developmental discrepancies.

Femoral Lengthening

Femoral lengthening by the Wagner method uses the same principles and concepts as tibial lengthening. Two 6.5-mm Schanz pins are placed into the proximal and distal femoral metaphyses over the anterolateral aspect of the thigh. Both cortices are engaged by the pins, and their position is checked radiographically (Fig. 28-8). Through a posterolateral incision in the thigh, placed midway between the two sets of pins, the femur is ex-

posed. With the distraction device in place, a transverse osteotomy is made in the femur exactly equidistant from the two sets of pins. The femoral osteotomy site is then distracted several millimeters and the fascia lata, lateral intermuscular septum, and periosteum are incised circumferentially. This permits the femoral osteotomy to be distracted rather easily for about 1 cm. The lateral retinaculum and fascia lata are generously incised at the level of the distal pin, and the knee is carried through the full preoperative range of motion. If this cannot be accomplished, further release of the retinaculum

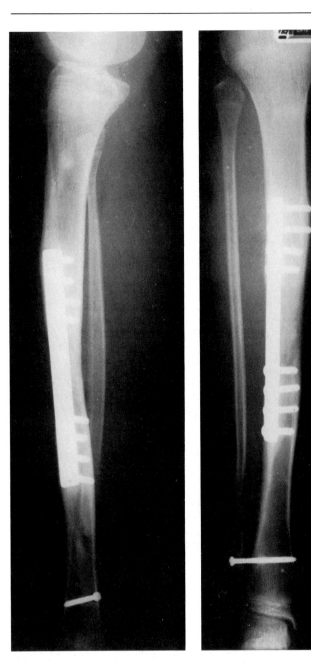

Fig. 28-4 Radiograph shows consolidation of the grafted area. The remodeled bone grafts are substantially mature.

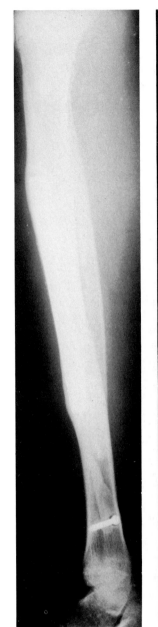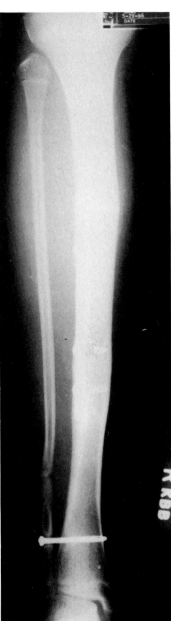

Fig. 28-5 Four of the eight original screws have been removed and the remaining four have been loosened.

and iliotibial tract is usually required. The correct alignment of the distracted fragments is then verified radiographically and the wound is closed.

Postoperatively I now use a continuous passive motion device designed to maintain full extension and at least 60 degrees of flexion. This is in keeping with Wagner's protocol. Range of motion is verified once or twice daily by a physical therapist during the lengthening process. The knob on the distraction device is turned one full turn daily (1.6 mm). Some patients are able to tolerate a half turn twice a day more comfortably. This is a highly individual issue. Assessment of

joint range of motion, neurovascular status, and blood pressure is done in the same manner as in tibial lengthening.

At the conclusion of the lengthening procedure, the distracted area almost always requires plating and bone grafting (Fig. 28-9). This is best accomplished with the patient in the prone position, with the posterior iliac crest serving as the bone donor site. I use the same incision used for the osteotomy. This requires that the pins and distraction device be carefully draped and meticulously excluded from the surgical incisions.

Postoperatively, the basic convalescent program is

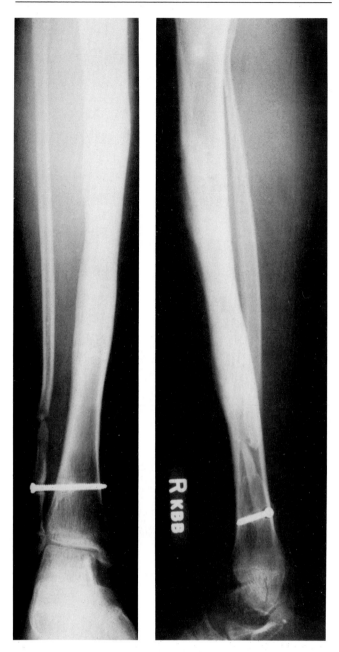

Fig. 28-6 All screws and the plate have been removed. The cortices of the bone in the distracted area are reasonably well formed.

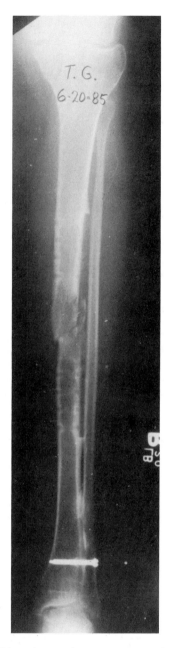

Fig. 28-7 This patient underwent one-step plate and screw removal four years after bone grafting and plating. The stress-shielding effect of the strong plate discouraged strong bone formation, and the tibia fractured shortly after weightbearing was begun.

the same as that in tibial lengthening. The emphasis is on regaining and increasing the knee's range of motion and thigh muscle strength. Removal of the plate and screws is the same as that in tibial lengthening.

Other Methods

Other methods of limb lengthening have been introduced recently.[13-16] The best-known are the Verona and the Ilizarov techniques.[16] Other variations include the method of femoral lengthening used by Barnes in the United States (W. Barnes, personal communication, 1983) and Klisic in Yugoslavia (P. Klisic, personal com-

munication, May 1987). These techniques employ different concepts, and their usefulness is not yet well established. I have no personal experience with any of these techniques, so my descriptions will be brief.

Elongation by means of physeal distraction has been practiced primarily in Italy. This technique uses two transfixion pins in the epiphysis and two in the metaphysis. No incision is made for osteotomy, but the physis is slowly distracted until it "gives." Distraction is then continued and the void created by the separated physis

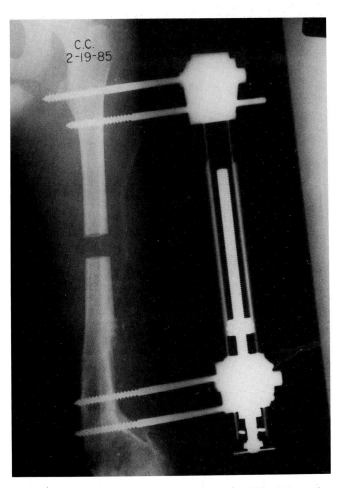

Fig. 28–8 Radiograph shows proper placement of the Schanz pins in the femur; osteotomy had been done and the fragments have been distracted 1 cm. Alignment is excellent.

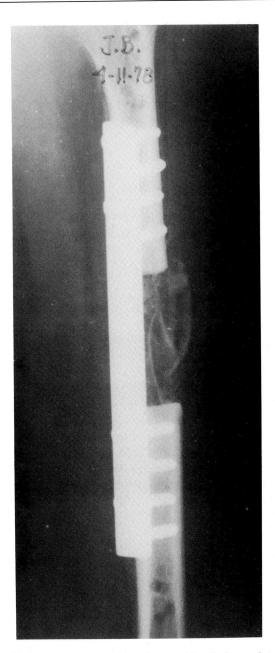

Fig. 28–9 After the desired length was achieved, the gap between the fragments was grafted with autogenous iliac bone and the fragments were fixed with a lengthening plate.

is steadily replaced by ossification of the proliferating physeal cartilage.

The advantages of this method are the absence of a major surgical wound and osteotomy and the rather predictable healing of the distracted area, therefore making internal fixation or bone grafting unnecessary. The disadvantages are substantial: (1) The procedure cannot be accomplished unless the physis is open. This excludes its use in acquired shortenings caused by physeal arrest. (2) The physis fuses at the conclusion of lengthening; thus, the procedure should only be done when the patient nears skeletal maturity, when the physis is still open. (3) It is only effective in the proximal tibia or distal femur because of the technical difficulty of placing transfixion pins in the distal tibial epiphysis. (4) The knee joint's range of motion is often difficult to maintain, and substantial long-lasting stiffness has been observed.

Ilizarov's technique employs a series of circular rings through which small, smooth Kirschner wires are placed, transfixing either the femur or the tibia both proximally and distally. Through a small incision in the proximal metaphysis, an incomplete "corticotomy" is done with a small osteotome. The final osteoclasis is done manually. Damage to the medullary contents must be avoided. Distraction is then carried out at the rate of 1 mm per day. Reparative bone can be seen early in the period of elongation and it is predictable enough to make internal fixation or bone grafting unnecessary. According to Ilizarov, the patient may be ambulatory (partial weightbearing) during the lengthening and consolidation process.

The advantages are self-evident. The disadvantages are the rather lengthy time required for consolidation (as long as 300 days), and the protracted period of pin care that is necessary. There may be other complications and problems of which I am not aware.

The method of femoral lengthening described by Barnes differs from other techniques in that it employs a sliding plate mechanism placed on the femur after a transverse osteotomy has been done in the proximal femur. The lengthening must be carried out at intervals thereafter (usually one to two weeks apart). This requires another operation to achieve elongation. No transfixion device is placed through the skin, the procedure is self-contained in the femur, and the plate serves as internal fixation until sufficient consolidation has occurred for weightbearing. The major disadvantage is the need for multiple and repeated (although relatively minor) surgical procedures.

Klisic of Yugoslavia prefers lengthening done in the metaphyseal area of the lower femur. He uses transfixion pins and a distraction device, as described by others.[13-16] The distal metaphysis is chosen because of its rich blood supply and the rapid healing of the distracted area. Grafting or internal fixation is rarely needed.

My experience during the past 15 years has been limited to the Wagner method. This does not mean that the other techniques do not have merit. Until they are proven to be more effective, more predictable, and less likely to produce problems and complications than Wagner's technique, I will continue my current program.

References

1. Barr JS, Stinchfield AJ, Reidy JA: Sympathetic ganglionectomy and limb length in poliomyelitis. *J Bone Joint Surg* 1950;32A:793–802.
2. Jones JM, Musgrove JE: Effect of arteriovenous fistula on the growth of bone: Preliminary report. *Mayo Clin Proc* 1949;24:405.
3. Pease CN: Local stimulation of growth of long bones: A preliminary report. *J Bone Joint Surg* 1952;34A:1–24.
4. Sofield HA, Blair SJ, Millar EA: Leg-lengthening: A personal follow-up of forty patients some twenty years after the operation. *J Bone Joint Surg* 1958;40A:311–322.
5. Wagner H: Operative Beinverlangerung. *Chirurg* 1971;42:260.
6. Coleman SS: Lower limb length discrepancy, in Lovell WW, Winter RB (eds): *Pediatric Orthopaedics*. Philadelphia, JB Lippincott, 1978.
7. Coleman SS: Simultaneous femoral and tibial lengthening for limb length discrepancies. *Arch Orthop Trauma Surg* 1985;103:359–366.
8. Codivilla A: On the means of lengthening in the lower limbs, the muscles and tissues which are shortened through deformity. *Am J Orthop Surg* 1905;2:353.
9. Abbott LC, Crego CH: Operative lengthening of the femur. *South Med J* 1928;21:823.
10. Anderson WV: Leg lengthening. *J Bone Joint Surg* 1952;34B:150.
11. Bost FC, Larsen LJ: Experiences with lengthening of the femur over an intramedullary rod. *J Bone Joint Surg* 1956;38A:567–584.
12. Westin GW: Femoral lengthening using a periosteal sleeve: Report of twenty-six cases. *J Bone Joint Surg* 1967;49A:836.
13. Monticelli G, Spinelli R: Distraction epiphysiolysis as a method of limb lengthening: I. Experimental study. *Clin Orthop* 1981;154:254–261.
14. Monticelli G, Spinelli R, Bonucci E: Distraction epiphysiolysis as a method of limb lengthening: II. Morphologic investigations. *Clin Orthop* 1981;154:262–273.
15. Monticelli G, Spinelli R: Distraction epiphysiolysis as a method of limb lengthening: III. Clinical applications. *Clin Orthop* 1981;154:274–285.
16. Ilizarov A: The Ilizarov technique. Presented at the 16th Pediatric Orthopedic International Seminar: Symposium on Leg Length Equalization. San Francisco, CA, May 23–24, 1988.

Assessment and Prediction in Leg-Length Discrepancy

C. F. Moseley, MD

Introduction

The actual treatment of a growing child with leg-length discrepancy must be preceded by a series of steps. These include clinical and radiologic assessment, analysis, prediction of the future, and goal-setting. Particular attention must be given to the assessment of past growth and the prediction of both future growth and the effects of surgical treatment.

Because the therapeutic goal must be stated in terms of the child's situation at maturity, it is necessary to predict the pattern of future growth on the basis of a rigorous analysis of past growth. This can be done fairly accurately and confidently, but the methods for doing so demand clear understanding and familiarity with the concepts involved and an awareness of possible pitfalls.

Clinical Assessment

Although a complete medical history should be obtained, it should be noted that historical information concerning the perceived growth patterns of the child, the heights of the parents and other family members, and the relative height of the patient compared with other children of the same age, although interesting, are not good predictors of future growth. Predictions are most reliable when they are based on leg-length and skeletal-age data, because these data are correlated in a known way and it is in these terms that the growth pattern is described.

It is self-evident that the assessment of the patient's leg-length discrepancy should include measurements of leg length. It must also, however, include all factors that contribute to the asymmetry because they may affect the therapeutic outcome.

With the patient supine, the true leg length is measured from the anterior superior iliac spine to the medial malleolus, and the apparent length from the umbilicus to the malleolus. The calculated discrepancies from the two techniques should be the same. Any difference is caused by pelvic obliquity. The measurement can be checked by squaring the legs with the pelvis and observing the relative levels of the medial malleoli. The legs should also be observed for angular deformities. With the patient standing, it is possible to assess the relative heights of the feet and the relative heights of the iliac crests. It is very useful to block-up the heel of the short leg until the optimum position has been reached. This makes apparent the total effect of all the factors contributing to the asymmetry.

The patient should also be examined for fixed pelvic obliquity and spinal imbalance, because these factors, if present, greatly influence the treatment goal. It may not be desirable to achieve leg-length equality and a level pelvis if fixed pelvic obliquity would then result in an unbalanced trunk. The patient's gait must be observed with respect to the disability resulting from the discrepancy or from other associated factors. In the presence of weakness or paralysis, for example, it is best to leave the weak leg 1 or 2 cm short to facilitate clearing the floor during swing phase. To confirm the appropriateness of the treatment goal, it is valuable to examine the gait while the patient wears a shoe with a temporary lift that equals the planned correction.

Radiologic Assessment

The radiologic assessment of the patient involves: (1) measurement of leg lengths, (2) determination of skeletal age, and (3) assessment of other contributing factors.

Three principal techniques are available for measuring leg length. The first is called a "teleoroentgenogram," an "orthoroentgenogram," or, simply, "three-foot legs" (Fig. 29–1). It involves a single exposure of the legs, including the hips and ankles, on a single film with a tube-to-film distance of 6 ft. It has the advantages of showing angular deformity and requiring only one exposure, but is subject to an inconsistent magnification error.

The "scanogram" (Fig. 29–2) obviates magnification error by exposing the hips, knees, and ankles separately, moving the tube and film so that the central X-ray beam always passes through the joint. Placement of a radiopaque rule behind the legs allows precise measurement of lengths without magnification error. The disadvantage of this technique is that movement of the patient between exposures may introduce error and, therefore, it is not reliable for children less than 6 years old who are likely to move.

The third method is computerized digital radiography. This technique minimizes radiation exposure, reduces mathematical error by having the computer calculate the length between designated landmarks, and can provide accurate measurements even in the presence of angular deformity.

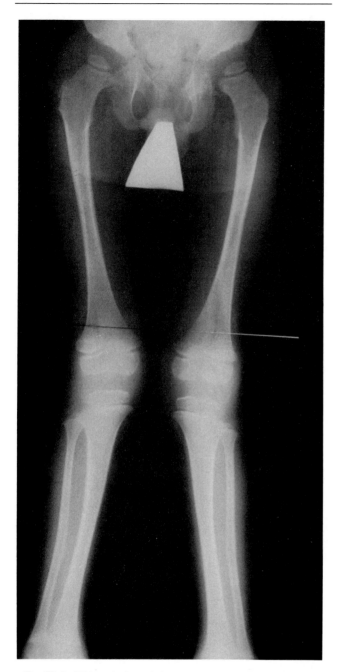

Fig. 29-1   This technique (teleoroentgenogram, orthoroentgenogram, or "three-foot legs") shows angular deformities but entails magnification error.

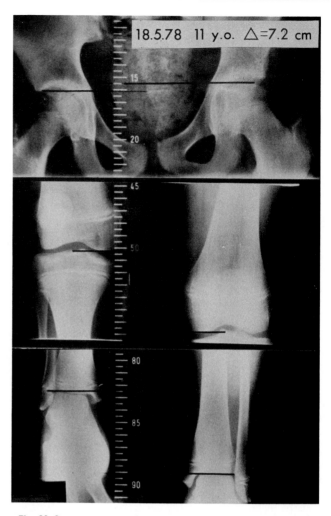

Fig. 29-2   In this scanogram, the hips, knees, and ankles are exposed separately so that the central X-ray beam passes through the joint, eliminating magnification error. The radiopaque rule permits lengths to be determined.

Many techniques have been described for determining skeletal age. Of the two principal ones, only that of Greulich and Pyle[1] is suitable for use in this context. The Greulich-Pyle atlas contains standard radiographs of the left hand and wrist of boys and girls of various skeletal ages. The skeletal age of the patient is determined by comparing the patient's radiograph with the standards and choosing the standard that most closely approximates it. Because the standards are sometimes more than a year apart, there is a significant error built into this technique. Also, not all children exactly follow the development pattern described by the atlas and some have congenital anomalies of the hand and wrist that make such a comparison difficult. Significant interobserver and intraobserver variations have been documented with this method.

The second method is that developed by Tanner and associates.[2] It uses the wrist radiograph in a different way to arrive at a more accurate determination. This method involves the assignment of a development score to each of 20 different bony landmarks in the hand and wrist. The skeletal age is derived from the total of the 20 scores. Although this technique has a smaller standard error, it is based on a population different from that in the atlas of Greulich and Pyle and has not been correlated with leg length. It cannot, therefore, be used in this context.

Radiographs can also be used to assess asymmetries of the feet and pelvis, obliquity of the pelvis, and spinal deformity and balance. It is sometimes useful to take an anteroposterior radiograph of the pelvis and hips with blocks under the heel on the short side to determine the true functional discrepancy, including the foot, and to assess the effect of correction on the lumbar spine.

Analysis and Prediction

Three methods are useful in the analysis of past growth, the prediction of future growth, and the planning of surgery. These three methods will be discussed in general terms, along with step-by-step instructions for their use.

In 1944 White and Stubbins[3] described a method based on a linear approximation of the true growth pattern. Menelaus[4] later published a series using this method with good results. This might be called the "rule-of-thumb method" because it is not quite as accurate as the others but is simpler and more convenient. It is useful if surgical correction is not imminent. To use it one only needs to remember that the distal femoral physis grows 10 mm/yr and the proximal tibial 6 mm/yr, and that girls finish growth at 14 years of age and boys at 16 years of age. The accuracy of this method is compromised by the fact that growth does not occur at a constant rate and does not stop abruptly.

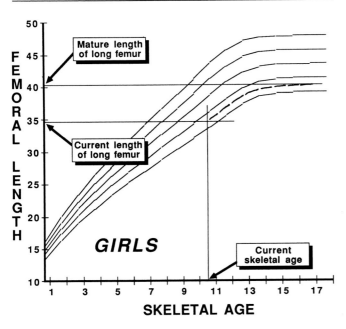

Fig. 29-3 The Green-Anderson growth chart is used to predict the length of the bone at maturity. The point representing the most recent visit is plotted using the length of the bone and the skeletal age. A line is drawn freehand from that point relative to the standard deviation lines until it plateaus and becomes horizontal. This represents the end of growth and the predicted length of the leg at maturity. Clinically, this procedure would also be done for the tibia. (Based on data from Anderson and associates.[5])

The "growth-remaining method" of Anderson and associates[5] uses a combination of graphs and calculations. The patient's growth data can be plotted on graphs showing the growth patterns of the femur and tibia of boys and girls, thus predicting the length of the long leg at maturity. A series of calculations then allows one to predict the discrepancy at maturity, and this in turn allows the use of the second graph showing the growth remaining in the epiphyses about the knee to determine the effect of epiphysiodesis. This method does not take into account the growth percentile of the child and depends on the accuracy of a single determination of skeletal age with its inherent inaccuracy.

The third method, or the "straight-line-graph method,"[6,7] uses a special graph derived from the growth data of Anderson and associates.[8] It represents the growth of the legs as straight lines and provides nomograms for using skeletal age data. The assessment of past growth, the prediction of future growth, and the prediction of the effect of surgery are all accomplished by plotting points and lines on the graph. This method automatically takes into account the child's growth percentile and minimizes the error inherent in skeletal age determination by averaging a number of determinations.

Step-by-Step Instructions

The Rule-of-Thumb Method

Required Information The distal femur grows 10 mm/yr. The proximal tibia grows 6 mm/yr. Girls stop growing at 14 years of age (calendar age, not skeletal age). Boys stop growing at 16 years of age.

Step 1 Calculate the longest time interval of data (date of most recent visit minus date of first visit).

Step 2 Calculate the years of growth remaining (age of maturity minus present age).

Step 3 Calculate the past growth of both legs (length at most recent visit minus length at first visit).

Step 4 Calculate the growth rates of both legs (past growth divided by time).

Step 5 Calculate the future growth of the legs (growth rate multiplied by years remaining).

Step 6 Predict the leg lengths at maturity (length at last visit plus future growth).

Step 7 Calculate the discrepancy at maturity (predicted length of long leg minus predicted length of short leg).

Step 8 Predict the amount of correction by epiphysiodesis (growth rate of plate multiplied by years remaining).

Step 9 Calculate the result of epiphysiodesis (discrepancy at maturity minus correction).

The Growth-Remaining Method

Requirements Green-Anderson graphs (or data) relating lengths of tibias and femurs to skeletal age and a Green-Anderson growth-remaining chart.

Step 1 Calculate the past growth of both legs (length at latest visit minus length at first visit).

Step 2 Calculate the discrepancy at last visit (length of long leg minus length of short leg).

Step 3 Calculate the growth inhibition (growth of long leg minus growth of short leg, multiplied by 100 and then divided by growth of long leg).

Step 4 Relate length of long leg to the population. We will call this the growth "percentage" since it is not, strictly speaking, the growth "percentile." To predict future growth by this method it is necessary to fit the patient into the Green-Anderson data, in other words, to answer the question: "How long is this patient's long leg compared to the mean for this skeletal age?" This can be done mathematically or graphically.

By calculation: (1) Determine the mean leg length for the population by finding the sum of the lengths of the tibia and femur for children of the appropriate sex from the Green-Anderson study. (2) Calculate this patient's growth "percentage" by multiplying the length of the long leg by 100 and dividing by the population mean.

By graph: Plot the lengths of the tibia and femur of the long leg on the Green-Anderson graphs relating bone length to skeletal age for boys or girls (Fig. 29–3).

Step 5 Predict the length of the long leg at maturity. This step can be done mathematically or graphically, depending on how the previous step was done. Both methods should give the same result.

By calculation: (1) Determine the mean length of the long leg at maturity for the population (of the appropriate sex) by reference to the Green-Anderson data. (2) Predict the length of the long leg at maturity (mean length of population multiplied by growth percentage and divided by 100).

By graph: For both tibia and femur, starting at the point plotted in the previous step, project a line (freehand) upward and to the right, maintaining a constant relationship to the percentile lines. These lines will plateau at the mature lengths of the bones, and the sum of these lengths gives the mature length of the leg.

Step 6 Calculate future growth of the long leg (length at maturity minus present length).

Step 7 Calculate the future increase in discrepancy (future growth of long leg multiplied by growth inhibition and divided by 100).

Step 8 Calculate the predicted discrepancy at maturity (present discrepancy plus future increase).

Step 9 Predict the amount of correction by epiphysiodesis. Refer to the Green-Anderson growth-remain-

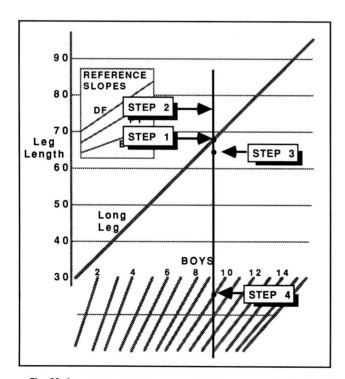
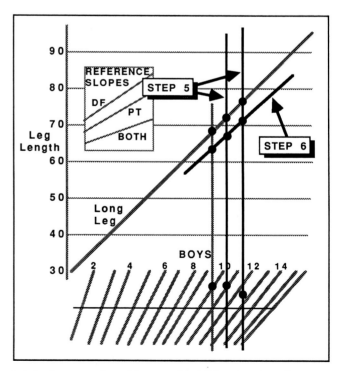

Fig. 29–4 The straight-line graph. **Left:** The points for leg lengths and skeletal age are plotted for one visit. **Right:** Data for subsequent visits and the growth line of the short leg.

ing graph. For the appropriate sex and skeletal age, determine the amount of growth reduction that would result from arresting growth above and below the knee.

The Straight-Line Graph

Requirements The straight-line graph.

Step 1 Plot the length of the long leg at the first visit. This point lies on the printed line for the long leg, at the appropriate length (Fig. 29–4, *left*).

Step 2 Draw the line for that visit. This is a vertical line that passes through the just-plotted point for the long leg and also through the skeletal age area for the appropriate sex. All points for this visit will be on this line (Fig. 29–4, *left*).

Step 3 Plot the point for the short leg. This point lies on the vertical line just plotted, at the appropriate length (Fig. 29–4, *left*).

Step 4 Plot the point for skeletal age. This point lies on the same vertical line. It is placed with reference to the sloping lines for skeletal age, and is interpolated between two of those lines if necessary (Fig. 29–4, *left*). Even if skeletal age is not available, it is worthwhile to plot the points for leg length. It will not contribute to predicting length at maturity but will help in plotting the line for the short leg.

Step 5 Repeat these steps for each visit. When all points have been plotted the graph will show a series of vertical lines, each representing an assessment of the child at one moment in time (Fig. 29–4, *right*).

Step 6 Draw the growth line of the short leg. This is the straight line that best fits the points previously plotted for the short leg (Fig. 29–4, *right*). It usually fits those points very accurately. If it does not, there is probably a measurement error, either in the radiographic technique (such as movement during the scan) or in the interpretation of the film (such as inconsistent landmarks). In the example shown in Figure 29–4, *right*, the straight line diverges from the growth line of the long leg, indicating growth inhibition and increasing discrepancy.

Step 7 Draw the growth percentile line. Draw the horizontal straight line that best fits the points previously plotted in the skeletal age area (Fig. 29–5). Because of the error inherent in the estimation of skeletal age, this line may not fit these points very closely. It must be drawn horizontally even if a sloping line appears to give a better fit. If there is a marked discrepancy between the positions of early skeletal age points compared to more recent points, then the more recent points should be considered to be more valid. Project this line to the right until it intersects the sloping line of mature skeletal age.

Fig. 29–5 The straight-line graph used to plot the growth percentile line and the maturity line. The position of the growth percentile line in this example shows that the leg lengths are longer than the mean. The points at which the growth lines of the two legs intersect the maturity line show the predicted lengths at maturity.

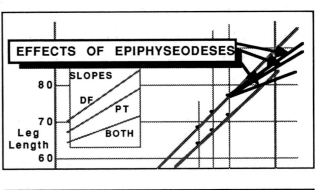
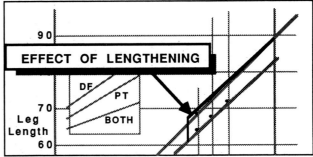

Fig. 29–6 The straight-line graph used to predict the effects of surgical correction. The predicted results of three types of epiphysiodesis are shown. In this example, a combined epiphysiodesis of the femur and tibia would overcorrect the discrepancy. It is not yet time for a single femoral or tibial epiphysiodesis.

Step 8 Draw the maturity line. From the point where the growth percentile line just drawn meets the sloping line of mature skeletal age, draw a vertical straight line to intersect the growth lines of the two legs (Fig. 29–5). This line represents the predicted situation at maturity. The two intersection points represent the predicted leg lengths at maturity, and, of course, the distance between them represents the anticipated discrepancy at maturity.

Step 9 Predict the effects of epiphysiodesis. Refer to the reference slopes for the three possible growth arrest procedures. From the point for the long leg at the last visit, draw three lines to the right, parallel to the three reference slopes (Fig. 29–6). Here is an easy way to draw parallel lines: (1) Place the long edge of a rectangular ruler (like those used for scoliosis) on the chosen reference slope. (2) Place the long edge of a second ruler against the left end of the first. (3) Holding the second ruler steady, slide the first ruler along it. As long as their edges are apposed, all lines drawn along the first ruler will be parallel to the reference slope. The three lines drawn parallel to the reference slopes will intersect the vertical maturity line at points that represent the lengths of the long leg at maturity after the corresponding epiphysiodesis. Exact equalization is indicated by a point of intersection the same as that of the short leg.

Step 10 Predict the effect of lengthening. From the vertical line of the last visit, draw a line parallel to that of the short leg, and elevated above it by exactly the amount of the lengthening. If the lengthening is exactly equal to the projected discrepancy at maturity, this line will meet the maturity line at exactly the same point as the growth line of the long leg. If, conversely, the lengthening is equal to the present discrepancy, it may

not. In the case of growth inhibition, it is necessary to overlengthen the leg of the growing child.

Summary

Successful treatment of patients with leg-length discrepancy requires rigorous assessment of the patient, usually over a period of time. This assessment involves not only the lengths of the legs, but all the factors that contribute to the asymmetry because they are all important in the selection of a treatment goal. Good results can be obtained with any of the three methods of prediction. Selection of a particular method must be based on convenience, accuracy, and user familiarity.

References

1. Greulich WW, Pyle SI: *Radiographic Atlas of Skeletal Development of the Hand and Wrist*, ed 2. Stanford, CA, Stanford University Press, 1959.
2. Tanner JM, Whitehouse RH, Marshall WA, et al: *Assessment of Skeletal Maturity and Prediction of Adult Height (TW2 Method)*. New York, Academic Press, 1975.
3. White JW, Stubbins SG Jr: Growth arrest for equalizing leg lengths. *JAMA* 1944;126:1146.
4. Menelaus MB: Correction of leg length discrepancy by epiphyseal arrest. *J Bone Joint Surg* 1966;48B:336.
5. Anderson M, Green WT, Messner MB: Growth and predictions of growth in the lower extremities. *J Bone Joint Surg* 1963;45A:1–14.
6. Moseley CF: A straight-line graph for leg-length discrepancies. *J Bone Joint Surg* 1977;59A:174–179.
7. Moseley CF: A straight line graph for leg length discrepancies. *Clin Orthop* 1978;136:33–40.
8. Anderson M, Messner MB, Green WT: Distribution of lengths of the normal femur and tibia in children from one to eighteen years of age. *J Bone Joint Surg* 1964;46A:1197.

Metaphyseal and Physeal Lengthening

Charles T. Price, MD

Introduction

New techniques for limb lengthening offer the advantage of lengthening without the need for bone grafting or internal fixation.[1-4] It remains to be seen whether the soft-tissue problems associated with lengthening will be decreased as a result of these newer techniques.

Limb lengthening without bone grafting was achieved by the Anderson technique of percutaneous osteotomy and gradual distraction, but many investigators noted that the osteogenic response was variable and unpredictable.[5-7] When union did occur, the new bone was often attenuated and poorly resistant to torsional stress.[6] As a consequence, routine grafting and plating, as advocated by Wagner, became popular.[8-11] However, the Wagner plate is a stress-shielding device and refracture may occur after plate removal.[8,11]

New Techniques

Distraction osteogenesis or callotasis popular today promotes better bone formation and eliminates the need for secondary grafting or internal fixation. These principles were first developed in Russia by Ilizarov at about the same time that Anderson was introducing his method in the United States. Because of language, social, and political barriers we did not become aware of Ilizarov's method until it gained popularity in Italy and Western Europe.[12]

The Ilizarov device is constructed from many small through-and-through transfixion pins attached to circular rings (Fig. 30–1). Stability depends on tension in the wires and criss-cross pin placement. Pin placement is demanding and construction of the frame can be complicated. Full rings with through-and-through pins are especially difficult for the femur and humerus. However, certain complicated angular corrections are possible with the Ilizarov device that are not possible with unilateral fixators. Segmental bone transfers and double-level lengthenings may also be easier with the Ilizarov device. The Ilizarov device has been modified and other devices have been developed as well.[3,13,14] De Bastiani and associates[2,15] developed a unilateral fixator using half pins, which allows distraction osteogenesis. This device, known as Orthofix, incorporates a telescopic body and very stiff pins tapered from 6 to 5 mm to maximize pin-bone rigidity. The telescopic body can

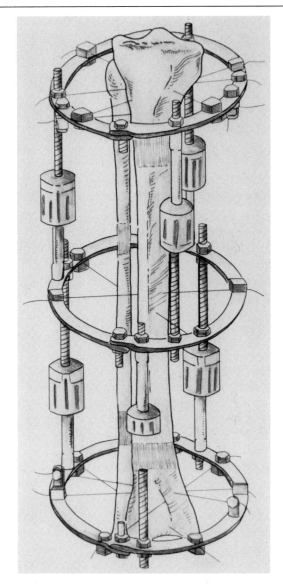

Fig. 30-1 Ilizarov device applied for double-level corticotomy or segmental transfer.

be released after osteogenesis occurs. This permits axial loading through bone and encourages corticalization.

I believe that the unilateral De Bastiani device is more appropriate for most lengthenings. It is simpler to apply, less bulky, and better tolerated by patients.

Regardless of the device chosen to guide the distraction, the steps of the procedure are designed to incorporate the biologic principles developed by Ilizarov.

Application of the Device

Whenever possible, the device is applied so that the osteotomy can be performed in metaphyseal bone. Osteogenesis is more rapid in the metaphyseal region. This is probably the result of the increased blood supply and increased diameter of the bone in this region. If the osteotomy is placed in the diaphysis, osteogenesis will still occur but may be delayed. The fixator must be aligned parallel to the shaft of the bone in order to avoid translation of the fragments as they are separated.

Osteotomy

Osteotomy or corticotomy is performed through a very limited opening. Care must be taken to preserve the periosteum and to protect, as much as possible, the intramedullary blood supply. For both femoral and tibial lengthening the approach is anterior. The proximal fibers of the rectus femoris muscle are separated to approach the femur. The periosteum is incised and elevated. An osteotome is used to divide the cortex by the method of Ilizarov. De Bastiani and associates modified this technique by predrilling holes in just the cortex before using the osteotome. The key is to perform a very gentle low-energy osteotomy in order to minimize inflammatory response and vascular disruption.

Waiting Period

The next step is a waiting period of seven to 15 days, while the osteotomy is held in its original or slightly compressed position. The duration of this waiting period has been determined by clinical experience. Skeletally immature patients require a shorter waiting period of seven to ten days, whereas skeletally mature patients need ten to 15 days. The waiting period is shorter if the Ilizarov device is used. This may be because the elasticity of the Ilizarov frame requires a brief period of distraction before the slack is out of the system and the bone begins to lengthen. This waiting period allows the inflammatory phase of healing to subside and the reparative phase to begin. In nondisplaced fractures it has been demonstrated that the reparative phase begins after four to 12 days.[16-18] Production of collagen and fibroblasts reaches a maximum at approximately one week.[19,20] The older the patient, the denser the bone; or the more trauma associated with the osteotomy, the longer the waiting period needs to be. At least partial weightbearing begins immediately after surgery and continues throughout the entire treatment period.

Distraction Period

Distraction is initiated at a rate of 1 mm/day in increments of 0.25 mm four times each day. Experimental evidence suggests that a distraction rate of 0.5 mm/day leads to premature consolidation, whereas rates of 1.5 mm/day or more produce local ischemia and exceed the rate of osteogenesis.[1,12] Ilizarov's experimental

observations are supported clinically by the poor osteogenic response noted with the techniques of Anderson and Wagner, in which lengthening proceeds at the rate of 1.5 mm/day.

The rhythm or frequency of lengthening is also important. In 1979 Leong and associates[21] recommended distraction at ". . . equally spaced time intervals to obtain repetitive load cycles and thereby reduce peak values of load and maintain similar stress relaxation patterns for each instantaneous load increase." Ilizarov's[1] studies of distraction frequency (once a day, twice a day, four times a day, and continuous motorized distraction) showed improved osteogenesis with increased frequency although the total amount of length gained remained constant at 1 mm/day. Continuous motorized distractor units are being developed by several companies, but at present it is most practical to initiate lengthening at the rate of 0.25 mm four times a day. After two or three weeks of lengthening it may be necessary to increase or decrease the rate of lengthening depending on the quality of bone formation. If callus formation is poor, or if the callus fractures during distraction, then a period of compression may be necessary before distraction is resumed.

It seems surprising that such prolific osteogenesis can occur under tension. Studies performed by Ilizarov[1] and by Aronson[22] have shown that the new bone trabeculae are oriented longitudinally in the direction of distraction. "Growth" occurs in the middle of the distraction gap by direct apposition. This bone formation occurs without the formation of cartilage or disorganized woven bone seen in fracture callus. This type of osteogenesis is pure intramembranous ossification. These observations suggest that intramembranous bone formation is stimulated by tensile forces. This concept is further supported by the observations that normal periosteal bone formation is intramembranous and that periosteum is a tissue known to be under tension.[23,24]

Ossification

After distraction has been completed and the immature bone has formed, it is necessary to achieve corticalization. This occurs with the Ilizarov device because there is some axial movement during weightbearing. Paley and associates[25] have shown that the Ilizarov device permits elastic deformation with axial loading. This may facilitate rapid transformation to lamellar bone. With the Orthofix device the telescopic body is locked and full weightbearing is encouraged. When radiographs show a smooth cortical surface, the telescopic body is released, so that axial load is transmitted through the bone, while torsion and angulation are prevented by the device.

Removal

The fixator is removed when radiographs show good bone consolidation. Total duration of lengthening, from initial surgery to removal of the device, is usually four to five weeks per centimeter gained in the tibia and five to six weeks per centimeter gained in the femur. The body of the fixator is removed and the pins are left in place for two to three days. Full weightbearing is encouraged. Should a fracture occur, the fixator can be reapplied without anesthesia.

Results

De Bastiani and associates[15] reported their results with 100 lengthenings by callus distraction. The increase in length obtained in nonachondroplastic patients averaged 11% (range, 9.5% to 12.0%) for the femur and 17% (range, 9.0% to 22.5%) for the tibia. This was comparable to gains in length reported with the Wagner technique. Their reported complication rate was only 14% (pin loosening in 2%, early consolidation in 7%, and fracture in 5%). This compared favorably with the 44.8% complication rate reported by Wagner.[8]

Cambras and associates,[13] using a modification of the Ilizarov technique, performed metaphyseal-diaphyseal corticotomy and lengthening in 38 patients ranging in age from 14 to 37 years. The mean increase in length was 6 cm (range, 3 to 15 cm). Complications occurred in 32% of patients (five superficial infections, two delayed consolidations, one neuropraxia, two persistent contractures, and two angular deformities). They achieved good results in 33 of their 38 patients.

Monticelli and Spinelli,[26] using a modified Ilizarov device, achieved the desired length in 42 of 43 patients. The average length gained was 7 cm (range, 4 to 10 cm). Major complications occurred in 16 patients (37%); these included two delayed ossifications, two deep pintract infections, one knee dislocation, and 11 residual ankle contractures. However, no patient required bone grafting and there were no refractures.

Dal Monte and Donzelli[4] performed the Ilizarov procedure in 13 patients with congenital tibial hypoplasia. The average correction was 36% of original length (range, 13% to 45%). There were 20 complications, including six contractures and one neuropraxia. There were no delayed consolidations and no fractures of the lengthened segment.

My early experience with the callus distraction technique of De Bastiani and associates included 18 completed lengthenings. The average gain in length was 28.7% (range, 10% to 50%). There were 18 major and minor complications, including one pin-tract infection, one pin loosening, two refractures, and 15 problems requiring additional anesthesia. These 15 procedures included one grafting and plating, four Achilles tendon lengthenings, three closed osteoclases for premature consolidation, and seven closed manipulations for angular deformity. Recent patients have been comfortable during manipulations without anesthesia. Despite these complications, all limbs achieved the desired length (Figs. 30–2 to 30–4).

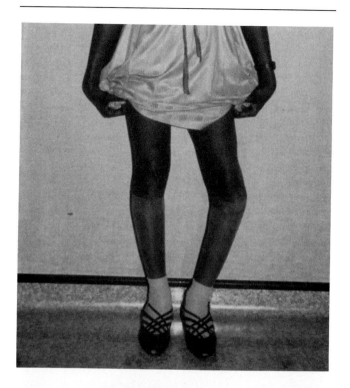

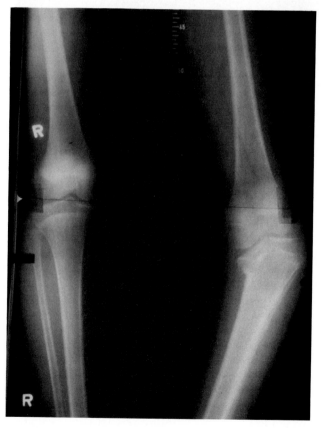

Fig. 30–2 Girl with varus deformity and 4.6-cm limb-length discrepancy after multiple osteotomies for infantile tibia vara. At this time she was 11 years 11 months old.

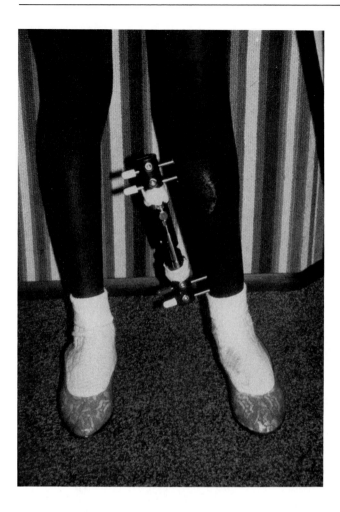

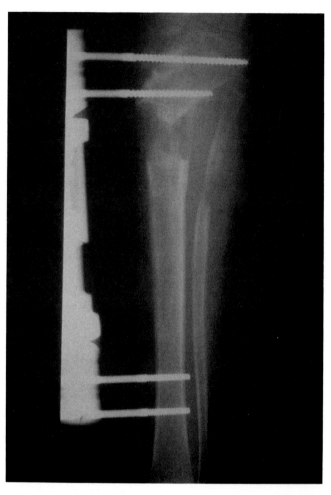

Fig. 30-3 Same patient shown in Figure 30–2 after osteotomy and lengthening by the technique of De Bastiani and associates. **Left:** Orthoflex external fixator. **Right:** Radiograph shows osteogenesis.

At this time, I believe that metaphyseal distraction osteogenesis is effective for correction of major limb-length discrepancies. The surgical indications and complications are similar to those of the Wagner technique. The principal advantage of metaphyseal lengthening is a reduced number of required surgical procedures.

Physeal Distraction

Lengthening through the physeal plate is attractive since this is where physiologic growth occurs, the area is highly vascular, and bone formation is rapid. The physeal region is wider than the diaphysis, so newly formed bone should be more resistant to fracture.

Physeal distraction is accomplished by percutaneously inserting pins proximal and distal to the physeal plate. Distraction begins in the immediate postoperative period. Many investigators report distraction at a rate of 1 mm/day until rupture of the growth plate occurs on the third or fourth day.[12,13,27,28] This rupture

is associated with a sudden diastasis of the growth plate and immediate pain that persists for two to five days. When the pain subsides, distraction continues in a manner similar to the cortical distraction discussed previously. Experimental and clinical studies have shown that this method of distraction by epiphysiolysis often allows growth to resume but may cause premature fusion of the physis with growth arrest after the completion of lengthening.[29–32] Several investigators have cautioned against this method of limb lengthening.[12,30] Ilizarov[1] abandoned physeal distraction in favor of cortical distraction, which is less painful and does not interfere with subsequent growth.

De Bastiani and associates[2] performed lengthening by physeal distraction at a slower rate of 0.5 mm/day. Their experimental work, as well as that of DePablos and Canadell,[31] has shown that this slower distraction rate gains length without disrupting the physeal plate. Increased thickness in the zone of hypertrophy occurs during lengthening but the physis reverts to a normal appearance after cessation of distraction.

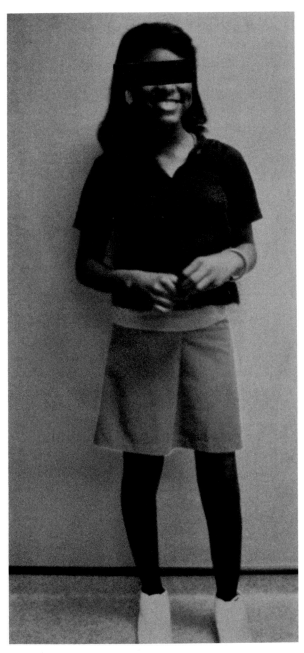

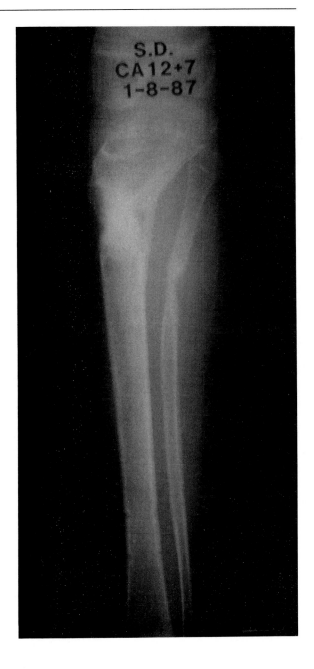

Fig. 30-4 Same patient shown in Figures 30–2 and 30–3. **Left:** Three months after removal of the fixator. **Right:** Radiograph shows excellent bone formation.

De Bastiani and associates[2] reported encouraging clinical results with slow physeal distraction in 40 patients with limb-length discrepancy. The average increase in length was 3.3 cm (10%), with a range of 1.5 to 7 cm (4.5% to 36%). Only five patients (12.5%) experienced complications. In all cases the lengthened physis resumed growth after completion of the procedure.

Despite encouraging reports on physeal distraction,[3,13,28,32] I believe that physeal distraction has very limited application. It should be reserved for older chil-

dren with less than two years of growth remaining because there is the risk of physeal rupture and growth arrest. Lengthening at the rate of 0.5 mm/day is a prolonged procedure when the discrepancy is major. Lengthening can be accomplished more quickly with corticotomy and callus distraction. Therefore, I reserve physeal distraction for children with 3- to 5-cm discrepancies who are too mature for epiphysiodesis or who refuse epiphysiodesis.

Additional problems with physeal distraction are encountered with regard to pin placement. Pin placement is very demanding because it is necessary to avoid the physeal plate and articular surfaces. The proximity of the pins to the joint restricts the range of motion and may be painful. In the distal femur the pins are intracapsular and septic arthritis is a potential complication.

Summary

The potential problems associated with physeal distraction and the relative success of callus distraction favor callus distraction as the procedure of choice for equalization of major limb-length discrepancies. Indications for lengthening are the same as in the Wagner procedure. The expected results and soft-tissue complications of callus distraction are similar to those of the Wagner technique. However, the number of procedures required and the osseous complications of lengthening appear to be reduced with these newer methods of limb lengthening.

References

1. Ilizarov G: Biologic principles of bone and soft tissue distraction neogenesis (regeneration—the theory of tension stress). Presented at the International Conference on the Ilizarov Techniques for the Management of Difficult Skeletal Problems, New York, Nov 1–3, 1987.
2. De Bastiani G, Aldegheri R, Renzi Brivio L, et al: Chondrodiastasis: Controlled symmetrical distraction of the epiphyseal plate. Limb lengthening in children. *J Bone Joint Surg* 1986;68B:550–556.
3. Monticelli G, Spinelli R: Distraction epiphysiolysis as a method of limb lengthening: III. Clinical applications. *Clin Orthop* 1981;154:274–285.
4. Dal Monte A, Donzelli 0: Tibial lengthening according to Ilizarov in congenital hypoplasia of the leg. *J Pediatr Orthop* 1987;7:135–138.
5. Coleman SS, Noonan TD: Anderson's method of tibial-lengthening by percutaneous osteotomy and gradual distraction: Experience with thirty-one cases. *J Bone Joint Surg* 1967;49A:263–279.
6. Gross RH: An evaluation of tibial lengthening procedures. *J Bone Joint Surg* 1971;53A:693–700.
7. Kawamura B, Hosono S, Takahashi T: The principles and technique of limb lengthening. *Int Orthop* 1981;5:69–83.
8. Wagner H: Operative lengthening of the femur. *Clin Orthop* 1978;136:125–142.
9. Hood RW, Riseborough EJ: Lengthening of the lower extremity by the Wagner method: A review of the Boston Children's Hospital Experience. *J Bone Joint Surg* 1981;63A:1122–1131.
10. Macnicol MF, Catto AM: Twenty-year review of tibial lengthening for poliomyelitis. *J Bone Joint Surg* 1982;64B:607–611.
11. Coleman S: Lower limb length discrepancy, in Lovell WW, Winter RB (eds): *Pediatric Orthopaedics*. Philadelphia, JB Lippincott, 1978, vol 2, pp 781–863.
12. Paley D: Current techniques of limb lengthening. *J Pediatr Orthop* 1988;8:73–92.
13. Cambras R, Puente J, Perez H, et al: Limb lengthening in children. *Orthopedics* 1984;7:468–476.
14. Mezhenina EP, Roulla EA, Pechersky AG, et al: Methods of limb elongation with congenital inequality in children. *J Pediatr Orthop* 1984;4:201–207.
15. De Bastiani G, Aldegheri R, Renzi-Brivio L, et al: Limb lengthening by callus distraction (callotasis). *J Pediatr Orthop* 1987;7:129–134.
16. Rhinelander FW, Baragry RA: Microangiography in bone healing: I. Undisplaced closed fractures. *J Bone Joint Surg* 1962;44A:1273–1298.
17. Enneking W: The repair of complete fractures of rat tibias. *Anat Rec* 1948;101:515.
18. Brand R, Rubin C: Fracture healing, in Albright JA, Brand RA (eds): *The Scientific Basis of Orthopaedics*, ed 2. Norwalk, Appleton & Lange, 1987, pp 327–329.
19. Udupa KN, Prasad GC: Chemical and histochemical studies on the organic constituents in fracture repair in rats. *J Bone Joint Surg* 1963;45B:770–779.
20. Stacher G, Firschein H: Collagen and mineral kinetics in bone after fracture. *Am J Physiol* 1967;213:863–866.
21. Leong JC, Ma RY, Clark JA, et al: Viscoelastic behavior of tissue in leg lengthening by distraction. *Clin Orthop* 1979;139:102–109.
22. Aronson J: The calcium dynamics of controlled mechanical distraction osteogenesis. Presented at the International Conference on the Ilizarov Techniques for the Management of Difficult Skeletal Problems, New York, Nov 1–3, 1987.
23. Lynch M, Taylor J: Periosteal division and longitudinal growth in the tibia of the rat. *J Bone Joint Surg* 1987;69B:812–816.
24. Warrell E, Taylor J: The role of periosteal tension in the growth of long bones. *J Anat* 1979;128:179–184.
25. Paley D, Fleming B, Pope M, et al: A comparative study of fracture gap motion and shear in external fixation. Presented at the Conference on Recent Advances in External Fixation, Riva Del Garda, Sept 28–30, 1986.
26. Monticelli G, Spinelli R: Leg lengthening by closed metaphyseal corticotomy. *Ital J Orthop Traumatol* 1983;9:139–150.
27. Monticelli G, Spinelli R: Limb lengthening by epiphyseal distraction. *Int Orthop* 1981;5:85–90.
28. Grill F: Distraction of the epiphyseal cartilage as a method of limb lengthening. *J Pediatr Orthop* 1984;4:105–108.
29. Monticelli G, Spinelli R, Bonucci E: Distraction epiphysiolysis as a method of limb lengthening: II. Morphologic investigations. *Clin Orthop* 1981;154:262–273.
30. Letts RM, Meadows L: Epiphysiolysis as a method of limb lengthening. *Clin Orthop* 1978;133:230–237.
31. DePablos J, Canadell J: Bone lengthening by physeal distraction: An experimental study. *Orthop Trans* 1986;10:370.
32. De Bastiani G, Aldegheri R, Renzi Brivio L, et al: Limb lengthening by distraction of the epiphyseal plate: A comparison of two techniques in the rabbit. *J Bone Joint Surg* 1986;68B:545–549.

CHAPTER 31

Principles of Physeal Bridge Resection

Stephen W. Burke, MD

Introduction

An etiologically diverse group of conditions can lead to growth plate closure. They have in common the fact that bone forms across the growth plate because of either malposition of bony fragments or physeal cartilage death. This, in turn, acts as a "tether," leading to either partial or total cessation of growth.

Although data are still accumulating, it seems clear that a rational approach to this problem is to remove the epiphyseal tether, allowing normal growth to resume. A number of different techniques and interposition materials are available. Although the advantages and disadvantages of each are evident, certain principles apply in all cases.

Accurate Prediction of Further Growth and Ultimate Discrepancy and Angular Deformity

It is generally agreed that a patient being considered for bridge resection should have at least two years or 2 cm of growth remaining[1-4] because less than 2 cm of discrepancy is generally well tolerated by patients. To carry this concept one step further, bilateral partial epiphyseal closure, as occurs in some cases of Blount's disease, might be better and more predictably handled by epiphysiodesis rather than by a bilateral attempt to restore growth. If bridge resection is performed bilaterally, a unilateral "success" would create an unacceptable leg-length discrepancy.

Although accurate determination of the amount of growth remaining primarily involves the use of a bone-age film, other factors must be considered. Regardless of the bone age, I would not expect any significant growth after a bridge resection in a postmenarchal girl. Similarly, a patient of relatively short stature may require more than two years of growth to make bridge resection a viable option.

Accurate measurement of the length and the amount of the deformity of the involved bone can be accomplished by a variety of techniques. True scanograms have the advantage of accurately assessing both length and alignment on one film.

Adequate Delineation of Bone Bridge

It is generally accepted that bridges larger than 50% are not amenable to resection. Therefore, accurate delineation of the bridge is essential.

Plain radiographs are useful in determining if a bridge is present; oblique views, in addition to standard anteroposterior and lateral views, are frequently helpful. As Bright[2] pointed out, it is often helpful to obtain radiographs with the beam orthogonal to the involved physis. This may require special positioning. Nonetheless, plain radiographs by themselves are not sufficiently accurate to determine the extent of the bone bridge. Several alternative specialized radiologic techniques are available.

Tomography

Tomography can be classified by the path that the beam takes relative to the imaged object. Tomography may be linear, circular, or hypocycloidal. The farther the beam moves, the more blurred the surrounding tissues and the more accurately delineated the area in question will be. Since hypocycloidal tomography involves the most movement of the beam, this is the most accurate, and for the purposes of bridge resection should be used exclusively.[2] Trying to make do with linear tomography can lead to erroneous conclusions and inappropriate operations.

Bone Scan

Several techniques have been described for evaluation of the growth plate by means of bone scans. Apex views[5] provide useful information. Computed tomographic radionuclide scanning is now available. My limited experience with these techniques suggests that they are less useful than other modalities, at least at present.

Computed Tomography

Computed tomography by itself is of limited use in the evaluation of a bone bridge. Unless the tomographic cut is directly through the growth plate and the bridge, the bridge will not be visualized. However, improved technology, using 1- to 2-mm cuts through the area in question and reformatting them in 5-mm sagittal and coronal segments, provides clear images of the bridge (Fig. 31–1). In many instances, these are superior to the visualization obtained by tomography and delineate the epiphyseal bridge more accurately.

Mapping the Bridge

It is important to appreciate the three-dimensional nature of the bridge. Specialized radiographic studies superimposed on cross-sectional diagrams of the involved physis, as described by Carlson and Wenger,[6] are useful. Serial sagittal and coronal images are obtained

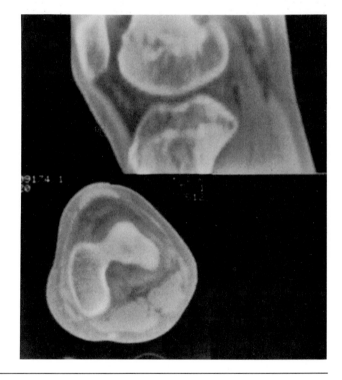

Fig. 31-1   A 12-year-old girl with a progressive valgus deformity of the left knee. **Top:** Anteroposterior radiograph. Note suggestion of lateral bar. **Bottom left:** Anteroposterior reconstruction from five-cut computed tomographic scan. Note lateral bar. **Bottom right:** Lateral reconstruction. Note posterior bar.

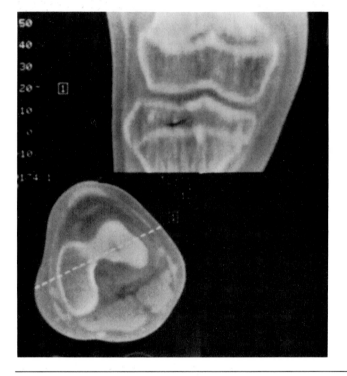

across the involved physis. A cross-sectional diagram of the physis is used, with lines representing the area of physeal closure seen on each anteroposterior and lateral section. The resulting cross-hatched area represents the physeal bridge (Fig. 31–2).

Accurate Atraumatic Resection of the Physeal Bridge and Realignment of the Extremity

When the bridge is resected, it is of paramount importance that the bar be removed without unnecessary damage to the residual viable growth plate. Hemostasis in the operative field by means of a tourniquet is generally advisable. Adequate illumination is essential and a head lamp is strongly recommended. For smaller joints, surgical loupes may be required.

To remove the bridge as expediently but as atraumatically as possible, sharp dental burrs and small sharp curettes to complete the removal are useful. Dental mirrors may help the surgeon to see into the recesses of the cavity.

The surgical exposure of the bridge depends somewhat on the nature of the bridge. Central bridges are best exposed through the metaphysis, either a metaphyseal window or the metaphyseal surface of an oste-

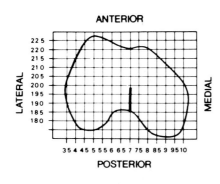
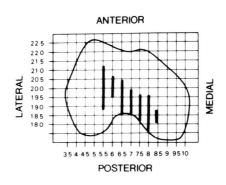
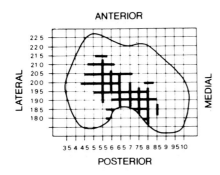
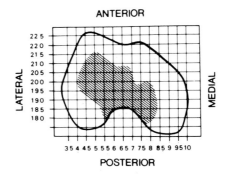

Fig. 31-2 Mapping technique. **Top left and top right:** Utilizing a cross-sectional schematic drawing, the area of apparent involvement seen on each sequential tomographic (or computed tomographic reformat) cut is plotted. **Bottom left:** Similar plotting for the orthagonal view. **Bottom right:** The cross-hatched area represents the bony bar. (Reproduced with permission from Carlson WO, Wenger DR: A mapping method to prepare for surgical excision of a partial physeal growth arrest. *J Pediatr Orthop* 1984;4:232–238.)

otomy if realignment of the extremity is indicated at the time of the procedure. The metaphyseal exposure should be located well away from the perichondrial ring to prevent inadvertent damage to the growth plate by perichondrial ring disruption.

In a peripheral or a combined peripheral-central bridge, entry through the perichondrial ring is required. To prevent a recurrent peripheral bridge, the perichondrial ring should be resected rather than reflected and reapproximated.

To minimize the damage to the intact physis, the growth plate should be identified through the physeal bridge and then exposed circumferentially, with the bar removed in a centrifugal pattern. After the growth plate is identified around the circumference of the bar, it should be undercut on both the epiphyseal and metaphyseal surfaces to ensure intimate contact with the interposition material. Obviously, overzealous undercutting may lead to further physeal damage and be counterproductive.[7]

Whether or not a realignment osteotomy is required at the time of bridge resection must be decided on a case-by-case basis. Generally, up to 30 degrees of de-

formity can be tolerated if it is in the plane of motion of the adjacent joint, whereas a deformity of more than 10 to 15 degrees probably requires realignment if it is not in the plane of the joint. Other factors that enter into the decision include the age of the child (the deformity is more likely to remodel in younger children with successful bridge resections) and the type of interposition material used (if the interposition material needs to be removed at maturity, any necessary correction of the residual deformity can be carried out at that time).

If simultaneous corrective osteotomy is contemplated, one must be aware that fixation—especially of the distal fragment—may be more difficult because of the bone removal necessitated by bridge resection. Fixation with pins and plaster or an external fixator may be helpful in this regard.

Prevention of Recurrent Bridge Formation

Prevention of recurrent bridge formation requires prevention of a hematoma in the cavity.[8] If a hematoma is allowed to form, it will heal into fibrous tissue and ultimately to bone, leading to recurrent bridge formation and recurrent deformity.

The first step in dealing with the cavity is to obtain hemostasis at the time of the bridge resection. This requires that the tourniquet be released and the cavity filled with thrombin-soaked Gelfoam or some other hemostatic material. After hemostasis has been obtained, this material should be removed before the interposition material is inserted. Insertion of some inert interposition material is necessary to prevent recurrent bridge formation. Three substances are in current clinical use: fat, medical elastomer 328 (Silastic), and Cranioplast. Additionally, cartilage has been used experimentally by several investigators. There are advantages and disadvantages to each (Table 31–1).

Fat is readily available, but is perhaps slightly less effective than Cranioplast or Silastic. It lends no inherent support to the bone, but has been shown histologically to remain viable for long periods. One problem with autologous fat is that some mechanism is needed to keep the fat within the cavity in intimate apposition to the bone. The solution seems to be to preserve the metaphyseal window when a metaphyseal approach is used. The window can then be sutured or wired back in place; this holds the fat down in the cavity. With peripheral bridges, in which a bone window is not feasible, construction of a suture stent is helpful.

Cranioplast and Silastic are protocol substances, requiring special consent before use. They appear to be equally effective, with Cranioplast perhaps lending more intrinsic support and stability to the bone than Silastic. Both of these substances require fixation to the epiphysis to prevent migration into the metaphysis, which has been associated with recurrent bridge formation. They both require removal at skeletal maturity.

Cartilage has been used as an interposition material only experimentally.[8,9] In laboratory animals, it is superior to fat, and seemingly does not require further surgery for its removal. The major problem is finding an adequate source that is free of the risk of immune reactions or diseases such as acquired immune deficiency syndrome or hepatitis.

Adequate Follow-up and Documentation

Radiographic measurements are clearly indicated in the follow-up of patients who undergo bridge resection. One difficulty is that bone surgery often stimulates all physes, making accurate determination of the effect of the bridge resection difficult. Metal markers in the form of either pins or wire sutures placed at the time of bridge resection make this follow-up determination much easier.

Follow-up to skeletal maturity is indicated, as premature closure of the physis may occur after several years of "normal" growth.[10,11]

Trying to compare the clinical results reported in published studies of bridge resection is difficult in that there is no way to control for the size of the bridge, the cause of the bridge, and other factors. Nevertheless, certain trends are evident. Good results are more likely with a newly formed bridge, a bridge caused by trauma, a central bridge, a smaller bridge, and a bridge in a younger child.[12]

Langenskiöld,[3] using fat as the interposition material in a series of 28 patients, reported good or excellent results in 15 patients, fair results in five, and poor results in eight. Williamson and Staheli[13] performed bridge resections with fat interposition in 22 patients. Mean growth was 81%. Results were excellent in 11 cases, good in five, fair in two, and poor in four. Ten of the fifteen angular deformities improved.

Bright,[11] who used Silastic in 100 patients, reported good or excellent results in 70 cases, fair results in 12, and poor results in 18. Complications included three wound infections, 13 recurrent bridges, and two reactions to the Silastic. Migration of the interposition material away from the physis accounted for most of the poor results.

Klassen and Peterson[14,15] used Cranioplast in 35 of 36 patients. They reported 25% to 95% growth in 23 patients, with ten actually having overgrowth. Three patients had normal growth. Recurrent bridges, generally associated with migration of the Cranioplast away from the physis, developed in six.

The various interposition materials seem to be equally

Table 31–1
Comparison of interposition materials*

Clinical Data	Materials			
	Fat	Silastic	Cranioplast	Cartilage
Availability	+++	Protocol	Protocol (?)	?
Efficacy	++, +++	+++	+++	++++
Stress raiser	++	++	+	++
Fixation required	No	Yes	Yes	No
Removal required	No	Yes	Yes	No

*Materials are rated as excellent = ++++, good = +++, fair = ++, and lowest = +.

effective, and the decision as to which one to use should be based on subjective considerations.

Conclusions

Resection of partial epiphyseal bridges is clearly efficacious in both laboratory experiments and clinical experience. Careful attention to detail in terms of remaining growth, delineation of extent of involvement, and careful surgical technique lead to predictable, satisfactory results in most patients.

References

1. Bright RW: Operative correction of partial epiphyseal plate closure by osseous-bridge resection and silicone-rubber implant: An experimental study in dogs. *J Bone Joint Surg* 1974;56A:655–664.
2. Bright RW: Physeal injuries, in Rockwood CA Jr, Wilkins KE, King RE (eds): *Fractures in Children*. Philadelphia, JB Lippincott, 1984, vol 3, 87–182.
3. Langenskiöld A: Surgical treatment of partial closure of the growth plate. *J Pediatr Orthop* 1981;1:3–11.
4. Langenskiöld A, Osterman K: Surgical treatment of partial closure of the epiphysial plate. *Reconstr Surg Traumatol* 1979;17:48–64.
5. Howman-Giles R, Trochei M, Yeates K, et al: Partial growth plate closure: Apex view on bone scan. *J Pediatr Orthop* 1985;5:109–111.
6. Carlson WO, Wenger DR: A mapping method to prepare for surgical excision of a partial physeal growth arrest. *J Pediatr Orthop* 1984;4:232–238.
7. Trueta J: *Studies on the Development and Decay of the Human Frame*. Philadelphia, WB Saunders, 1968.
8. Österman K: Operative elimination of partial premature epiphyseal closure: An experimental study. *Acta Orthop Scand*, 1972; 47 (suppl) 1–79.
9. Lennox DW, Goldner RD, Sussman MD: Cartilage as an interposition material to prevent transphyseal bone bridge formation: An experimental model. *J Pediatr Orthop* 1983;3:207–210.
10. Botte M, Sutherland DH, Mubarak SJ: Treatment of partial epiphyseal arrest by resection of the osseous bridge and interposition with silicone rubber. *Orthop Trans* 1985;9:37.
11. Bright RW: Partial growth arrest: Identification, classification and results of treatment. *Orthop Trans* 1982;6:65–66.
12. Talbert RE, Wilkins KE: Physeal bar resection: Factors contributing to success. *Orthop Trans* 1987;11:524.
13. Williamson RV, Staheli LT: Partial epiphyseal growth arrest: Treatment by bridge resection and fat interposition. *Orthop Trans* 1987;11:443.
14. Klassen RA, Peterson HA: Excision of physeal bars: The Mayo Clinic experience. *Orthop Trans* 1982;6:65.
15. Peterson HA: Partial growth plate arrest and its treatment. *J Pediatr Orthop* 1984;4:246–258.

Congenital Hip Dislocation: Techniques for Primary Open Reduction Including Femoral Shortening

Dennis R. Wenger, MD

Introduction

Ideally, congenital dislocation of the hip is diagnosed in infancy and treated with a Pavlik harness.[1] In North America, 6- to 18-month-old children are usually treated with skin traction followed by closed reduction. A few require open reduction by either an anterior[2,3] or medial (Ludloff) approach.[4] Most investigators recommend anterior open reduction and capsulorrhaphy in children more than 18 months of age. Traditionally, these procedures are performed after a two- to three-week period of skin traction in the hospital.[2,3]

Over the last decade, primary open reduction and femoral shortening without prior traction have become an accepted method of treatment of older children with congenital dislocation of the hip, especially children who are older than 4 years.[5-7] After gaining experience, some have used this method in children 3 years of age and older.[8] The use of this method is justified because expensive in-hospital traction is avoided, there is predictable maintenance of reduction, and the avascular necrosis rate is low. I agree with this approach and, in difficult social circumstances (families who were unable to cooperate with closed reduction for economic reasons, travel distance, or because home traction was impossible), I have used this method in children 2 years of age and older with predictable results. However, most 2- to 4-year-old children who have congenital dislocation of the hip can be treated by closed or open reduction after traction. The surgeon's philosophy and experience will determine the treatment choice for this age group.

Although primary open reduction and femoral shortening have become the favored method for treating congenital dislocation of the hip in older children in North America, other effective methods are available. Morel and Briand[9] described a successful technique for closed reduction using prolonged, longitudinal, internal-rotation traction to set the femur on a "reduction axis." This is followed by cast immobilization and then Salter innominate osteotomy. This requires several months of hospitalization. Although effective, such methods are not economically or culturally practical in North America.

This chapter describes an approach to treatment of congenital dislocation of the hip in the older child, emphasizing technical points that provide predictable maintenance of reduction. This approach is based on my surgical experience treating this condition in older children during the last 12 years. The gross pathologic anatomy of the deformed capsule is presented, followed by a detailed description of capsular exposure, excision, and repair. Capsulorrhaphy is emphasized because, in my experience, failure to correct soft-tissue deformity is one of the major reasons for resubluxation or redislocation after open reduction for congenital dislocation of the hip (Figs. 32–1 and 32–2). Techniques are presented for performing the associated femoral and acetabular bony procedures that allow early return to more normal hip anatomy and biomechanics.

Pathologic Anatomy

The completely dislocated hip in the older child becomes fixed in a position superior to the original true acetabulum. The degree of superior migration varies. The dislocated hip can be in a position of (1) severe subluxation (the inferior head still adjacent to the labrum), (2) dislocation with formation of a false acetabulum just superior to the true acetabulum, or (3) severe dislocation with the femoral head positioned high in the abductor musculature without formation of a false acetabulum. The extent of proximal migration determines the degree of pathologic deformation of the capsule and the extent of soft-tissue reconstruction required to correct the deformity.

The capsular abnormality in congenital dislocation of the hip must be recognized and corrected to achieve satisfactory results from open reduction. Acetabular redirection and femoral osteotomy are widely understood methods of bony correction, perhaps because the techniques can be illustrated clearly and documented radiographically. In contrast, the soft-tissue abnormalities and methods for their surgical correction are not well described. As a result, surgeons often produce a hip that appears to be reduced postoperatively (Fig. 32–1, *top right*), but the hip subluxates with weight-bearing or redislocates (Fig. 32–1, *bottom*). The bony correction can appear faultless on the radiograph.

Soft-Tissue Abnormalities

The dislocated hip leads to adaptive enlargement of the hip capsule. In the completely dislocated hip, the capsule is nearly twice the normal size (Fig. 32–3). The ligamentum teres hypertrophies as a result of having become in part a weightbearing structure. In older children, this ligament occasionally avulses from the fem-

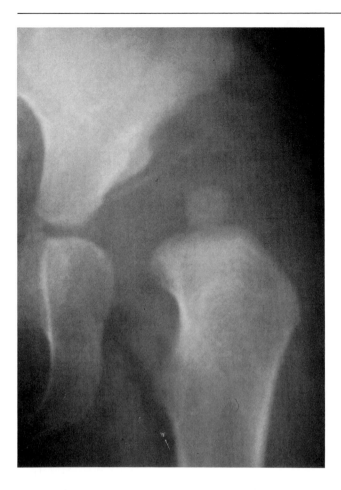

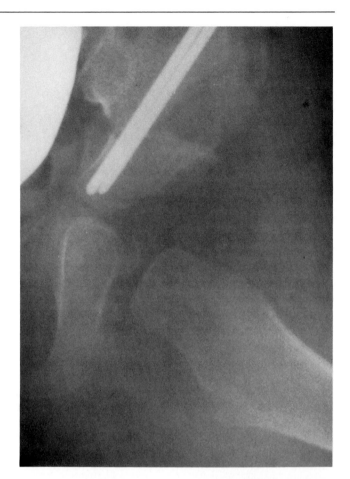

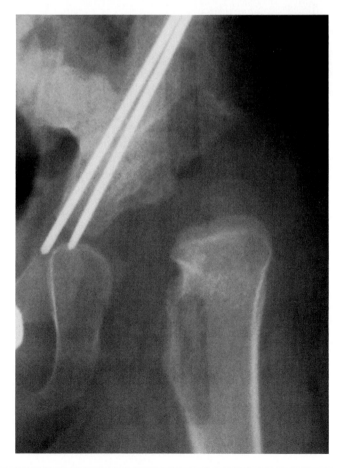

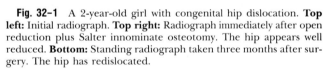

Fig. 32-1 A 2-year-old girl with congenital hip dislocation. **Top left:** Initial radiograph. **Top right:** Radiograph immediately after open reduction plus Salter innominate osteotomy. The hip appears well reduced. **Bottom:** Standing radiograph taken three months after surgery. The hip has redislocated.

oral head, retracting and reattaching to the inferior capsule, forming a mass of repair tissue in the inferior capsule that may impede reduction.

Superolaterally, the fibrocartilaginous labrum is flattened and the attached hypertrophied capsule protrudes into the overlying abductor muscle mass. The overlying muscle adheres to the displaced capsule. If the surgeon fails to separate the capsule from the adherent overlying muscles adequately, reduction is difficult and the chance is increased for postoperative redislocation. In a dislocation with a high femoral head position, the abductor muscles have contracted and, despite prior traction or femoral shortening, these contracted muscles and fascia can make it difficult to pull the proximal femur distal enough to reduce the femoral head fully. In rare cases, this requires either release of the piriformis insertion or release of the anterior-most gluteus minimus fibers, or both, to allow adequate distal movement of the femoral head after femoral shortening.

The mid and inferior portions of the capsule are constricted by the overlying psoas tendon. The transverse acetabular ligament, crossing the base of the horseshoe-shaped true acetabulum, is contracted and thickened. Perhaps this is because of the tug of the thickened capsule and ligamentum teres that have become weightbearing structures.

Bony Abnormalities

The well-described bony abnormalities in congenital dislocation of the hip[10] include a smaller-than-normal acetabulum that is narrowed at the base by capsular constriction. The acetabulum is deficient and often anteverted. The femur is anteverted; however, the anatomic neck shaft angle is rarely abnormal in typical congenital dislocation of the hip with no associated neurologic condition. The femoral head is often flattened medially because of weightbearing in the dislocated position. Also, the enlarged intervening ligamentum teres contributes to medial head deformation.

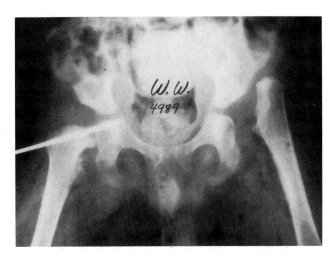

Fig. 32–2   Pelvic radiograph in an 18-month-old child with bilateral congenital hip dislocation treated by anterior open reduction. The transarticular pin was used because the surgeon did not understand how to correct the soft-tissue abnormalities.

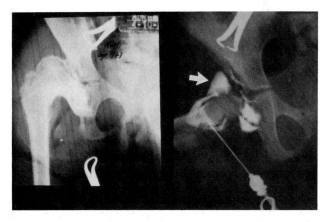

Fig. 32–3   Right hip arthrograms before (**left**) and after (**right**) manipulative reduction in a 5-year-old child with congenital hip dislocation. Note the large dye pool caused by capsular enlargement (arrow). Failure to close this pouch surgically may lead to redislocation.

Anterior Open Reduction

I will describe a technique for primary open reduction, including femoral shortening and acetabuloplasty, to serve as a guide for surgical correction in the child 4 years of age and older.[11] The older child typically requires the combined procedures. However, for younger children, the surgeon may elect to do only open reduction and only one, or none, of the associated bony procedures.

Patient Positioning

Place the patient on a radiolucent segment of the operating table to allow the use of an image intensifier, if needed. Place the trunk in a 45-degree lateral position by placing a large sandbag under the chest (Fig. 32–4). Do not place the sandbag behind the buttocks,

because it will prevent proper hip preparation and make clear radiographic imaging difficult.

Adductor Tenotomy and Skin Incision

If the surgeon elects open reduction after traction without associated femoral shortening, the first step of the procedure is percutaneous adductor longus tenotomy. With femoral shortening, adductor tenotomy is unnecessary because tension is reduced in all muscle groups, including the adductors.

In my early experience with primary open reduction that included femoral shortening, I used a single, long-curved anterolateral hip incision that provided exposure for open reduction, acetabuloplasty, and femoral shortening through a single incision. The exposure was

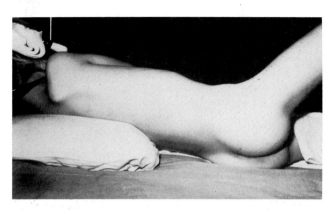

Fig. 32-4 Patient positioning for right-sided congenital hip dislocation surgery. Placing the sandbag behind the thorax rather than behind the hip allows better hip preparation and intraoperative radiographs.

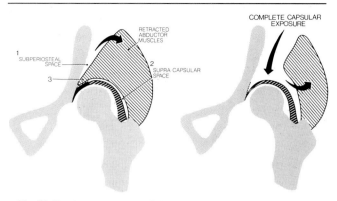

Fig. 32-5 Clear exposure of the capsule requires development of the subperiosteal space lateral to the ilium (1) and the supracapsular space (2). The dense tissue at the junction of the lateral periosteum and hip capsular origin (3) must be incised to expose the capsule.

excellent; however, despite careful skin closure and a running subcuticular skin suture, a large, unsightly scar resulted. Two separate incisions greatly improved wound cosmesis. The first is a relatively transverse anterolateral hip incision placed 1 cm below the iliac crest, anterosuperior iliac spine, and inguinal ligament.[2,3]

Capsular Exposure

After the skin incision is made, identify the lateral femoral cutaneous nerve and the interval between the sartorius and tensor fascia muscles. Then, carefully split the iliac crest apophyseal cartilage to allow later anatomic repair. Strip the iliac crest subperiosteally, first laterally and then medially, and identify both the direct and reflected heads of the rectus femoris tendons.

Use the subperiosteal elevation of the muscle from the medial wall of the ilium to extend the dissection distally and allow separation of muscles that have an intrapelvic origin (psoas, iliacus) from those with their origin outside the pelvis (rectus).

Laterally, the subperiosteal stripping must be carried as distally as possible. In patients with a false acetabulum, the periosteum of the ilium and the distorted hip capsule have condensed into a single layer that must be stripped from the wing of the ilium and false acetabulum (when present), down to the level of the true origin of the capsule.

The direct and reflected heads of the rectus tendon must be freed and transected. Retract them distally to the intertrochanteric level, then develop a plane just above the hip capsule and free the capsule from the attached, overlying abductors. Clear the space above the hip capsule as far posteriorly as possible, and then connect the already widely opened subperiosteal space on the lateral wall of the ilium to the space above the hip capsule using a scalpel or curved scissors (Fig. 32-5). This cut should extend far posteriorly, providing complete exposure of the displaced hip capsule to a point posterior to the true acetabulum.

Next, flex the hip to relax the psoas muscle and longitudinally incise the fascia on its deep surface at the pelvic brim. To facilitate exposure of the underlying tendon, rotate the psoas muscle with a blunt right-angle retractor. Then, partially release the retractor's "toe-in" to allow the underlying tendon to shift laterally, maintaining most of the muscle mass medially. Pass a gallbladder-type, right-angle hemostat around the tendon only and perform an intramuscular tenotomy. Use caution with this maneuver because the femoral nerve, which lies on the anterior surface of the psoas muscle, can be easily mistaken for the psoas tendon.

Capsulotomy

Figure 32-6 demonstrates a method for capsulotomy and subsequent corrective capsulorrhaphy. Open the widely exposed capsule with a scalpel, making the first cut parallel to the acetabular rim and a few millimeters below the labrum. Extend the cut posteriorly to a point behind the femoral head. Next, make a second capsular cut at a right angle to the first and aligned with the femoral neck (Fig. 32-6, *top left*). The length of this perpendicular cut determines the size of the triangle of redundant superolateral capsule that will later be excised (Fig. 32-6, *bottom left*) in preparation for capsular repair. In a completely dislocated hip, the right-angle cut is usually 1 cm in younger children (less than 4 years old) and about 1.5 cm in older children.

As soon as the dislocated femoral head is well exposed, Kocher clamps are attached to temporarily retract the two triangular flaps formed by the T-shaped incision. Using the ligamentum teres as a guide, open the capsule distally and medially to the depths of the true acetabulum. Next, transect the ligamentum teres from the femoral head and, with a Kocher clamp attached to provide tension, follow the ligament distally and medially to its insertion into the transverse acetab-

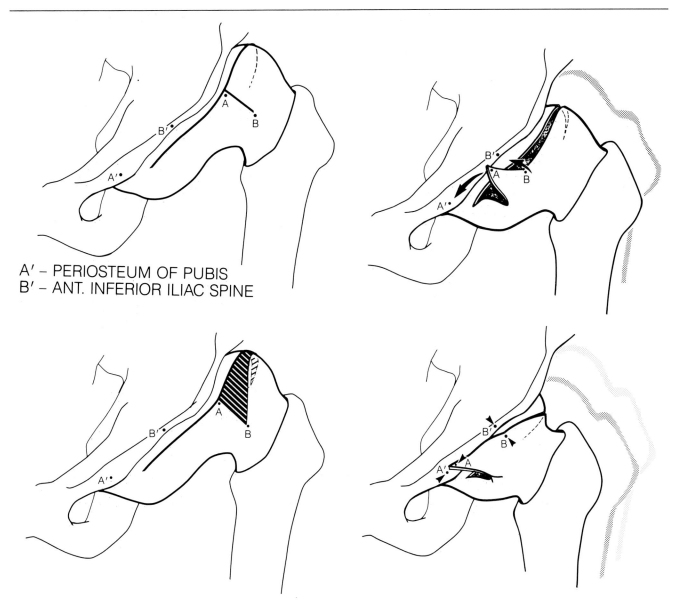

A' — PERIOSTEUM OF PUBIS
B' — ANT. INFERIOR ILIAC SPINE

Fig. 32–6 Left-sided congenital hip dislocation surgery. **Top left:** T-shaped capsular incision. The superior cut, extending posteriorly to a point behind the dislocated femoral head, should later be extended to behind the true acetabulum. **Bottom left:** The cross-hatched area depicts the portion of capsule that should be excised. **Top right:** Distal and medial advancement of the capsule converts the right angle defect (created by capsular excision) into a straight line. **Bottom right:** Point B is sutured to B' (anterior inferior iliac spine) and A to A' (periosteum of the pubis).

ular ligament at the base of the true acetabulum. Transect this ligament and excise the ligamentum teres along with any associated fatty tissue in the acetabular base. Clear any tissue or fat from the acetabulum with a rongeur. Palpate the inferomedial capsular area and incise with a scalpel any obstructions to reduction, such as a residual transverse ligament or capsular folds. Complete anteroinferior freeing of the constricted capsule provides adequate space for subsequent complete reduction of the femoral head. If the child has had prior traction, reduce the femoral head and proceed with capsulorrhaphy at this time. If not, proceed with femoral shortening.

Femoral Shortening

Make a separate lateral incision beginning at the tip of the greater trochanter and extending distally for a distance that provides adequate exposure for shortening. In younger children this may be nearly to the midshaft of the femur. This longer incision allows careful palpation of the entire greater trochanter. Also, the vastus lateral is freed adequately from the femoral shaft to allow subsequent femoral shortening. The lateral shaft exposure includes a transverse and very proximal periosteal incision at the lowermost point of the greater trochanteric apophysis to provide clear visualization of

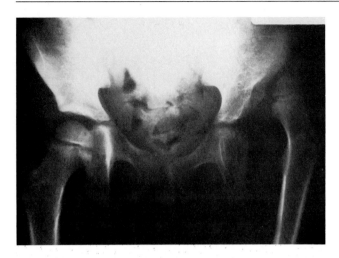

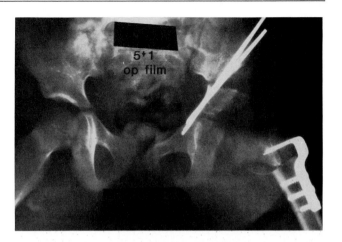

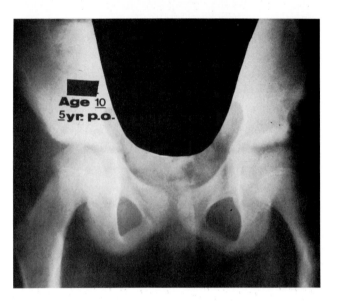

Fig. 32-7 Left-sided congenital hip dislocation in a 5-year-old girl. **Top left:** Initial radiograph. **Top right:** Hip reduced by open reduction and femoral shortening plus innominate osteotomy. **Bottom:** Pelvic radiograph five years after surgery.

the anterior femoral neck. Also, the lesser trochanter can be palpated behind the femur. Palpation of the greater trochanteric apophysis, calcar of the femoral neck, and lesser trochanter identifies landmarks for accurate placement of the initial guide pin and chisel, thus minimizing X-ray exposure.

To prepare for derotation, estimate existing femoral anteversion by grasping the proximal tibia with the knee flexed 90 degrees. With the other hand, palpate the femoral neck within the lateral incision and then the femoral head in the anterior incision. This provides an excellent estimate of anteversion.

Anteversion can be determined by computed tomographic analysis; however, this is unnecessary when the femoral neck can be palpated intraoperatively. In congenital dislocation of the hip, the femur is usually anteverted 40 to 60 degrees as compared with the normal 10 to 20 degrees.

I find the neck shaft angle more difficult to determine intraoperatively; however, my experience has shown that the angle is nearly normal (130 to 140 degrees) in congenital dislocation of the hip and should not be altered with the femoral shortening. Only femoral derotation and shortening are required.

Technique With AO Infant Blade Plate

After trying a variety of fixation devices, including cross-pin fixation, the Coventry plate, and the Wagner bifurcating plate, I have selected the infant-size AO blade plate as the most reliable device for predictable fixation and maintenance of correction. The blade plate can be used for most children more than 3 years old and is usually large enough for children who are 5 to 6 years old despite its description as "infant-size" (Fig. 32-7).

To avoid producing varus, the initial guide pin is introduced transversely at the distal extent of the greater trochanteric apophysis, and the inserting chisel is placed parallel to and immediately below the pin (Fig. 32-8). Direct the guide pin and chisel somewhat anteriorly,

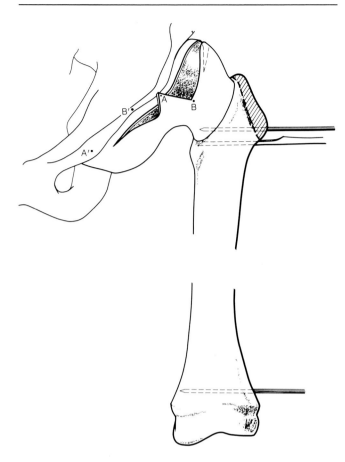

Fig. 32-8 Placement of the initial (proximal) guide and seating chisel at right angles to the shaft of the femur and centrally into the anteverted femoral neck.

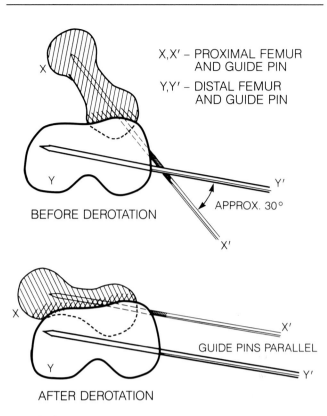

X,X' – PROXIMAL FEMUR
AND GUIDE PIN

Y,Y' – DISTAL FEMUR
AND GUIDE PIN

BEFORE DEROTATION

APPROX. 30°

AFTER DEROTATION

GUIDE PINS PARALLEL

Fig. 32-9 Diagrammatic cross section of the proximal and distal femur at the points of guide pin insertion. After derotation, fix the osteotomy with the guide pins parallel.

according to the estimated femoral anteversion, seeking the center of the femoral neck in the transverse plane. Anteroposterior and frog-leg image-intensifier views confirm the correct chisel position in both planes.

To quantitate the degree of anteversion correction more accurately, place a second transverse guide pin in the distal femur just above the femoral condyles (Fig. 32–8). Introduce this pin at a right angle to the femur in the frontal plane but in cross section, forming an angular difference in the transverse plane between this pin in the distal femur and the previously placed proximal pin (Fig. 32–9). This angle should be the degree of anteversion correction.

This method for determining anteversion correction is more accurate than marking the osteotomy site with longitudinal bone cuts, because medial displacement of the distal femoral fragment with the blade plate can distort the markings. In my early experience, I produced 40 to 60 degrees of derotational correction but found that iatrogenic posterior hip dislocation could be produced by excessive derotation. Now, I derotate about 30 degrees, changing the anteversion from an initial 40 to 60 degrees to 10 to 30 degrees after derotation.

Use a power saw to make the initial osteotomy; cut 1 cm below and parallel to the inserting chisel (Fig. 32–10, *top left*). Allow the bone ends to overlap, reduce the femoral head into the true acetabulum, and estimate the degree of shortening required to provide a pressure-free reduction. Clear the periosteum from the distal femoral segment and complete the shortening osteotomy, removing a 1.5- to 3-cm segment as determined by the degree of overlap with reduction (Fig. 32–10, *bottom left*). Insert the blade plate into the proximal segment and rotate the distal fragment laterally until the proximal and distal guide pins are parallel in a transverse plane (Fig. 32–9). Then fix the distal femoral segment to the plate (Fig. 32–10, *top right*).

Technique for Younger Children: Anterior AO Mandibular Plate

Under special circumstances, the surgeon may need to perform femoral shortening in a child whose femur is too small for the AO infant blade plate. In these cases, I prefer the four-hole AO mandibular plate placed anteriorly, bridging the shortening osteotomy at the intertrochanteric level. Originally, I used the third-tubular plate; however, it was too large for small children and did not have dynamic compression screw holes. In contrast, the more compact mandibular plate allows dynamic compression with screw tightening.

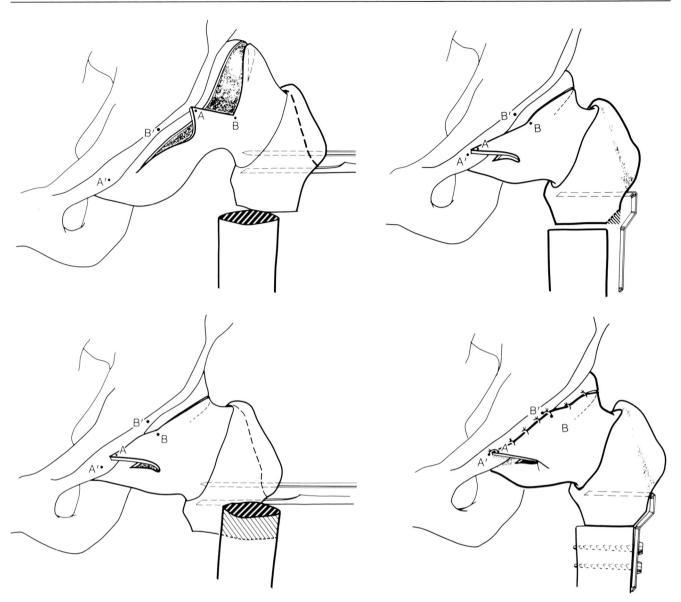

Fig. 32–10   Technique. **Top left:** Perform the osteotomy 1 cm below the inserting chisel. **Bottom left:** Reduce the hip and allow the bone ends to overlap to determine the degree of shortening required. **Top right:** Replace the chisel with the AO blade plate. **Bottom right:** After appropriate derotation, fix the fragments with blade plate. Then repair the capsule using No. 1 nonabsorbable sutures.

With direct placement of the anterior plate, the surgeon can perform the osteotomy at the desired intertrochanteric level and maintain two screws proximal to the osteotomy without entering or damaging the greater trochanteric apophysis (Fig. 32–11). This cannot be achieved with a right-angle blade plate in a young child.

To simplify application of the four-hole plate, clear the proposed site and position the plate at the anterior femoral neck, centered over the intertrochanteric line, with the proximal half of the plate medial to the greater trochanteric apophysis (Fig. 32–12, *top left*). Drill the two proximal holes and attach the plate before performing the osteotomy. (These holes are drilled from front to back; therefore, be careful with the depth gauge

and tap because the sciatic nerve lies posteriorly.) Remove the distal-most of the proximal screws, rotate the plate 90 degrees, and perform the shortening osteotomy (Fig. 32–12, *top right* and *bottom left*). Finally, replace and tighten the proximal screws, rotate and position the shortened femur, and attach the plate to the distal fragment (Fig. 32–12, *bottom right*). Prior proximal plate attachment greatly simplifies the mechanics of plate positioning, derotation, shortening, and distal screw insertion.

Capsulorrhaphy

At this point in the procedure, the femoral head is at the level of the acetabulum and capsular excision

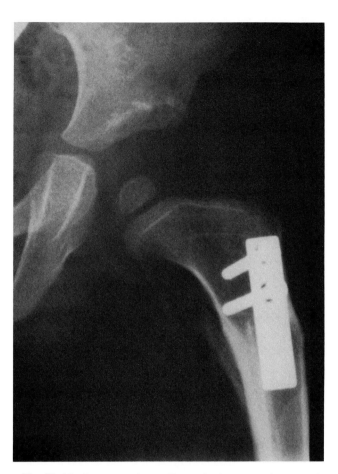

Fig. 32-11 Postoperative radiograph demonstrating anterior placement of the straight mandibular plate in a younger child treated by open reduction and femoral shortening.

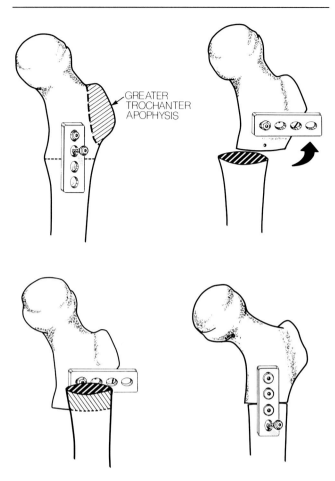

Fig. 32-12 Technique for younger children. **Top left:** Four-hole AO mandibular plate positioned medial to the greater trochanteric apophysis and centered at the lesser trochanter level. **Top right:** Second screw removed and plate rotated. **Bottom left:** Shortening osteotomy performed. **Bottom right:** Plate attached after derotation.

and repair can proceed. I prefer the excisional method, described by Salter,[2] that requires excision of the redundant superolateral pouch of capsule. Unless this excess capsule is obliterated, the hip may redislocate. Proper excision and repair leaves no space into which the head could redislocate.

The previously performed T-shaped capsular incision produced two triangular flaps. The superolateral flap should be excised (Fig. 32–6, *bottom left*) and the inferomedial flap (point A) pulled medially and sutured to the periosteum of the pubis (point A′) (Fig. 32–6, *top right* and *bottom right*) using nonabsorbable sutures. Similarly, point B on the capsule, which is the lower extent of the incision parallel to the femoral neck, should be pulled proximally and medially by hip flexion and internal rotation (Fig. 32–6, *top right* and *bottom right*) and sutured to point B′. Each suture started in the lateral capsule should be advanced about 1 cm anteriorly before being placed in the medial capsular remnant. This maintains the femur in internal rotation and stabilizes the reduction. The sutures are placed at 5- to 7-mm intervals, held temporarily with hemostats, and

then tied sequentially from posterolateral to anteromedial with an assistant holding the hip in mild flexion and internal rotation while the psoas muscle is retracted to allow clear visualization of the medial capsular sutures (Fig. 32–10, *bottom right*). After all sutures have been placed and tied, assess the security of the repair, which should resemble a secure hernia repair.

Acetabuloplasty

Salter[2] and Salter and Dubos[3] provide excellent descriptions of acetabuloplasty. This chapter discusses indications for acetabuloplasty in association with femoral shortening.

In my early experience, I combined open reduction capsulorrhaphy and Salter innominate osteotomy following traction for treatment of routine congenital dislocation of the hip in patients more than 2 years old. Subsequently, I began to perform primary femoral derotational shortening in most cases, to avoid traction,

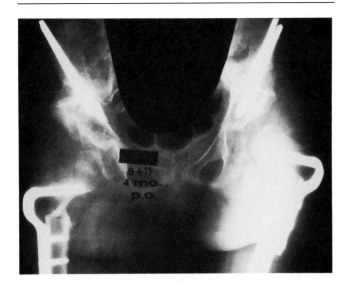

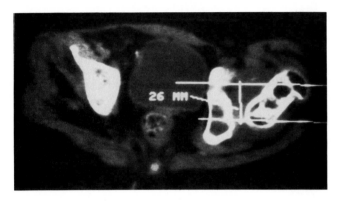

Fig. 32–13   Top: Pelvic radiograph four months after bilateral open reduction, femoral shortening, and acetabuloplasty in a 6-year-old girl. The left hip has redislocated. **Bottom:** Computed tomographic scan demonstrates iatrogenic posterior dislocation caused by excessive derotation plus capsulorrhaphy.

and found that, after femoral shortening and capsulorrhaphy, many children had a very stable reduction without innominate osteotomy. Correction of the femoral anteversion made the acetabular mal-direction less apparent in this younger group. Therefore, I stopped performing routine Salter innominate osteotomies in younger children, usually under the age of 3 to 4 years, but continue to use it in older children.

Acetabular Procedures in Young Children

In children 2 to 4 years old, I complete the reduction, shortening, and capsulorrhaphy sequence and then perform a minimal "augmentation acetabuloplasty." This procedure is performed by transversely directing a curved osteotome 1.5 cm into the iliac bone above the labrum, beginning anteriorly and proceeding posteriorly to the posterior margin of the hip joint. The sciatic notch is not cleared. The osteotome extends medially to a level above the medial

margin of the femoral head and does not curve distally into the triradiate cartilage. The acetabular rim and labrum are gradually mobilized enough to allow distal rotation of this fragment, probably hinging on the acetabular growth cartilage. The triangular fragment of bone, previously excised from the femur, is then driven into the newly created space. No fixation pins are used. This minimal procedure moves the labrum somewhat distally and slightly improves the anterolateral coverage without requiring the surgeon to clear the sciatic notch, take a graft from the iliac crest, or use pins that require later removal. In addition to the modest immediate improvement of the acetabular rim position, the acetabular cut may stimulate growth in the underlying acetabulum growth cartilage. The acetabular "augmentation" may not be needed in the younger child with excellent acetabular coverage after derotational shortening.

Acetabular Procedures in Older Children

In children more than 4 years old, the deficient, maldirected acetabulum covers the femoral head poorly despite derotational femoral shortening. In these patients, I perform a standard Salter innominate osteotomy at the time of open reduction, capsulorrhaphy, and femoral shortening (Fig. 32–7).

Cast Immobilization

After a one-stage hip reduction is completed, suction drainage tubes are placed in each wound and the wounds are closed, ending with a cosmetic subcuticular suture. The child is placed in a single hip spica cast with the hip flexed and abducted 30 degrees. If derotational femoral osteotomy has not been done, the limb is rotated 30 degrees internally to protect the capsulorrhaphy; however, if the femur has been derotated, the leg is placed in a neutral position. If the limb is internally rotated too much in a patient whose femur has been derotated, the femoral head will appear inferiorly subluxated on radiographs. At its worst, too much internal rotation will produce posterior dislocation.

The hip spica cast is maintained for six weeks and then changed, as a day-surgery procedure with the patient under general anesthesia, to either Petrie casts or a second more loosely fitting hip spica cast for another four to six weeks. For 2-year-old children, and especially for overweight children, Petrie casts are awkward and may produce excessive stress at the osteotomy site. Therefore, I use a second hip spica cast after six weeks for this younger group.

The second cast is removed ten to 12 weeks after surgery, with a subsequent nighttime abduction brace used only for a patient with bothersome residual dysplasia. The abduction brace should be of the A-frame type to encourage hip extension and abduction, not the typical Lorenz-type brace that encourages hip flexion and external rotation. Once the hip extension and in-

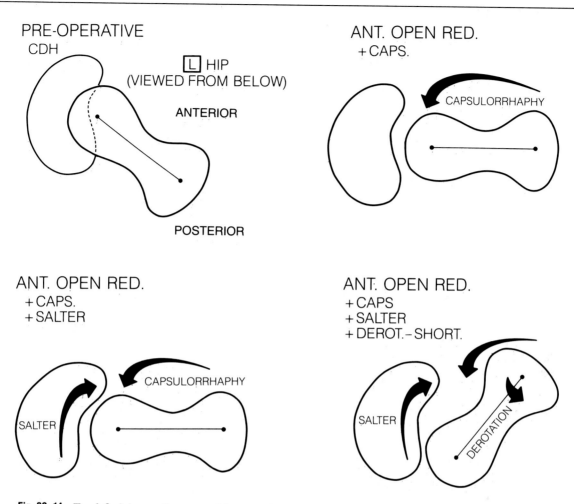

Fig. 32-14 **Top left:** Schema of anteverted femur and acetabulum in untreated congenital hip dislocation. **Top right:** Redirection of femoral neck by snug anterior capsulorrhaphy. **Bottom left:** Capsulorrhaphy plus Salter innominate osteotomy. **Bottom right:** Capsulorrhaphy plus Salter innominate osteotomy plus full femoral derotation. Combined in excess this sequence can produce posterior dislocation.

ternal rotation position has been adopted and encouraged by capsulorrhaphy, the flexion-abduction, external rotation position, which is highly desired after closed reduction, should be avoided.

Timing of Bilateral Surgery

I treat bilateral dislocations using two surgical procedures at one- to two-week intervals and remove half of the cast for the second procedure. The other half of the cast is kept in position during the second operation to protect the first reduction. At the end of the second operation, I remove the remainder of the cast and apply a new double hip spica cast.

Pitfalls in the Combined Technique

Combining open reduction, femoral shortening, capsulorrhaphy, and acetabuloplasty into one operation has great potential for early reestablishment of more normal mechanics; however, the production of many loose parts requires surgical skill for correct reassem-

bly. Excessive derotation combined with an overly snug anterior capsulorrhaphy can lead to iatrogenic posterior dislocation (Fig. 32-13).

Certain adjustments in technique must be made in making the transition from the open reduction plus Salter osteotomy technique to the combined procedure including femoral shortening. Figure 32-14 demonstrates sequentially the potential for producing iatrogenic posterior dislocation with the combined method for congenital hip dislocation reduction. Posterior dislocation can result from the combination of (1) full derotation, (2) acetabular redirection by Salter innominate osteotomy that improves anterior coverage but decreases posterior coverage, and (3) excessive internal rotation produced by the capsulorrhaphy. Each procedure by itself increases hip stability; however, combining these procedures to excess can lead to iatrogenic posterior dislocation. This problem can be avoided by derotating the femur only 30 degrees, even when it is anteverted as much as 60 degrees, and by slightly decreasing the amount of lateral-to-medial suture advancement in the capsulorrhaphy to decrease modestly the amount of internal rotation produced.

The potential problem of iatrogenic posterior dislocation does not detract from the value of the combined procedure but emphasizes that experience and judgment are required to combine all elements successfully in a single operation.

Summary

Combining primary open reduction, femoral shortening, capsulorrhaphy, and acetabuloplasty in a single operation allows predictable treatment of congenital dislocation of the hip in older children without the time and expense of preliminary traction. In addition to the bony abnormalities of congenital hip dislocation, the complex pathologic anatomy of the hypertrophied capsule and associated soft tissues must be recognized and corrected. Failure to treat all components of this condition often leads to reduction that is apparently satisfactory in the intraoperative and early postoperative periods but is followed by hip subluxation or redislocation with weightbearing. Correcting all components of the congenital hip dislocation deformity in a single operation provides the best opportunity for early return of normal hip mechanics and function in the older child.

References

1. Mubarak S, Garfin S, Vance R, et al: Pitfalls in the use of the Pavlik harness for treatment of congenital dysplasia, subluxation, and dislocation of the hip. *J Bone Joint Surg* 1981;63A:1239–1248.
2. Salter RB: Innominate osteotomy in the treatment of congenital dislocation and subluxation of the hip. *J Bone Joint Surg* 1961;43B:518–539.
3. Salter RB, Dubos JP: The first fifteen years' personal experience with innominate osteotomy in the treatment of congenital dislocation and subluxation of the hip. *Clin Orthop* 1974;98:72–103.
4. Weinstein SL, Ponseti IV: Congenital dislocation of the hip. *J Bone Joint Surg* 1979;61A:119–124.
5. Ashley RK, Larsen LJ, James PM: Reduction of dislocation of the hip in older children: A preliminary report. *J Bone Joint Surg* 1972;54A:545–550.
6. Dega W, Król J, Polakowski L: Surgical treatment of congenital dislocation of the hip in children: A one-stage procedure. *J Bone Joint Surg* 1959;41A:920–934.
7. Klisic P, Jankovic L: Combined procedure of open reduction and shortening of the femur in treatment of congenital dislocation of the hips in older children. *Clin Orthop* 1976;119:60–69.
8. Schoenecker PL, Strecker WB: Congenital dislocation of the hip in children: Comparison of the effects of femoral shortening and of skeletal traction in treatment. *J Bone Joint Surg* 1984;66A:21–27.
9. Morel G, Briand JL: Progressive gradual reduction of the dislocated hip in the child after walking age, in Tachdijian M (ed): *Congenital Dislocation of the Hip*. New York, Churchill Livingstone, 1982, pp 373–384.
10. Ponseti IV: Morphology of the acetabulum in congenital dislocation of the hip: Gross, histological and roentgenographic studies. *J Bone Joint Surg* 1978;60A:586–599.
11. Wenger DR: *Treatment of Congenital Dislocation of the Hip in the Older Child*, videotape. Chicago, American Academy of Orthopaedic Surgeons, 1985.

AIDS and Hemophilic Arthropathy

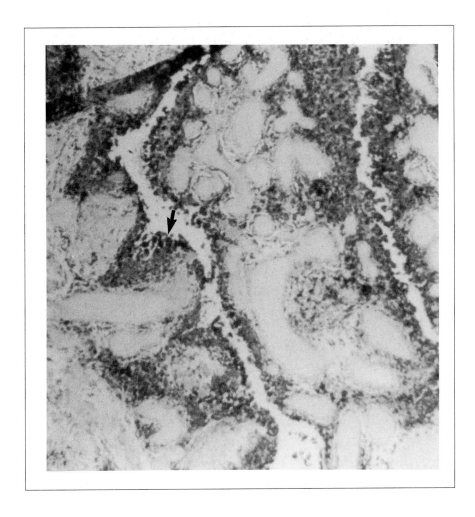

Acquired Immune Deficiency Syndrome Associated With Hemophilia in the United States

Jeanette K. Stehr-Green, MD

Bruce L. Evatt, MD

Dale N. Lawrence, MD

As of Jan 4, 1988, 463 cases of acquired immune deficiency syndrome (AIDS) associated with hemophilia have been reported in the United States. Although these cases compose less than 1% of all AIDS cases reported in the United States, the surveillance and study of AIDS in this population continue to be important because of the following:

(1) More cases will probably occur. Some 15,000 to 18,000 persons in the United States have a coagulation disorder.[1] Although heat treatment of concentrated clotting factors, the development of serologic methods of screening blood for human immunodeficiency virus (HIV), and the self-deferral of high-risk blood donors have minimized further risk of HIV infection in persons with hemophilia, many were infected before the introduction of these interventions. Studies from hemophilia treatment centers suggest that 33% to 92% of persons with hemophilia A and 14% to 52% of persons with hemophilia B have the HIV antibody.[2-8]

(2) The natural history of HIV infection in persons with hemophilia may differ from that in other risk groups. The route and frequency of exposure to HIV among persons with hemophilia (through commercially produced concentrated clotting factors) differed from those in homosexual and bisexual men, intravenous drug users, and transfusion recipients. These risk groups may also differ in terms of important, but as yet undetermined, cofactors for the development of AIDS, such as coexisting infections.

(3) Persons with hemophilia may be a source of infection for other individuals. Sex partners and offspring of persons with hemophilia are also at risk for HIV infection. Counseling and public health interventions are needed to prevent the further spread of infection.

(4) The safety of the blood supply needs to be monitored. Hemophiliacs continue to receive blood products. Although steps to prevent further HIV infection in this population have been initiated, it is important to monitor the effectiveness of these interventions through surveillance for seroconversion of seronegative patients.

To further inform the orthopaedic surgeon about hemophilia-associated AIDS, we will review the surveillance of AIDS in persons with hemophilia, HIV transmission to sex partners and offspring, and current information on the safety of blood products used by these patients. In addition, because the orthopaedic surgeon may be involved in activities that result in exposure to HIV-infected blood and body fluids, we have included recommendations for prevention of HIV transmission in the health-care setting.

Update of Surveillance for Hemophilia-Associated AIDS

HIV infection can result in a spectrum of clinical manifestations that range from asymptomatic (with only laboratory evidence of infection) to severe immunodeficiency with life-threatening secondary infections or cancers. National surveillance of AIDS encompasses only the severe manifestations thought to be very specific for HIV infection. Because the case definition is precise and can be consistently interpreted, surveillance can be useful in following epidemiologic trends in severe HIV-related disease. In August 1987, the case definition was revised to broaden the range of specific AIDS-indicative diseases (including HIV dementia and HIV wasting syndrome) to include indicator diseases that are presumptively diagnosed and to eliminate exclusions resulting from concurrent existence of other causes of immunodeficiency in the presence of laboratory evidence of infection with HIV (Table 33–1).[9,10]

Between Jan 1, 1981, and Jan 4, 1988, 463 cases of hemophilia-associated AIDS were reported to the Centers for Disease Control (CDC). The number of cases diagnosed each year has steadily increased, nearly doubling through 1985 and increasing more modestly (50%) in 1986 (Fig. 33–1). Cases have been reported from 46 states, Puerto Rico, and Guam; 36% of the patients resided in California, New York, New Jersey, and Pennsylvania. No cases have been reported from Delaware, Idaho, Montana, or Arkansas. The geographic distribution of cases probably reflects the geographic distribution of the population with hemophilia: 40% of the 25 federally funded hemophilia treatment centers in the United states are located in California, New York, New Jersey, and Pennsylvania.

All but 12 (3%) of the patients with hemophilia-associated AIDS were male. Median age at diagnosis was 31 years (range, 3 to 86 years). A significant decline in the median age of patients diagnosed each year was not found. The CDC reported that 391 (84%) of the 463 patients were white, 30 (6%) were black, 32 (7%) were

Table 33-1
CDC surveillance case definition for AIDS-indicator diseases

Diseases	1985	1987
Parasitic		
Pneumocystis carinii pneumonia	Yes	Yes*
Chronic cryptosporidiosis	Yes	Yes
Toxoplasmosis of brain	Yes	Yes*
Chronic isosporiasis	Yes†	Yes†
Strongyloidiasis, disseminated	Yes	No
Fungal		
Esophageal candidiasis	Yes	Yes*
Bronchial or pulmonary candidiasis	Yes†	Yes
Cryptococcosis, extrapulmonary	Yes	Yes
Histoplasmosis, disseminated	Yes†	Yes†
Coccidiodomycosis, disseminated	No	Yes†
Bacterial		
Mycobacterium avium, intracellulare or *kansasii*, disseminated	Yes	Yes
Mycobacterium tuberculosis, extrapulmonary	No	Yes†
Any other mycobacterial disease, disseminated	No	Yes*†
Salmonella septicemia, recurrent	No	Yes†
Serious bacterial infections, recurrent	No	Yes†‡
Viral		
Cytomegalovirus	Yes	Yes
Chronic/disseminated *Herpes simplex*	Yes	Yes
Cancer		
Kaposi's sarcoma	Yes§	Yes*§
Lymphoma of brain	Yes§	Yes§
Non-Hodgkin's B-cell lymphoma	Yes†	Yes†
Other		
Chronic interstitial pneumonitis	Yes†‡	Yes*‡
Progressive multifocal leukoencephalopathy	Yes	Yes*
HIV encephalopathy	No	Yes†
HIV wasting syndrome	No	Yes†

*Can be presumptively diagnosed.
†With laboratory evidence of HIV infection.
‡In children only.
§In patient less than 60 years old without laboratory evidence of HIV infection, or at any age with laboratory evidence of HIV infection.

Hispanic, seven (2%) were of Asian/Pacific Island descent, and three (1%) were of American Indian/Alaskan Native descent.

Most patients with hemophilia-associated AIDS had hemophilia A, were severely affected by their coagulation disorder, and had received commercially produced concentrated clotting factors (Table 33–2). These findings parallel those of HIV serosurveys from hemophilia treatment centers: patients receiving concentrated clotting factor products (composed of blood components from hundreds to thousands of donors) had a higher seroprevalence rate of HIV than did those receiving cryoprecipitate (from a single donor); of those receiving concentrated factor products, seropositive patients received larger and more frequent doses of concentrate than did seronegative patients.[3-8] Since persons with severe hemophilia receive larger and more frequent doses of clotting factor, they would be expected to have a higher risk for HIV infection (and, therefore, a higher risk for developing AIDS) than those with less severe hemophilia.

The larger number of AIDS patients with hemophilia A reflects in part the larger number of persons with hemophilia A in the United States and the greater prevalence of severe disease requiring more frequent exposure to blood products in these patients. However, processes used to manufacture factors VIII and IX differ and may result in a differential degree of inactivation of HIV. One purification process for factor IX includes the use of ethanol, a substance that effectively inactivates HIV, suggesting that some factor IX products may have been associated with a lower degree of HIV contamination and, thus, a lower risk for HIV infection and AIDS.[11,12]

Of the 463 patients, 359 (78%) have been reported to have one condition indicative of AIDS, 79 (17%) had two conditions, 19 (4%) had three conditions, and six (1%) had four or more conditions. Except for Kaposi's sarcoma, the distribution of specific AIDS-indicative diseases in patients with hemophilia-associated AIDS was similar to that in other risk groups (Table 33–3). More than 60% of the patients had *Pneumocystis carinii* pneumonia, regardless of risk group. The higher frequency of Kaposi's sarcoma in homosexual men has been noted previously.[13,14] Cofactors, such as amyl nitrite use, cytomegalovirus infection, and oncogenic viral infection, have been proposed but remain unclarified.[13,15-20]

As of Jan 4, 1988, 270 (58%) of the 463 patients with hemophilia-associated AIDS were known to have died: this case-fatality rate is similar to that for other risk groups. Of those who died, 84% died within one year of AIDS diagnosis. It is important to realize that AIDS case reports are usually submitted after the diagnosis of the initial indicator disease leading to the diagnosis of AIDS. Follow-up reports on the occurrence of additional diseases or death are less likely to be submitted. Therefore, the cumulative incidences of particular diseases and the fatality rate must be considered to be minimal estimates, and population-based studies should be used to obtain more accurate estimates.

National AIDS surveillance suggests that approximately 3% of all men with hemophilia in the United States have developed AIDS. However, studies from hemophilia centers suggest that the cumulative incidence of AIDS in seropositive patients has reached 25% in some populations (J.K. Stehr-Green, unpublished data). The total number of patients with HIV-related illnesses, including illnesses not meeting the case definition for AIDS, exceeds these figures substantially.

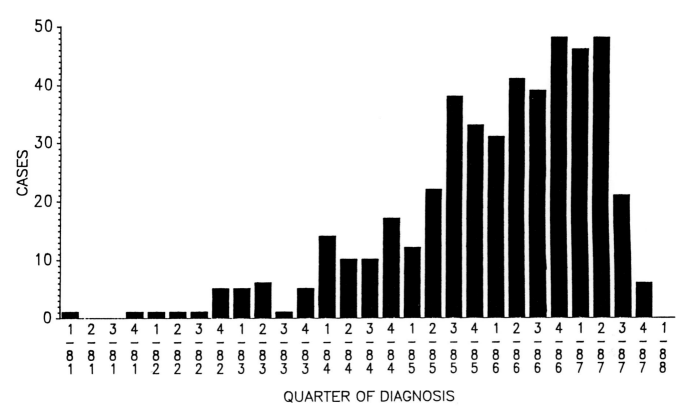

Fig. 33–1 Hemophilia-associated AIDS cases by quarter of diagnosis, United States, January 1981 to December 1987.

HIV Transmission to Sex Partners and Offspring of Patients With Hemophilia

Transmission of HIV Infection to Sex Partners

HIV is transmitted through sexual contact, perinatally from infected mother to neonate, and through infected blood and blood components. Although homosexual activity has been the primary mode of sexual transmission in the United States, heterosexual transmission has become a well-established route of HIV infection, not only in Africa but in the United States and other countries as well. Heterosexual transmission from infected patients with hemophilia has also been documented, ranging from 6% to 18% of tested sex partners (Table 33–4).[21-26]

As of Jan 8, 1988, AIDS had been diagnosed in 16 female sex partners of men with hemophilia.[24] None of the women reported risk factors for HIV infection other than heterosexual relations with their partners. Eight cases (50%) were diagnosed in 1987. Nine of the women (56%) have died. In only four cases were HIV-related symptoms reported in the infected male partner before AIDS was diagnosed in the woman.

Seropositivity among heterosexual partners in general (hemophilia- and nonhemophilia-related transmission) has been associated with the failure to use condoms and the total number of sexual contacts with the infected partner that included ejaculation, oral sex, and anal intercourse.[25-27] In a 1986 study, the "most dominant" risk factor for heterosexual HIV transmission was the immunologic status of the infected male partner as determined by his T-helper cell count.[25] Infected male partners with low T-helper cell counts (<350 cells/ml) were more likely to have seropositive sex partners than were male partners with relatively high T-helper cell counts (≥350 cells/ml). However, heterosexual transmission of AIDS can still occur, even in the absence of these identified risk factors.

Longitudinal studies suggest that the seroprevalence rate in sex partners of men with hemophilia is increasing despite general increased public knowledge of the risk of heterosexual transmission of HIV and means of prevention.[24] A statewide survey of persons with hemophilia in Michigan suggests at least some lack knowledge about HIV transmission or deny the problem as it relates to their own lives: only 50% of survey respondents had discussed AIDS with their sex partners, 28% claimed that there was no need for precautions, and only 15% used condoms consistently when engaging in sexual intercourse.[28] Because of the study design, the investigators were unable to correlate the HIV serologic status of the respondent (an important correlate

Table 33-2
Findings in patients with hemophilia-associated AIDS in the United States, Jan 1, 1981, to Jan 4, 1988

Findings	Patients	
	No.	%
Coagulation disorder (No. = 463)		
Hemophilia A	410	89
Hemophilia B	34	7
von Willebrand's disease	11	2
Other	8	2
Severity of hemophilia* (No. = 438)		
Severe	325	74
Moderate	59	13
Mild	54	12
Blood products (No. = 423)		
Concentrated clotting factors only	248	59
Single-donor products only†	13	3
Concentrated factors and single-donor products	162	38

*For patients with hemophilia A and B only: severe, ≤1% of normal level of clotting factor; moderate, 2% to 5% of normal level; mild, >5% of normal level.
†Single-donor products include cryoprecipitate, fresh frozen plasma, and packed red blood cells.

for the use of condoms[29]) with sexual attitudes and behaviors. Nevertheless, with the high rate of seroprevalence in this population, it is apparent that a problem does exist. Furthermore, a 1987 survey of hemophilia treatment centers in the United States reported that only 34% of the 2,276 sex partners of HIV-infected men with hemophilia were known to have been serologically tested for HIV.[30] Of these women, 280 (12%) were known to have been pregnant since January 1985; only 170 of these (61%) had been tested for HIV antibody. These findings further emphasize the need of appropriate counseling and health care for these patients and their families.

Perinatal Transmission of HIV Infection

Transmission of HIV from an infected mother to her baby has been documented in the sex partners of men with hemophilia[31,32] as well as in other HIV-infected persons.[33-36] Evidence suggests that perinatal transmission occurs by three modes[37]: (1) transplacental passage of the virus in utero; (2) exposure to infected maternal blood and vaginal fluids during labor and delivery; and (3) postpartum ingestion of breast milk containing the virus. Transmission during pregnancy or during labor and delivery is suggested by the occurrence of infection in infants who had no contact with their infected mothers after birth.[34,38] Isolation of HIV from breast milk[39] and a case report of infection in a breast-fed child whose mother was not infected until after delivery (through a postpartum blood transfusion)[40] suggest breast-feeding as a mode of transmission. However, the proportion of perinatally acquired HIV infection attributable to each of these modes of transmission is unknown.

The rate of perinatal transmission of HIV from an infected pregnant woman to her child is largely unknown but may be as high as 50%.[37] The issue is clouded

Table 33-3
Comparison of AIDS-indicator diseases*

Disease	% of Patients Whose AIDS Was Associated With		
	Hemophilia	Homosexuality or Bisexuality	Intravenous Drug Abuse
Pneumocystis carinii pneumonia	63	63	67
Esophageal candidiasis	18	9	15
Cryptococcosis, extrapulmonary	11	6	12
Chronic cryptosporidiosis	6	4	2
Mycobacterium avium-intracellulare	8	4	4
Cytomegalovirus, disseminated	4	5	2
Lymphoma	4	NA	NA
Toxoplasmosis of brain	3	2	2
Chronic/disseminated *Herpes simplex*	2	3	3
Histoplasmosis, disseminated	2	NA	NA
Kaposi's sarcoma	1	27	3
Chronic interstitial pneumonitis	1	—	—
Progressive multifocal leukoencephalopathy	1	NA	NA

*As of Jan 4, 1988, for hemophilia-associated AIDS and as of Feb 9, 1987, for AIDS associated with homosexuality, bisexuality, or intravenous drug abuse.[13]

Table 33-4
HIV-seroprevalence rate in female sex partners of seropositive men with hemophilia

Investigators	Years	No. Tested	Seropositive	
			No.	%
Kreiss et al[21]	1984	21	2	10
Allain[22]	1986	148	10	7
Andes et al[23]	?	34	2	6
Lawrence et al[24]	1984–1987			
Initial evaluation		56	5	9
Reevaluation		11	2	18
Goedert et al[25]	1986	24	4	17
Padian et al[26]	1985–1986	19	4	21

in that HIV infection is usually diagnosed by the detection of IgG antibody to HIV. Maternal IgG antibody is passively transferred through the placenta and cannot be distinguished from IgG actively produced by an infected child. As a result, a positive serologic test in a neonate (using IgG) may simply reflect passively transferred antibody from the infected mother. Detection of IgM (which does not cross the placenta) has been used to distinguish maternal infection from neonatal infection in other diseases, but IgM antibody to HIV has been detected inconsistently, and testing is not reliable at this time. Therefore, serial IgG-antibody testing during the first 12 to 15 months after birth (to determine if antibody disappears), antigen detection, viral culture, or DNA probes must be used to detect active HIV infection in the infant.

The risk factors associated with transmission have not been defined, but possibilities include maternal viral titers, level of immune suppression in the mother, co-existing infections, and substance abuse.[37] It appears that both symptomatic and asymptomatic women can transmit HIV. One study reported that women with low T-helper cell counts were more likely to transmit the virus.[41]

Prospective studies suggest that maternal HIV infection is probably not associated with markedly adverse prenatal or neonatal infant outcomes,[37,42] although an increase in spontaneous abortions has been reported by some researchers.[37] It is not known whether pregnancy increases an infected woman's risk of developing clinical manifestations of HIV infection or AIDS.[37] Nevertheless, pregnancy in the HIV-seropositive patient seems risky for both the mother and the child, and precautions should be taken to prevent pregnancy.

Safety of Blood and Blood Components

Donor Screening

In 1984, after a retrovirus was identified as the cause of AIDS, tests were developed to detect antibody to

HIV. The initial tests included modifications of the enzyme-linked immunosorbent assay (ELISA), Western blot technique, immunofluorescence, and radioimmunoprecipitation. In January 1985, the CDC recommended that, in conjunction with self-deferral of high-risk blood donors, all blood used for transfusion or manufactured blood products be screened for HIV using an ELISA.[43] In March 1985, the US Food and Drug Administration (FDA) licensed the ELISA as a screening test in blood and plasma centers.

Early studies by the Atlanta Region of the American Red Cross and CDC demonstrated a specificity of 99.8% and positive predictive value of 86.3% using the ELISA.[44,45] Clinical data submitted by the manufacturers to the FDA indicate that the sensitivity and specificity of the seven licensed anti-HIV-ELISA kits exceed 99%.[46] The specificity is increased to approximately 99.8% if an initially reactive test is repeated. False-positive and false-negative reactions have been observed. False-positive reactions usually occur in uninfected persons who have immunologic disturbances or who have had multiple transfusions. False-negative test results are observed in persons who have recently become infected with HIV and who have not developed detectable antibody.

Use of the Western blot greatly increases the specificity of diagnosis of HIV infection; however, it has been more difficult to standardize, and only one licensed Western blot kit is currently available. The Western blot examines patterns of antibodies to specific HIV antigens (viral proteins of specific molecular weights, such as p24, p31, gp41) rather than the presence of antibody to antigen derived from disruption of the whole virus as in the ELISA. For a test to be considered positive, antibody must be reactive with multiple virus-protein bands, that is, p24, p31, and either gp41 or gp160.[46] If fewer bands are present, the test is considered indeterminate; if no bands are present, the test is interpreted as negative. An indeterminate Western blot pattern may occur in a person recently infected with HIV or in an HIV-infected person who has advanced immunodeficiency; however, in clinical trials, as many as 15% to 20% of persons at low risk for HIV infection have had indeterminate Western blot patterns. To distinguish between the infected and uninfected patient with an indeterminate initial test, the Western blot should be repeated within six months. In the patient with recent infections, repeat testing often results in a positive blot pattern. Repeat testing of the truly uninfected person will show no change.

As noted above, antibody screening tests can give negative results in patients recently infected with HIV who have not developed antibodies to the virus at the time of blood donation. Most persons exposed to HIV develop detectable antibody response within six to 12 weeks of infection[47]; however, delayed seroconversions (longer than six months after infection) have been reported.[48] This period from infection to development of antibody creates a "window" during which infection cannot be readily detected but transmission of infection can occur. One prospective clinical study of repeat donors over a 21-month period suggests the probability of blood donation in this "window" to be about one in 84,000.[49] Although this risk is small, it varies depending on the prevalence of HIV infection in the community. The improvement of ELISA kits[50] and use of tests that measure the presence of viral antigen, rather than antibody, may help prevent transmission through blood donation during this window period.

Safety of Factor Concentrates

In 1984, HIV was found to be heat-labile in vitro. Studies demonstrated that HIV, which had been added to factor concentrate test samples, was effectively inactivated at 60 C to 68 C without significantly altering the plasma recovery or half-life of clotting factors.[51,52] Studies of small numbers of seronegative patients documented a lack of HIV seroconversion with American-made heat-treated factor VIII concentrates.[53,54] In October 1984, the CDC and the National Hemophilia Foundation recommended use of heat-treated factor concentrates to prevent further infection with HIV.[55]

Since then, the CDC has evaluated about 75 reports of HIV seroconversion associated with heat-treated factor concentrates. As of March 1988, only 18 reports met the criteria for association of seroconversion with heat-treated factor concentrates. Ten of the 18 were associated with concentrates produced before the initiation of donor screening; of these, most occurred in patients receiving concentrate produced by a single manufacturer. To determine the risk of seroconversion in patients receiving unscreened, heat-treated products, the CDC surveyed 13 hemophilia treatment centers located in Western Europe, Canada, and Australia.[56] Centers outside the United States were chosen because they had used heat-treated products longer. These hemophilia treatment centers reported that 1,300

patients were seronegative when unscreened heat-treated concentrates were introduced. In 23 patients, seroconversion occurred after the change to heat-treated products. Only three documented seroconversions could be attributed to the heat-treated factor product. These three patients represented 0.2% of the 1,300 patients at these centers.

Eight reports have met the criteria for an association between seroconversion and the use of donor-screened, heat-treated products. All patients had received non-screened products in the past; however, timing of the seroconversions allowed an association with screened, heat-treated products. One seroconversion occurred in the United States in a patient with an inhibitor to factor VIII who had received extremely large doses of concentrate (J.M. Jason, personal communication). The implicated product had been heated in the dry state at 60 C for 24 hours. Seven of the seroconversions were reported from Canada (R. Remus, personal communication). The seroconversions occurred at one hemophilia treatment center and were noted in the late spring and summer of 1987. The investigators demonstrated a statistical association between seroconversion and receipt of one batch of concentrate produced by a single manufacturer. This product, which was not made by the company involved in the seroconversion in the United States, had been heated in the dry state at 60 C for 30 hours. The company has now withdrawn these products from the market.

Because of these seroconversions and the continued high risk for non-A/non-B hepatitis, manufacturers continue to improve the safety of factor products. Detergent-treated products, products with varying lengths of heat treatment, and monoclonal-antibody-purified products have been introduced and licensed. The limited experience with these products prevents assessment of the safety of these products relative to products currently in use, but preliminary studies suggest that some may be effective against non-A/non-B hepatitis. Unfortunately, the higher cost of these products may limit their availability.

HIV Transmission in the Health-Care Setting

Recommendations for the Health-Care Professional

Because HIV infection can be transmitted by exposure to infected blood or blood components, health-care workers whose activities involve contact with the infected patient's blood or body fluids are also at risk for HIV infection. Seroconversions in health-care workers after exposure to an HIV-infected patient have been reported; however, prospective studies suggest the risk is relatively small.[57] In a study conducted by the CDC, 883 health-care workers were tested for antibody to HIV after a documented exposure to HIV as of July 1987. Of the 883, a total of 708 had percutaneous (needlestick) exposures, and 175 had exposure through mucous membranes or open wounds. Of 396 workers for whom only a convalescent-phase serum sample was obtained ≥ 90 days postexposure, one worker was seropositive. Heterosexual transmission could not be ruled out for this patient. In the 425 workers for whom both acute- and convalescent-phase serum samples were tested, seroconversions were documented in three (0.7%) after the exposure. All three had percutaneous exposures, and none had other documented risk factors for HIV infection. In a similar study, 332 health-care workers with a total of 453 needlestick or percutaneous exposures were tested at the National Institutes of Health for HIV antibody as of April 1987; 103 workers had percutaneous exposures and 229 had mucous-membrane exposures. There were no instances of seroconversion. In a smaller study of 129 workers at the University of California, results were similar (no seroconversions).

The risk for HIV transmission in the health-care setting appears to be small, but transmission is possible. Health-care workers need to adhere rigorously to infection-control precautions to minimize the risk of exposure to blood and body fluids. Furthermore, since medical histories and examinations cannot reliably identify all patients infected with HIV, these precautions should be used consistently for all patients, especially those in the emergency-care settings in which the risk of contact with blood is increased and the infection status of the patient is usually not known.[57]

Guidelines

(1) All health-care workers should routinely use appropriate barrier precautions to prevent skin and mucous-membrane exposure to blood and body fluids. The type and extent of protection will vary with the situation and anticipated exposure. Gloves should be worn when exposure to blood and body fluids, mucous membranes, or nonintact skin is possible, when items or surfaces soiled with blood or body fluids are handled, and when venipuncture and other vascular-access procedures are performed. Gloves should be changed after contact with each patient. If the procedure is likely to generate droplets or splashes of blood, masks, protective eyewear, and gowns or aprons should be worn.

(2) Skin surfaces should be washed immediately if they become contaminated with blood or body fluids. Hands should be washed when gloves are removed.

(3) Care should be taken to prevent injuries caused by needles and other sharp instruments. Needles should not be recapped, bent, broken, or manipulated by hand after use. Disposable needles and syringes, scalpel blades, and other sharp items should be placed directly into a puncture-resistant container after use.

(4) Resuscitation equipment should be readily available so mouth-to-mouth resuscitation can be avoided.

(5) Health-care workers who have exudative lesions

or weeping dermatitis should refrain from all direct patient care and from handling patient-care equipment until the condition resolves.

The use of appropriate barrier precautions should be reemphasized for health-care workers who participate in invasive procedures, defined as surgical entry into tissues, cavities, or organs or repair of major traumatic injuries. These procedures include not only obvious surgical manipulations in the operating room or emergency room but also cardiac catheterization and angiographic procedures, vaginal and cesarean deliveries and other invasive obstetric procedures, and dental manipulations during which oral, perioral, or tooth structures are cut or removed. In addition to gloves and surgical masks, protective eyewear or face shields should be worn for procedures that commonly result in the generation of droplets or bone chips or splashing of blood or other body fluids. Gowns or aprons made of materials that provide an effective barrier should be worn during invasive procedures that are likely to result in splashing of blood or other body fluids.

Summary

Persons with hemophilia and other coagulation disorders were at risk for infection with HIV as a result of receiving blood products, particularly concentrated clotting factors. Because these products are now donor-screened and heat-treated to inactivate HIV, the risk of further infection in this population has been minimized. However, before the introduction of these interventions, many persons with hemophilia had been infected. As of Jan 4, 1988, 463 cases of hemophilia-associated AIDS had been reported to the Centers for Disease Control. Most patients had severe hemophilia and received commercially produced concentrated clotting factors. These patients may constitute as many as 25% of those hemophilic men known to be infected with HIV.

Through heterosexual and perinatal transmission, the partners and offspring of persons with hemophilia can become infected with HIV. The seroprevalence rate for female sex partners of men with hemophilia may be as high as 21%, and 16 AIDS cases have already been reported. Counseling and public health interventions are needed to prevent the further spread of HIV infection in sex partners and offspring of these patients and to prevent the associated morbidity and fatalities.

Because HIV infection can be transmitted by exposure to infected blood or blood components, health-care workers whose activities involve contact with infected blood or body fluids are also at risk for HIV infection. Prospective studies suggest this risk is very low; nevertheless, health-care workers need to adhere rigorously to infection-control precautions to minimize the risk of exposure to blood and body fluids. These precautions include wearing gloves, masks, protective eyewear, and gowns depending on the type of exposure anticipated. These precautions should be used with all patients.

References

1. *Study To Evaluate the Supply-Demand Relationship for AHF and PTC Through 1980*, US Dept of Health, Education, and Welfare, publication No. 77–1274. Government Printing Office, 1977.

2. Jason J, McDougal JS, Holman RC, et al: Human T-lymphotropic retrovirus type III/lymphadenopathy-associated virus antibody: Association with hemophiliacs' immune status and blood component usage. *JAMA* 1985;253:3409–3415.

3. Jason JM, Holman RC, Kennedy MS, et al: Longitudinal assessment of persons with hemophilia exposed to HTLV-III/LAV. Presented at the 26th Interscience Conference on Antimicrobial Agents and Chemotherapy, New Orleans, Sept 29, 1986.

4. Ragni MV, Tegtmeier GE, Levy JA, et al: AIDS retrovirus antibodies in hemophiliacs treated with factor VIII or factor IX concentrates, cryoprecipitates, or fresh frozen plasma: Prevalence, seroconversion rate, and clinical correlations. *Blood* 1986;67:592–595.

5. Goedert JJ, Sarngadharan MG, Eyster ME, et al: Antibodies reactive with human T cell leukemia viruses in the serum of hemophiliacs receiving factor VIII concentrate. *Blood* 1985;65:492–495.

6. Kreiss JK, Kitchen LW, Prince HE, et al: Human T cell leukemia virus type III antibody, lymphadenopathy, and acquired immune deficiency syndrome in hemophiliac subjects: Results of a prospective study. *Am J Med* 1986;80:345–350.

7. Gjerset GF, McGrady G, Counts RB, et al: Lymphadenopathy-associated virus antibodies and T cells in hemophiliacs treated with cryoprecipitate or concentrate. *Blood* 1985;66:718–720.

8. Waskin H, Smith KJ, Simon TL, et al: Prevalence of HTLV-III antibody among New Mexico residents with hemophilia. *West J Med* 1986;145:477–480.

9. Centers for Disease Control: Revision of the case definition of acquired immunodeficiency syndrome for national reporting—United States. *MMWR* 1985;34:373–375.

10. Centers for Disease Control: Revision of the CDC surveillance case definition for acquired immunodeficiency syndrome. *MMWR* 1987;36(suppl):3S–15S.

11. Martin LS, McDougal JS, Loskoski SL: Disinfection and inactivation of the human T lymphotropic virus type III/lymphadenopathy-associated virus. *J Infect Dis* 1985;152:400–403.

12. Piszkiewicz D, Kingdom H, Apfelzweig R, et al: Inactivation of HTLV-III/LAV during plasma fractionation, letter. *Lancet* 1985;2:1188–1189.

13. Selik RM, Starcher ET, Curran JW: Opportunistic diseases reported in AIDS patients: Frequencies, associations, and trends. *AIDS* 1987;1:175–182.

14. Centers for Disease Control: Update: Acquired immunodeficiency syndrome—United States. *MMWR* 1986;35:757–766.

15. Goedert JJ, Neuland CY, Wallen WC, et al: Amyl nitrite may alter T lymphocytes in homosexual men. *Lancet* 1982;1:412–416.

16. Marmor M, Friedman-Kien AE, Laubenstein L, et al: Risk factors for Kaposi's sarcoma in homosexual men. *Lancet* 1982;1:1083–1087.

17. Newell GR, Mansell PW, Wilson MB, et al: Risk factor analysis among men referred for possible acquired immune deficiency syndrome. *Prev Med* 1985;14:81–91.

18. Haverkos HW, Pinsky PF, Drotman DP, et al: Disease manifestation among homosexual men with acquired immunodeficiency syndrome: A possible role of nitrites in Kaposi's sarcoma. *Sex Transm Dis* 1985;12:203–208.

19. Giraldo G, Beth E, Huang ES: Kaposi's sarcoma and its relationship to cytomegalovirus (CMV): III. CMV, DNA and CMV early antigens in Kaposi's sarcoma. *Int J Cancer* 1980;26:23–29.

20. Drew WL, Conant MA, Miner RC, et al: Cytomegalovirus and Kaposi's sarcoma in young homosexual men. *Lancet* 1982;2:125–127.

21. Kreiss JK, Kitchen LW, Prince HE, et al: Antibody to human T-lymphotropic virus type III in wives of hemophiliacs: Evidence for heterosexual transmission. *Ann Intern Med* 1985;102:623–626.

22. Allain JP: Prevalence of HTLV-III/LAV antibodies in patients with hemophilia and in their sexual partners in France, letter. *N Engl J Med* 1986;315:517–518.

23. Andes WA, Rangan SR, deShazo RD, et al: The risks of heterosexual transmission of HIV in hemophiliac couples. Presented at the 1987 Annual Conference of the National Hemophilia Foundation, Omaha, Oct 7–11, 1987.

24. Lawrence DN, Jason JM, Holman RC, et al: Risk of human immunodeficiency virus transmission to sex partners of U.S. hemophilic men. *Am J Hematol*, in press.

25. Goedert JJ, Eyster ME, Biggar RJ: Heterosexual transmission of human immunodeficiency virus: Association with severe T4-cell depletion in male hemophiliacs. Presented at the Third International Conference on AIDS, Washington DC, 1987.

26. Padian N, Marquis L, Francis DP, et al: Male-to-female transmission of human immunodeficiency virus. *JAMA* 1987;258:788–790.

27. Fischl MA, Dickinson GM, Scott GB, et al: Evaluation of heterosexual partners, children, and household contacts of adults with AIDS. *JAMA* 1987;257:640–644.

28. Wasserman K, Wilson PA: Psychosocial impact of AIDS. Presented at the 1987 Annual Conference of the National Hemophilia Foundation, Omaha, Oct 7–11, 1987.

29. Clemow LP, Lerner AR, Saidi P: Impact of HIV-antibody testing on the use of condoms and on behavioral and emotional coping responses among hemophiliacs. Presented at the 1987 Annual Conference of the National Hemophilia Foundation, Omaha, Oct 7–11, 1987.

30. Centers for Disease Control: HIV infection and pregnancies in sexual partners of HIV-seropositive men—United States. *MMWR* 1987;36:593–595.

31. Ragni MV, Urbach AH, Kiernan S, et al: Acquired immunodeficiency syndrome in the child of a haemophiliac. *Lancet* 1985;1:133–135.

32. Ragni MV, Spero JA, Bontempo FA, et al: Recurrent infections and lymphadenopathy in the children of a hemophiliac: A survey of children of hemophiliacs positive for human immunodeficiency virus antibody. *Ann Intern Med* 1986;105:886–887.

33. Rubinstein A, Sicklick M, Gupta A, et al: Acquired immunodeficiency with reversed T₄/T₈ ratios in infants born to promiscuous and drug-addicted mothers. *JAMA* 1983;249:2350–2356.

34. Scott GB, Buck BE, Leterman JG, et al: Acquired immunodeficiency syndrome in infants. *N Engl J Med* 1984;310:76–81.

35. Scott GB, Fischl MA, Klimas N, et al: Mothers of infants with the acquired immunodeficiency syndrome. *JAMA* 1985;253:363–366.

36. Cowan MJ, Hellmann D, Chudwin D, et al: Maternal transmission of acquired immune deficiency syndrome: Evidence for both symptomatic and asymptomatic carriers. *Pediatrics* 1984;73:382–386.

37. Rogers MF: Transmission of the human immunodeficiency virus infection in the United States, in Silverman BK, Waddell A (eds): *Report of the Surgeon General's Workshop on Children with HIV Infection and Their Families*. US Dept of Health and Human Services publication No. HRS-D-MC 87–1. US Government Printing Office, 1987.

38. Lapointe N, Michaud J, Pekovic D, et al: Transplacental transmission of HTLV-III virus, letter. *N Engl J Med* 1985;312:1325–1326.

39. Thiry L, Sprecher-Goldberger S, Jonckheer T, et al: Isolation of AIDS virus from cell-free breast milk of three healthy virus carriers, letter. *Lancet* 1985;2:891–892.

40. Ziegler JB, Cooper DA, Johnson RO, et al: Postnatal transmission of AIDS-associated retrovirus from mother to infant. *Lancet* 1985;1:896–898.

41. Nzilambi N, Ryder RW, Behets F: Perinatal HIV transmission in two African hospitals. Presented at the Third International Conference on AIDS, Washington DC, 1987.

42. Selwyn PA, Schoenbaum EE, Feingold AR, et al: Pregnancy outcomes and perinatal transmission of HIV in IV drug users. Presented at the 115th Annual Meeting of the American Public Health Association, New Orleans, Oct 19, 1987.

43. Centers for Disease Control: Provisional Public Health Service inter-agency recommendations for screening donated blood and plasma for antibody to the virus causing acquired immunodeficiency syndrome. *MMWR* 1985;34:1–5.

44. Ward JW, Grindon AJ, Feorino PM, et al: Laboratory and epidemiologic evaluation of an enzyme immunoassay for antibodies to HTLV-III. *JAMA* 1986;256:357–361.

45. Centers for Disease Control: Update: Public Health Service workshop on human T-lymphotropic virus type III antibody testing--United States. *MMWR* 1985;34:477–478.

46. Centers for Disease Control: Update: Serologic testing for antibody to human immunodeficiency virus. *MMWR* 1988;833–845.

47. Centers for Disease Control: Public Health Service guidelines for counseling and antibody testing to prevent HIV infection and AIDS. *MMWR* 1987:36:509–514.

48. Ranki A, Valle SL, Krohn M, et al: Long latency precedes overt seroconversion in sexually transmitted human-immunodeficiency-virus infection. *Lancet* 1987;2:589–593.

49. Kleinman S: Risk of HIV transmission by anti-HIV negative blood. Presented at the Third International Conference on AIDS, Washington DC, 1987.

50. Lelie PN, Reesink HW, Huisman JG: Earlier detection of HIV and second-generation antibody assays, letter. *Lancet* 1987;2:343.

51. McDougal JS, Martin LS, Cort SP, et al: Thermal inactivation of the acquired immunodeficiency syndrome virus, human T lymphotropic virus-III/lymphadenopathy-associated virus, with special reference to antihemophilic factor. *J Clin Invest* 1985;76:875–877.

52. Levy JA, Mitra G, Mozen MM: Recovery and inactivation of infectious retroviruses from factor VIII concentrate. *Lancet* 1984;2:722–723.

53. Rouzioux C, Chamaret S, Montagnier L, et al: Absence of antibodies to AIDS virus in haemophiliacs treated with heat-treated factor VIII concentrate, letter. *Lancet* 1985;12:271–272.

54. Felding P, Nilsson IM, Hansson BG, et al: Absence of antibodies to LAV/HTLV-III in haemophiliacs treated with heat-treated factor VIII concentrate of American origin, letter. *Lancet* 1985;2:832–833.

55. Centers for Disease Control: Update: Acquired immunodeficiency syndrome (AIDS) in persons with hemophilia. *MMWR* 1984;33:589–591.

56. Centers for Disease Control: Survey of non-US hemophilia treatment centers for HIV seroconversions following therapy with heat-treated factor concentrates. *MMWR* 1987;36:121–124.

57. Centers for Disease Control: Recommendations for prevention of HIV transmission in health-care settings. *MMWR* 1987;36(suppl):3S–18S.

Nonsurgical Management of Hemophilic Arthropathy

Walter B. Greene, MD

Campbell W. McMillan, MD

Introduction

Injury to a blood vessel initiates a fascinating symphony of reactions to restore hemostasis. This highly integrated process not only permits safe surgery, but also protects us from the many bumps of everyday activity. The clotting process may be divided into vascular, platelet, and plasma phases[1-4] that overlap to some extent.

The vascular phase includes the clinically evident vasoconstriction and the less evident exposure of tissue elements that (1) promote adhesion and aggregation of platelets, (2) release tissue thromboplastin to activate the extrinsic coagulation pathway, and (3) activate factor XII to initiate the intrinsic coagulation pathway. The major components of the platelet phase include (1) platelet adhesion to the vascular tissues (assisted by factor VIII-related von Willebrand factor), (2) platelet aggregation, (3) release of platelet thromboplastin to activate the intrinsic coagulation pathway, and (4) clot retraction initiated by platelet thrombosthenin.

The plasma phase of restoring hemostasis is initially directed toward coagulation but is later directed toward fibrinolysis. Two sequences of reactions, one initiated outside the vessel and one initiated within the vessel, produce the enzyme thrombin, the key to formation and stabilization of a fibrin clot (Fig. 34–1). In the extrinsic pathway, tissue thromboplastin activates factor VII, which, in the presence of ionic calcium, activates factor X. The intrinsic pathway begins with sequential activation of factors XII, XI, and IX. Activated factor IX, in the presence of ionic calcium and phospholipids,[2] activates factor X in a reaction tremendously accelerated by activated factor VIII (factor VIII is activated by thrombin and activated factor X). Activated factor X, whether derived from the intrinsic or the extrinsic pathway, combines with factor V, ionic calcium, and platelet thromboplastin to convert prothrombin to thrombin. Thrombin then acts to cleave peptides from fibrinogen, creating fibrin monomers. The unstable fibrin polymer that then forms is subsequently stabilized by activated factor XIII working in concert with ionic calcium. When the clot is no longer needed, fibrinolytic activity ensues.

Overview of Clotting Deficiencies

Although any of the 13 recognized plasma coagulation factors may be deficient or absent, musculoskel-etal problems are primarily limited to deficient factor VIII coagulant activity, known as classic hemophilia or hemophilia A, and deficient factor IX activity, known as Christmas disease or hemophilia B. Factor VIII deficiency constitutes about 75% of all inherited clotting disorders and affects 60 to 80 persons per million population.[5] Factor IX deficiency, the next most common inherited clotting disorder, constitutes about 12% of the total and affects ten to 15 persons per million population.[5] The other clotting deficiencies are not only less frequent but also differ from classic hemophilia and Christmas disease on clinical grounds. Musculoskeletal bleeding, particularly into the joints, characterizes the clinical problems seen in patients with factor VIII and factor IX deficiencies. The other inherited coagulation disorders are characterized by mucosal hemorrhages such as epistaxis and menorrhagia and rarely involve joint hemorrhage except after major trauma. Why some coagulation defects cause joint problems and others do not has not been satisfactorily explained, but since the other inherited coagulation disorders rarely present major musculoskeletal problems, our discussion will be limited to factor VIII and factor IX deficiencies.

Clinical Assessment of Hemostasis and Diagnosis of Coagulation Disorders

Suspected coagulation abnormalities can be effectively screened by pertinent questions during the history-taking and selected laboratory tests. Both major forms of hemophilia are characterized by excessive hemorrhage from surface wounds and recurrent bleeding into musculoskeletal sites, particularly the joints. Both factor VIII and factor IX deficiencies are transmitted by a sex-linked recessive gene, and, therefore, both disorders are largely restricted to males. A history of affected males on the maternal side of the family combined with a typical history of hemorrhage should lead to confirmation by laboratory tests. Screening laboratory tests for coagulation problems include (1) platelet count combined with inspection of the blood smear, (2) Ivy bleeding time to assess platelet function, (3) plasma prothrombin time (PT) to assess the extrinsic and common pathways of coagulation, and (4) plasma partial thromboplastin time (PTT) to assess the intrinsic and common pathways of coagulation.[1] The PTT is the screening test abnormal in both classic hemophilia and

EXTRINSIC PATHWAY   INTRINSIC PATHWAY

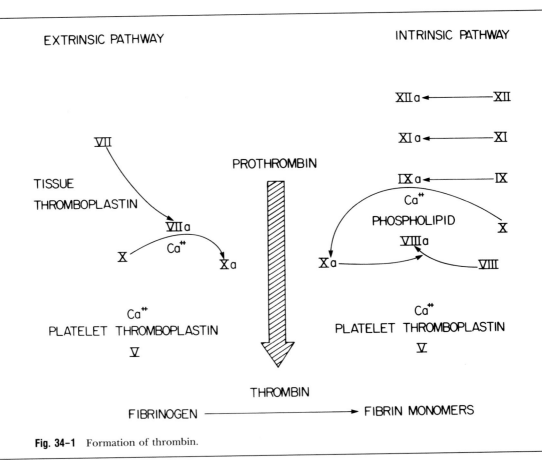

Fig. 34-1   Formation of thrombin.

Christmas disease. Specific factor assays are utilized to establish the specific deficiency and its degree.

Factor VIII and factor IX activities are quantitated in units with 1 unit equal to the activity in 1 ml of pooled, normal plasma. Factor VIII and factor IX concentrations are commonly designated as percent activity, representing units per deciliter. Therefore, factor VIII and factor IX activities in a normal person should be 100% but a range from 50% to 200% is within normal limits. The other coagulation factors are also quantitated in this manner with the exception of fibrinogen, which is directly measurable and therefore expressed in milligrams per deciliter.

Deficiencies of either factor VIII or factor IX are commonly graded as follows: severe, less than 1% activity; moderate, 1% to 5% activity; and mild, more than 5% activity. The degree of deficiency correlates with the tendency toward musculoskeletal hemorrhages. In patients with severe deficiency, muscle or joint hemorrhages develop spontaneously or as a result of minimal trauma. In patients with mild deficiency, a hemarthrosis rarely develops unless significant trauma occurs. Patients with moderate deficiency have intermediate symptoms but tend to have significantly less joint arthropathy than those with severe disorders.

Role of the Comprehensive Center

In the mid-1970s the Maternal and Child Division of the US Department of Health, Education and Welfare sponsored regional comprehensive hemophilia clinics. These clinics were typically staffed by a hematologist, orthopaedic surgeon, physical therapist, specially trained nurse, dentist, social worker, psychiatrist, vocational rehabilitation counselor, and genetic counselor. With the advent of the acquired immune deficiency syndrome (AIDS), infectious disease consultation was also provided. The comprehensive center works with local community health providers to give periodic examinations, teach patients how to transfuse themselves, and to provide information to help patients prevent or deal with disabling complications. Annual assessment during the past decade has shown that these comprehensive clinics have reduced the time the patient is away from work or school and have reduced medical expenses per patient per year. Those of us who have been involved in the fragmented approaches of the past are convinced that the comprehensive clinics are vastly superior. When the comprehensive clinic is combined with treatment by interested and knowledgeable physicians in the patient's community, the patient with hemophilia receives optimal medical therapy.

Replacement Therapy in Hemophilia

Without appropriate replacement of the missing clotting factor, neither acute bleeding episodes nor surgery can be effectively managed. Whole blood and plasma were the mainstays of transfusion therapy until the discovery of cryoprecipitate by Pool and Shannon[6] in 1965. They found that one half the factor VIII in a standard bag of fresh-frozen plasma could be recovered in about 25 ml of cryoprecipitate when the bag was slowly thawed at 5 C. Cryoprecipitate greatly reduced the volume requirements necessitated by plasma transfusions. Subsequently, Wagner and associates[7] and Brinkhous and associates[8] reduced volume requirements even more by using agents such as glycine to extract and concentrate factor VIII from cryoprecipitate. With concentrates, the amount of factor VIII normally found in a patient's total blood volume can be delivered in a 50-ml syringe. Effective treatment of acute hemorrhages was possible with cryoprecipitate but the development of concentrates made elective surgery and home transfusion therapy feasible.

Factor IX concentrates differ from factor VIII preparations in that factor IX is not exclusively present in the preparation. Four vitamin K-dependent factors (factors VII, IX, X, and prothrombin) are concentrated from plasma fractions and labeled as prothrombin complex concentrates.[9,10] The label on each bottle does indicate coagulation activity in factor IX units, but the package insert for prothrombin complex concentrate also lists the activities of the other three factors.

The development of concentrates has also increased the transmission of blood-borne diseases. Plasma from many donors was pooled in the preparation of both factor VIII and factor IX concentrates. In the 1970s, hepatitis was the recognized complication of transfusion therapy. Many patients with severe hemophilia had hepatitis-associated antibodies although, fortunately, few developed chronic hepatitis.[11] In the early 1980s, AIDS was clearly identified in hemophiliacs.[12] Donors whose blood is used to prepare the concentrates are now screened for hepatitis B and human immunodeficiency virus (HIV). In addition, the products are heat-treated. With heat treatment and pasteurization there is reasonable, although not absolute, certainty that the HIV has *not* been transmitted by concentrates infused since 1985.[13,14] Vaccination for hepatitis B is also recommended for seronegative patients.

Other possible complications of replacement therapy include hemolysis and thrombosis. In patients with blood types A, AB, or B, hemolysis may develop when large quantities of factor VIII or factor IX are administered. This occurs because the anti-A and anti-B antibodies cannot be eliminated totally from concentrates.[15] Thrombosis is unusual after administration of factor IX concentrates but one must always be aware of the possibility.[16] Current products appear to be less hazardous in this regard.

Transfusion replacement options are limited in hemophiliacs in whom an inhibitor to the appropriate clotting factor develops. Inhibitors are antibodies that are largely, although not exclusively, found in severely deficient subjects. The problem occurs in about 15% of patients with classic hemophilia.[17] Although factor IX inhibitors may occur in patients with Christmas disease, the prevalence in this disorder is much less than that in factor VIII deficiency.[18] Low-titer inhibitors may develop at any time, but once a patient has received 100 transfusions, the likelihood of a high-titer inhibitor developing is remote.[19]

Patients with inhibitors do not bleed more frequently than or differently from other hemophiliacs. Rather, these patients are resistant to conventional replacement therapy since the antibody inhibits or ties up the infused product. The potency of a patient's inhibitor status is defined in Bethesda units per milliliters of plasma. Inhibitors of less than 10 Bethesda units/ml may be treated with factor VIII replacement therapy although the dose must be appropriately increased to overwhelm the antibodies.[20] Inhibitor titers of 10 to 20 Bethesda units/ml sometimes can be treated with high doses of factor VIII. Inhibitor activities of more than 20 Bethesda units/ml are difficult to treat and, at present, therapy is not effective enough to allow elective surgery. Clinical experiments to induce immune tolerance in patients with high-titer inhibitors are ongoing,[21-23] but because of their high cost, the risk of HIV transmission, and the somewhat uncertain response, we would agree with others[20] that these measures should be reserved for extreme situations.

Although complications may develop with replacement therapy, factor VIII and factor IX concentrates have provided unmistakable benefits to patients with hemophilia. This was demonstrated from 1983 to 1985 when the risk of AIDS to hemophiliacs became fully evident. At that time, some persons with hemophilia tried to avoid transfusion therapy for "minor" bleeding. These minor bleeding episodes frequently progressed to major hemorrhages that required hospitalization and ultimately the patient required more transfusions.

Guidelines for Replacement Therapy

By definition, a unit of factor VIII is that activity of factor VIII in 1 ml of fresh-frozen plasma. Per kilogram of body weight, each unit of factor VIII infused will produce a 2% increase in the plasma VIII level. For example, we would treat an acute hemarthrosis by raising the factor VIII level to 50%. In a 50-kg person with severe hemophilia, the dose of factor VIII concentrate would be 25 units × 50 kg or 1,250 units. The activity of factor VIII falls off exponentially with an initial half-time of about four to six hours followed by a steady-state half-time of 12 hours (Fig. 34–2). In practical terms, the half-life of factor VIII is 12 hours (assuming no inhibitor activity), and 12 hours after infusion of 25 units/kg of body weight the typical patient in the above example would have a factor VIII level of 25%.

For factor IX deficiency, the guidelines for bolus replacement therapy are approximately the same, although for different reasons. One unit of factor IX per kilogram of body weight increases the plasma level by only 1%. However, because the half-time of factor IX is 18 to 24 hours and because patients with factor IX deficiency do not seem to require the same peak concentration used in factor VIII deficiency, the total amount transfused for acute hemorrhages tends to be equivalent in the two clotting disorders. For example, a 50-kg patient with factor IX deficiency would receive 25 units/kg or 1,250 units of prothrombin complex concentrate for an acute hemarthrosis. The initial increase in factor IX is less than in factor VIII deficiency, but at the more critical time of 24 to 48 hours the coverage is roughly equivalent (Figs. 34–2 and 34–3). Therefore, in practical terms, the recommended units per kilogram of body weight for bolus replacement therapy of factor VIII deficiency are equivalent to those for factor IX deficiency.

Home Transfusion Therapy

After the development of effective concentrates, home transfusion therapy became a reality.[24] Quick ad-

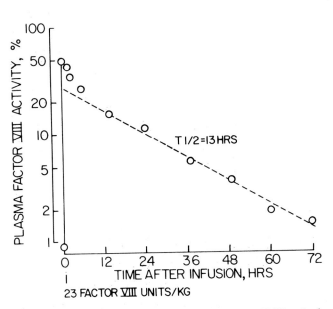

Fig. 34-2   Fall-off curve after infusion of factor VIII (23 units/kg of body weight) in a patient with severe classic hemophilia. This patient's half-time of 13 hours demonstrates typical variation in the individual person.

ministration of the appropriate clotting factor stops minor hemorrhages before they become major problems. Active encouragement by physicians and specially trained nurses makes it feasible to institute home replacement therapy in 75% to 80% of preschool patients with severe hemophilia. We advocate a transfusion of 25 units/kg of body weight for routine treatment of muscle or joint hemorrhage. Patients or parents are instructed to call if there is any evidence of nerve compression, retroperitoneal bleeding, or bleeding that does not respond to the initial injection. Unfortunately, home transfusion therapy has not eliminated hemophilic arthropathy.

Pathophysiology of Hemophilic Arthropathy

The pathophysiology of hemophilic arthropathy begins with the hemarthrosis. Blood breakdown products must be absorbed by the synovium. Iron seems to be the most damaging element. In a study of normal patients undergoing surgery shortly after traumatic hemarthrosis, synovial biopsy specimens demonstrated iron in both the synovial cells and subsynovial macrophages.[25] The synovial cells contained siderosomes (secondary lysosomes thought to contain iron ferritin granules) as well as free-lying electron-dense granules thought to represent hemosiderin. As soon as four days after the onset of a single hemarthrosis, the synovium demonstrates focal areas of villous proliferation.

In the joint of a hemophiliac who experiences several bleeding episodes within a short period, the synovium becomes inflamed and hypertrophic.[26-28] The hypertrophic synovium is characterized by villous formation, markedly increased vascularity, and chronic inflammatory cells (Fig. 34–4, *top*). The zone of synoviocytes lining the villus is thicker, being four or five cells deep. Hemosiderin deposits accumulate in the outer border of the synovial villi (Fig. 34–4, *bottom*). Inflammatory cells congregate around the vessels and hemosiderin deposits. Electron microscopy shows that many of the siderosomes contain iron and that these iron-positive cells are in the process of disintegration.[28] The synoviocyte can absorb a limited amount of iron; once that quantity is exceeded, however, the cell disintegrates and releases lysosomes that not only destroy articular cartilage but also inflame the synovial tissue.[29-31] The hypervascular synovium in a person with a clotting deficiency is friable and tends to ooze blood into the joint. This perpetuates synovial inflammation and joint destruction.

Blood breakdown products also affect the chondrocyte. Experimental studies demonstrate that even in the early stage of joint disease the chondrocytes contain siderosomes and have cellular changes consistent with cell disruption.[32] Chondrocytes in growing animals are particularly susceptible to intramuscular iron-dextran

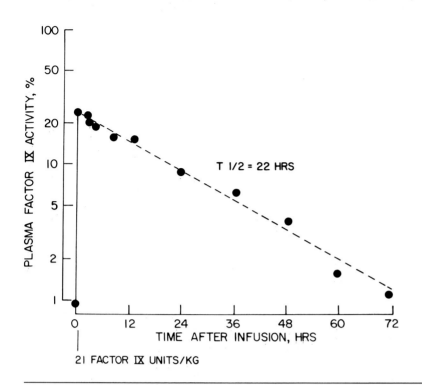

Fig. 34-3 Fall-off curve after infusion of factor IX (21 units/kg of body weight) in a patient with severe factor IX deficiency.

injections.[33] The severe damage seen in hemophilic arthropathy typically occurs at an early age. Initially we thought the problem was psychological—that children with hemophilia failed to restrict their activities appropriately and therefore experienced one joint bleeding episode after another. However, we now believe that there is a physiologic as well as a psychological reason for the rapid joint destruction so often seen in children with hemophilia. The physiologic basis is the susceptibility of chondrocytes in a growing person to iron deposition within the cell (Fig. 34–5). With disintegration of the chondrocyte, not only are lysosomes released to destroy cartilage matrix, but the factory making the cartilage matrix (the chondrocyte) is also destroyed.

In advanced hemophilic arthropathy, the synovium loses its marked villous formation and is largely replaced by fibrous tissue.[26,28] A layer of synovial cells stained with hemosiderin deposits is present but the synovial folds are obliterated (Fig. 34–6). This is associated with loss of joint motion and loss of distensibility of the joint. Because the joint folds are obliterated, a hemarthrosis in a joint with advanced arthropathy does not cause the marked distension typically seen in the earlier phases of hemophilic arthropathy; however, the amount of pain is approximately the same.

In advanced arthropathy the articular cartilage appears grossly and histologically similar to osteoarthritis except that a brown pannus usually covers the articular surface, and iron deposits within the chondrocyte have been demonstrated on specimens obtained during total joint arthroplasty.[28,34] Necrosis of the chondrocyte associated with siderosome formation has been observed in these specimens. Fissures and clefts in the articular surface, decreased staining for glycosaminoglycans, clusters of cartilage cells, and uneven wearing of the articular cartilage are otherwise similar to the histologic changes seen in osteoarthritis (Fig. 34–7).

As a general rule, recurrent hemarthrosis of the same joint within a short period sets the stage for hemophilic arthropathy; however, anyone who has worked in a hemophilia clinic can recall individuals in whom a relentless hypertrophic synovitis developed after only one or two joint bleeding episodes. This individual susceptibility raises the question of an autoimmune reaction,[30] but this association has not been defined.

In summary, the unique aspect of the pathophysiology of hemophilic arthropathy is the destructive effect that iron has on both the chondrocyte and the synoviocyte. This "double whammy" may result in rapid joint erosions, particularly in the child.

Roentgenographic Evaluation

Radiographic changes in the early stages of hemophilic arthropathy are similar to those in rheumatoid arthritis, whereas later changes are more typical of osteoarthritis. Radiographic findings in hypertrophic synovitis include soft-tissue swelling, osteopenia, and overgrowth of the epiphysis. Later bony changes include

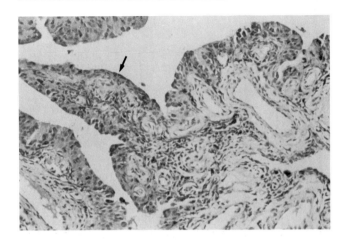

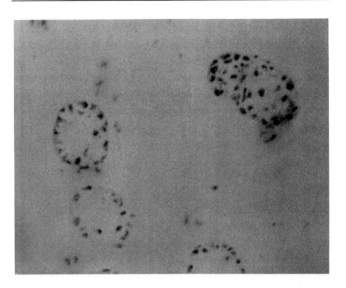

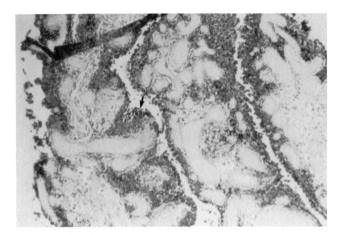

Fig. 34-5 Cartilage shaving from patellar erosions in an 11-year-old with factor IX hemophilia. The patient had had only nine months of difficulty with this knee. Chondrocytes demonstrate disintegration with iron deposition around the periphery (Perls' stain).

Fig. 34-4 **Top:** Knee synovium from an 8-year-old boy with hemophilia who had an 18-month history of hypertrophic synovitis and recurrent hemarthrosis. Note villous formation, markedly increased vascularity, and chronic inflammatory cell infiltrates. The arrow points to a typical villus. **Bottom:** Perls' stain demonstrates that iron in this tissue is concentrated in the area of synovial lining cells. The arrow indicates the area of synovial lining.

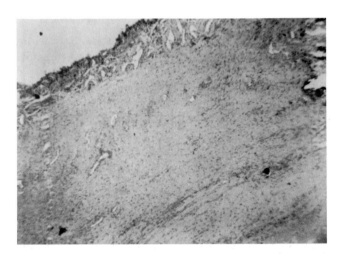

Fig. 34-6 Synovectomy specimen from an 18-year-old patient with hemophilia. Synovium consists largely of fibrous tissue. (Reproduced with permission from Greene WB, Wilson FC: The management of musculoskeletal problems in hemophilia: Part II. Pathophysiologic and roentgenographic changes in hemophilic arthropathy, in Evarts CM (ed): American Academy of Orthopaedic Surgeons *Instructional Course Lectures, XXXII.* St. Louis, CV Mosby, 1983, pp 217–223.)

subchondral cysts, marginal erosions, subchondral surface irregularity, widening of the intercondylar notch of the femur, squaring of the patella, enlargement of the radial head, and widening of the trochlear notch of the olecranon. With progression of the arthropathy, articular cartilage narrowing becomes obvious. Some patients develop marked deformity and angulation changes.

At present, two radiographic classifications are commonly used to stage hemophilic arthropathy. In the United States the classification system developed by Arnold and Hilgartner[30] is usually used. In this system grade 0 is a normal joint, grade 1 demonstrates soft-tissue swelling, grade 2 is characterized by osteopenia and overgrowth of the epiphysis, grade 3 has changes in the bony contours such as squaring of the patella and subchondral cyst, grade 4 has narrowing of the articular cartilage, and grade 5 is extensive joint de-

struction with fibrous ankylosis. The eight-part, 13-point radiographic classification described by Pettersson and associates[35] has been recommended by the Orthopaedic Advisory Committee of the World Federation of Hemophilia. In a recent comparison of the Arnold and Pettersson classification systems, Greene and associates[36] found that the Pettersson classification was more difficult to use but was better for staging advanced

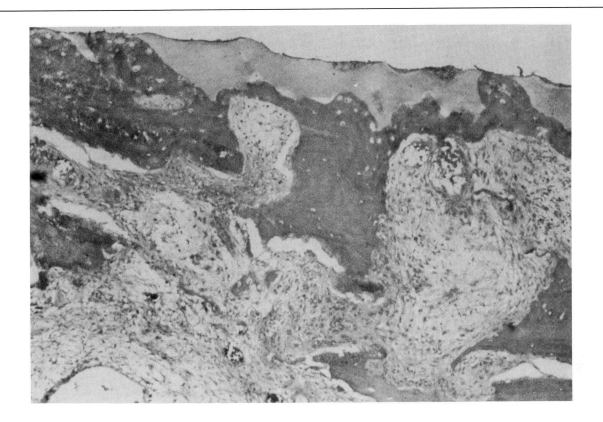

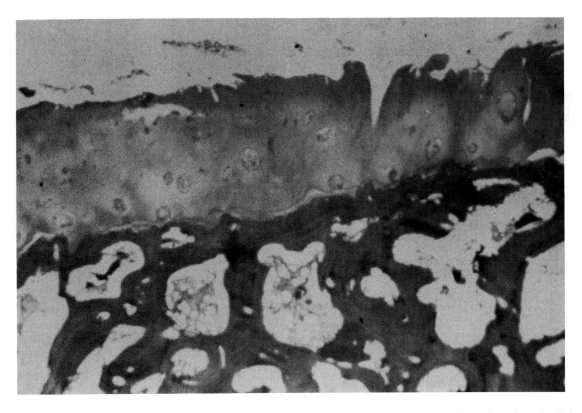

Fig. 34–7 Tissue from radial head excision in a 26-year-old patient with hemophilia. **Top:** Central portion of radial head. Articular cartilage and tidemark are completely destroyed, and fibrous tissue overlies bone. **Bottom:** Peripheral portion of radial head. Vascular invasion in cartilage with some cartilage cell clusters and fibrillation. (Reproduced with permission from Greene WB, Wilson FC: The management of musculoskeletal problems in hemophilia: Part II. Pathophysiologic and roentgenographic changes in hemophilic arthropathy, in Evarts CM (ed): American Academy of Orthopaedic Surgeons *Instructional Course Lectures, XXXII*. St. Louis, CV Mosby, 1983, pp 217–223.)

arthropathy. In this study, a four-part, seven-point classification system demonstrated equivalent accuracy but was simpler to use than the Pettersson system (Table 34–1).

Role of the Orthopaedic Surgeon

Although home transfusion therapy has been extremely helpful, it has not been a panacea for eliminating hemophilic arthropathy, even with the most compliant patient. Other therapies discussed below are necessary if hemophilic arthropathy is to be prevented. An "aggressive" nonsurgical program is especially beneficial in hemophilia since the surgical options are costly, complicated, and at best temporizing. The orthopaedic surgeon, who understands joint mechanics and rehabilitation, needs to be involved from the beginning.

Learning To Live With the Disease: Recreation, Sports, and Prophylactic Exercise

Like others, children with hemophilia enjoy play and recreation even though some sports may be detrimental to their joints. Working with patients from an early age and their parents is helpful in guiding children with hemophilia to live within the limits of their disease. Our goal is to encourage maximum activity as long as that activity does not routinely precipitate a bleeding episode. This attitude not only has psychological benefits, but we think that it is physiologically sound. Sports help to maintain muscle strength. Since one aspect of muscle function is to absorb stress, good muscle strength helps protect the joint.

Swimming at an early age is encouraged. Swimming exercises most muscle groups, it has a low index of injury when compared with other sports,[37] and after development of severe joint problems it may be the

Table 34–1
Seven-point classification of hemophilic arthropathy

Classification	Score
Subchondral irregularity	
Absent	0
Mild (≤50% of joint surface)	1
Pronounced	2
Joint space narrowing	
Absent	0
≤50%	1
>50%	2
Joint margin erosion	
Absent	0
Present	1
Joint surface incongruity	
Absent	0
Mild	1
Pronounced	2

only athletic activity a patient can enjoy. Unless a patient is having difficulty with recurrent hemarthrosis and synovitis, sports with relatively little contact—such as softball, kickball, and even soccer—are permitted, particularly in the grade-school years. An adolescent without significant arthropathy may play tennis even on an interscholastic competitive level. We also encourage teenagers to consider golf. Contact sports such as tackle football are discouraged.

One of the keys to allowing greater participation in recreational sports is the use of home transfusion therapy. In that way, the minor muscle hemorrhages that occasionally develop with soccer or other such sports can be aborted before major problems occur.

Any physical therapy program, particularly when prescribed on a prophylactic basis, has limited success when applied to a chronic problem. Most people, and particularly children, become bored with regimented exercises. On the other hand, a specific exercise program is more efficient than recreational activities in muscle strengthening. We have found that limited therapy goals that target the most vulnerable area are more likely to succeed in a person with a chronic disease. An exercise program that can be done at home, without expensive equipment, and that can be completed within 15 minutes is more likely to be sustained than a more extensive program that interferes excessively with daily living.

For several reasons we think that the knee muscles should be targeted in patients with hemophilia. In this disease, the knee is the most frequently and most severely affected joint. Reasons for its vulnerability include its weightbearing function, its lack of intrinsic bony stability compared with the hip and ankle, and the three-dimensional movements and stresses occurring at this joint. The knee extensor and flexor muscles not only provide movement but also decelerate movement and absorb weightbearing forces acting across the joint.[38] If repeated bleeding episodes occur in the knee, the hypertrophic synovitis is accompanied by a rather dramatic thigh atrophy. This muscle weakness makes the knee even more vulnerable to stresses, resulting in further joint bleeding episodes. More such episodes exacerbate the synovitis and a vicious cycle is created that ultimately causes joint destruction. Strickler and Greene[39] measured knee flexor and extensor torque in 59 patients with hemophilia and showed a dramatic reduction in their muscle strength. In our adult patients (most of whom had some degree of knee arthropathy), the knee extensor torque averaged 52.5 ft-lb compared to normal men whose knee extensor torque averaged approximately 150 ft-lb.[40] Our patients also had a marked reduction in knee flexor strength although the difference was not as great.

When they are about 7 years old, our patients with hemophilia are instructed in an exercise program for the knee flexors and extensors. The patients are encouraged to do the exercises for 15 minutes each day.

Greene and Strickler[40] developed a modified isokinetic strengthening program that in 32 patients with severe hemophilia produced in six months a 22% increase in extensor strength and a 25% increase in flexor strength. Greater increase in muscle strength was obtained in patients who exercised three or more days per week and in those without joint narrowing. These modified isokinetic exercises eliminated the need for special equipment and allowed the exercises to be done at home. Isokinetic strengthening also permits maximal muscle tension through a full arc of motion, but the muscle tension can also be decreased to allow acceptable patellofemoral compressive forces. Since the patella is frequently involved in hemophilic arthropathy, the possibility of modulating patellofemoral forces may be beneficial for these patients.

Adolescence causes difficulty in normal children. At this time of "normal defiance," the teenager with hemophilia may start living beyond the safe and acceptable limits of the disease. A good doctor-patient relationship developed before these years minimizes the stress of adolescence. We have also been impressed that summer camps designed for children with hemophilia often ease the transition through adolescence. At these camps children with hemophilia, who are often the only affected persons in their own communities, have fun and can share their frustrations with other children who have similar problems. The camp places the disease in perspective.

Acute Hemarthrosis

The joints that commonly bleed in persons with hemophilia include the knee, ankle, and elbow. In small children the ankle is frequently the target joint because it is vulnerable to the jumping from heights that is part of play at this age. After the age of 5 years, the knee joint assumes a more prominent role and overall is the joint in our clinic population that has the highest frequency of hemarthrosis. The elbow joint also becomes more of a problem after 5 years of age and, similar to fracture patterns, the nondominant elbow is more often affected. The shoulder and hip joints may also be affected by hemarthrosis, but in this era of home therapy they rarely progress to significant arthropathy. Even before the days of effective transfusion, it was rare to have joint bleeding in other areas except after major trauma.

In severe hemophilia, hemarthroses may occur spontaneously or after minimal trauma. A prodrome of pain is frequently perceived before joint swelling is obvious. The physical signs of a minor hemarthrosis include increased warmth, swelling, and some limitation of motion. Minor joint bleeding can be handled at home if transfusion therapy has been instituted. As soon as possible the patient or parents should transfuse the appropriate concentrate. For factor VIII deficiency we like to infuse an amount that produces factor levels that are 50% of normal, although some groups advocate transfusing only to the 30% level. For hemarthrosis involving weightbearing joints, we encourage the patient to use crutches until the pain has fully subsided and until 90 degrees of knee motion or full ankle dorsiflexion has been achieved. Ice packs and mild analgesics are useful adjuncts in controlling pain.

Major joint bleeding must be treated aggressively if hemophilic arthropathy is to be prevented. Major hemarthroses occur after significant trauma or as a recurrent hemarthrosis in a joint recently affected. The large amount of blood in the joint causes several problems. First, the degree of swelling makes the joint very painful and difficult to move. Second, the large bulk of blood in the joint makes recurrent bleeding and synovitis more likely. Our treatment for a major hemarthrosis starts with the usual transfusion of 25 units/kg of body weight, but a simple transfusion is not enough. Therapy continues with aspiration, splinting as needed, protection of the joint until rehabilitation is under way, and, most importantly, repeated transfusion until a later hemorrhage has become unlikely.

Aspiration is critical. Removing most of the blood significantly reduces the risk of synovitis or recurrent hemorrhage. Joint aspiration also dramatically reduces the severe pain associated with a major hemarthrosis. We routinely perform the procedure in our outpatient clinic. Routine sterile precautions should practically eliminate introducing septic complications. In fact, the risk of hematogenous septic arthritis may be reduced by removing the pool of blood, which is a potential culture medium. Published case reports indicate that septic joints in hemophiliacs have largely followed major hemarthroses that were either not treated or treated only by simple transfusion on a delayed basis.[41-43]

Splinting or slings protect the joint after aspiration. These devices make the patient more comfortable but should be used for no longer than 24 to 48 hours, as prolonged immobilization of the joint is detrimental. After the splint is discarded, crutches are used in ankle and knee hemorrhages until joint motion has been satisfactorily regained.

Despite initial transfusion, aspiration, and splinting, the joint is still more susceptible to hemorrhage five to seven days after a major hemarthrosis because some of the blood has already been absorbed by the synovium and some cannot be removed by aspiration. In our experience, another hemorrhage so soon after a major hemarthrosis makes development of a hypertrophic synovitis joint more likely. A short period of prophylactic transfusions gives further protection. We repeat our initial transfusion every 48 hours until we think the joint has completely recovered. Transfusion on this schedule maintains the factor VIII or factor IX level above 1% (more than 1 unit/dl) and prevents spontaneous recurrent hemorrhage caused by minimal trauma. Typically, two prophylactic transfusions are given after a major hemarthrosis, although occasionally we continue therapy longer. This program gives the joint six days of factor coverage, a period that usually allows rehabilitation of joint function and gives the synovium time to absorb the blood remaining after aspiration.

In advanced hemophilic arthropathy, a hemarthrosis can only expand or distend the joint a limited amount. In these joints, treatment is usually limited to transfusion and splinting as needed. Aspiration in this situation is more difficult and frequently yields only 5 to 10 ml of bloody fluid.

Although results are difficult to document, we have been happy with our treatment program for major hemarthrosis. In our experience it certainly has been easier to prevent the synovitis and joint destruction that frequently follows a major hemarthrosis than it is to treat an established thick, boggy synovium that is causing recurrent joint hemorrhages and joint destruction.

Subacute Hemarthropathy

The state of synovial hypertrophy with or without recurrent hemarthrosis was termed "subacute hemarthropathy" by Arnold and Hilgartner.[30] We adopted this terminology and further defined subacute hemarthropathy as either three bleeding episodes in a joint within six weeks or persistent synovial hypertrophy six weeks after the last apparent joint bleeding episode. The involved joint is typically swollen but not particularly painful unless there was a recent acute hemarthrosis. The loss of joint motion is surprisingly mild, being in the range of 10 to 30 degrees. Joint swelling primarily results from synovial hypertrophy, although a mild joint effusion is also present. The synovial fluid is typically bloody with a hematocrit of 10% to 20%, probably caused by the constant oozing of blood from the hypervascular, friable synovium.

Our present treatment protocol for subacute hemarthropathy involves two stages, but both stages are based on prophylactic transfusion therapy. In stage I, transfusions are given three times a week for the first three weeks and then twice a week for the next three weeks. In both factor VIII deficiency and factor IX deficiency, the replacement dose is 25 units/kg of body weight. The aim of transfusion therapy is to provide enough factor replacement so that a spontaneous hemorrhage is unlikely, thus allowing the synovitis to resolve. Transfusions given three times a week maintain, for all practical purposes, factor levels above 1%. When transfusions are given twice a week, there are times when the factor levels fall below 1% but this regimen has the advantage of decreasing cost as well as the number of venipunctures. At the end of stage I the patient's

condition is reevaluated. If synovial hypertrophy is still present, the patient moves to stage II of our treatment protocol.

Stage II involves prophylactic transfusions for a minimum of four additional months. Transfusions are given either two or three times a week. Synovectomy is considered only after this protocol is completed. Many of our patients do not undergo synovectomy until they have had several more months of therapy. We realize that in certain patients prolonged observation may not be beneficial, but the dilemma is that some joints show a dramatic reduction in the synovitis with no consistent therapy and with therapy most patients demonstrate some decrease in the synovial hypertrophy. Because rehabilitation after synovectomy is particularly difficult in patients with hemophilia and because any surgery in a patient with hemophilia entails a large cost and prolonged hospitalization, we have been cautious in proceeding with this operation.

Previously, our nonsurgical treatment for subacute hemarthropathy included three weeks of cast immobilization (if joint narrowing was not present) and a seven-day course of prednisone. Although we did not see complications from either casts or steroids, both have been discontinued because we did not think they added to the success of our prophylactic transfusion regimen.

In a previous evaluation of this nonsurgical treatment in 20 children with 34 affected joints (W.B. Greene, C.W. McMillan, M. Wanen, and W. Dykstra, unpublished data), the hemarthroses in the affected joint averaged 3.6 per month before therapy and 1.7 per month after treatment. Good results were demonstrated in 17 joints, fair results in seven, and poor results in ten. Poor results were associated with breakthrough bleeding and severe synovial hypertrophy in the knee joint.

Other approaches to hypertrophic synovitis in hemophilia have included osmic acid, rifampicin, and radioactive gold. Osmic acid[44] and rifampicin[45] have been shown to be ineffective. Ahlberg and Pettersson[46] found intra-articular injections of radioactive gold to be efficacious if radioactive changes were minimal, but Martin-Villar[44] found that radioactive gold was ineffective in the patients monitored for more than one year. These treatments are presently not available for use in the United States but newer radioactive agents may be helpful. Nonsurgical synovectomy by means of chemicals or radioactive compounds is more difficult in hemophilic arthropathy because most joint problems in this disease begin in childhood, a time when these agents have more potential for teratogenic complications.

The best treatment for subacute hemarthropathy remains to be found. Many of the anti-inflammatory drugs used in rheumatoid arthritis are not available. Passive prophylactic treatment may be helpful but also fails frequently. A more effective way to decrease the synovial inflammation and a better definition of the optimal time for synovectomy are just two of the unsolved problems in subacute hemarthropathy.

Chronic Arthropathy

In the later stage of hemophilic arthropathy, joint deformities and pain become clinical problems. Nonsurgical treatment can be helpful in these conditions and is mandatory for the 15% with inhibitor antibodies. Also, nonsurgical treatment may gain additional time for those who will eventually require reconstructive surgery. Patients with hemophilia typically develop chronic arthropathy symptoms by the second or third decade, a time when they are still too young for total joint replacement. If function can be maintained until later years, the patient is certainly a better candidate for total joint arthroplasty.

General management includes physiotherapy and analgesics. The physical therapy program should be tailored to maintain strength and motion across affected joints. With severe arthritic changes, isokinetic or isotonic strengthening is not feasible and may precipitate joint bleeding. These patients are better handled by isometric strengthening. Although aspirin and steroid medications are contraindicated, other anti-inflammatory drugs may provide pain relief. Our experience has primarily been with naproxen. Gastrointestinal bleeding may occur but naproxen is certainly safer than aspirin. The use of potentially addicting analgesics must be avoided since problems with drug abuse can occur easily in any patient with severe arthropathy.

Specific problems may be helped by appropriate orthopaedic management. Although not as common today, knee flexion contracture is still seen in patients with hemophilia, particularly in those with inhibitor antibodies. Since the flexed knee causes both increased quadriceps demand and increased patellofemoral compression,[47] ambulation is markedly compromised by this deformity. Our goal is to maintain the knee flexion contracture at 15 degrees or less because greater contractures markedly increase stresses transmitted across the joint.

If the knee flexion contracture is of recent onset (one to four weeks), then bony changes and posterior subluxation of the tibia are of less concern. In severe contractures (more than 25 degrees), our treatment starts with inpatient traction. A special skin wrap is applied so that the amount of traction will be equivalent to that utilized with skeletal pins. Insertion of skeletal traction is painful and in hemophiliacs requires costly factor replacement. In addition, most hemophiliacs with severe knee contractures have inhibitor antibodies, a condition that precludes skeletal traction. The skin wrap

involves (1) application of tincture of benzoin to the calf, (2) careful placement of Elastoplast tape around the leg, extending from the malleoli to the proximal tibia, (3) a medial and lateral moleskin strip placed along the calf, (4) coverage of the moleskin wrap by cotton Webril, and (5) a final wrap of Conform bandage. The moleskin strips are secured to a wooden block placed beyond the foot through which traction (approximately 10% of body weight) is suspended. If traction causes the moleskin to slip, then the shearing force is transmitted across the Elastoplast tape and not directly onto the patient's skin. By sequential adjustments of the knee, contractures of 45 degrees or more can be diminished within one week. An open thigh cylinder that allows further extension but blocks any flexion is used for a brief time after traction. With hypertrophic synovitis and/or bony changes, the risk of recurrent hemarthroses and contractures is further minimized by a period of brace protection. For knee arthropathy we use a polypropylene long leg orthosis with drop-lock or dial-lock knee hinges. The foot portion of the brace is trimmed so that only the heel is incorporated. This allows full ankle joint mobility.

In patients with long-term knee flexion contractures, correction by simple traction or wedging casts only accentuates posterior subluxation of the tibia. Jordan[48] perfected and popularized the Quengel cast to allow correction of both posterior subluxation and flexion contracture. The key to the Quengel cast is special offset hinges that correct the tibial subluxation and a toggle stick that permits windlass correction of the flexion deformity. The technique we use in applying the Quengel casting has been previously described.[49] These patients also undergo subsequent treatment with an open thigh cylinder cast and an orthotic device.

Reverse dynamic slings have also been described for knee flexion contractures of long duration.[50] The advantage claimed for the slings is a period of hospitalization shorter than that required for cast techniques. Our experience with this treatment is limited, but our clinical impression is that reverse slings accentuate the external tibial torsion that may develop with chronic knee arthropathy in a child who has hemophilia.

Shoe modifications may be extremely helpful in patients with chronic hemarthropathy. In these patients, knees and ankles (and occasionally the hips) are frequently involved. The entire limb must be assessed to give the patient the best balance and function. An equinus deformity is the most common problem in chronic hemarthropathy of the ankle. Simple elevation of the heel to accommodate the equinus deformity may make a dramatic difference in function. In severe arthritis of the ankle and subtalar joint, the use of shoes with shock-absorbing soles and a rockerbottom slope from the heel to the forefoot decreases weightbearing forces transmitted from heel strike to midstance. In a severe equinovarus deformity, special form-fitted shoes to accommodate the deformity may make a pantalar arthrodesis unnecessary (Fig. 34–8).

Muscle Hemorrhage

In patients with severe factor VIII or factor IX deficiency, muscle hemorrhages are common. Like joint bleeding, muscle hemorrhage may occur spontaneously or after minimal trauma. Characteristic sites include the iliopsoas, quadriceps, calf, anterior compartment of the leg, and volar compartment of the forearm. Aronstam and associates[51] documented the clinical features of lower-extremity muscle bleeding in children with severe hemophilia. The site of bleeding involved the quadriceps muscle in 44%, the posterior calf muscles in 35%, the adductors in 7%, and the anterior calf muscles in 7%. Clinical symptoms progressed from "stiffness" to pain on movement to pain at rest. In this study, in which

most bleeding episodes were treated within three hours, the mean time for complete restoration of muscle or joint movement was 3.5 days.

For minor muscle hematomas, home transfusion therapy is effective. A single infusion to achieve 30% to 50% levels is usually adequate if treatment is quick. We also encourage the patient with lower-extremity bleeding to remain on crutches until full range of motion has been regained. Proper teaching of home transfusion therapy should instruct the patient or parents to recognize complications that may be associated with more severe muscle hemorrhages. In particular, patients are encouraged to call with any evidence of neurologic dysfunction. In this event, the patient is admitted to the hospital and given transfusion therapy to maintain factor levels at 50% or higher. Subsequent orthopaedic management depends on the specific muscle involved and the reliability of coagulation control. If compartment syndrome develops in a hemophiliac

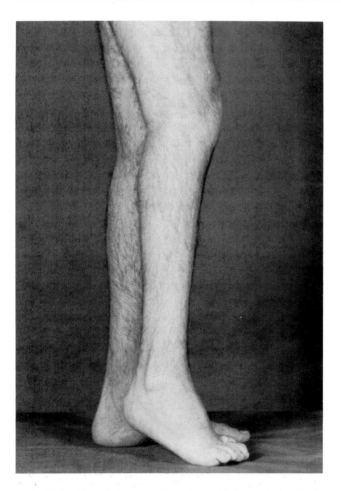 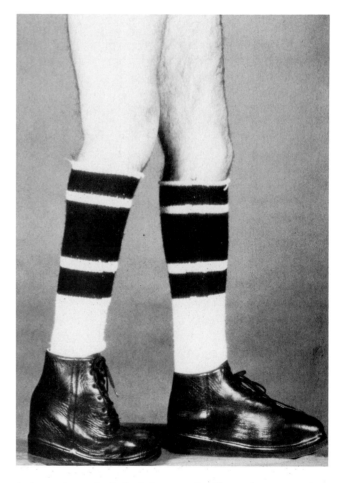

Fig. 34–8 Left: A 25-year-old patient with hemophilia who had chronic hemarthropathy in both knees and ankles and severe equinus contracture in the right ankle. The patient had previously used long leg braces. **Right:** Special form-fitted shoes allowed more effective walking without a brace. (Reproduced with permission from Greene WB, Wilson FC: The management of musculoskeletal problems in hemophilia: Part III. Nonoperative management of hemophilic arthropathy and muscle hemorrhage, in Evarts CM (ed): American Academy of Orthopaedic Surgeons *Instructional Course Lectures, XXXII.* St. Louis, CV Mosby, 1983, pp 223–233.)

without inhibitor antibodies, routine orthopaedic surgical management should be undertaken. Basically this means measurement of compartment pressure and immediate fasciotomy if it is increased.

Patients with inhibitor antibodies are at increased risk for problems related to a muscle hematoma. A high-titer inhibitor limits home transfusion and surgical options. Although one patient with a high-titer inhibitor who underwent surgical release of an acute volar compartment has been described,[52] clotting adequate to allow surgical therapy may not always be possible. Patients with inhibitor antibodies must be taught to seek medical attention early so that the different transfusions possible in such cases can be started before the muscle hemorrhage has progressed to a compartment syndrome. In addition, nonsurgical techniques such as splinting, elevation, and compression dressings can be used to minimize the joint contractures that may develop as fibrous tissue repairs the injured muscle.

Iliacus Hematoma

Although sometimes termed retroperitoneal hemorrhage, this common problem has actually been shown by Goodfellow and associates[53] to represent a hemorrhage into the iliacus muscle. The iliacus muscle is confined between the pelvic wall and the overlying iliacus fascia. A relatively small hematoma in this muscle causes significant pain in the groin and anterior thigh region. Further expansion of the hematoma may cause a femoral nerve palsy. The patient's hip is held in a flexed position, and the pain is markedly increased by attempts at extension. A hip joint hemorrhage presents a similar picture but may be differentiated on clinical examination by rotating the hip with the leg flexed. In that position the iliacus muscle is relaxed and with an iliacus hemorrhage the hip rotation will be relatively normal. Computed axial tomography is often helpful in defining the location and extent of any muscle hemorrhage, but is particularly useful in this instance (Fig. 34–9).

Patients using home therapy are encouraged to treat groin or anterior thigh pain expeditiously. Early treatment aborts continuing hemorrhage into the iliacus muscle and probably decreases the possibility of a pelvic pseudotumor. In large iliacus hematomas, femoral nerve palsies are common, with an incidence of 60% reported in the 1970s.[54] If femoral nerve palsy is present, the patient is treated with bedrest and continuous infusion to maintain at least 50% levels for seven to 14 days. The femoral nerve palsy routinely resolves although several months may elapse before the quadriceps regains enough strength to extend the knee against gravity. Appropriate physical therapy enhances rehabilitation.

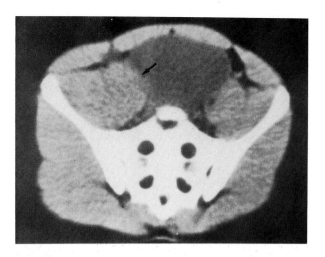

Fig. 34–9   Computed axial tomographic scan of the pelvis of a 14-year-old patient with hemophilia who had left-sided iliacus hematoma and complete femoral nerve palsy. Note the marked enlargement of the left iliacus and psoas muscle that is highlighted by the arrow. (Reproduced with permission from Greene WB, Wilson FC: The management of musculoskeletal problems in hemophilia: Part III. Nonoperative management of hemophilic arthropathy and muscle hemorrhage, in Evarts CM (ed): American Academy of Orthopaedic Surgeons *Instructional Course Lectures, XXXII.* St. Louis, CV Mosby, 1983, pp 223–233.)

Gastrocsoleus Hemorrhage

Muscle hemorrhage that does not resolve quickly is usually followed by limited joint motion. Gastrocsoleus bleeding is likely to lead to equinus contractures, particularly if there is a delay in transfusions. Patients who have gastrocsoleus hemorrhages lasting more than 12 hours benefit from cast therapy. After a single-dose transfusion, we immobilize these patients with a compressive dressing and posterior plaster splint that positions the ankle in as much dorsiflexion as possible. After 48 hours, the patient is reexamined. If an equinus contracture is still present, a short leg walking cast is applied with the ankle held in maximum dorsiflexion. The walking cast minimizes contractures of the organizing hematoma and aids ambulation when the calf muscles are unable to tolerate unprotected weightbearing. The cast is changed every few days until the patient can achieve neutral dorsiflexion with the knee held in full extension. Appropriate stretching exercises are then used to gain further dorsiflexion. With this aggressive program, fixed equinus contractures should not develop.

Serial wedging casts are rarely needed with appropriate initial management. One patient had a 30-degree equinus contracture after a gastrocsoleus hemorrhage that went untreated for six months. We used six weeks of serial long leg casting and four weeks of short leg casting. Frequent cast changes were accompanied by closing wedges, done every two or three days. This treatment produced 5 degrees of dorsiflexion, which was maintained for more than seven years.

The Next Decade

The structures of factor VIII and factor IX molecules have been elucidated, and purified recombinant DNA factor VIII concentrate is now undergoing clinical trials. Such products will allow transfusion without risk of viral transmission. We hope these recombinant techniques will eventually reduce the economic burden that modern treatment now imposes on patients with hemophilia. Joint bleeding will still occur. Hemophilic arthropathy will still develop, although its frequency and severity should be reduced. An orthopaedic surgeon who understands the disease and its effect on the musculoskeletal system will still be needed to keep major hemorrhages from producing established joint disease. Orthopaedic surgeons will no doubt be more involved with elective surgery in patients with hemophilia not only for problems caused by their bleeding disorder but also for "routine" injuries that will become more prevalent as these patients are able to lead more normal lives. Unfortunately, hemophilia with inhibitor antibodies will probably still have limited transfusion possibilities. For patients in this group, the orthopaedic surgeon will need to combine advances in rehabilitation with lessons learned from the era when only nonsurgical treatment was available.

References

1. McMillan CW: Hemostasis: General consideration, in Miller DR, Baehner RB, McMillan CW, et al (eds): *Smith's Blood Diseases of Infancy and Childhood.* St. Louis, CV Mosby, 1984, pp 761–783.

2. McMillan CW: Evolution of modern concepts of hemostasis: A backward glance at the discoveries that made modern practice possible. *Am J Pediatr Hematol Oncol* 1981;3:97–103.

3. Sadler JE, Davie EW: Hemophilia A, hemophilia B, and von Willebrand's disease, in Stamatoyannopoulos G, Nienhuis AW, Leder P, et al (eds): *The Molecular Basis of Blood Diseases.* Philadelphia, WB Saunders, 1987, pp 575–630.

4. Walz DA: Perspectives of blood coagulation, in Lusher JM, Barnhart MI (eds): *Acquired Bleeding Disorders in Children: Abnormalities of Hemostasis.* New York, Masson Publishing USA, 1981, pp 1–11.

5. May RB, McMillan CW: Bleeding disorders in the newborn, in Conn HF, Conn RB (eds): *Current Diagnosis.* Philadelphia, WB Saunders, 1977, pp 1045–1098.

6. Pool JG, Shannon AE: Production of high-potency concentrates of antihemophilic globulin in a closed-bag system: Assay in vitro and in vivo. *N Engl J Med* 1965;273:1443–1447.

7. Wagner RH, McLester WD, Smith M, et al: Purification of antihemophilic factor (factor VIII) by amino acid precipitation. *Thromb Diath Haemorrh* 1964;11:64–74.

8. Brinkhous KM, Shanbrom E, Roberts HR, et al: A new high-potency glycine-precipitated antihemophilic factor (AHF) concentrate. *JAMA* 1968;205:613–617.

9. Lusher JM, Shapiro SS, Palascak JE, et al: Efficacy of prothrombin-complex concentrates in hemophiliacs with antibodies to factor VIII: A multicenter therapeutic trial. *N Engl J Med* 1980;303:421–425.

10. Tullis JL, Melin M, Jurigian P: Clinical use of human prothrombin complexes. *N Engl J Med* 1965;273:667–674.

11. Hasiba U, Eyster ME, Gill FM, et al: Liver dysfunction in Pennsylvania's multitransfused hemophiliacs. *Dig Dis Sci* 1980; 25:776–782.

12. Evatt BL, Ramsey RB, Lawrence DN, et al: The acquired immunodeficiency syndrome in patients with hemophilia. *Ann Intern Med* 1984;100:499–504.

13. Spire B, Dormont D, Barré-Sinoussi F, et al: Inactivation of lymphadenopathy-associated virus by heat, gamma rays, and ultraviolet light. *Lancet* 1985;1:188–189.

14. Levy JA, Mitra GA, Wong MF, et al: Inactivation by wet and dry heat of AIDS-associated retroviruses during factor VIII purification from plasma. *Lancet* 1985;1:1456–1457.

15. Seeler RA, Telischi M, Langehennig PL, et al: Comparison of anti-A and anti-B titers in factor VIII and IX concentrates. *J Pediatr* 1976;89:87–89.

16. Blatt PM, Lundblad RL, Kingdon HS, et al: Thrombogenic materials in prothrombin complex concentrates. *Ann Intern Med* 1974;81:766–770.

17. Shapiro SS: Antibodies to blood coagulation factors. *Clin Haematol* 1979;8:207–214.

18. McMillan CW, Greene WB, Blatt PM, et al: The management of musculoskeletal problems in hemophilia: Part I. Principles of medical management of hemophilia, in Evarts CM (ed): American Academy of Orthopaedic Surgeons *Instructional Course Lectures, XXXII.* St. Louis, CV Mosby, 1983, pp 210–216.

19. Strauss HS: Acquired circulating anticoagulants in hemophilia A. *N Engl J Med* 1969;281:866–873.

20. Roberts HR: Induction of immune tolerance to factor VIII: A plea for caution. *JAMA* 1988;259:84–85.

21. Brackmann HH, Egli H: Treatment of hemophilia patients with inhibitors, in Seligsohn U, Rimon A, Horoszowski H (eds): *Hemophilia.* London, Castle House, 1981, pp 113–119.

22. Brackmann HH, Gormsen J: Massive factor-VIII infusion in haemophiliac with factor-VIII inhibitor, high responder. *Lancet* 1977;2:933.

23. Ewing NP, Sanders NL, Dietrich SL, et al: Induction of immune tolerance to factor VIII in hemophiliacs with inhibitors. *JAMA* 1988;259:65–68.

24. Hilgartner MW: Home care for hemophilia: Current state of the art. *Scand J Haematol* 1977;30(suppl):58–64.

25. Roy S, Ghadially FN: Ultrastructure of synovial membrane in human hemarthrosis. *J Bone Joint Surg* 1967;49A:1636–1646.

26. Swanton MC: Hemophilic arthropathy in dogs. *Lab Invest* 1959;8:1269–1277.

27. Hoaglund FT: Experimental hemarthrosis: The response of canine knees to injections of autologous blood. *J Bone Joint Surg* 1967;49A:285–298.

28. Stein H, Duthie RB: The pathogenesis of chronic haemophilic arthropathy. *J Bone Joint Surg* 1981;63B:601–609.

29. Hilgartner MW, Arnold WD, Granda JL: Acid phosphatase levels of synovial tissue and fluid in patients with hemophilia, in *Proceedings of the XIV International Congress of Hematology.* Sao Paulo, Grafica Chieregati, 1972.

30. Arnold WD, Hilgartner MW: Hemophilic arthropathy: Current concepts of pathogenesis and management. *J Bone Joint Surg* 1977;59A:287–305.

31. Mainardi CL, Levine PH, Werb Z, et al: Proliferative synovitis in hemophilia: Biochemical and morphologic observations. *Arthritis Rheum* 1978;21:137–144.

32. Roy S: Ultrastructure of articular cartilage in experimental hemarthrosis. *Arch Pathol* 1968;86:69–76.

33. Brighton CT, Bigley EC Jr, Smolenski BI: Iron induced arthritis in immature rabbits. *Arthritis Rheum* 1970;13:849–857.

34. Hough AJ, Banfield WG, Sokoloff L: Cartilage in hemophilic

arthropathy: Ultrastructural and microanalytical studies. *Arch Pathol Lab Med* 1976;100:91–96.

35. Pettersson H, Ahlberg A, Nilsson IM: A radiologic classification of hemophilic arthropathy. *Clin Orthop* 1980;149:153–159.

36. Greene WB, Yankaskas BC, Guilford WB: Comparison of radiologic classification of hemophilic arthropathy with clinical parameters. *J Bone Joint Surg*, in press.

37. Chambers RB: Orthopaedic injuries in athletes (ages 6 to 17): Comparison of injuries occurring in six sports. *Am J Sports Med* 1979;7:195–197.

38. Winter DA, Robertson DG: Joint torque and energy patterns in normal gait. *Biol Cybern* 1978;29:137–142.

39. Strickler EM, Greene WB: Isokinetic torque levels in hemophiliac knee musculature. *Arch Phys Med Rehabil* 1984;65:766–770.

40. Greene WB, Strickler EM: A modified isokinetic strengthening program for patients with severe hemophilia. *Dev Med Child Neurol* 1983;25:189–196.

41. Houghton GR: Septic arthritis of the hip in a hemophiliac: Report of a case. *Clin Orthop* 1977;129:223–224.

42. Wilkins RM, Wiedel JD: Septic arthritis of the knee in a hemophiliac: A case report. *J Bone Joint Surg* 1983;65A:267–268.

43. Hofmann A, Wyatt R, Bybee B: Septic arthritis of the knee in a 12-year-old hemophiliac. *J Pediatr Orthop* 1984;4:498–499.

44. Martin-Villar J: Long term evaluation of 49 cases of haemophilic arthropathy treated with synoviorthesis with [198]Au. Presented at the Symposium on the Co-ordinated Management of Musculoskeletal Manifestations of Haemophilia, London, Dec 4, 1981.

45. Mariani G, Sadun R: Intra-articular rifampicin for treatment of chronic synovitis, presented at the Symposium on the Co-ordinated Management of Musculoskeletal Manifestations of Haemophilia, London, Dec 4, 1981.

46. Ahlberg A, Pettersson H: Synoviorthesis with radioactive gold in hemophiliacs: Clinical and radiological follow-up. *Acta Orthop Scand* 1979;50:513–517.

47. Perry J, Antonelli D, Ford W: Analysis of knee-joint forces during flexed-knee stance. *J Bone Joint Surg* 1975;57A:961–967.

48. Jordan HH: *Orthopedic Appliances*. Springfield, Charles C Thomas, 1963, pp 21–29.

49. Greene WB, Wilson FC: The management of musculoskeletal problems in hemophilia: Part III. Nonoperative management of hemophilic arthropathy and muscle hemorrhage, in Evarts CM (ed): American Academy of Orthopaedic Surgeons *Instructional Course Lectures, XXXII*. St. Louis, CV Mosby, 1983, pp 223–233.

50. Stein H, Dickson RA: Reversed dynamic slings for knee-flexion contractures in the hemophiliac. *J Bone Joint Surg* 1975; 57A:282–283.

51. Aronstam A, Browne RS, Wassef M, et al: The clinical features of early bleeding into the muscles of the lower limb in severe haemophiliacs. *J Bone Joint Surg* 1983;65B:19–23.

52. Madigan RR, Hanna WT, Wallace SL: Acute compartment syndrome in hemophilia: A case report. *J Bone Joint Surg* 1981;63A:1327–1329.

53. Goodfellow J, Fearn CB, Matthews JM: Iliacus haematoma: A common complication of haemophilia. *J Bone Joint Surg* 1967;49B:748–756.

54. Houghton GR, Duthie RB: Orthopedic problems in hemophilia. *Clin Orthop* 1979;138:197–216.

Surgical Management of Hemophilic Arthropathy

Lisa T. DeGnore, MD

Frank C. Wilson, MD

With the development of clotting factor concentrates in the 1960s and the advent of cryoprecipitate and heat-treated factor concentrates in the 1980s, hemophiliacs have acquired near-normal life expectancies, with the result that medical care has focused more on the quality of life for these patients. Previously, hemophilia was a crippling childhood disorder with 75% of its victims disabled by the age of 16 years.[1] With the marked decrease in mortality rates, elective surgery has become relatively commonplace for those patients in whom intractable bleeding, severe arthropathy, or both develop despite replacement therapy. However, even with hemostatic control, the rate of surgical complications is higher for hemophiliacs than for the general population.[2,3] Moreover, the appearance of the human immunodeficiency virus (HIV) and its prevalence among hemophiliacs whose condition was diagnosed before 1984 pose newer and more difficult problems for the orthopaedist, the solutions to which remain elusive.[4-6]

Preoperative Considerations

Indications and Contraindications

The indications for surgical treatment of joint disease in hemophiliacs are similar to those for patients with normal clotting mechanisms, namely, either disabling joint destruction or intractable bleeding, or both. Surgical approaches are contraindicated in patients with acute hepatitis, although chronic hepatitis, present in most adult hemophiliacs, does not necessarily preclude surgery. The presence of a high-titer inhibitor is, with a few exceptions, an absolute contraindication to surgery, while a low or moderate titer is a relative one.[7-11] More recently the acquired immune deficiency syndrome (AIDS) has posed new therapeutic and ethical dilemmas for responsible physicians.[6-12]

Requisites

Surgery requires close cooperation among the orthopaedist, hematologist, psychiatrist, physical therapist, dentist, social worker, vocational counselor, and financial counselor—all of whom must possess special knowledge of hemophilia.

Factor availability—at least a three-week supply—must be assured before the hospital admission. Given the cost factors involved, financial counseling is also needed for most patients. Laboratory facilities for accurate factor and inhibitor assays, complete blood banking capabilities, and the capacity for liver function tests and HIV determinations are necessary before surgery is undertaken.

Finally, psychiatric consultation is often advisable, because drug addiction and the need for emotional support are greater in these patients.

In general, patients should be admitted several days before surgery and tested for the presence of an inhibitor; a formal fall-off study is performed if the patient's response to factor VIII is not well known to the surgical team. Factor VIII therapy is begun the day before surgery and monitored closely. Because the risk of a postoperative hemolytic reaction increases with A, B, or AB blood types, a factor concentrate with the lowest isoantibody titer should be used in these patients.

Intraoperative Considerations

Hematologic Factors

The dosage of factor VIII varies with the age and weight of a patient, the results of the fall-off study, or levels obtained during continuous infusion. For example, a patient in whom factor VIII has a half-life of 12 hours (as indicated by a fall-off study) will require less factor than one in whom the half-life is six hours. The factor level is brought to 100% and confirmed by the laboratory before the incision is made.

Anesthetic Factors

The anesthesiologist involved in the care of the hemophiliac must be aware of the need to preserve patent veins; central venous access may be necessary (performed after adequate factor coverage), and a second vein should always be identified. Before intubation, regional anesthesia, or intramuscular injection, adequate correction of coagulation defects must be made.

Technical Factors

To minimize risk and cost, as many indicated procedures as feasible should be performed under the same anesthetic; however, contaminated procedures should never be coupled with clean ones. For example, joint replacement and dental procedures are incompatible because of the risk of seeding the prosthesis with oral bacteria.

Where and when appropriate, a tourniquet is used; it should be released before closure.

The need for meticulous hemostasis is obvious. Snug, layered closure is used, with suction drainage as indicated.

Throughout the procedure, care must be taken to protect the members of the operating team from transmission of HIV and the hepatitis virus. Exposure occurs primarily through contact with blood products; for the anesthesiologist, oral secretions are a concern. Sharp instruments should not be left on the operating table; double gloves, impermeable gowns, and disposable drapes should be used. As both viruses are relatively easy to kill, surgical equipment may be disinfected with a standard solution such as 10% sodium hypochlorite. If a member of the operating team is inadvertently pricked or cut, the wound should be washed immediately with iodine, soap, and water. If the injured person has been immunized for hepatitis B (and has adequate titers), or is positive for hepatitis B surface antigen or antibody, no further treatment is necessary. Otherwise, two doses of hepatitis B immune globulin should be given, 5 ml immediately and 5 ml after one month.

After closure, well-padded splints or bivalved casts are used for immobilization. Rigid circumferential dressings should be avoided. The limb must be easily available to identify postoperative hemorrhage or a developing compartment syndrome.

The incidence of infection with HIV among patients with severe hemophilia has been reported to range from 75% to 90%; it is generally closer to 90% among patients seen by orthopaedists, since these patients have had more bleeding episodes and received more factor therapy.[6] Of our 49 patients undergoing major orthopaedic procedures since 1973, 37 (76%) were seropositive by electroimmunoassay and Western blot tests, five (10%) were seronegative, and seven (14%) refused testing (and were presumed to be seropositive), for an overall infection rate of 90%. Of the 37 known to be seropositive, five (14%) progressed to stage V or stage VI (full-blown AIDS) in the Walter Reed classification within an average of 5.3 years after surgery (range, 1.5 to 9 years), and of these, four died an average of 4.1 years after surgery (range, 2.3 to 6.0 years).[12] Thus, strict precautions must be observed when exposure to blood or secretions is likely. Should the blood or secretions from an HIV-positive patient accidentally come into contact with the blood or the mucous membranes of a health-care worker, the worker should be tested immediately, at six weeks, 12 weeks, six months, and one year.[13,14] If the patient is HIV-negative, and this result is confirmed by Western blot test, the health care worker need be tested only initially and after 12 to 24 weeks.

Postoperative Considerations

Factor Levels

After procedures involving bone, our current regimen is to maintain the factor VIII level, by continuous infusion, at 75% to 100% for days 1 through 5, at 50% to 74% for days 6 through 10, and at 25% to 49% for days 11 through 15. Thereafter, factor VIII is administered in a bolus as needed for physical therapy. The difficulty of achieving the desired levels is suggested by the levels actually attained at our institution, where factor levels for joint replacement averaged 105%, 75%, and 58%, respectively, for these intervals.

For soft-tissue procedures, each of the above intervals is reduced by several days. A recent publication by the National Hemophilia Foundation[15] suggested maintaining factor VIII levels at 75% to 100% for the first two days postoperatively and then decreasing the level to 30% for the remaining postoperative course. We have no experience with this regimen.

Factor VIII levels are assayed throughout hospitalization: in the recovery room, twice daily until they are stable, then daily until the infusion is discontinued. A sudden decrease in factor VIII level may indicate the development of an inhibitor and must be investigated.

Monitoring for Hemolysis

The presence of an inhibitor may also be signaled by a sudden drop in the hematocrit; however, this finding more often suggests hemolysis. Daily hematocrits are obtained, and a physical examination is performed immediately if a decrease is noted. If no obvious source of bleeding is found, further laboratory investigation is necessary: red cell abnormalities (e.g., spherocytosis), a positive direct Coombs test, increases in bilirubin, plasma-free globin, urine hemosiderin, and a decrease in serum haptoglobin help confirm hemolysis. Prompt identification of the causes and treatment of hemolysis are essential.

Pain Control

As many hemophiliacs have increased tolerance to oral narcotics, more potent analgesic drugs are often necessary; however, tranquilizers and psychiatric counseling may potentiate the efficacy of narcotics. Aspirin should be avoided because of the associated irreversible platelet inhibition. It should be remembered that a sudden increase in postoperative pain may indicate a bleeding complication requiring increased factor VIII administration.

Rehabilitation

Rehabilitation is begun promptly after surgery. After knee replacement, continuous passive motion is started in the recovery room at 0 to 30 degrees and, usually, progresses by 5- to 10-degree increments twice daily in cycles of one hour of movement followed by two hours of rest.[16] When 70 degrees of flexion is reached, and the patient can perform straight leg raising, active-assistive exercises are begun at the bedside. Protected weightbearing starts when the patient can actively extend to within 15 degrees of full extension. Factor replacement may be necessary after discharge, especially following synovectomy, to prevent hemarthroses during rehabilitation.

Complications

Several complications are unique to surgery on hemophiliacs: bleeding, thrombosis, hemolytic anemia, hepatitis, and infection.

Bleeding

Excessive bleeding in the postoperative period is usually attributable to a low titer of factor VIII, the appearance of an inhibitor, injury while being moved or ambulating, or the development of coagulopathy. Bleeding is frequently signaled by acute pain and swelling in a joint or wound seepage; rarely, it is signaled by a compartment syndrome. In patients who develop an inhibitor or acute coagulopathy, bleeding may occur as a wound hematoma or as diffuse oozing from mucous membranes (including the gastrointestinal tract); conversely, there may be a sudden drop in the hematocrit without an overt source of bleeding.

Inhibitor formation occurs in 15% to 20% of the hemophilic population and presents the most therapeutically challenging cause of postoperative bleeding.[17] Patients with a low-titer inhibitor (less than 20 Bethesda units) may be treated with aggressive factor replacement.[17] When factor requirements become excessive or a high-titer inhibitor is present, activated prothrombin complex concentrate (APCC) or animal factor VIII concentrates are used.[7-11,17-20] The mechanism for the efficacy of APCC has not been fully elucidated, monitoring of levels is impossible, and it is less effective than factor VIII in patients without an inhibitor.[19] Several APCC products are in current use, predominantly Autoplex and Feiba.[9,17-19] A major concern with this therapy is cost; a full course of therapy may run $80,000 per week, which, coupled with the inherent risks of hepatitis, thrombosis, and disseminated intravascular coagulation, explains why these products are used only for life-threatening hemorrhages. Nilsson and associates[8] discussed plasma adsorption as another treatment for inhibitors, but the value of this procedure has not been confirmed.

Thrombosis

Although rare in patients with coagulation defects, thrombosis can occur with the use of APCC products or in severe liver dysfunction.[9,17,18] When APCC products are used in patients with an inhibitor, daily platelet counts and fibrinogen levels must be obtained. An acute decrease signals thrombosis, and a decrease of platelets to less than 50,000 μl must be treated by stopping the infusion and close monitoring.[9,18]

Hemolytic Anemia

This complication is usually seen within the first five days postoperatively. If not prevented by the use of type-specific concentrates with a low titer of antibodies, hemolysis is managed by replacement with washed, packed, type-O red cells and type-specific cryoprecipitate.

Hepatitis

Hepatitis is the most common complication of factor VIII therapy. Of patients with severe hemophilia, 75% to 85% have transient increases in liver transaminases; these increases usually correlate with histologic liver disease.[21] The incidence of clinically apparent liver dysfunction is, however, only 18% to 25%. Strict donor screening and heat treatment in the preparation of factor concentrate and cryoprecipitate reduce the risk of this complication, but non-A/non-B, delta, and other types of viral hepatitis are serologically undetectable. Treatment of a patient who develops acute liver dysfunction is supportive.

Infection

In 290 orthopaedic procedures (including 175 synovectomies, 93 arthroplasties, and 22 arthrodeses) reported in the literature from 1972 to 1987, eight (3%) postoperative infections were listed.[2,5,22-42] Of these, five (two knee replacements and three arthrodeses) were superficial and resolved with dressing changes and antibiotics.[2,26,40] Three knee replacements developed deep infections.[23-25] Of these, two required removal of the prosthesis and arthrodesis; both fusions were reported to be successful, and the third resolved with repeated aspiration and intravenous antibiotics.[23-25]

With the increased incidence of seropositivity for the HIV antibody in the hemophilic population, the effect of a disturbed immune system on surgical wound healing must be considered. However, methods of detecting HIV were not available until 1984. Thus, the effect of HIV status on the previously reported infections is unknown. As our experience with HIV in hemophiliacs grows, and our testing and reporting systems become standardized, we will be able to determine more precisely the effect of HIV infection on wound healing.

Surgical Experience With Specific Procedures

Synovectomy

Storti and associates[43] reported in 1969 that synovectomy was an effective means of controlling recurrent hemarthroses in hemophilic joints. Since that time, others have reported successful control of hemarthroses for periods averaging six years, presumably from the removal of hypertrophied, vascularized, friable synovium that contains an increased level of proteolytic enzymes. There is no conclusive evidence that synovectomy significantly slows progression of the arthropathy, despite the reduction in destructive enzyme levels.[22]

Our indications for synovectomy are hemarthroses occurring on an average of once a month for six months or more, despite adequate factor replacement, and associated with persistent synovial hypertrophy. Since synovectomy appears to be less effective in stage IV or stage V joint disease, the operation is performed primarily on younger hemophiliacs.

We have performed 34 synovectomies: 16 of the knee, 15 of the elbow with radial head excision, and three of the ankle. The average follow-up was 4.8 years (range, seven months to 12 years). Three patients were lost to follow-up. The average number of bleeding episodes preoperatively was 26 per year in the target joint. Four joints (two ankles, one elbow, and one knee) had no postoperative bleeding episodes after an average follow-up of 4.2 years. Overall, there was an average decline in the number of bleeding episodes after surgery to four per year.

During the first postoperative week, patients undergoing synovectomy of the knee were usually kept on a continuous passive motion machine. As rehabilitation progressed, the time in the machine was gradually decreased to 12 to 18 hours per day.[16] Two patients were unable to tolerate this regimen and required manipulation under anesthesia in the second postoperative week. Patients who underwent knee synovectomy gained an average of 2 degrees of extension but lost 11 degrees of flexion. After elbow synovectomy, patients gained an average of 1 degree of flexion but lost 5 degrees of extension, 1 degree of pronation, and 5 degrees of supination. After ankle synovectomy, patients lost an average of 8 degrees of dorsiflexion and 1 degree of plantarflexion.

There were four other complications. On the 17th postoperative day, a small wound hematoma developed in one patient. The hematoma responded to aspiration and increased factor VIII infusion. The second patient had mild hemolytic anemia that was managed successfully by the administration of low-antibody titer factor VIII. The third had an acute hemarthrosis on the eighth postoperative day while on the continuous passive motion machine. The hemarthrosis responded to increased administration of factor VIII, aspiration, and splinting. The fourth patient required ankle arthrodesis 10.5 years after synovectomy because of the progression of his arthropathy.

Joint Replacement

Although the procedure is often performed in younger patients, the indication for total joint replacement in hemophiliacs is basically the same as for the general population: disabling, end-stage arthropathy. As experience with surgery on hemophiliacs has grown, several groups have confirmed the value of replacement arthroplasty in relieving pain and disability, at least in the short term.[23-26] Long-term benefits are less clear, since the follow-up for most groups averages less than six years.[23-26] The late failure rates for these relatively young and active (once disabling pain is removed) patients will be defined in years to come.

Our experience with joint replacement includes 34 procedures in 21 patients: 24 knee replacements (11 total condylar, 11 Walldius, one spherocentric, and one revision), five hip replacements (four cemented and one uncemented), three elbow replacements, one Neer total shoulder replacement, and one shoulder hemiarthroplasty. We reviewed 24 total knee replacements in 16 patients followed for an average of 63 months (range, 15 to 150 months). Before surgery and during the follow-up period, these patients were rated on a 100-point scale that allowed 40 points for pain, 30 for stability, 20 for motion, and 10 for strength. The average improvement was from 55 points preoperatively to 73 points postoperatively. The greatest improvement occurred in the area of pain relief: the stability rates did not change, motion ratings improved only slightly, and muscle strength decreased slightly. The results of knee replacement in nonhemophiliacs at our institution were similar: overall ratings improved from 51 to 79 points, with less improvement in pain and more in stability.[44] Although not numerically rated, our results after other joint replacements in hemophiliacs were generally comparable to those in patients with other forms of arthritis.

In the 34 joint replacements, there were 20 complications. Three patients had knee hemarthroses, seven, ten, and 12 days after surgery. The bleeding episodes at ten and 12 days occurred while the patients were in physical therapy; the other occurred at rest in a patient with low factor VIII titers. All were treated with boluses of factor VIII and resolved without wound compromise. Three patients developed acute hemolytic anemia that responded to infusions of low-antibody titer factor VIII. Two peroneal nerve palsies followed knee replacement: one occurred 12 days after an acute hemarthrosis and the other on the first postoperative day, probably from failure to resect enough bone to correct a preexisting flexion contracture. In two patients, late loosening of the prosthesis occurred: one is asymptomatic 6.5 years after hip replacement; the second underwent revision of the tibial component three years after spherocentric knee replacement, but persistent pain and bleeding led to revision of the patellar component and quadricepsplasty at another institution. The patient described earlier who developed an inhibitor (400 Bethesda units) nine days after knee replacement later had a hemarthrosis, infection, and wound dehiscence, which led to removal of the prosthesis and arthrodesis. Konyne (an APCC product) was used to control hemostasis during the arthrodesis; however, on the third postoperative day, the patient developed a pulmonary embolus, and the Konyne was discontinued. The patient recovered without further thromboses or bleeding episodes. The wound healed after a small split-thickness skin graft was applied. Despite these many complications, fusion was achieved, and this patient was walking and pain-free 9.6 years after discharge. His total hospitalization lasted 217 days and cost $80,000 in 1978. There were five other infections and another wound dehiscence that healed uneventfully.

Two patients who underwent knee replacement developed early infections; both were seropositive for the HIV antibody but without clinical symptoms (stages I to III). One patient, in whom an infected intravenous site seeded several joints, was treated successfully with antibiotics. In the patient with the inhibitor, the knee prosthesis was seeded with *Staphylococcus epidermidis* during the second postoperative week. This patient underwent removal of the prosthesis at three months and compression arthrodesis without sequelae and was asymptomatic almost ten years later.

There were four late infections in our 34 joint replacements. In three patients, the prosthetic joints were seeded shortly after the diagnosis of stages V and VI AIDS. In the first patient, a hip prosthesis that was five years old was seeded with *Staphylococcus aureus* one month after an episode of abdominal sepsis. The prosthesis was removed and antibiotic therapy instituted; however, the patient died one month later of overwhelming infection, liver failure, and encephalopathy. In the second patient, a pyarthrosis developed in an 18-month-old knee replacement. Cultures showed *S epidermidis* and *Haemophilus parainfluenzae*; the infection resolved with aspiration and intravenous antibiotics, but the patient died of *Pneumocystis* pneumonia nine months later. A third late infection occurred in an elbow prosthesis 11.5 years after surgery. The patient developed a β-hemolytic streptococcus pyarthrosis that also resolved with repeated aspiration and antibiotics. The fourth late infection with *S epidermidis* occurred in a patient with stage I to III HIV infection four years after knee replacement. The patient refused removal and arthrodesis; after 2.3 years, the patient had intermittent drainage from the knee and minimal movement.

Although our early infection rate after knee replacement was higher for hemophiliacs than for nonhemophiliacs, 8% vs 1.8%, there was no obvious correlation with clinical HIV infection (F.C. Wilson and L.T. DeGnore, unpublished data). Late infection, however, coincided with disintegration of the immune system and the onset of clinically apparent AIDS.

Arthrodesis

As with most other arthritic joints, the primary indication for arthrodesis in hemophilic joints is prosthetic failure; however, arthrodesis is preferred for disabling ankle arthropathy because of the uncertain results of ankle arthroplasty. We have performed three arthrodeses: one of the knee was for the wound dehiscence mentioned earlier; the other two were primary knee and ankle arthrodeses. All joints fused, and the patients were asymptomatic an average of 3.7 years after surgery. Despite the dictum that external pin fixation is contraindicated in hemophiliacs because of the risk of pin-tract bleeding, skeletal compression pins were used for a knee arthrodesis without occurrence of this complication.

Cost-Benefit Analysis

To determine the cost-effectiveness of surgery on hemophiliacs, we reviewed data for patients who underwent joint replacement and synovectomy. Over the past eight years at our hospital the cost of factor VIII and factor IX has averaged $0.07 to $0.11 per unit. An average bolus treatment for one bleeding episode in a 70-kg adult costs $90 to $110; patients with severe hemophilia usually require several treatments per week. While hospital charges have increased in the past eight years, we are reporting costs at the time of surgery.

The total hospital and professional costs for four hemophiliacs undergoing joint replacement averaged $24,741; $15,129 of this (61%) was for factor VIII replacement. In 1982 (comparable time frame) the average joint replacement in a nonhemophiliac cost $11,086. For ten synovectomies for which records were available, perioperative costs averaged $14,866, of which $7,080 (48%) was for factor VIII replacement. Comparable data on synovectomies of other joints were not available.

These impressive costs are offset by the sharp decline in postoperative requirements for factor VIII replacement. For joint replacement, the cost for factor replacement during the year before surgery averaged $3,726. In the first three postoperative years, factor VIII therapy for bleeding episodes into the surgically treated joint averaged $92 per year. In ten patients who underwent synovectomy, replacement therapy during the preoperative year averaged $6,095; these costs averaged $330 for each of the first three years after surgery.

Summary

We reviewed the preoperative, intraoperative, and postoperative care of hemophilic patients, our experience with specific surgical procedures, and provided a cost-benefit analysis of joint replacement and synovectomy. The advent of factor VIII concentrates to control bleeding has enabled us to offer surgical options to hemophiliacs similar to those offered to patients with normal coagulation mechanisms. The appearance of the AIDS virus, however, has further complicated the care of hemophiliacs with severe arthropathy.

References

1. Wilson FC, Mahew DE, McMillan CW: The management of musculoskeletal problems in hemophilia: Part IV. Surgical management of musculoskeletal problems in hemophilia, in Evarts CM (ed): American Academy of Orthopaedic Surgeons *Instructional Course Lectures, XXXII.* St. Louis, CV Mosby, 1983, pp 233–241.

2. Houghton GR, Duthie RB: Orthopedic problems in hemophilia. *Clin Orthop* 1979;138:197–216.

3. Willert H-G, Horrig C, Ewald W, et al: Orthopaedic surgery in hemophilic patients. *Arch Orthop Trauma Surg* 1983;101:121–132.

4. Centers for Disease Control: Acquired immunodeficiency syndrome (AIDS) in persons with hemophilia. *MMWR* 1984; 33:2679–2680.

5. Allain J-P, Laurian Y, Paul DA, et al: Long-term evaluation of HIV antigen and antibodies to p24 and gp41 in patients with hemophilia: Potential clinical importance. *N Engl J Med* 1987;317:1114–1121.

6. Hilgartner MW: AIDS and hemophilia, editorial. *N Engl J Med* 1987;317:1153–1154.

7. White GC II, Taylor RE, Blatt PM, et al: Treatment of a high titer anti-factor-VIII antibody by continuous factor VIII administration: Report of a case. *Blood* 1983;62:141–145.

8. Nilsson IM, Jonsson S, Sundqvist S-B, et al: A procedure for removing high titer antibodies by extracorporeal protein-A-sepharose adsorption in hemophilia: Substitution therapy and surgery in a patient with hemophilia B and antibodies. *Blood* 1981;58:38–44.

9. Abildgaard CF, Penner JA, Watson-Williams EJ: Anti-inhibitor coagulant complex (Autoplex) for treatment of factor VIII inhibitors in hemophilia. *Blood* 1980;56:978–984.

10. Blatt PM, White GC, McMillan CW, et al: Treatment of anti-factor VIII antibodies. *Thromb Haemostasis* 1977;38:514–523.

11. Brackmann HH: Induced immunotolerance in factor VIII inhibitor patients, in Hoyer LW (ed): *Factor VIII Inhibitors.* New York, Alan R Liss, 1984, pp 181–195.

12. Redfield RR, Wright DC, Tramont EC: The Walter Reed staging classification for HTLV-III/LAV infection. *N Engl J Med* 1986;314:131–132.

13. Centers for Disease Control: Update: Human immunodeficiency virus infections in health-care workers exposed to blood of infected patients. *MMWR* 1987;36:3032–3034.

14. Centers for Disease Control: Recommendations for prevention of HIV transmission in health-care settings. *MMWR* 1987;36(suppl 2S):3S–18S.

15. Andes WA, Aledort LM: *Surgery in Hemophilia.* New York, National Hemophilia Foundation, 1987, pp 1–11.

16. Green WB: Use of continuous passive slow motion in the postoperative rehabilitation of difficult pediatric knee and elbow problems. *J Pediatr Orthop* 1983;3:419–423.

17. Sjamsoedin LJM, Heijnen L, Mauser-Bunschoten EP, et al: The effect of activated prothrombin-complex concentrate (FEIBA) on joint and muscle bleeding in patients with hemophilia A and antibodies to factor VIII: A double-blind clinical trial. *N Engl J Med* 1981;305:717–721.

18. Hutchinson RJ, Penner JA, Hensinger RN: Anti-inhibitor coagulant complex (Autoplex) in hemophilia inhibitor patients undergoing synovectomy. *Pediatrics* 1983;71:631–633.

19. Blatt PM, Ménaché D, Roberts HR: A survey of the effectiveness of prothrombin complex concentrates in controlling hemorrhage in patients with hemophilia and anti-factor VIII antibodies. *Thromb Haemost* 1980;44:39–42.

20. Colvin BT, Ainsworth M, Buckley C: Experience with highly purified porcine factor VIII in a patient with haemophilia A and a factor VIII inhibitor. *Clin Lab Haematol* 1983;5:55–59.

21. Spero JA: Histologic liver disease and hemophilia. *Hemophilia* 1980;2:1–2.

22. Post M, Watts G, Telfer M: Synovectomy in hemophilic arthropathy: A retrospective review of 17 cases. *Clin Orthop* 1986; 202:139–146.

23. Goldberg VM, Heiple KG, Ratnoff OD, et al: Total knee arthroplasty in classic hemophilia. *J Bone Joint Surg* 1981; 63A:695–701.

24. McCollough NC III, Enis JE, Lovitt J, et al: Synovectomy or total replacement of the knee in hemophilia. *J Bone Joint Surg* 1979;61A:69–75.

25. Rana NA, Shapiro GR, Green D: Long-term follow-up of prosthetic joint replacement in hemophilia. *Am J Hematol* 1986;23:329–337.

26. Small M, Steven MM, Freeman PA, et al: Total knee arthroplasty in haemophilic arthritis. *J Bone Joint Surg* 1983;65B:163–165.

27. Smith MA, Savidge GF, Fountain EJ: Interposition arthroplasty in the management of advanced haemophilic arthropathy of the elbow. *J Bone Joint Surg* 1983;65B:436–440.

28. Handelsman JE: The knee joint in hemophilia. *Orthop Clin North Am* 1979;10:139–173.

29. Post M, Telfer MC: Surgery in hemophilic patients. *J Bone Joint Surg* 1975;57A:1136–1145.

30. Nilsson IM, Hedner U, Ahlberg A, et al: Surgery of hemophiliacs—20 years' experience. *World J Surg* 1977;1:55–66.

31. Hoskinson J, Duthie RB: Management of musculoskeletal problems in the hemophilias. *Orthop Clin North Am* 1978;9:455–480.

32. Hofmann P, Brackmann HH, Pichotka H: Orthopaedic surgery in hemophiliacs in *Proceedings of the First International Symposium on Hemophilia Treatment.* Tokyo, Kyoritsu Printings, 1980, pp 133–153.

33. Greer RB III: Operative management of hemophilic arthropathy: An overview. *Orthopedics* 1980;3:135–138.

34. Pietrogrande V, Dioguardi N, Mannucci PM: Short-term evaluation of synovectomy in haemophilia. *Br Med J* 1972;2:378–381.

35. Houghton GR, Dickson RA: Lower limb arthrodeses in haemophilia. *J Bone Joint Surg* 1978;60B:387–389.

36. Storti E, Ascari E: Long-term evaluation of synovectomy in the treatment of recurrent hemophilic hemarthrosis, in Brinkhous KM, Henker HC (eds): *Handbook of Hemophilia.* New York, American Elsevier, 1975, part II, pp 735–750.

37. Rothwell AG, Faed JM: The performance of multiple joint procedures at one operation in a patient with haemophilia. *Aust NZ J Surg* 1979;49:476–479.

38. Le Balc'h T, Ebelin M, Laurian Y, et al: Synovectomy of the elbow in young hemophilic patients. *J Bone Joint Surg* 1987; 69A:264–269.

39. Montane I, McCollough NC III, Lian EC-Y: Synovectomy of the knee for hemophilic arthropathy. *J Bone Joint Surg* 1986; 68A:210–216.

40. Small M, Steven MM, Freeman PA, et al: Total knee arthroplasty in haemophilic arthritis. *J Bone Joint Surg* 1983;65B:163–165.

41. Surace A, Pietrogrande V: Total replacement of knee and elbow in hemophilia: Three cases. *Int Surg* 1983;68:85–88.

42. Gamba G, Grignani G, Ascari E: Synoviorthesis versus synovectomy in the treatment of recurrent haemophilic haemarthrosis: Long-term evaluation. *Thromb Haemost* 1981;45:127–129.

43. Storti E, Traldi A, Tosatti E, et al: Synovectomy, a new approach to haemophilic arthropathy. *Acta Haematol* 1969;41:193–205.

44. Oglesby JW, Wilson FC: The evolution of knee arthroplasty: Results with three generations of prostheses. *Clin Orthop* 1984;186:96–103.

Management of Soft-Tissue Sarcomas in the Adult

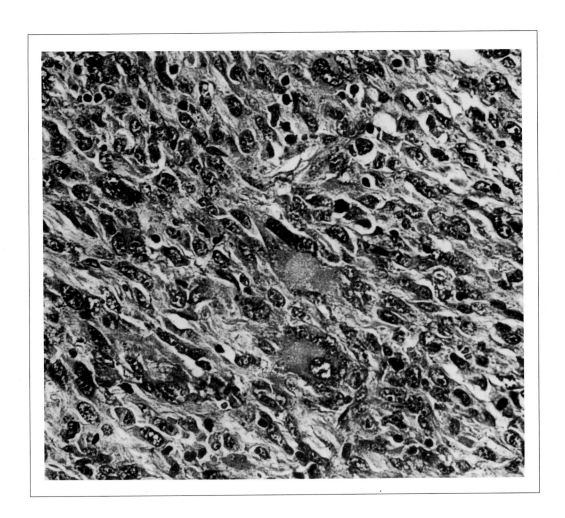

The Evaluation of a Soft-Tissue Mass in the Extremities

Thomas A. Lange, MD

A soft-tissue mass in an extremity presents a diagnostic challenge for the evaluating surgeon. The concerned patient needs, and deserves, the surgeon's best judgment as to whether the mass can be observed or should be excised. To avoid the pitfalls of observing an aggressive or malignant tumor or of "shelling out" a seemingly benign mass only to learn later of its malignant histologic features, I recommend the use of an algorithm[1] in the decision-making process (Fig. 36–1).

The History

A patient with a soft-tissue tumor usually seeks a physician's advice because of a recently noticed lump or mass. A careful history may aid in determining the etiology. A history of thigh-muscle trauma, for instance, may suggest the diagnosis of myositis ossificans (a well-known imposter of a malignant soft-tissue tumor).[2] A patient with a calf tumor who also has rheumatoid arthritis probably has a Baker's cyst that has penetrated into the gastrocnemius muscle. The diagnosis is easily confirmed by aspiration, and malignancy can be ruled out by cytologic examination.

Infection or an abscess may lead to a mass for which the causative agent or incident is remote. This has occurred in infants in whom immunization injections in the thigh led to development of a sterile abscess (Fig. 36–2) and occasionally in adults in whom bacteria seeded a muscle hematoma.

Obviously, the history alone does not dictate the management, but it certainly should be considered in the evaluation of soft-tissue masses.

Physical Examination

In performing the physical examination, one should look for symmetry of the extremities, edema formation, deformity of normal contours, changes in skin color, and the presence of increased superficial veins. The range of motion of the joints proximal and distal to the lesion should be recorded.

Palpation should include the soft tissue of the entire extremity, including the superficial proximal lymph-node bed. The skin temperature over the mass should be noted in relation to its vascularity. Specifically, one attempts to determine the size, mobility, compressibility, and depth of the mass. The information from this tactile examination is enhanced by using a lubricating jelly on the patient's skin to reduce the friction between the examiner's fingers and the patient's skin. This "low-friction" or "slippery skin" examination allows a much more accurate assessment of the mass, especially its boundaries and size. The compressibility or firmness of a mass dictates the sequence of studies to be obtained, as indicated by the algorithm (Fig. 36–1).

Xeroradiography vs Soft-Tissue Radiography

Virtually all soft-tissue masses in the extremities require a radiograph. For palpably large, deep, but soft lesions such as intramuscular lipomas, a xeroradiograph or soft-tissue radiograph can be diagnostic (Fig. 36–3, left). The xeroradiograph in particular provides high contrast between soft tissues of different densities.[3] Although commonly used for mammography, it may be used for extremity masses equally well. If xeroradiography is not available, other radiographic techniques suitable for soft tissues may provide similar information. An intramuscular lipoma is readily outlined by denser muscle fibers and fascia. The contrasting tissue densities seen in soft-tissue radiographs or xeroradiographs usually allow the extent of these unique lesions to be determined fairly accurately. Computed tomography of such a lesion, however, provides even more exquisite detail and contrast and confirms the preoperative diagnosis of a benign intramuscular lipoma (Fig. 36–3, right). Other soft or compressible masses may contain 1- to 2-mm calcific densities or phleboliths. These may also be detected in the soft tissues by xeroradiographic or soft-tissue radiographic techniques. This finding should suggest the diagnosis of an intramuscular hemangioma (Fig. 36–4, left). This specific lesion may be further characterized by magnetic resonance imaging, which often reveals extensive high-signal vascular channels throughout a muscle (Fig. 36–4, right).[4] Before magnetic resonance imaging was available, triple-phase bone scans best verified the vascular nature of these benign neoplasms. With the above-noted exceptions, screening radiographs of most soft-tissue tumors will not provide any diagnostic clues and it is necessary to resort to additional techniques and studies.

Transillumination

A superficial lesion that seems on palpation to be a ganglion or cyst can be transilluminated. If light ap-

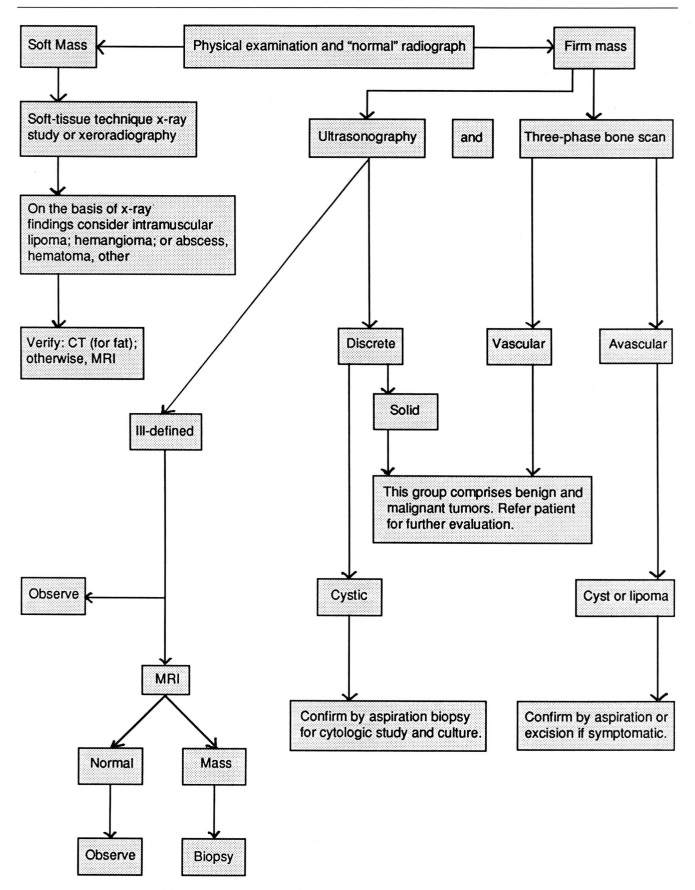

Fig. 36-1 Sequence of special studies to evaluate a soft-tissue mass when the radiographic appearance is normal. (Reproduced with permission from Lange TA: Workup for diagnosing a mass in an extremity. *Consultant* 1987;27:62–73.)

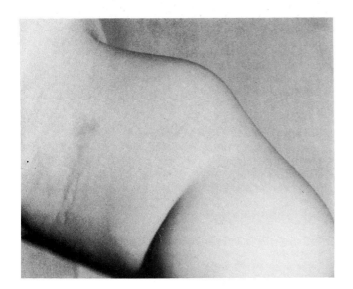
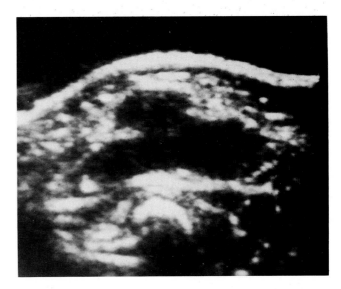

Fig. 36-2   A 2-year-old girl with a two-week history of an enlarging left thigh mass. **Left:** On physical examination the mass was minimally tender and relatively firm. The child was afebrile. **Right:** The transverse-image ultrasonogram revealed a hypoechoic (low echo) dumbbell-shaped mass that had penetrated the muscle fascia. An abscess was suspected and confirmed by aspiration.

pears to fill the lesion to the extent that it is palpable, its cystic nature can be confirmed by aspiration. The aspirate should be sent for cytologic study to rule out cystic degeneration of a malignancy. Some cystic soft-tissue sarcomas have been mistakenly treated initially as benign cysts. Cytopathologic study of the aspirate avoids delay in the proper diagnosis of a synovial sarcoma masquerading as a cyst. For this reason, aspiration of presumed cysts should probably precede excisional biopsy if there is any question of malignancy.

Ultrasonography

Most malignant soft-tissue tumors are located deep to muscle fascia and are firm and relatively immobile. Radiographically, the tumor density is usually the same as that of muscle and therefore cannot be seen except for distortion of surrounding soft-tissue planes. In such instances, my first study after the standard radiograph is ultrasonography.

My associates and I[5] recently reviewed our experience with ultrasound as the primary screening study in 50 patients with extremity soft-tissue masses that had not previously undergone biopsy. All lesions later underwent biopsy to allow correlations between the ultrasonographic results and assignment to the broad diagnostic categories of benign or malignant. The ultrasonographic findings divided the lesions into one of two groups—those easily defined by an echo pattern distinct from surrounding soft tissues (called "discrete") and those lesions not discernible ("indiscrete")

on the basis of the ultrasonographic patterns. One significant finding was that all 15 lesions that could not be defined by ultrasound were benign masses such as hematomas, intramuscular hemangiomas, or lipomas. These tumors usually felt soft or "compressible." On the other hand, all 14 malignant tumors were identified within the group of 35 lesions that were "discrete" or well demarcated by ultrasound. Thus, this screening study defines those tumors, whether cystic or solid, that demand further study and biopsy (Table 36-1).

Ultrasound may not consistently distinguish between cystic and solid tumor masses. It is sensitive to particulate matter floating within a cyst, recording it as echoes. Thus, because of the internal echoes produced, an abscess with thick proteinaceous pus or a complex Baker's cyst with rice bodies may appear to be solid. Although we found on biopsy that 14 of the lesions were fluid-filled, only seven were correctly identified as cysts preoperatively by the radiologist because the other seven lesions produced internal echoes. This limitation in identifying cysts does not detract from the value of ultrasound as a screening study since cystic lesions, especially those about the knee, may also be malignant.

Other benefits of ultrasound include its general availability and low cost compared with many other studies. Since it does not use radiation and is noninvasive, it is safe and comfortable for use in children. In addition to classifying the lesion into one of two major groups (potentially malignant vs benign), ultrasound gives information about the size and depth of the mass relative to tissue planes. Not the least important is the advantage to the physician who now has an image of the lesion

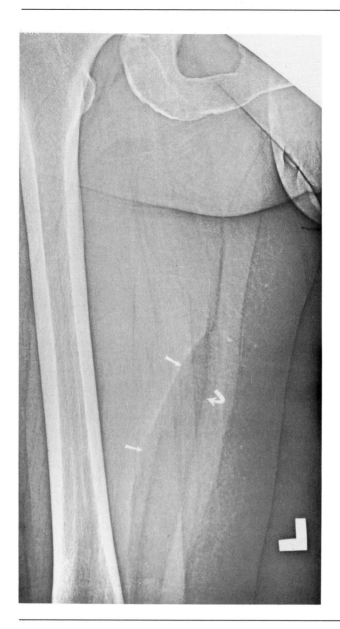

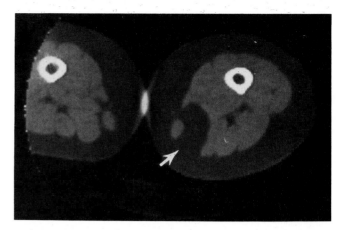

Fig. 36-3   Intramuscular lipoma. **Left:** An anteroposterior xeroradiograph depicts a fat density within the adductor muscles. The lesion is identified by arrows. **Right:** Computed tomographic scan of the thigh demonstrates the fat density (arrow) in a cross-sectional view of the adductor muscles.

Table 36-1
Comparison of ultrasonographic and biopsy findings*

Findings	Specimens				
	Benign		Malignant		Total
	Solid	Cystic	Solid	Cystic	
Surgical and biopsy	23	13	13	1	50
Ultrasonographic					
Discrete	9	12	13	1	35
Cystic	—	7	—	1†	8
Solid	9	5	13	—	27
Ill defined	14	1	—	—	15

*Adapted from Lange and associates.[5]
†Ultrasound suggested a central cystic component in this case. At surgery, a central hematoma was found in a rhabdomyosarcoma.

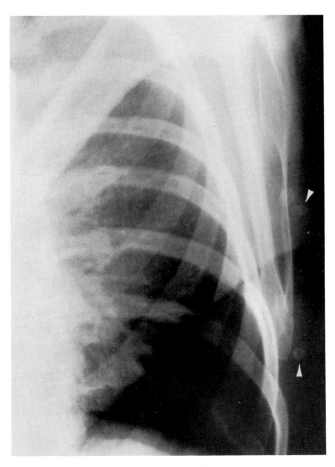
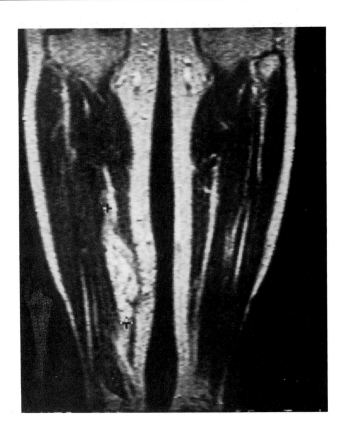

Fig. 36-4 Intramuscular hemangioma. **Left:** A tangential radiographic view of the scapula reveals multiple phleboliths in the soft tissues overlying the scapula. These small spherical mineral densities (arrows) are a frequent indication of transmural hemangioma. **Right:** Intramuscular hemangioma in the lower leg seen by magnetic resonance imaging. This study revealed extensive posterior tibial muscle involvement and militated against attempting resection.

that was previously invisible on the radiograph and merely a palpable entity. Doppler ultrasound used to evaluate the vascularity of soft-tissue masses produced findings that correlated with gross pathologic categories. The findings were that avascular lesions are benign, inflammatory lesions are moderately vascular, and malignant tumors are highly vascular (R. Leithiser, unpublished data).

Triple-Phase Bone Scans

A readily available, minimally invasive study that can yield a wealth of data is the triple-phase technetium Tc 99m methylene diphosphonate bone scan.

In order to gain the most information possible from the study, three phases are recorded after the radionuclide is injected. These include: (1) the flow study—a series of immediate images of the lesion or region of interest at five-second intervals (Fig. 36–5, *top*); (2) the

blood-pool image—obtained one to five minutes after injection (Fig. 36–5, *bottom left*); and (3) the skeletal image—the standard two- to four-hour delayed views of the bone (Fig. 36–5, *bottom right*).

Most solid tumors show some increase in vascularity on either the flow study or the early blood-pool image.[6] The exceptions are most lipomas and benign cysts. These early phases showing the vascular nature of the tumor are an important addition to the standard delayed "skeletal" images. In special cases such as myositis ossificans, extraosseous osteogenic sarcoma, synovioma with calcification, and myxoid liposarcoma, increased radionuclide activity is seen in the soft-tissue mass in the skeletal phase as well. The information from the triple-phase radionuclide study supplements the ultrasound information by providing a biologic perspective, that is, the vascularity of the mass in question. For example, a lesion that is avascular or "cold" on the flow and blood-pool images of the bone scan but is discrete on ultrasound is probably a cyst or ganglion. By con-

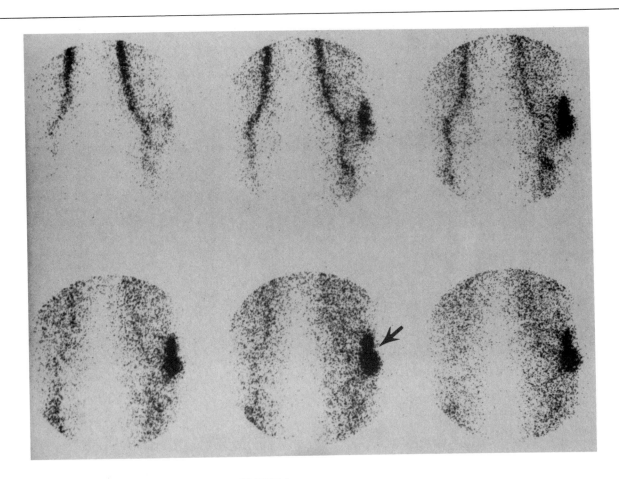

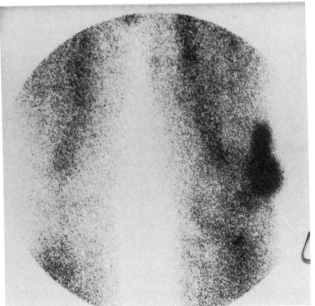

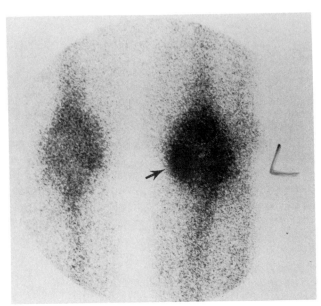

Fig. 36–5   Bone scan flow study. **Top:** Initial views reveal the tumor to be hypervascular. The large femoral arteries dominate the left upper picture; however, by the time the fifth image was obtained a few seconds later, the mass was well defined by the radionuclide material (arrow). **Bottom left:** The blood-pool image, obtained a few minutes after the radionuclide injection, shows that the tumor is significantly more vascular than the surrounding soft tissues. Less vascular tumors may only show up in this phase. **Bottom right:** The conventional delayed image, usually obtained two or three hours after radionuclide injection, shows that most of the radioactive material is cleared from the soft tissues and has been taken up by the bone. The very dark area on the medial aspect of the left knee (arrow) is caused by mild degenerative arthritis of the knee joint and is not related to the tumor. The region of the tumor adjacent to the large L has no increased uptake in the skeletal phase.

trast, a lesion that is relatively vascular according to early radionuclide scans but is ill-defined or not visualized with ultrasound may be an intramuscular hemangioma.

The skeletal phase of the bone scan is also informative, demonstrating the physical relationship of the bone to an overlying soft-tissue tumor, an important aspect to consider in surgical planning.[7] Specifically, if the bone underlying a malignant soft-tissue tumor is "hot" on the bone scan, the surgeon should consider this evidence of direct contact or invasion of bone. This information suggests aggressive biologic behavior on the part of the tumor and should be confirmed by computed tomography or magnetic resonance imaging.

Biopsy

By the time these screening studies are completed and the results analyzed, one has a strong sense of whether a mass in the extremity is malignant or not. That is, any mass that is both "discrete" (well-defined or measurable) on ultrasonography and vascular on the three-phase bone scan is potentially malignant. At this point magnetic resonance imaging of the lesion is done in preparation for biopsy and to enhance surgical planning (Fig. 36–6). Magnetic resonance imaging has certain advantages over computed tomography in the evaluation of many soft-tissue tumors.[8,9]

Biopsy of any lesion suspected of being malignant on the basis of the above screening studies should be done in a way that does not jeopardize an opportunity to do a radical resection later.[10] When a needle biopsy is performed, care must be taken to take the biopsy specimen from a site that will not compromise the intended resection and that can be included in the specimen for the pathologist.[11] In my experience, a biopsy done with a disposable fine needle does not significantly detract from the images obtained with subsequent localizing studies such as magnetic resonance imaging or arteriography.

Open-biopsy incisions, when necessary, should be longitudinal and should be located at the distal pole of the lesion. Poor planning of biopsy sites, attempted debulking of large lesions, and large postoperative hematomas may preclude limb salvage in patients with extremity sarcomas.[12] Hematoma contamination of tissue planes by tumor cells is minimized when (1) the incision and soft-tissue dissection for the biopsy are small, (2) hemostasis is meticulous, and (3) wound drainage is provided with an exit hole close to and in the plane of the incision.

Frozen sections are routine to assure that fresh viable tumor tissue, and not reactive muscle or necrotic tumor, is available for permanent study. They also indicate when to preserve tissue for electron microscopy or submit cultures of the material.

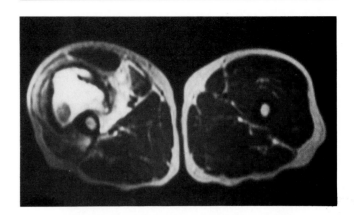

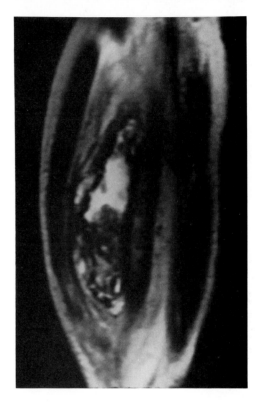

Fig. 36–6 Magnetic resonance imaging of a large, complex mass in the quadriceps of a 54-year-old man. **Top:** Axial view shows a high-intensity signal. **Bottom:** Sagittal section reveals the lesion to be extensive longitudinally and adjacent to the femur. Its pathologic cause was an infected hematoma.

Conclusions

Although soft-tissue masses of the extremity are not as easy to see as bone tumors on a radiograph, these lesions can be initially evaluated by such readily available techniques as ultrasonography and three-phase bone scans. This screening work-up, done on an outpatient basis, enables the physician to determine quickly the urgency of biopsy and definitive care. Soft-tissue masses that appear discrete on ultrasound examination and vascular in the bone-scan vascular phases are those lesions that require further studies. Localization provided by magnetic resonance imaging, and occasionally by arteriography, and an accurate biopsy appropriately placed on the extremity will allow limb salvage as an alternative to amputation when a soft-tissue tumor is determined to be malignant. Accepted surgical techniques in tumor surgery, along with appropriate preoperative and/or postoperative adjuvant therapies, allow 50% to 80% of the limbs with malignant soft-tissue neoplasms to be saved.[13,14] For this degree of success to occur, the physician who first sees a patient with a soft-tissue mass must play a critical role in the initial assessment.

Summary

A soft-tissue mass in an extremity may present a diagnostic dilemma for the evaluating surgeon. A decision either to observe or remove the mass is required. An algorithm can assist in the decision-making process.

A careful history may aid in determining the etiology. A history of thigh-muscle trauma, for instance, may suggest myositis ossificans as the diagnosis of a malignant soft-tissue tumor. A large, firm mass that is fixed to deep structures or located within muscle should prompt the following studies: (1) plain radiographs of the extremity; (2) an ultrasound study of the mass; and (3) a three-phase technetium 99m methylene diphosphonate bone scan.

References

1. Lange TA: Workup for diagnosing a mass in an extremity. *Consultant* 1987;27:62–73.

2. Jackson DW, Feagin JA: Quadriceps contusions in young athletes: Relation of severity of injury to treatment and prognosis. *J Bone Joint Surg* 1973;55A:95–105.

3. Wolfe JN: Xeroradiography of the bones, joints, and soft tissues. *Radiology* 1969;93:583–587.

4. Kaplan PA, Williams SM: Mucocutaneous and peripheral soft-tissue hemangiomas: MR imaging. *Radiology* 1987;163:163–166.

5. Lange TA, Austin CW, Seibert JJ, et al: Ultrasound imaging as a screening study for malignant soft-tissue tumors. *J Bone Joint Surg* 1987;69A:100–105.

6. Lange TA: Imaging technique for a soft-tissue mass in the extremity. *Iowa Orthop J* 1986;6:125–128.

7. Enneking WF, Chew FS, Springfield DS, et al: The role of radionuclide bone-scanning in determining the resectability of soft-tissue sarcomas. *J Bone Joint Surg* 1981;63A:249–257.

8. Petasnick JP, Turner DA, Charters JR, et al: Soft-tissue masses of the locomotor system: Comparison of MR imaging with CT. *Radiology* 1986;160:125–133.

9. Totty WG, Murphy WA, Lee JKT: Soft-tissue tumors: MR imaging. *Radiology* 1986;160:135–141.

10. Mankin HJ, Lange TA, Spanier SS: The hazards of biopsy in patients with malignant primary bone and soft-tissue tumors. *J Bone Joint Surg* 1982;64A:1121–1127.

11. Simon MA: Current concepts review: Biopsy of musculoskeletal tumors. *J Bone Joint Surg* 1982;64A:1253–1257.

12. Leibel SA, Tranbaugh RF, Wara WM, et al: Soft tissue sarcomas of the extremities: Survival and patterns of failure with conservative surgery and postoperative irradiation compared to surgery alone. *Cancer* 1982;50:1076–1083.

13. Simon MA, Enneking WF: The management of soft-tissue sarcomas of the extremities. *J Bone Joint Surg* 1976;58A:317–327.

14. Eilber FR, Morton DL, Eckhardt J, et al: Limb salvage for skeletal and soft tissue sarcomas: Multidisciplinary preoperative therapy. *Cancer* 1984;53:2579–2584.

CHAPTER 37

Preoperative Staging Techniques for Soft-Tissue Neoplasms

John T. Makley, MD

A potential soft-tissue malignancy requires concerned diligence on the part of the orthopaedic oncologist. The initial task is to identify, as accurately as possible, the anatomic extent of the neoplasm. This includes identifying local compartmental barriers, the neoplasm's relationship to important neurovascular arrangements, its proximity to regional skeletal structures, and whether these structures have maintained their integrity. The many preoperative staging studies should provide the information needed to determine the local extent of the neoplasm and to identify possible regional or metastatic disease. This knowledge is vital in planning the therapeutic approach to be used. Accurate preoperative definition of the anatomic extent of disease and the delineation of the neoplasm's surgical margins have a direct bearing on the ultimate outcome.[1-3] Our highly sophisticated imaging techniques, which include arteriography, computed axial tomography (CT), radioactive isotopic scans, and the more recent magnetic resonance imaging (MRI), enhance the clinician's ability to define these characteristics.

Unfortunately, a soft-tissue neoplasm is often discovered late in its course and becomes enormous before the patient seeks medical attention. Plain radiographs are seldom helpful but may on occasion suggest a presumptive diagnosis or further staging studies. Calcified densities within a soft-tissue mass, for example, might lead one to suspect a benign vascular tumor, synovial chondromatosis, myositis ossificans, or a more ominous synovial sarcoma. A large soft-tissue mass emanating from a bony lesion in a younger person certainly suggests Ewing's sarcoma. However, the osseous involvement may be so subtle that it is overlooked, falsely suggesting a primary soft-tissue sarcoma. Soft-tissue radiographic techniques often provide more information than do those for bone. For example, xerography, a technique once used frequently, can delineate soft-tissue lesions better than plain films can.

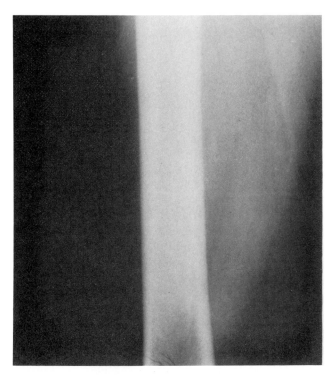 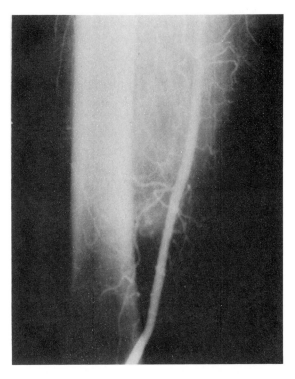

Fig. 37-1 Plain film **(left)** gives a vague impression of a soft-tissue mass along the femur, whereas a late-phase arteriogram **(right)** clearly shows the mass pushing the major vessel to the side. Note that the mass is outlined by the smaller vessels.

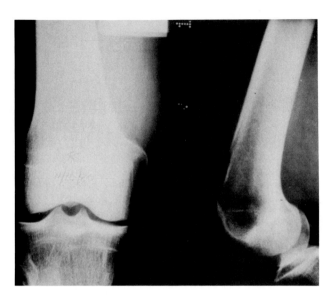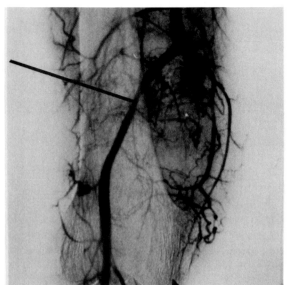

Fig. 37-2   Leiomyosarcoma in a 60-year-old man. **Left:** There is a slowly enlarging mass behind the knee. **Right:** Arteriogram demonstrates significant luminal narrowing as well as venous obstruction of the smaller vessels.

Arteriography

Arteriography was a widely used imaging technique before the development of CT and MRI. Despite its invasiveness, it remains a useful tool and is the best way to delineate tumor-vessel relationships. It must be used carefully, particularly in patients with known allergies or renal insufficiency. The contrast material may cause further renal injury. Adequate hydration must be maintained. With newer digital subtraction techniques, however, much less dye is needed to obtain reasonably good views of the vascular anatomy of the neoplasm and its environment.

Simple anteroposterior views often are not sufficient to delineate the complex vascular relationships between the bulk of the neoplasm and the major vascular channels. Lateral and oblique views should be requested. Delayed views showing the venous phase often produce a spectacular two-dimensional view of the tumor (Fig. 37–1). Although the arteriogram cannot prove malignancy, it is often suggestive and at times can be specific (as in venous leiomyosarcomas).[4] In such cases the arteriogram often shows narrowing of the vessel that is encased by the tumor. Sometimes a venous-phase arteriogram shows tumor actually obstructing the lumen (Figs. 37–2 and 37–3).

The arterial catheter also offers a portal for local administration of chemotherapeutic agents. Several protocols used for soft-tissue sarcomas employ intra-arterial agents before surgical intervention. Certainly, preoperative embolization of feeder vessels, particularly in vascular metastatic tumors, helps prevent ex-cessive hemorrhage during surgery. The venogram can be useful in specific situations such as suspected inter-muscular or intramuscular hemangioma (Fig. 37–4).

Since 5% to 20% of soft-tissue sarcomas metastasize to local lymph nodes, lymphangiography helps to as-certain nodal involvement in lesions of the lower ex-tremity. This technique requires a considerable amount of time and is very difficult to accomplish. The pro-cedure has been discarded in most institutions because radiologists believe that CT scanning is more sensitive in detecting node involvement. At my institution, clin-ically suspect nodes draining the regional area of a sus-pected neoplasm often undergo biopsy at the time of definitive surgery, particularly if they have been con-firmed by CT scan.

Arteriography offers a number of advantages: it (1) delineates vascular structures during the arterial phase, (2) delineates the neoplasm's longitudinal dimensions during the venous phases, (3) provides arterial access for local chemotherapy, (4) permits arterial emboliza-tion of the neoplasm, and (5) may provide diagnostic clues. On the other hand, it (1) is an invasive technique (rarely indicated in young children), (2) often requires a large dye load (contraindicated in patients with renal compromise), (3) cannot determine whether a tumor is benign or malignant, (4) may cause allergic reactions, and (5) is painful, often requiring anesthesia in children and sedation in adults.

Radioisotope Imaging

The first radioisotopic imaging techniques used the bone-seeking isotopes of fluorine and strontium. The

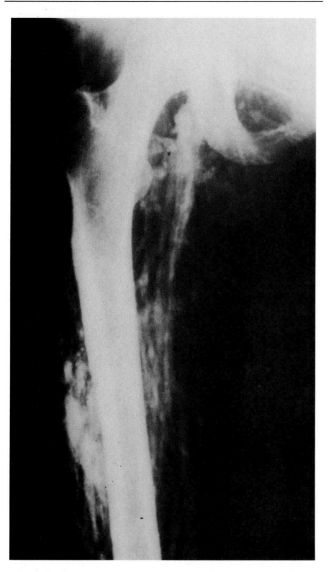

Fig. 37–3 Venogram shows large vascular spaces and pooling along the vastus lateralis, which was involved in an intramuscular hemangioma.

later development of technetium Tc 99m made this staging study useful and readily available. Technetium Tc 99m has an affinity for the mineralization front in bone similar to that of tetracycline. Experience has shown that it is specific for bone and permits an entire skeletal survey for detection of osseous lesions. Thus, this has become the most sensitive indicator for bone metastasis, especially in tumors with a predilection for bone metastases such as breast, lung, kidney, and prostate tumors. False-positive results do occur and findings must be correlated with the clinical situation and confirmed histopathologically before any firm treatment decision can be made. The proximity of a soft-tissue neoplasm to the bone has grave implications for the patient for whom a limb-sparing operation is contemplated. Bone involvement by the tumor has been shown

to produce a positive scan.[5–9] Obtaining the best information may require multiple views, not just routine whole-body imaging.

Since most neoplasms have a vascular component, the early phase of the technetium Tc 99m scan often shows the neoplasm quite well because of blood pooling.[7] Conversely, however, in those tumors with a minimal vascular component, such as desmoid tumors, the scan may be of little value. The later phase of the bone scan may show whether the tumor has produced a local bony reaction. According to Enneking and associates,[5] bone scans identified neoplastic involvement of contiguous bone with 92% accuracy.

The use of gallium as an isotopic medium to label inflammatory cells, particularly lymphocytes, made new scanning information available. Because most malignant soft-tissue neoplasms have an accompanying inflammatory response, especially when necrosis occurs, a gallium scan is almost always positive in such cases. Thus, a positive gallium scan and positive early (blood-pooling stage) and late technetium Tc 99m scans usually indicate malignancy[8] (Fig. 37–4). Occasionally, disagreeing scans (for example, a positive gallium scan and a negative technetium Tc 99m scan) indicate a benign lesion. This occurs in nodular fasciitis (pseudosarcomatous fasciitis), a lesion characterized by a prominent inflammatory component. The gallium scan is especially "hot" in lymphomas and may be useful in staging these neoplasms. Another isotopic scanning technique that is beginning to be helpful in staging consists of radioactive tagging of monoclonal antibodies specific for certain neoplasms. It is especially useful, even spectacular, in detecting metastatic disease such as that from neuroblastoma and osteosarcoma.

Computed Tomography

Computed tomography has greatly enhanced the accuracy of preoperative staging studies. Constructing cross-sectional images of the torso and extremities provides a much better way to delineate the anatomy of lesions, including soft-tissue tumors.[7,10–12] The CT scan passes multiple rotating beams of radiation through tissues. Sophisticated computer programming provides a good contrasting image. The contrast is probably best with calcified tissues, and thus bony detail is delineated effectively. Destruction of medullary bone by various neoplasms can be visualized remarkably well. Also, there is excellent contrast between fatty tissue and muscle. When a lipoma occurs within muscle of the thigh, the CT scan is almost diagnostic. However, when a neoplasm occurs in the muscle of an extremity, the contrast may not be as good because some neoplasms have densities similar to that of muscle. The advancing margin of a neoplasm is often difficult or impossible to delineate by conventional CT scanning.[11] The addition of

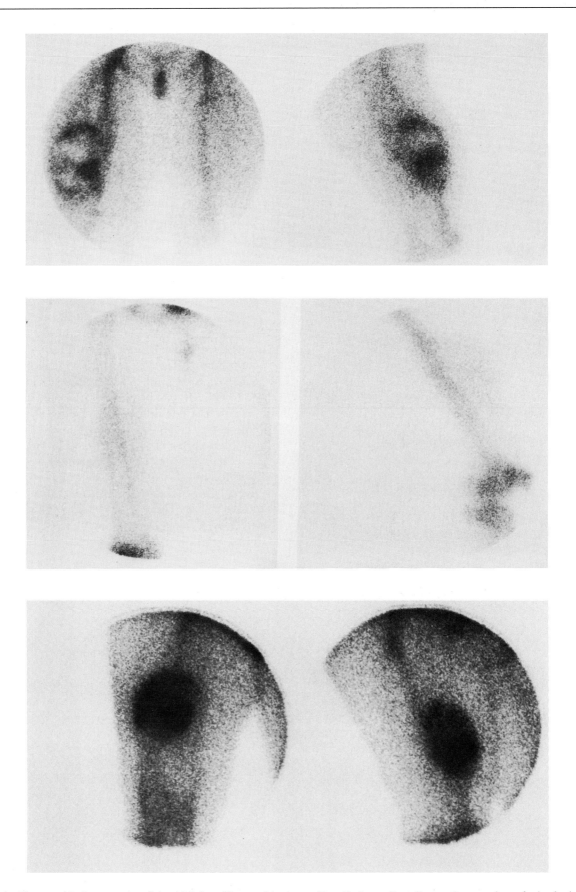

Fig. 37–4   Pleomorphic liposarcoma of the thigh in a 28-year-old woman. **Top:** Early pooling. **Center:** Increased uptake in the late phase of a technetium Tc 99m scan. **Bottom:** Positive gallium scan at 24 hours.

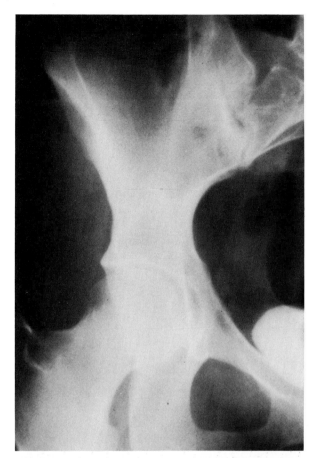

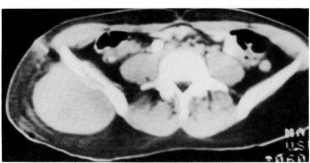

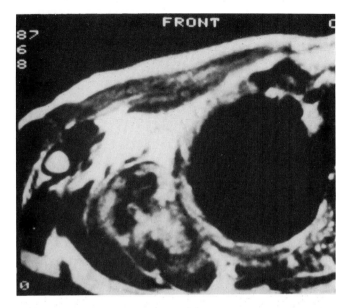

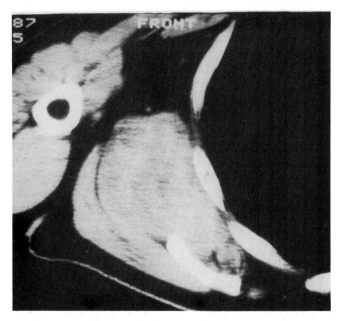

Fig. 37–5 Ewing's sarcoma. **Top:** Anteroposterior pelvic view was interpreted as normal despite the clinical presence of a large soft-tissue mass in the buttock. **Bottom:** Computed tomographic scan clearly demonstrates the large mass emanating from the ilium.

Fig. 37–6 Benign aggressive desmoplastic fibroma. **Top:** Magnetic resonance imaging shows a mottled, multidense mass with ill-defined borders in the axillae and chest wall. **Bottom:** Computed tomographic scan also demonstrates this ill-defined mass with variable densities within the lesion.

intravenous contrast material, however, accentuates the vascular anatomy and can improve the image of a lesion appreciably.[10]

Lesions of the pelvis and retroperitoneal areas were difficult to evaluate until the CT scan was developed. Contrast of soft-tissue lesions around the pelvis is quite good in many instances. In the case of a young woman who had a mass in the buttock, the plain film was interpreted as normal but the CT scan showed a huge soft-tissue mass emanating from the ilium (Fig. 37–5). Additionally, the CT scan is often helpful in demon-

strating nodal involvement. It is considered to be more sensitive than lymphangiography.

CT scanning does, however, have inherent disadvantages and they must be weighed carefully. Radiation exposure is proportional to the number of cuts obtained. The average radiation dose from CT is approximately 1 rad to the irradiated tissue. Chest CT has become almost routine in the preoperative evaluation of a suspected sarcoma since metastatic lesions as small as 2 to 3 mm can be seen. Although this is far better

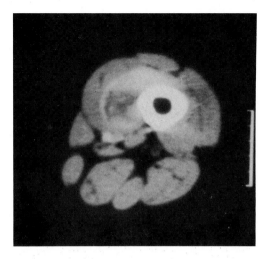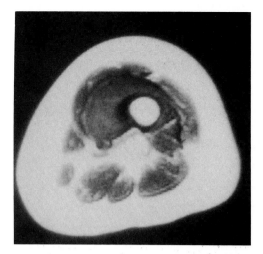

Fig. 37-7 Liposarcoma. **Left:** Computed tomographic scan demonstrates the mass around the bone in the anterior compartment. **Right:** Magnetic resonance imaging shows more clearly the tumor-muscle demarcation representing the pseudocapsule.

resolution than that obtainable by routine chest films, it also presumes adequate overlapping of CT scans. The cost-effectiveness of CT scanning of the chest for follow-up of possible lung metastases after initial treatment remains controversial. Many centers use preoperative CT scanning as a baseline, followed by routine monthly anteroposterior and lateral radiographs. Should a possible lesion appear, a follow-up CT scan is obtained. Finally, when metallic objects are in the plane of the CT beam, severe distortion of the image results, often negating useful information.

The advantages of CT scanning are (1) cross-sectional reconstructions, (2) excellent contrast between bone and soft tissue and between fat and muscle, (3) utility in guiding thin-needle biopsy, and (4) utility in screening suspected metastases to lung, nodules, and lymph nodes. Its disadvantages are (1) the possible high dosage of radiation, (2) the poor contrast between neoplasm and muscle, (3) the fact that longitudinal reconstruction is generally not available, (4) possible allergic reaction to the contrast dye, and (5) expense.

Magnetic Resonance Imaging

Remarkable multiplanar views of affected areas can be obtained with MRI. Steady improvements in this technique have made MRI the most important means of determining the anatomic extent of a soft-tissue neoplasm.[9,10,13-21]

The technical complexities of this technique are beyond the scope of this discussion, but a brief overview of the basics may be helpful. The technique depends on the ability of a strong external electromagnetic field to align protons. When a radiofrequency pulse is applied, these protons change orientation. As they return to their original position, they re-emit detectable radiofrequency signals that permit the position of the proton to be determined. The density of protons and their relaxation times can be calculated by varying the frequency, rate, and direction of the radiofrequency pulses. This produces images that can be reconstructed by computer in multiple planes.[14] Because of the many variable external factors, MRI offers potentially greater specificity than almost any other technique.

MRI probably reflects the tissue constituents of a given soft-tissue lesion better than other methods of imaging. This was shown by Sundaram and associates,[19] who noted that low-signal (T_2) lesions tended to show more collagenized tissue consistent with scarring or acellular areas. In their review, they showed that five of six low-signal T_2 lesions were benign (Fig. 37–6). The reverse did not hold true for malignant tumors, however, since both benign and malignant neoplasms may have high T_2 signals. Neoplasms of soft tissue are particularly well demarcated from surrounding fat, muscle, vascular structures, joints, or bone.[17] On the other hand, the contrast with bone and calcifying tissues is not as great as that with the CT scan. Although an angiogram contrasts tumor and vascular structures better and a bone scan delineates bone and tumor relationships better, MRI is by far the best staging study for evaluation of a soft-tissue neoplasm (Fig. 37–7). The use of surface coils often enhances the image, even demonstrating the advancing edematous pseudocapsule of the tumor.[13,17] Newer developments may make the invasiveness of arteriography unnecessary and provide three-dimensional views of the vascular anatomy of a given soft-tissue neoplasm.[22]

MRI is helpful in the evaluation of soft-tissue neoplasms because it (1) requires no radiation or injection of contrast dye, (2) provides multiplanar views, (3) delineates the tumor from the surrounding tissue, and (4) makes it possible to determine the intraosseous extent of the tumor. However, it has the disadvantages of being (1) costly, (2) time-consuming, (3) poor at providing detail of bone and calcified tissue, (4) contraindicated in patients with intracranial clips or pacemakers, and (5) unsuitable for patients with claustrophobia.

Summary

Preoperative staging studies need not be limited to one of the techniques discussed since each has its own specific advantages and disadvantages in the overall evaluation of soft-tissue neoplasms. Among orthopaedic oncologists, however, it is apparent that MRI is becoming the preoperative staging study of choice. It is by the careful, judicial use of one or all of these techniques that optimal diagnostic information is obtained and the patient given the best treatment alternatives.

References

1. Collin C, Hajdu SI, Godbold J, et al: Localized operable soft tissue sarcoma of the upper extremity: Presentation, management, and factors affecting local recurrences in 108 patients. *Ann Surg* 1987;205:331–339.
2. Collin C, Hadju SI, Godbold J, et al: Localized, operable soft tissue sarcoma of the lower extremity. *Arch Surg* 1986;121:1425–1433.
3. Lawrence W Jr, Donegan WL, Natarajan N, et al: Adult soft tissue sarcomas: A pattern of care survey of the American College of Surgeons. *Ann Surg* 1987;205:349–359.
4. Ekelund L, Rydholm A: The value of angiography in soft tissue leiomyosarcomas of the extremities. *Skel Radiol* 1983;9:201–204.
5. Enneking WF, Chew FS, Springfield DS, et al: The role of radionuclide bone-scanning in determining the resectability of soft-tissue sarcomas. *J Bone Joint Surg* 1981;63A:249–257.
6. Hudson TM, Bertoni F, Enneking WF: Scintigraphy of aggressive fibromatosis. *Skeletal Radiol* 1985;13:26–32.
7. Hudson TM, Schakel M II, Springfield DS, et al: The comparative value of bone scintigraphy and computed tomography in determining bone involvement by soft tissue sarcomas. *J Bone Joint Surg* 1984;66A:1400–1407.
8. Kirchner PT, Simon MA: The clinical value of bone and gallium scintigraphy for soft tissue sarcomas of the extremities. *J Bone Joint Surg* 1984;66A:319–327.
9. Pearlman AW: Preoperative evaluation of liposarcoma by nuclear imaging. *Clin Nucl Med* 1977;2:47–51.
10. Levine E, Lee KR, Neff JR, et al: Comparison of computed tomography and other imaging modalities in the evaluation of musculoskeletal tumors. *Radiology* 1979;131:431–437.
11. Rosenthal DI: Computed tomography of orthopedic neoplasms. *Orthop Clin North Am* 1985;16:461–470.
12. Weinberger G, Levinsohn EM: Computed tomography in the evaluation of sarcomatous tumors of the thigh. *AJR* 1978;130:115–118.
13. Beltran J, Simon DC, Katz W, et al: Increased MR signal intensity in skeletal muscle adjacent to malignant tumors: Pathologic correlation and clinical relevance. *Radiology* 1987;162:251–255.
14. Bland KI, McCoy DM, Kinard RE, et al: Application of magnetic resonance imaging and computerized tomography as an adjunct to the surgical management of soft tissue sarcomas. *Ann Surg* 1987;205:473–481.
15. Brady TJ, Rosen BR, Pykett IL, et al: NMR imaging of leg tumors. *Radiology* 1983;149:181–187.
16. Levin DN, Herrmann A, Spraggins T, et al: Musculoskeletal tumors: Improved depiction with linear combinations of MR images. *Radiology* 1987;163:545–549.
17. Pettersson H, Gillespy T III, Hamlin DJ, et al: Primary musculoskeletal tumors: Examination with MR imaging compared with conventional modalities. *Radiology* 1987;164:237–241.
18. Sartoris DJ, Resnick D: MR imaging of the musculoskeletal system: Current and future status. *AJR* 1987;149:457–467.
19. Sundaram M, McGuire MH, Schajowicz F: Soft tissue masses: Histologic basis for decreased signal (short T2) on T2-weighted MR images. *AJR* 1987;148:1247–1250.
20. Vanel D, Lacombe M-J, Couanet D, et al: Musculoskeletal tumors: Follow-up with MR imaging after treatment with surgery and radiation therapy. *Radiology* 1987;164:243–245.
21. Chang AE, Matory YL, Dwyer AJ, et al: Magnetic resonance imaging *versus* computed tomography in the evaluation of soft tissue tumors of the extremities. *Ann Surg* 1987;205:340–348.
22. Alfidi RJ, Masaryk TJ, Haacke EM, et al: MR angiography of peripheral, carotid, and coronary arteries. *AJR* 1987;149:1097–1109.

A Clinicopathologic Comparison of Malignant Fibrous Histiocytoma and Liposarcoma

Suzanne S. Spanier, MD

James Floyd, MD

Introduction

The pathologic classification of neoplasms provides information by which the behavior of newly diagnosed cases, with features similar to those for which the outcome is known, can be predicted. Thus, it provides the basis for treatment. For many years classification was done by light microscopy, aided only by histochemical stains. The pathologist determined how closely the neoplasm resembled a given normal tissue. As new ways of probing cells and clinical follow-up on patient cohorts become available, the pathologist's thinking about histogenesis and diagnostic groupings undergoes change.[1-3] Diagnostic categories are not static: as newly recognized neoplasms are defined and described, others may be moved from one diagnostic category to another.

About 15 years ago electron microscopy added a new dimension to the sorting process and forced changes in diagnostic groupings. Now the first application of immunohistochemical techniques using monoclonal antibodies to specific cell structures or products is adding another dimension. The malignancy grade, an essential part of the diagnosis, adds yet another. These new techniques are time-consuming, often require special handling of unfixed tissues, and are very expensive. A legitimate question is whether the added cost and effort are worthwhile. Do revised diagnostic groupings really have clinical meaning? In an attempt to answer this question, we compared two recently separated sarcomas that were often classified together in the past.

Not so long ago, liposarcoma was one of the most commonly diagnosed soft-tissue sarcomas.[4,5] Today, malignant fibrous histiocytoma, almost unheard of 15 years ago, is by far the most commonly diagnosed sarcoma[6] and true liposarcoma is considered uncommon.[7] One reason for this change was that the clinical follow-up of patients with clearly lipomatous tumors—many of which had been classified as liposarcoma—showed that some tumors with characteristic histologic and clinical patterns, did not metastasize. These are now considered benign.[3,7-12] Electron microscopy has further diminished the number of newly diagnosed cases by demonstrating other histogenic differentiation in some instances.[4,7] As new entities are introduced, old ones are reassessed.[7,12,13]

Present-Day Criteria

Malignant fibrous histiocytoma (MFH) is a descriptive term used to designate sarcomas displaying evidence of functional differentiation along both histiocytic and fibroblastic lines. By light microscopy, histiocytes are identified by their indented or folded nuclei, abundant cytoplasm, evidence of phagocytosis, formation of Langhans' and foreign-body giant cells, and lipid-accumulating xanthoma (foam) cells. Fibrogenesis is demonstrated by collagen production. Furthermore, these features may vary, both qualitatively and quantitatively, creating a spectrum of tumors with quite dissimilar appearances.

Ultrastructurally, they contain variable amounts of rough endoplasmic reticulum, lysosomes, phagosomes, and lipid droplets. Cytoplasmic lipid is membrane-bound. Because these features are nonspecific, the major use of electron microscopy is to establish the lack of organelles or products whose presence would indicate another classification. Immunohistochemical techniques can be helpful if a panel of monoclonal antibodies with appropriate controls is used. MFHs contain vimentin, one of five major classes of intermediate microfilaments identified in studies of the structural proteins and cytoplasmic filaments of neoplasms. Vimentin has so far been found exclusively in sarcomas and is thus believed to be a mesenchymal marker. MFHs do not, however, contain the epithelial cytokeratins or markers for muscle or melanoma. Variable amounts of the histiocytic markers α_1-antitrypsin and α_1-antichymotrypsin have been demonstrated in MFH, but their usefulness is limited by their nonspecificity.[14,15] Thus, a positive reaction for α_1-antitrypsin or α_1-antichymotrypsin and vimentin in the absence of positive reactions to other panel antibodies supports, but does not prove, histiocytic differentiation.

In the past, liposarcoma was often diagnosed on the basis of cytoplasmic vacuoles resembling fat or by a fat stain demonstrating intracytoplasmic lipid. It is now known that cytoplasmic vacuoles are nonspecific and often related to cell degeneration. Moreover, cytoplasmic lipid is found in a variety of normal and neoplastic mesenchymal cells, including MFH, and is not specific for lipoblasts.[16] Liposarcoma is now diagnosed only when there is convincing evidence that the neoplastic cells are committed to synthesizing and storing fat. By light microscopy the classic signet-ring lipoblast and the multivacuolated "mulberry" form are recognized. Ultrastructural analysis has contributed greatly to a descriptive understanding of the stages by which lipoblasts develop and, thus, is helpful in the identifi-

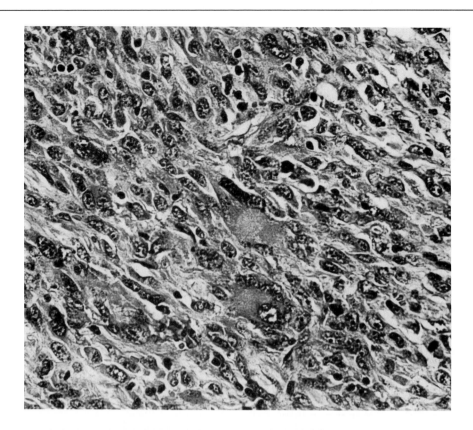

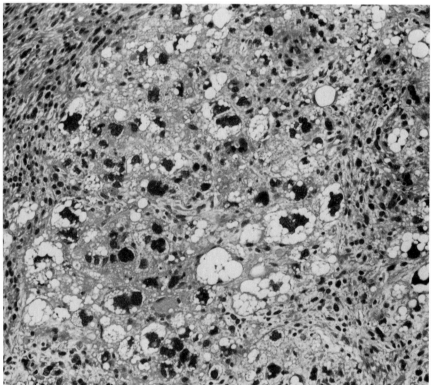

Fig. 38–1 Grade IV pleomorphic neoplasms. **Top:** Malignant fibrous histiocytoma composed of cells resembling histiocytes. The cells have abundant cytoplasm and nuclei that are round to oval and frequently indented. Bizarre, large, multinucleated cells with nonmirror-image nuclei and phagocytosed debris appear toward the center. Metastases to lung occurred despite local control. **Bottom:** Liposarcoma composed of a background of spindle cells with hyperchromatic oval nuclei. Although this neoplasm can resemble malignant fibrous histiocytoma, it can be distinguished by its large, lacy, multivacuolated "mulberry" lipoblasts. This 5-cm lesion metastasized to the lung, mesentery, and small bowel despite local control.

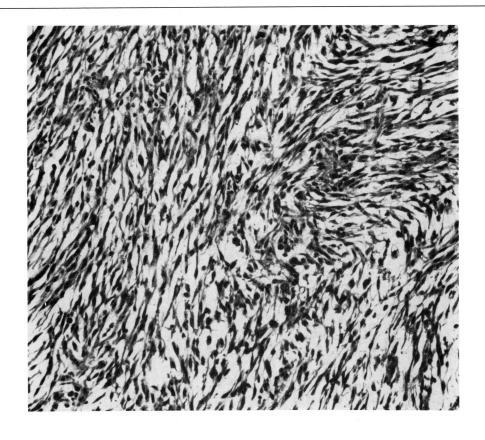

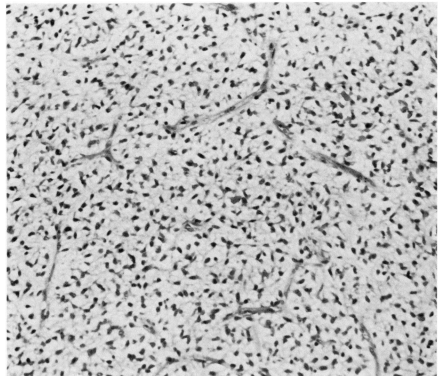

Fig. 38-2 Myxoid neoplasms. **Top:** Grade III malignant fibrous histiocytoma features stellate and spindle cells resembling fibroblasts. They are arranged in a fasicular pattern and embedded in a myxoid matrix. The background vascular pattern is not apparent. This tumor metastasized after two local recurrences. **Bottom:** Grade II liposarcoma. The lipoblasts are embedded in a myxoid matrix. The round to oval nuclei are uniform and mitoses are not evident. A fine, plexiform capillary network is a prominent background feature. The patient remains disease-free six years after wide excision.

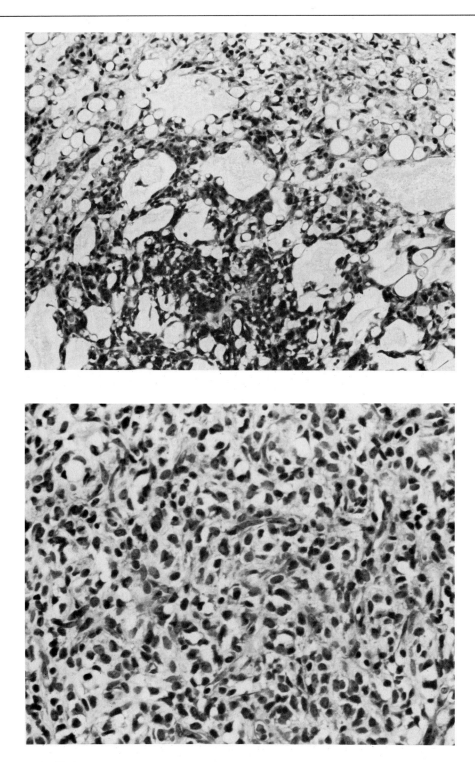

Fig. 38-3 Liposarcoma. **Top:** Part of this grade III liposarcoma with round cells could be classified as myxoid liposarcoma. It contains many signet-ring lipoblasts. Toward the lower left, the cellularity is markedly increased by clusters of poorly differentiated cells with enlarged hyperchromatic nuclei. The production of fat and mucin is diminished. The patient is well three years after wide excision and irradiation. **Bottom:** In this grade IV round cell liposarcoma, cellularity is markedly increased and fat production is decreased. The nuclei are enlarged and hyperchromatic. Despite local control, metastases to skull and liver occurred within two years.

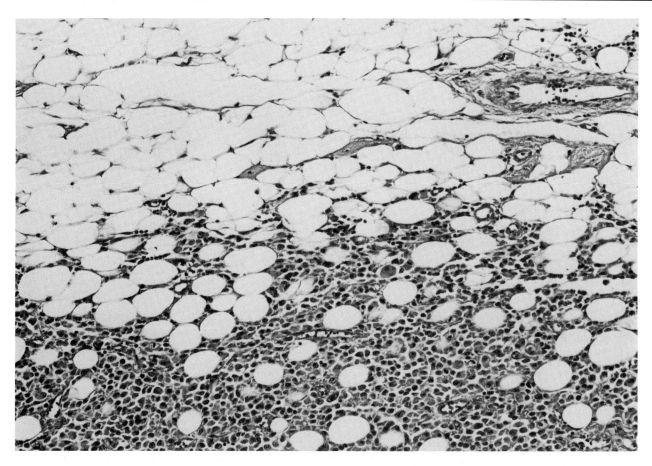

Fig. 38-4 Grade IV dedifferentiated liposarcoma. Although the portion of this neoplasm shown at the top is indistinguishable from lipoma or atypical lipoma, the portion shown at the bottom reveals a transition to a markedly cellular, poorly differentiated lesion in which fat production is almost nonexistent. The patient had a ten-year history of a very slowly enlarging thigh mass followed by sudden rapid growth. Most of the surgical specimen consisted of benign-appearing lipoma. Less than 10% was composed of undifferentiated cells. Multiple pulmonary metastases occurred within six months.

cation of the immature lipoblast.[1] Major ultrastructural features include cytoplasmic glycogen, micropinocytic vesicles, and discontinuous external laminae. However, the critical feature for designating a cell as a lipoblast is the presence of cytoplasmic nonmembrane-bound lipid droplets.[1,2,4] No antibody specific to lipoblasts has been developed and immunohistochemistry is not particularly helpful.

Histologic Grade

The histologic grade of a neoplasm is an assessment of its malignancy potential. It is expressed on a scale of 1 to 3 or 1 to 4 with the higher numbers assigned to the most malignant tumors. In MFH, grade is based on cellularity, mitotic rate, anaplasia (lack of differentiation), and necrosis. In liposarcoma, it is based on cellularity, mitotic rate, pleomorphism, and, in myxoid tumors, the degree of round cell differentiation.

Histologic Subtypes

Both MFH and liposarcoma have recognized subtypes that can be confused histologically.

Pleomorphic Subtypes

Malignant Fibrous Histiocytoma As its name implies, pleomorphic MFH has a wide range of appearances. The histologic findings may range from almost purely fibroblastic areas, which may have a storiform or fasicular pattern, to areas dominated by bizarre, multinucleated giant cells in which phagocytosed material may sometimes be found within the cytoplasm. Grotesque giant cells are a hallmark of this type (Fig. 38-1, *top*).

Liposarcoma Pleomorphic liposarcoma is characterized by the presence of multivacuolated, mulberry-type lipoblasts and spindle cells. The mitotic rate may be somewhat increased. This lesion may have large areas of extremely anaplastic cells indistinguishable from

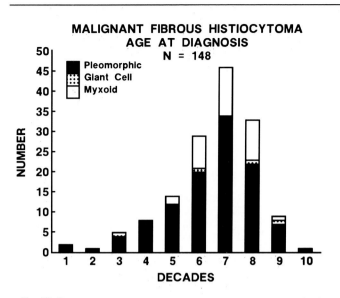

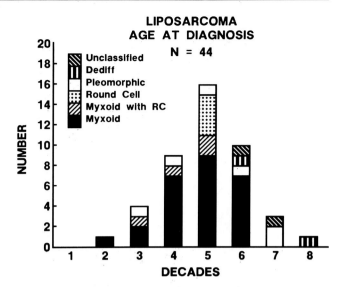

Fig. 38-5 Distribution of neoplasm subtypes by decade of life at the time of diagnosis for malignant fibrous histiocytoma **(left)** and liposarcoma **(right)**.

Table 38-1
Tumor sites

Malignant Fibrous Histiocytoma		Liposarcoma	
Site	No.	Site	No.
Subcutaneous	42	Thigh	
Thigh		Anterior	14
Anterior	31	Posterior	12
Medial	16	Medial	6
Posterior	10	Buttock	3
Arm		Popliteal fossa	3
Posterior	7	Anterolateral leg	2
Anterior	5	Volar foot	2
Buttock	7	Calf	1
Chest wall	4	Paraspinous	1
Miscellaneous	26		

pleomorphic MFH[7] and hence may require electron microscopy for differentiation (Fig. 38–1, *bottom*).

Myxoid Subtypes

Malignant Fibrous Histiocytoma Myxoid MFH is a less common variant only recently separated from myxoid liposarcoma.[17] It is distinguished by prominent areas of myxoid change in the stroma in which spindle and stellate cells, usually without visible histiocytic function, are embedded. The background vascularity is not prominent, and lipoblasts are not found (Fig. 38–2, *top*). An inflammatory infiltrate is often a striking accompaniment. Portions of the neoplasm may be indistinguishable from the pleomorphic type; if more than 50% of

the tumor contains pleomorphic elements, it is classified as pleomorphic.[17]

Liposarcoma Myxoid liposarcoma has a background featuring a prominent, anastomosing, fine capillary network in which the lipoblasts are embedded in a hyaluronidase-sensitive, mucicarmine-positive, myxoid intercellular matrix. Cellularity, lipoblast size and shape, and amount of cytoplasmic fat and glycogen vary markedly, not only from tumor to tumor but also within different areas of the same tumor. Mitoses are uncommon, and nuclear hyperchromatism and pleomorphism are not characteristic (Fig. 38–2, *bottom*).

In some tumors of this type there are clusters or sheets of poorly differentiated cells with enlarged, densely staining atypical nuclei—so-called round cells. These tumors are either assigned a higher grade or designated as myxoid with round cell areas (Fig. 38–3, *top*).[7]

Round Cell Liposarcoma In some tumors of the myxoid type the round cells predominate. Cellularity is markedly increased, fat production is poor, and lipoblastic cells are difficult to find. There is little intercellular matrix, the vascular network is not evident, and glycogen is scant. Some pathologists classify these tumors as a high-grade myxoid type[7] whereas others use the designation "round cell type" (Fig. 38–3, *bottom*).

Uncommon Subtypes

MFH and liposarcoma both have other rare subtypes. MFH has a "giant cell type," also termed "malignant giant cell tumor of soft parts." It is distinguished by its multinodular growth pattern and the presence of many multinucleated osteoclast-like giant cells. Histologi-

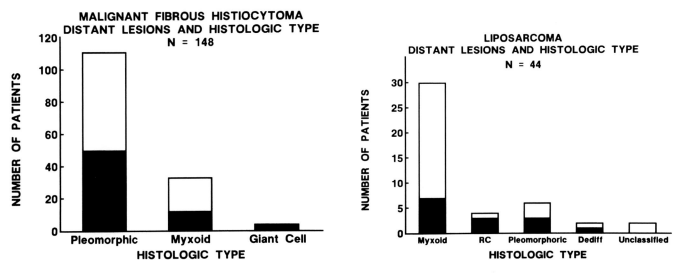

Fig. 38-6   Histologic tumor types by total number of patients (top of column) and number in whom distant lesions developed (top of solid area of column) for malignant fibrous histiocytoma (**left**) and liposarcoma (**right**).

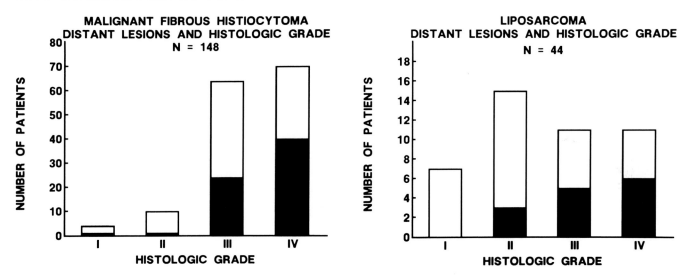

Fig. 38-7   Tumor grade by total number of patients (top of column) and number in whom distant lesions developed (top of solid area of column) for malignant fibrous histiocytoma (**left**) and liposarcoma (**right**).

cally, it appears more "malignant" than the giant cell tumor of bone; unlike the giant cell tumor of bone, it is a high-grade tumor.[18] The "inflammatory malignant fibrous histiocytoma" is very rare in the musculoskeletal system. Xanthoma cells predominate, and an intense inflammatory infiltrate may be present.[19] The "angiomatoid malignant fibrous histiocytoma" is a recently described subtype. It is a low-grade neoplasm with a predilection for the subcutaneous tissues of children.[20] The "dedifferentiated liposarcoma" is another recently described entity.[7] It is composed of well-differentiated liposarcoma or atypical lipomatous tissue in which there are areas of high-grade anaplastic cells (Fig. 38–4).

Clinical Findings

In an attempt to determine how well these diagnostic regroupings define clinically cohesive patient cohorts, we reviewed cases treated at the University of Florida. The minimum follow-up was two years. There were 148 cases of MFH and 44 cases of liposarcoma. The populations studied were comparable to those reported in other centers.[6,7,12,13,17]

Epidemiologic Factors

Pleomorphic MFH was about five times as common as the myxoid form. The peak incidence for both types

Table 38–2
Effect of primary tumor size on distant lesions

Tumor Size (cm)	Malignant Fibrous Histiocytoma		Liposarcoma	
	With Distant Lesions	Without Distant Lesions	With Distant Lesions	Without Distant Lesions
<5	2	23	1	4
5 to 10	6	24	0	9
11 to 15	16	5	2	9
16 to 20	4	4	2	3
>20	10	2	1	2
Unknown	0	2	1	0

Table 38–3
Sites of distant lesions

Sites	Distant Lesions	
	Initial	Later
Malignant fibrous histiocytoma		
Lung	50	7
Lymph nodes	10	7
Bone	4	2
Retroperitoneum	1	1
Other soft tissue	1	1
Other	1	0
Liposarcoma		
Lung, parenchyma	5(4)*	3
Small bowel, mesentery, intra-pelvic, intra-abdominal	4	5 (1)*
Retroperitoneum	3	1
Bones and skull	1	5 (1)*
Neck	2	4 (1)*
Liver	0	4
Other soft tissue	3	2

*Numbers in parentheses indicate liposarcomas other than the myxoid/round cell types.

was in the seventh decade of life (Fig. 38–5, *left*). In contrast, the myxoid form was by far the most common type of liposarcoma. Although the overall peak incidence was in the fifth decade of life, there was a relationship between age and tumor type. The myxoid/round cell spectrum was more common in younger patients whereas the other types predominated in elderly patients (Fig. 38–5, *right*). There was no significant difference between men and women with regard to histogenic type. Both were rare in blacks: seven MFHs and two liposarcomas.

Anatomic Location

More than 25% of MFHs occurred in the subcutaneous tissues. Of the deeper sites, the thigh was favored; the thigh and subcutaneous sites accounted for two thirds of the cases. In liposarcoma the thigh alone accounted for 75% of cases. There was a special predilection for the anterior compartment. Most were located in or below the buttock (Table 38–1). True liposarcoma in the subcutaneous tissues is extremely rare[3,7,21] and was not encountered in our study.

Tumor Type and Histologic Grade

In MFH, most of the tumors were high-grade, but low-grade forms of both the pleomorphic type and the myxoid type did occur. In contrast, in liposarcoma, there was a strong relationship between tumor type and histologic grade. This was not surprising because of the way grade is defined. One half of our liposarcomas were low-grade: grades I and II tumors were exclusively myxoid; grades III and IV tumors consisted of the myxoid with round cell areas, the round cell and the pleomorphic types. Thus, specification of the liposarcoma subtype provided some degree of prognostic information.

Factors Affecting Distant Lesions

Histologic Type There was a relationship between histologic type and the development of metastases. Metastases developed in approximately 50% of patients with pleomorphic MFH compared with approximately 33% of those with myxoid MFH[17] (Fig. 38–6, *left*). The same pattern was seen in liposarcoma: fewer than 25% of those with the myxoid type had distant lesions whereas more than 50% of those with the other types had distant involvement. It is important to remember that patients with myxoid liposarcoma have a better prognosis than those with myxoid malignant fibrous histiocytoma (Fig. 38–6, *right*).

Histologic Grade In MFH, metastases developed in only 14% of patients with grades I or II tumors whereas they developed in 38% of those with grade III tumors and in 57% of those with grade IV tumors (Fig. 38–7, *left*). Similarly, in liposarcoma, distant lesions developed in fewer than 20% of those with grades I or II tumors but in 50% of those with grades III or IV tumors (Fig. 38–7, *right*).

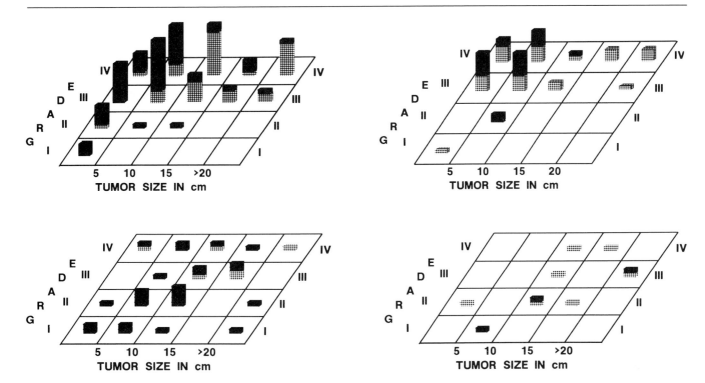

Fig. 38-8 Tumor size and grade by recurrence. Solid areas indicate no metastases; textured areas indicate neoplasms that metastasized. **Top:** Malignant fibrous histiocytomas with no recurrences **(left)** and with local recurrences **(right)**. **Bottom:** Liposarcomas with no recurrences **(left)** and with local recurrences **(right)**.

Tumor Size Of the 98 patients never having local recurrences, only 14% with tumors measuring less than 10 cm had metastases, whereas 73% of those with tumors larger than 10 cm had metastases. The pattern was the same in the 34 patients who had no local recurrence of liposarcoma. Only 12% of those with tumors smaller than 15 cm had distant lesions whereas 38% of those with tumors larger than 15 cm did (Table 38–2). Patients with tumors larger than 15 cm also fared poorly in the study by Evans.[7]

Local Recurrence Of the 98 patients with MFH who had no local recurrence, 39% had metastases. In contrast, metastases developed in 56% of the 50 patients with clinical recurrences. The same pattern occurred in liposarcoma: distant lesions occurred in fewer than 20% of the 34 patients who had no recurrences but in 70% of the ten patients with recurrences.

Sites of Distant Lesions

Metastases developed in 66 patients with MFH initially detected in 67 sites. In MFH of any subtype, the lung was overwhelmingly favored: it was the first site in 76% and was eventually involved in 86%. Regional lymph nodes were the next most favored site: they were the initial sites in 15% and were eventually involved in 26%. Bones accounted for less than 10%. Retroperitoneal or other soft tissues were involved only four times (Table 38–3).

In liposarcoma, distant lesions were initially detected in 18 sites in 14 patients. Unusual sites were favored.[7] Although lung lesions eventually developed in 57%, the lung was the first site in only five of these 14 patients. Further, most of the initial lung lesions were caused by variants other than the myxoid/round cell types. Preferred sites of the myxoid/round cell types were small bowel and mesentery, retroperitoneum, other intra-abdominal and intrapelvic sites, bones and skull, neck, liver, and other soft tissues (Table 38–3). In five of six patients who had clinically unsuspected retroperitoneal and intra-abdominal disease, unanticipated bowel perforation was the cause of death. By the time of death 12 of the 14 patients had involvement of intra-abdominal or retroperitoneal sites. In contrast to its occurrence in MFH, metastasis to lymph nodes, although often suggested clinically, was never proved.

This peculiar pattern of distant lesions has led some to ask whether these lesions represent multicentric rather than metastatic disease.[3,16,22] What is important is that chest radiographs and physical examination detect almost all metastases in patients with MFH whereas chest radiographs alone are inadequate in patients with high-grade or recurrent myxoid/round cell liposarcoma. The addition of a bone scan and an abdominal computed tomographic scan will detect almost all distant lesions.

Should every patient with myxoid/round cell liposarcoma undergo abdominal computed tomography? Figure 38–8 delineates the patients at risk for distant lesions. In both liposarcoma and MFH, the tumor's size and histologic grade were the most important factors in patients without local recurrences (Fig. 38–8, *top left* and *bottom left*). Although there were relatively few low-grade MFHs, most were smaller than 10 cm and only one metastasized. Of the high-grade tumors, most of those smaller than 10 cm also failed to metastasize. The MFHs that did metastasize were high-grade and larger than 10 cm. This pattern was the same in liposarcoma. Although the tumors tended to be larger, they were also of lower grades. The tumors associated with distant lesions were both high-grade and large. In patients with local recurrences, more tumors metastasized and smaller tumors metastasized more frequently (Fig. 38–8, *top right* and *bottom right*). This supports the idea that the distant lesions seen in liposarcoma are metastases. It should be noted that the outcome in both MFH and liposarcoma can be altered by achieving local control.

Summary

The diagnosis of MFH depends on the demonstration of histiocytic and fibroblastic functions. MFHs may phagocytose fat; therefore, lipid stains are useless. By electron microscopy, cytoplasmic lipid is membrane-bound. Immunohistochemical staining for vimentin and histiocytic markers may be helpful. Liposarcoma is diagnosed only when there is convincing evidence of synthesis and storage of fat by the tumor cells. By electron microscopy, cytoplasmic lipid is nonmembrane-bound.

Both MFH and liposarcoma have subtypes. In MFH, the pleomorphic forms are the most common. Myxoid MFH is less common; all other types are rare. In liposarcoma, the myxoid types are by far the most common. The myxoid types of both MFH and liposarcoma may contain other elements that vary in degree and geographic distribution and that can raise the histologic grade. About 50% of liposarcomas are low-grade tumors; these are almost always purely myxoid. Low-grade myxoid liposarcoma has a much better prognosis than other types. Myxoid liposarcoma has a better prognosis than myxoid MFH.

The peak incidence of MFH is in the seventh decade of life whereas that of liposarcoma is in the fifth decade. A substantial number (roughly 25% to 30%) of MFHs occur in the subcutaneous tissue. Clinically they are almost invariably mistaken for ganglion cysts. Liposarcoma, however, is likely to occur in or below the buttocks. Most are in the anterior thigh. Subcutaneous liposarcoma is extremely rare. A tumor in this area is likely to be either a more malignant myxoid MFH or one of the benign atypical lipomatous tumors.

In both MFH and liposarcoma, the development of distant lesions is related to the tumor's histologic grade and size and to local recurrence.

Favored metastatic sites of MFH are lung and lymph nodes. Favored sites of distant lesions in the myxoid/round cell types of liposarcoma are intra-abdominal, retroperitoneal, other soft-tissue areas (especially in the neck), and bone. Lymph node involvement is very rare.

Because myxoid/round cell liposarcomas have a marked propensity to involve intra-abdominal sites, abdominal computed tomography and bone scan are recommended in the initial evaluation and follow-up of high-risk patients (those with high-grade tumors larger than 15 cm and those with local recurrence of intermediate- or high-grade tumors of any size).

References

1. Bolen JW, Thorning D: Benign lipoblastoma and myxoid liposarcoma: A comparative light- and electron-microscopic study. *Am J Surg Pathol* 1980;4:163–174.
2. Rossouw DJ, Cinti S, Dickersin GR: Liposarcoma: An ultra-structural study of 15 cases. *Am J Clin Pathol* 1986;85:649–667.
3. Stout AP: Liposarcoma: The malignant tumor of lipoblasts. *Ann Surg* 1944;119:86–107.
4. Desal U, Ramos CV, Taylor HB: Ultrastructural observations in pleomorphic liposarcoma. *Cancer* 1978;42:1284–1290.
5. Pack GT, Pierson JC: Liposarcoma: A study of 105 cases. *Surgery* 1954;36:687–712.
6. Weiss SW, Enzinger FM: Malignant fibrous histiocytoma: An analysis of 200 cases. *Cancer* 1978;41:2250–2266.
7. Evans HL: Liposarcoma: A study of 55 cases with a reassessment of its classification. *Am J Surg Pathol* 1979;3:507–523.
8. Enzinger FM: Benign lipomatous tumors simulating a sarcoma, in *Management of Primary Bone and Soft Tissue Tumors*. Chicago, Year Book Medical Publishers, 1977, pp 11–24.
9. Enzinger FM, Harvey DA: Spindle cell lipoma. *Cancer* 1975; 36:1852–1859.
10. Shmookler BM, Enzinger FM: Pleomorphic lipoma: A benign tumor simulating liposarcoma. A clinicopathologic analysis of 48 cases. *Cancer* 1981;47:126–133.
11. Evans HL, Soule EH, Winkelmann RK: Atypical lipoma, atypical intramuscular lipoma, and well differentiated retroperitoneal liposarcoma: A reappraisal of 30 cases formerly classified as well differentiated liposarcoma. *Cancer* 1979;43:574–584.
12. Orson GG, Sim FH, Reiman HM, et al: Liposarcoma of the musculoskeletal system. *Cancer* 1987;60:1362–1370.
13. Campbell DA Jr, Eckhauser FE, Oehler JR, et al: Liposarcoma of the lower extremity. *Surgery* 1980;88:453–460.
14. du Boulay CEH: Demonstration of alpha-1-antitrypsin and alpha-1-antichymotrypsin in fibrous histiocytomas using the immuno-peroxidase technique. *Am J Surg Pathol* 1982;6:559–564.
15. Silva FG, Taylor WE, Burns DK: Demonstration of alpha-1-antitrypsin in yet another neoplasm, letter. *Hum Pathol* 1984; 15:494–495.
16. Enzinger FM, Winslow DJ: Liposarcoma: A study of 103 cases. *Virchows Arch Pathol Anat* 1962;335:367–388.
17. Weiss SW, Enzinger FM: Myxoid variant of malignant fibrous histiocytoma. *Cancer* 1977;39:1672–1685.
18. Guccion JG, Enzinger FM: Malignant giant cell tumor of soft parts: An analysis of 32 cases. *Cancer* 1972;29:1518–1529.
19. Kyriakos M, Kempson RL: Inflammatory fibrous histiocytoma: An aggressive and lethal lesion. *Cancer* 1976;37:1584–1606.
20. Enzinger FM: Angiomatoid malignant fibrous histiocytoma: A

distinct fibrohistiocytic tumor of children and young adults simulating a vascular neoplasm. *Cancer* 1979;44:2147–2157.

21. Hassan MA: Subcutaneous liposarcoma of forearm followed by liposarcoma of omentum. *Br J Surg* 1970;57:393–396.

22. Georgiades DE, Alcalais CB, Karabela VG: Multicentric well-differentiated liposarcomas: A case report and a brief review of the literature. *Cancer* 1969;24:1091–1097.

Preoperative Intra-arterial Doxorubicin and Low-Dose Radiation for High-Grade Soft-Tissue Sarcomas of the Extremities

William K. Dunham, MD

Jeffrey L. Myers, MD

Robert J. Sollaccio, MD

Merle M. Salter, MD

Robert P. Castleberry, MD

Wanda K. Bernreuter, MD

John J. Ward, MD

Theoretical Considerations

Combination therapy offers the most successful outcome in the treatment of high-grade soft-tissue sarcomas.[1-4] Although the best combination of treatments using radiation, medical oncology, and surgery has not yet been defined, modest gains in terms of local control of the tumor, quality of life, and survival have been made.

Attempts to find the right combination of therapeutic methods have been based on common sense rather than on scientific studies. The rarity of sarcomas of the extremities is one justification for this, but this approach is less than ideal. What are the logical reasons for the treatment combination of preoperative intra-arterial chemotherapy and radiation therapy that we are describing? We administer the adjuvant chemotherapy preoperatively rather than postoperatively because the tumor is in an undisturbed state and its blood supply and anatomy are unaffected by manipulation, clot, or hematoma. Agents used to kill tumor cells reach their destination with less disturbance and with a more complete distribution. We use the arterial route because it offers the most direct delivery of chemotherapeutic drugs at the highest concentration to the tumor interface. One preliminary study, however, indicates that intravenous administration of chemotherapy may be as effective as intra-arterial administration.[5] We use doxorubicin because it is one of the most effective antisarcoma drugs available and it appears to have a valuable radiation-sensitizing effect.[6,7] Although the exact mechanism of radiation sensitization is unknown, it is believed that doxorubicin renders hypoxic cells more sensitive to radiation. It is the hypoxic cell population in tumors that is the most radiation-resistant. This treatment technique, like any other that might be chosen, has constraints. It must allow wound healing because surgery remains an essential component of the therapy. The gain from the adjuvant therapy must strongly outweigh the risk of complications and side effects.

Empirical evidence collected by the surgeons using this particular technique indicates that preoperative treatment makes the sarcoma more operable, that is, more surgically accessible.[5,8] The tumor is more easily defined by physical examination, a more definitive margin of the neoplasm can be palpated at the time of surgery, and the tumor appears to be less fixed to surrounding structures. The center of the mass remains firm, but the periphery is softer and better defined.

In the radiographic assessment of tumors with mineralized areas, the mineral density usually increases with treatment; this reflects necrotic calcification. In soft-tissue neoplasms, the outline of the tumor often becomes more definable on plain radiographs (that is, muscle planes reappear). Imaging studies (computed tomography and magnetic resonance imaging) do not distinguish between reactive and neoplastic tissue and occasionally show a more poorly defined margin after treatment. Magnetic resonance imaging, which is very sensitive to reactive changes as well as to neoplastic change, may at times show a slight increase in the amount of abnormal-appearing tissue near the periphery of the tumor after preoperative treatment. Although tumor growth during therapy may be suspected, it has been demonstrated that this increase is often the result of necrotic and/or reactive change.[9,10] Jaffe and associates,[11,12] who used intra-arterial cisplatin to treat osteosarcoma, regarded the disappearance of neoplastic vascularity as evidence of tumor response to the drug. They referred to a carapace, or shell, that tends to form at the periphery of bone tumors preoperatively treated with intra-arterial cisplatin.

Picci and associates[13] showed that there are predictable areas of residual tumor in osteosarcomas treated preoperatively with intra-arterial drugs (methotrexate and cisplatin). One of these areas is the peripheral aspect of the osteosarcoma. Although this is not surprising in that the periphery is the most viable and replicating edge of the sarcoma, it warns us against believing that the periphery of the tumor is sterile.

We believe that the periphery of a preoperatively treated tumor is much easier to dissect away from vital structures at the time of surgery. The tumor margin is more easily defined and the abnormal tissue can be distinguished from the normal tissue visually and tactilely.

The obvious advantage of using preoperative chemotherapy to kill tumor cells is that fewer vital structures need to be sacrificed to control the tumor locally. This allows the surgeon to approach the tumor more closely; fewer limbs, therefore, have to be amputated to maintain local tumor control.

Lastly, preoperative treatment allows an in vivo assessment of the effectiveness of the drug through the study of specimens. Rosen and associates[14] successfully used this assessment to select effective chemotherapeutic agents in osteosarcoma. This approach has not yet been accomplished in soft-tissue sarcomas.

Development of the Technique

Our technique[8,15] is that initiated and developed by Eilber and associates[16–18] at UCLA. By early 1987, they had treated 375 patients with high-grade soft-tissue sarcomas of the extremity. The control group of 55 patients had a local recurrence rate of 25% after surgical and radiation techniques. In 1975, Eilber and associates began a prospective trial using intra-arterial doxorubicin followed by rapid-fraction radiation therapy (3,500 cGy). Three of 77 patients required amputation. Limb-salvage was possible in the other 74. Local tumor recurrence was noted in four patients. Because the complications were high in this group, with 17% requiring a second surgical procedure, a second prospective trial was begun in 1981 and completed in 1984.

This trial consisted of an identical regimen of intra-arterial doxorubicin followed by only 1,750 cGy of radiation. Of 137 patients in the study, 17 had local recurrences. Complications occurred in only 34 and only seven required a second surgical procedure. In 1984 Eilber and associates increased the radiation dosage to 2,800 cGy. After a median follow-up of 24 months, only five of the 97 patients had local recurrences, only ten needed a second operation for complications, and two required primary amputation. Eilber and associates believed they had a definite dose-response curve to the radiation.[5]

At least two other reported series using approximately 100-mg doses of intra-arterial doxorubicin followed by radiation and wide resection have produced similar results. Goodnight and associates[19] described 25 patients with sarcoma who were treated with the technique. After a median follow-up of 32 months, there were no local recurrences and 21 of the 25 had functional limbs. Mantravadi and associates,[20] in a study of 32 patients with high-grade soft-tissue sarcomas, reported successful limb-salvage in 30 patients and local recurrence in only one. We believe that the combination of intra-arterial doxorubicin as a sensitizing agent administered directly into the vessels supplying the sar-

coma, low-dose radiation, and a wide resection two weeks later is as good as, if not better than, any current recommended treatment protocol.

Clinical Experience and Results

We treated 61 patients with high-grade soft-tissue sarcomas, stages II-A and II-B, between August 1979 and August 1987. A standard policy was used for maximizing limb-salvage and local disease control. This approach consisted of preoperative regional intra-arterial chemotherapy with 100 mg of doxorubicin infused over a period of 80 hours. Patients treated before February 1985 received 3,000 cGy in ten fractions starting one to three days after intra-arterial doxorubicin was discontinued. Thirty-seven patients were treated during this period. The remaining 24 patients received 1,750 cGy in five fractions. Thirty-one patients were treated with postoperative adjunctive doxorubicin and six were treated with multidrug regimens. Twenty-four patients had no postoperative chemotherapy. The eligible patients had a high-grade soft-tissue sarcoma of the limb or limb girdle (excluding those of the retroperitoneum or head and neck). Six additional patients with small foci of metastatic sarcoma and symptomatic primary lesions were treated according to this protocol. The objective in these six patients was local tumor control and preservation of quality of life. They were included in the analysis of wound problems but excluded from the analysis of survival. Sixty-eight patients with high-grade bone sarcomas were also included in the analysis of the morbidity of the technique.

Pathologic Factors

All tumors underwent an initial biopsy, 46 incisional and 15 excisional. We reviewed the pathology reports and slides for all patients. Four to 34 (mean, 14) slides were available in each case. All patients had high-grade soft-tissue sarcoma as defined by Enneking and associates.[21] All lesions were staged according to the Musculoskeletal Tumor System by means of the history, physical examination, radiographs, bone scan, computed tomographic scans of the primary tumor and the lungs, and, in the latter part of the study, magnetic resonance imaging of the primary tumor. The resection was graded as wide, marginal, or intracapsular (lesional). The pathologist graded the surgical procedure and reported this and the tumor response grade on the final pathology report. If there was normal tissue at all of the extremes of the specimen, the resection was graded as wide. If reactive tissue in the form of inflammatory tissue or fibrotic pseudocapsule was identified at the periphery of the tumor, the resection was graded as marginal. If tumor was present at any margin, the resection was graded as intracapsular or lesional.[22]

All tumor-containing slides were scanned at low magnification and the relative cross-sectional area showing complete necrosis was recorded as a percentage of total area examined. Necrosis was defined as an area in which no basophilic staining of tumor nuclei could be identified. The result was expressed as a tumor response grade: grade I, less than 75% necrosis; grade II, 75% to 90% necrosis; grade III, 90% to 99% necrosis; and grade IV, 100% necrosis.[23-25]

Surgical Treatment

Surgery was performed approximately two weeks after completion of the preoperative treatment. A three-dimensional resection through normal tissue surrounding the neoplasm, including an en bloc resection of the biopsy tract with a 2-cm margin, was performed. If a major neurovascular bundle came close to the lesion, as was the usual case, the neurovascular bundle was dissected away from the tumor at its adventitial border. After this was completed, the rest of the resection was accomplished through normal-appearing muscle. If a questionable area was encountered, frozen sections were examined to confirm that the margin was tumor-free.

After excision, the wound was closed with minimal tension. If a vital structure or bone was exposed to the skin or subcutaneous tissue, muscle flaps were turned into the area to facilitate closure. If there was any undue tension in the skin, split-thickness skin grafts were placed over the transposed muscle. Suction catheters and five to seven days of extremity elevation were used to facilitate wound healing.

Patient Characteristics

The study included 61 patients with stage II high-grade soft-tissue sarcomas. Sixteen had stage II-A sarcomas and 45 had stage II-B sarcomas. The median follow-up on these patients was 38 months (range, four to 97 months). The average age was 48 years (range, 16 to 84 years). There were 31 women and 30 men.

The location of the tumor was distal to the knee in 12 cases, between the knee joint and the inguinal ligament in 32 cases, and in the inguinal area in two cases. In the upper extremity, there were eight cases between the elbow and the hand, five cases between the elbow and the shoulder, and two cases involving the shoulder girdle.

Types of Soft-Tissue Sarcoma

The four major types of soft-tissue sarcoma included in this study were malignant fibrous histiocytoma (20 cases), liposarcoma (14 cases), synovial cell sarcoma (nine cases), and malignant peripheral nerve sheath tumor (five cases). The other 13 types of sarcomas are shown in Table 39-1.

Limb-Salvage Results

The limb-salvage rate in this group of patients was 90%, with 55 of 61 patients retaining viable, useful extremities. By the functional evaluation system of the

Table 39-1
Types of soft-tissue sarcoma

Types	No. of Patients
Malignant fibrous histiocytoma	20
Liposarcoma	14
Synovial cell sarcoma	9
Malignant peripheral nerve sheath tumor	5
Clear cell sarcoma	3
Fibrosarcoma	2
Spindle cell sarcoma	1
Epithelial sarcoma	1
Alveolar soft parts sarcoma	1
Leiomyosarcoma	1
Rhabdomyosarcoma	1
Hemangiopericytoma	2
Hemangioendothelioma	1
Total	61

Musculoskeletal Tumor Society, there were 34 excellent, 18 good, and three fair results.[26] Three patients underwent initial amputation, two early in our experience because of wound necrosis and one because of an infected biopsy site that precluded vascular grafting. Three patients with local recurrences underwent later amputation. This 90% limb-salvage rate was achieved even though the patients were unselected and included all with stage II soft-tissue sarcomas of the extremities.

Pathologic Results

Tumor size was recorded in 42 cases and ranged from 1.5 to 20.0 cm (mean, 9.4 cm) in greatest dimension. Surgical procedures were considered wide in 45 cases, marginal in 12, and intralesional in four. The tumor response grade was grade I in 35 of 46 cases, grade II in six cases, grade III in four cases, and grade IV in one case. No residual tumor was identified in the resected specimens from the remaining 15 patients.

Six tumors recurred locally 1.0 to 6.4 years after resection (three wide, two marginal, and one intralesional). In two of the six there was no residual tumor in the initial specimen. In four cases the tumor response was grade I. There was no local recurrence in patients with more than 75% tumor necrosis (grade II or above). Tumor response grade did not correlate with overall survival. Of 12 patients who were either alive with metastatic disease or dead of disease at the end of the study, eight had grade I responses, one had a grade II response, two had grade III responses, and one had a grade IV response. This suggests that the grade of tumor response or necrosis may not be useful in selecting adjuvant therapy in soft-tissue sarcomas. Interestingly, metastases and tumor death were more common in patients who underwent marginal resection (four of 12) or intralesional resection (two of four). In contrast, only six of 45 patients who underwent wide excision had distant metastases. Fifteen of 61 patients (25%) had more than 75% tumor necrosis after preoperative chemotherapy and radiation. This was slightly lower than the 37% of cases with 80% or more necrosis reported by Eilber and associates.[5] The discrepancy may reflect differences in sampling techniques or differences in the relative distribution of histologic tumor types or tumor grades (that is, grade II vs grade III tumors). As in previous studies, no relationship was found between radiation dosage and tumor response.[23-25]

Local Recurrence

The local recurrence rate in this series was 10% (six of 61 cases). Three of the six local recurrences were treated with amputations at the joint above the level of recurrence. Three others were treated with a second local resection. These local recurrences occurred an average of 26 months after initial treatment (range, ten to 74 months). The average follow-up after local recurrence in these patients was 36 months (range, 12 to 62 months). None of the patients with local recurrence suffered systemic relapse. This high rate of survival in patients who had local recurrences and subsequent treatment was remarkable but has been reported in other series.[2]

Survival

Of these 61 patients, 13 had pulmonary metastases; at the end of the study, nine of these 13 had died, and three were alive with disease. One patient had a solitary metastasis after 27 months, underwent a resection, and showed no evidence of disease 50 months later. The survival rate was 79% and the rate of recurrence-free survival was 52%. The metastasis-free survival, which should be the most meaningful in this study, was 70% (Fig. 39–1). Systemic chemotherapy in the form of doxorubicin was offered to our adult patients. Of the 37 given this drug as an adjuvant, seven either died or had progressive disease. Twenty-four patients declined systemic adjuvant chemotherapy; five of these had progressive recurrence of the sarcoma. Six young patients were given a multidrug chemotherapy protocol consisting of doxorubicin, dactinomycin, cisplatin, cyclophosphamide, vincristine, and bleomycin. There were no systemic relapses in this small group with a mean follow-up of 21 months (range, six to 40 months). We cannot make any statement concerning the efficacy of systemic chemotherapy.

Morbidity

Of the entire group of 130 patients with high-grade sarcoma in an extremity (bone and soft tissue, stages II and III) treated with this technique, 23 (18%) had delayed wound healing, and nine (7%) required a sec-ond surgical procedure to achieve wound healing. Seventeen patients (13%) had burns from the doxorubicin.

Technical Considerations

Using this technique requires the services of an interested, interventional radiologist who is experienced in catheter placement in the femoral and axillary arteries. The arterial puncture site should be kept as far as possible from the infusing catheter tip. A successful 80-hour infusion is best achieved by leaving the catheter tip in a large vessel, either the common iliac or femoral artery in the lower extremity and the axillary or brachial artery in the upper extremity.

For infusion of upper-extremity tumors on the left side, a femoral approach is used; the catheter is threaded up to and left in the axillary artery. For tumors in the right upper extremity, the right axillary artery is entered. The femoral approach is not used for right upper-extremity tumors because the infusion catheter would have to remain under the right carotid artery in the brachiocephalic trunk for the 80 hours of infusion. Catheters in this position have been associated with stroke and should, therefore, be avoided. The most difficult tumor location for catheter placement is the right upper arm. A retrograde right axillary approach is used. The puncture site is inches from the infusing tip.

In the lower extremities, an antegrade femoral puncture is used when the tumor is distal to the mid-thigh. If the tumor is more proximal or if the patient is obese, the approach is contralateral and retrograde. The catheter is placed over the aortic bifurcation and then down into the femoral artery. For tumors in the foot or lower leg, the catheter tip is placed beyond the branching of the profunda femoris in the superficial femoral artery.

Arteriographic examination of the tumor is done at the time of catheter placement primarily to look for encasement of major vessels.

Next, an infusion port is placed on the catheter hub. The catheter is connected to a constant-rate infusion pump and the doxorubicin is infused continuously for 80 hours. Nurses accustomed to managing infusion pumps and chemotherapy are necessary. The doxorubicin is diluted (10 mg in 500 ml of 5% dextrose in water) and infused for eight hours. This is repeated ten times. Careful monitoring of the infusion site and the circulation in the involved leg, as well as the leg in which the arterial puncture was done, is essential. During the 80 hours of infusion the patient is limited to strict bedrest. Sitting is not allowed if the tumor is in the lower extremity or if the catheter is placed in the femoral artery. The patient is allowed to roll side-to-side and is encouraged to do this every couple of hours. In upper-extremity tumors, a shoulder immobilizer is used and

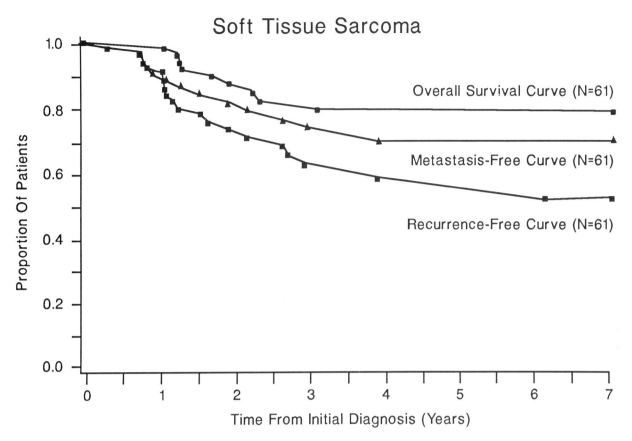

Fig. 39-1   Overall survival curve, metastasis-free curve, and recurrence-free curve in 61 patients with soft-tissue sarcoma.

the patient is allowed to elevate the head of the bed 45 degrees.

During the past year, we used a pulsator connected to the infusion pump. Our goal was to increase mixing and to prevent layering or streaming of the chemotherapy agent, thus reducing the number of skin burns. We were unimpressed with this device and have discontinued its use.

Radiation Therapy

After the infusion of intra-arterial doxorubicin is complete, the catheter is removed and the patient is transferred to the Radiation Oncology Department for treatment planning. This process includes a technique called simulation whereby treatment portals are designed with the aid of computed tomography and/or magnetic resonance imaging. The tumor boundaries are identified and 6- to 8-cm margins are added proximal and distal to the lesion. When possible, a small strip of subcutaneous tissue is spared from irradiation to minimize disruption of dermal lymphatics. When this is not feasible, the radiation treatment encompasses all normal tissue lateral and medial to the lesion. The location of the tumor dictates the beam energy (usually 4 or 10 MeV) selected for treatment. The higher the beam

energy, the greater the penetrating ability and the skin-sparing effect. For example, a deep-seated lesion requires a beam with greater penetration, that is, a high-energy photon beam. The fields are set up by an isocentric technique and a midline dose of 350 cGy/ day delivered through appositional fields. A total of 1,750 cGy is delivered in five fractions over five to seven calendar days.

Morbidity

This technique resulted in a low incidence of major complications and morbidity. The doxorubicin does enter the circulation with undetermined amounts being bound in the infused extremity and tumor. Hair loss may occur, but less often than with intravenous infusion. A modest leukopenia may develop but has not led to any delay in subsequent treatment. The patient usually suffers some mild anorexia by the end of the 80 hours of infusion, but vomiting has not been a problem.

The main long-term side effect of doxorubicin is cardiac toxicity. This occurs at a cumulative dose of 500 to 600 mg/m² of body surface. The initial 100 mg of doxorubicin must be added to any systemic postoperative drugs given when the total allowable dose is calculated. Two of our young female patients had mild congestive heart failure two years after treatment. Both of these patients responded to medical management. One was still taking medication at the end of the study.

Catheter dislodgement, extravasation, and arterial thrombosis have not been a significant problem in our experience. However, there are significant complications from this technique and they fall into two main groups: problems related to wound healing and burns from the arterial infusion of doxorubicin. Our experience with regard to complications involved a larger group of 131 patients, including patients with stage III sarcomas and those with high-grade bone sarcomas treated with the same technique. In four patients the wound did not heal and required amputation. Two cases occurred very early (in 1980 and 1981) before close coordination among our treatment team was developed. The other two cases of wound necrosis were in bone tumors. One occurred in a popliteal arterial graft that clotted. The second patient had an internal hemipelvectomy with sacrifice of the hypogastric artery. A muscle flap should have been used initially. Only in the two soft-tissue sarcomas do we attribute the amputation primarily to the preoperative treatment. Additional surgical procedures to achieve wound healing were necessary in nine patients (7%). Hematoma evacuations were required in three patients and secondary debridements with muscle flap or skin graft in two patients.

Wounds required a week or two longer to heal than normally expected. The larger the tumor removed, the more likely wound problems are to develop.[23] Tumors removed from areas such as the proximal tibia, where there is minimal muscle or soft tissue, are more likely to lead to problems. Fourteen patients, in addition to the nine described above, had delayed wound healing (more than three weeks), for a total incidence of 17%.

The other significant complication from this treatment is burning of the skin and subcutaneous tissues by arterial doxorubicin.

For unknown reasons, the doxorubicin sometimes begins to stream to a particular subcutaneous skin artery. The concentration becomes high in these areas and the patient begins to feel a burning sensation in the skin. Within several hours the skin becomes red and demarcated and a so-called hot spot is apparent. Our management has been to discontinue the infusion for two hours and then begin again. If the area enlarges or if the symptoms return or increase, the catheter is pulled back 2 or 3 inches. This usually solves the problem, although other hot spots may develop after the catheter is retracted. If this continues, infusion must be stopped. We had to discontinue the infusion after 60 mg in one retrograde axillary puncture.

These cutaneous burns occurred in 17 of our 131 patients (13%). There were ten mild burns and seven severe burns. No burns required surgical procedures or caused loss of a limb. The mild burns resemble a first-degree sunburn, although the subcutaneous tissue

may remain thickened. The seven patients who sustained severe burns had painful, indurated, red blotches that slowly, over a period of one to two months, changed into thickened, brownish, but painless areas that left an area of the subcutaneous tissue and skin scarred. The patients with mild burns were left with slightly thickened, indurated areas in the subcutaneous tissue. Eilber and associates[5] reported a 20% incidence of subcutaneous fibrosis resulting from these burns.

Our patients had no pathologic fractures of bone in the treated area. Such fractures have been reported[5] and usually lead to amputation. One of our patients developed osteomyelitis in the ischial tuberosity after delayed healing of a thigh wound.

References

1. Consensus Conference: Limb-sparing treatment of adult soft-tissue sarcomas and osteosarcomas. *JAMA* 1985;254:1791–1794.
2. Lawrence W Jr, Donegan WL, Natarajan N, et al: Adult soft tissue sarcomas: A pattern of care survey of the American College of Surgeons. *Ann Surg* 1987;205:349–359.
3. Collin C, Hadju SI, Godbold J, et al: Localized operable soft tissue sarcoma of the upper extremity: Presentation, management, and factors affecting local recurrence in 108 patients. *Ann Surg* 1987;205:331–339.
4. Collin C, Hadju SI, Godbold J, et al: Localized, operable soft tissue sarcoma of the lower extremity. *Arch Surg* 1986;121:1425–1433.
5. Eilber F, Giuliano A, Huth J, et al: Neoadjuvant chemotherapy, radiation and limited surgery for high grade soft tissue sarcoma of the extremity. Presented at the Innisbrook Conference on Sarcoma, Tarpon Springs, Florida, Oct 8–10, 1987.
6. Fu KK: Biological basis for the interaction of chemotherapeutic agents and radiation therapy. *Cancer* 1985;55:2123–2130.
7. Durand RE: Adriamycin: A possible indirect radiosensitizer of hypoxic tumor cells. *Radiology* 1976;119:217–222.
8. Dunham WK Jr, Omura GA, Urist MM, et al: Treatment adjuvant to surgery for primary high-grade sarcoma of the extremities, in Enneking WF (ed): *Limb Salvage in Musculoskeletal Oncology*. New York, Churchill Livingstone, 1987, pp 298–313.
9. Bernreuter WK, Koehler RE, Dunham WK, et al: MR, CT and radionuclide scans of bone and soft-tissue neoplasms. *Radiology*, in press.
10. Shirkhoda A, Jaffe N, Wallace S, et al: Computed tomography of osteosarcoma after intraarterial chemotherapy. *AJR* 1985;144:95–99.
11. Jaffe N, Spears R, Eftekhari F, et al: Pathologic fracture in osteosarcoma: Impact of chemotherapy on primary tumor and survival. *Cancer* 1987;59:701–709.
12. Jaffe N, Knapp J, Chuang V, et al: Osteosarcoma: Intra-arterial treatment of the primary tumor with cis-diammine-dichloroplatinum II (CDP). Angiographic, pathologic, and pharmacologic studies. *Cancer* 1983;51:402–407.
13. Picci P, Bacci G, Campanacci M, et al: Histologic evaluation of necrosis in osteosarcoma induced by chemotherapy: Regional mapping of viable and nonviable tumor. *Cancer* 1985;56:1515–1521.
14. Rosen G, Caparros B, Huvos AG, et al: Preoperative chemotherapy for osteogenic sarcoma: Selection of postoperative adjuvant chemotherapy based on the response of the primary tumor to preoperative chemotherapy. *Cancer* 1982;49:1221–1230.
15. Denton JW, Dunham WK, Salter M, et al: Preoperative regional

chemotherapy and rapid fraction irradiation for sarcomas of the soft tissue and bone. *Surg Gynecol Obstet* 1984;158:545–551.

16. Eilber FR, Mirra JJ, Grant TT, et al: Is amputation necessary for sarcomas? A seven-year experience with limb salvage. *Ann Surg* 1980;192:431–438.

17. Eilber FR, Morton DL, Eckardt J, et al: Limb salvage for skeletal and soft tissue sarcomas: Multidisciplinary preoperative therapy. *Cancer* 1984;53:2579–2584.

18. Eilber FR, Guiliano AE, Huth J, et al: Limb-salvage of high grade soft tissue sarcomas of the extremity: Experience at University of California, Los Angeles. *Cancer Treatment Symp* 1985;3:49–57.

19. Goodnight JE Jr, Bargar WL, Voegeli T, et al: Limb-sparing surgery for extremity sarcomas after preoperative intraarterial doxorubicin and radiation therapy. *Am J Surg* 1985;150:109–113.

20. Mantravadi RV, Trippon MJ, Patel MK, et al: Limb salvage in extremity soft tissue sarcoma: Combined modality therapy. *Radiology* 1984;152:523–526.

21. Enneking WF, Spanier SS, Goodman MA: A system for the sur-

gical staging of musculoskeletal sarcoma. *Clin Orthop* 1980; 153:106–120.

22. Enneking WF, Spanier SS, Malawer MM: The effect of the anatomic setting on the results of surgical procedures for soft parts sarcoma of the thigh. *Cancer* 1981;47:1005–1022.

23. Eilber FR, Guiliano AE, Huth J, et al: High-grade soft-tissue sarcomas of the extremity: UCLA experience with limb salvage. *Prog Clin Biol Res* 1985;205:59–74.

24. Huth JF, Mirra JJ, Eilber FR: Assessment of in vivo response to preoperative chemotherapy and radiation therapy as a predictor of survival in patients with soft-tissue sarcoma. *Am J Clin Oncol* 1985;8:497–503.

25. Willett CG, Schiller AL, Suit HD, et al: The histologic response of soft tissue sarcoma to radiation therapy. *Cancer* 1987; 60:1500–1504.

26. Enneking WF: A system for the functional evaluation of the surgical management of musculoskeletal tumors, in Enneking WF (ed): *Limb Salvage in Musculoskeletal Oncology*. New York, Churchill Livingstone, 1987, pp 5–16.

Clinical Research Database System

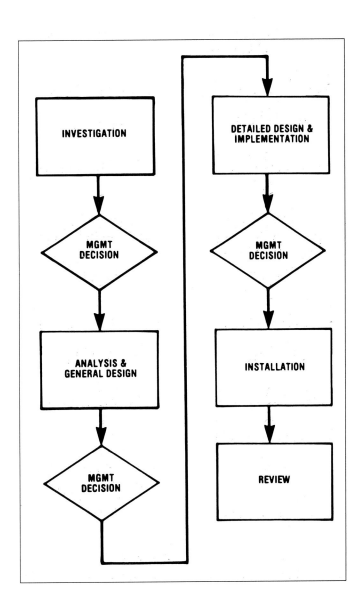

Clinical Research Database System for Orthopaedic Surgery

Erwin A. Aguilar, PharmD

Timony F. Swoop, MBA

Eugene J. Dabezies, MD

Robert D. D'Ambrosia, MD

Introduction

Historically, the orthopaedist concentrated on the treatment of musculoskeletal disorders and paid little attention to record-keeping. Because of pressures from many areas, however, practice patterns and requirements are changing. It is now increasingly necessary to keep detailed records and to document the outcome for third-party, legal, and governmental inquiries.[1-4]

Because of both internal and external pressures, we created a clinical research database system to establish a record system that was both accurate and available for quick retrieval. This system enables us to study the various facets of diagnosis and treatment of orthopaedic disease.[1]

The development of such a system was simplified by the recent advances in microprocessor technology that have made the personal computer feasible and affordable. We describe a microcomputer system that is invaluable in supporting clinical research and also has great potential in orthopaedic health-care delivery and research.[1]

Our first step was to seek the advice of a professional computer consultant to help us identify our needs and goals. This consultative process is described below.

The Consultative Process

Webster's Dictionary defines systems analysis as "the act, process, or profession of studying an activity typically by mathematical means in order to define its goals or purposes and to discover operations and procedures for accomplishing them most efficiently." Today, this usually involves computer applications. Our consultant applied systems analysis techniques to the problem of recording, messaging, and retrieving data at the LSU Medical Center Department of Orthopaedics.

Any complex system, and any organizational structure that implements a complex system, such as the orthopaedic department of a medical school, is made up of interrelated parts that function separately. The interrelationships among the parts of the system lie in the sharing of the resources used. One of the resources that must be shared in any viable system is information.

An information system is formed through the coordinated functioning of people, equipment, procedures, data, and other resources to provide uniform, reliable, and accurate information. In effect, the organizational system is tied together by its informational elements. Information can be seen as the bonding agent that permits systems to function cohesively.

An effective information system is synergistic, which means simply that when an information system functions as it should, it produces results with a greater value than the total value produced by its separate, individual parts.

The Systems Approach

The systems approach is prospective—a way of identifying and viewing complex, interrelated functions as integral elements of systems. Although there is a concern for the individual parts of a system, emphasis is on the integration of components to produce the end products of the systems themselves. For example, the medical record can be considered one of the components of a functioning system. Another component is the need to retrieve information to support research projects. These two components can be viewed and studied separately. The systems approach suggests that we view them collectively in terms of a goal to be met.

Systems analysis is the application of the systems approach to the study and solution of problems. Systems analysis, then, is a mental approach—a way of thinking about a problem, analyzing its components, and structuring a solution. The systems approach, as applied to an orthopaedic department of a medical school, means seeing the organization itself as a system, analyzing its goals and objectives, and understanding uses for the information that will be the end product of the problem's solution.

Figure 40–1 reflects the typical diagram overview of the Systems Development Life Cycle, which shows the relationships between major phases and management checkpoints. Our focus here is on the "Investigation" aspect of the cycle. Note that three different points in this process require a management decision. Not only is this not accidental, it is highly significant, indicating that the management must participate in the decision-making process for the system to be effective.

Recognition of Need

Before an investigation can begin, the need or problem must be recognized. In the case of our system, the overriding problem was our inability to collect and use previous case and treatment histories to support var-

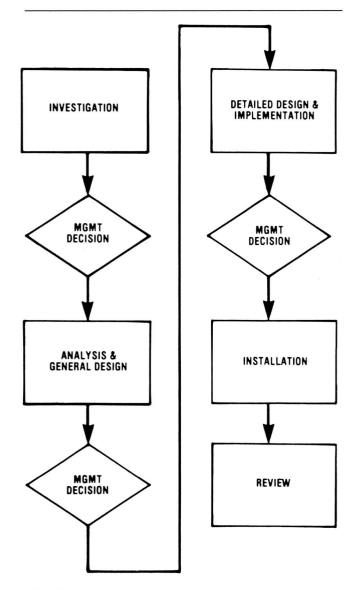

Fig. 40-1 Typical diagrammatic overview of the Systems Development Life Cycle, showing the relationships between major phases and management checkpoints.

INVESTIGATION PHASE

1. Initial Investigation
2. Feasibility Study

ANALYSIS AND GENERAL DESIGN PHASE

3. Existing System Review
4. New System Requirements
5. New System Design
6. Implementation and Installation Planning

DETAILED DESIGN AND IMPLEMENTATION PHASE

7. Technical Design
8. Test Specifications and Planning
9. Programming and Testing
10. User Training
11. System Test

INSTALLATION PHASE

12. File Conversion
13. System Installation

REVIEW PHASE

14. Development Recap
15. Post-Implementation Review

Fig. 40-2 Tasks of the Systems Development Life Cycle.

ious research projects and a general analysis of previous casework.

Figure 40–2 further breaks down the Systems Development Life Cycle into 15 separate tasks. The first phase, "Investigation," is broken into two distinct steps—"Initial Investigation" and "Feasibility Study."

Defining the Problem

One of the first steps in any initial investigation is to define the problems that led to the request for assistance. Whether this is done internally or, as in our case, externally by an outside consultant, this definition should be stated in such a way that it is clearly understood and agreed to by both the users and the systems analysts doing the initial investigation. The definition arrived at will sometimes differ from the initial description by the user. The "user" is the surgeon or professor who will use the system. One of the purposes of systems analysis is to separate the symptoms from the problems. In so doing, the actual problem may be found to differ from the perceived problem, leading to a restatement.

The purpose of having a separate task called "Initial Investigation" is to enable the systems analyst to arrive at some preliminary feasible solution for the problem rather quickly. In our case, the initial investigation required time sufficient to understand the problem to be addressed, interviews to determine how the existing data collection and analysis systems worked, identification of transaction volume and case study volume, and relatively short interviews with the using physicians to determine what they wanted from the system.

A preliminary determination of feasibility can be made at this stage. The end result of this activity is an understanding of the request at a level sufficient to make a preliminary recommendation on a course of action to be followed. This is done to maximize output and minimize the investment of time by both the consultant and the physicians. In this case, it was evident at a rather early stage that there was significant justification to proceed further. As in most cases, however, it was also determined that there were conflicting requirements for meeting objectives.

Feasibility Study

Something that is "feasible" can be accomplished. Feasibility also implies practicality. The term "feasibility study" in this context includes some additional meanings: (1) When the feasibility study is completed, the original problem or need should have been understood and alternative solutions should have been considered. (2) The feasibility study should offer at least two, perhaps more, prospective solutions to the stated need or problem. (3) When an information system is considered, the feasibility study involves a number of separate, related considerations, including financial, technical, and human factors. All appropriate factors connected with any given system should be evaluated. (4) This stage of the feasibility study should conclude with a clear-cut recommendation. At this time the physicians should have enough information for them to make reasonable decisions about the cost and effectiveness of the system to be developed.

The Process

The feasibility study is a classic, although miniature, systems analysis study.

A major portion of any feasibility study involves gaining a clear understanding of how the existing system functions. To accomplish this, we investigated the physical model of the existing system and developed a logical model. The physical model of any system tends to identify the aspects of the system that depend on how the processing is currently being done—the people who are involved in the processing, the forms used, and so on. From this, the systems analyst attempts to develop a logical model. The logical model then concentrates on what the system does as opposed to how it does it. Our systems analyst gained a complete understanding of how the system operated and what it did by means of in-depth interviews with all the physicians, using various techniques for data retrieval, and investigating sample forms and input and output devices.

After learning how the existing system of research data gathering operated and understanding the techniques used for data input and data analysis, the consultant tried to develop a systems approach that would solve our problems.

A long-standing guideline for systems development is known as the "80-20 Rule." Eighty percent of the benefits of a system can be achieved for 20% of the cost; the remaining 80% of the cost goes into providing the last 20% of the benefits. The point is that the scope of the project should be firmly established in terms of the clinical objectives to be met, the major outputs to be produced, and the main processing functions to be included. These objectives represent 80% of the benefits.

Feasibility Report

At this stage the following information was available and presented to the physicians for their decisions: (1) A narrative explanation of the purpose and scope of the project, including the reasons for undertaking it, the areas of the organization and the functions included, and how this project contributed to the objectives of the physicians. (2) A brief description of the existing system, what changes were anticipated, and the expected results. (3) A concise, specific statement of anticipated benefits, including dollar values where appropriate. (4) Preliminary cost estimates for the development and operation of the system. (5) An impact statement describing any changes in policy or procedure thought to be needed in the computer center or elsewhere in the hospital.

We believe that the physicians had a clear understanding of what the problem was, what we proposed as its solution, and the technical and policy requirements necessary to effect this solution. This then became the first major decision point in the process of systems development.

What Is a Database?

A database is a collection of related information organized in such a manner that useful information can be extracted quickly. The effectiveness of a database is derived from the fact that a single comprehensive collection of information can provide data to be used for a variety of organizational purposes.[5]

Definitions

The components of a database system are as follows[6]: *Data elements*—Individual facts, observations, or items of information. The patient's name, sex, and telephone number, for example, are separate data elements. *Field*—A named physical storage location for a single data element. The first name of an individual is an example of a field. *Record*—A collection of facts about a single entity within the database, including the data elements for the fields that relate to a specific patient. *File*—A collection of records that describes all the data in a category. For example, all information about tibial fractures would be in the "lower leg" file. To organize this matrix, records are arranged to correspond to rows and fields to columns.[6]

More precisely, a database is a collection of files that describe the total information required for a specific application. A database management system is a computer program designed to define, create, manipulate, and summarize the collected information.[6]

It is analogous to a filing system in which the database

management system corresponds to a filing cabinet; the file is the folder, the record is the collected information, data elements are the individual facts, and the field is the location of each data element (Fig. 40–3).

Method

Our objective was to design a computer-based information processing system that would help us (1) solve problems of data collection and processing of clinical information, (2) record the results of clinical research, (3) develop an educational tool that could be used in residency training, and (4) evaluate our experience with the patient. In addition, we wanted to have capabilities for word processing, slide-making, and graphics.

To develop these objectives, we went through the steps of professional consultation, allocation of financial resources, design of the database system, identification of personnel requirements, design of data-collection sheets, and implementation.

Our computer consultant helped us establish a budget so that financial resources would be adequate and wisely used. He also defined the personnel needed. He interviewed and hired the director of the computer center. Because of his previous experience and training, the director could operate all aspects of the system. Other staff included two research associates working in the outpatient clinics to complete the data-collection sheets, two university students on a part-time basis (equaling 40 hours a week) to assist the director, and a faculty liaison for appropriate orthopaedic guidance.

The most time-consuming process was designing the

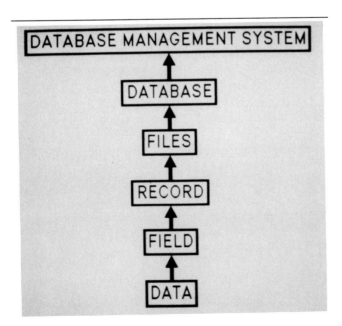

Fig. 40-3 Database system flow chart.

data-collection sheets. Because we had no previous forms to serve as guides, we elected to devise five separate collection sheets arbitrarily based on body regions. It took about 50 hours per sheet to design the forms for the forearm and hand, the arm, the pelvis and femur, the leg, and the spine. In addition, we have now developed a special-project sheet for total hip arthroplasty, femoral intramedullary nailing, and total knee arthroplasty.

We next established a target date for implementing data collection and agreed to run the system for six months before making any modifications.

Mechanics of the System

Stages of Data Recording and Processing

Because data constitute the link between treatment and evaluation of results, the management and handling of such data merit careful consideration (Fig. 40–4).[7] The general purpose of data recording is to establish in writing a mechanism for assuring the preservation of the data collected in the course of surgery and subsequent follow-up studies. A major factor in the design of our data files was that we wanted a system that could be used for rapid searches.[1,7–13]

Forms

We had to produce the forms needed for both hospital and outpatient use. To obtain quality information, we had to compromise. Not only was it too expensive to collect all information, but in developing a comprehensive system such as this, there was a real danger of information overload. The forms, then, had to contain only selected information.

The information is divided into three categories (Fig. 40–5). First is the identifier, which gives such information as name, age, and address. The second category is the diagnostic and surgical procedures, and the third category is used for follow-up in the outpatient clinic. The items in each form are coded with a yes or no selection, a multiple-choice selection, or a worded answer.

Implementation

We initially had hoped that the residents and faculty would fill out the data-collection sheets. It soon became obvious, however, that the sheets were not being completed, making it necessary to bring in other personnel to ensure that the sheets were completed. Data collection is now initiated by responsible personnel who are trained so that they know hospital procedures and orthopaedic terminology.

We continue to have several sources of problems. The history, physical findings, and diagnosis sections are often not completed. Missing data in the way of associated injuries and current conditions must be identi-

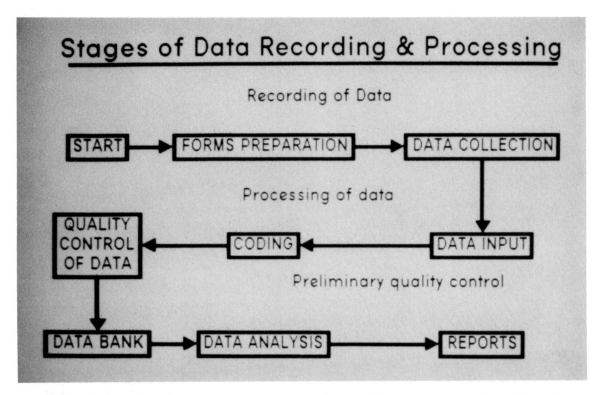

Fig. 40-4 Some basic procedures relating to various aspects of data recording and processing. (Reproduced with permission from Guzman M, Sibriani R, Flores R: Methods for evaluating the impact of food and nutrition programmes: Data recording and processing. *Food Nutr Bull* 1984;6(suppl 8):233–251.)

fied. Inconsistency in wording of the diagnosis at admission, inaccurate radiographic interpretations, and incomplete classification of the fracture are other sources of error. Another problem is misrepresentation by the patient, who sometimes gives incorrect information, such as an address, or fails to mention previous problems. All such factors adversely affect the database.

Data Collection

Charts are abstracted and forms are filled out and returned to the computer center for processing. Every time a patient is seen at the outpatient clinic, a new form is generated. Following this procedure allows us to have a chronologic set of forms for every patient.

Once the patient is discharged from the hospital, the data-collection sheet is removed from the chart and returned to the computer center. At each outpatient clinic, data sheets are collected and brought to the computer center, where they are reviewed to be certain that the information is accurate and that the forms are completed appropriately.

Diagnostic Coding

Because CPT coding was not adequate, we set up a diagnostic convention based on ICD·9·CM coding, which lists appropriate diagnoses. We thus have a consistent diagnosis and classification that can be entered

into the database system. This diagnostic terminology manual has proved to be an invaluable aid in all aspects of our database.

The diagnostic terminology manual is a list of diagnostic classifications with line diagrams. It also helps ensure that a correct and complete diagnosis will be recorded in the chart.

The information is then entered into the three respective categories of identification, diagnoses and procedures, and outpatient follow-ups. Using a disk subsystem enables us to keep a complete record. When a cartridge is filled, we add a new cartridge and continue to record data. This design allows for continued expansion of information but, at a later date, will make searching through the various disks a tedious task. This was a compromise we made to keep the system affordable.

The director of the computer center is responsible both for the quality of the data and for entering this information into the database system.

Data Input

First, the general data for the patient are entered into the identifier file. This information should include the reason for admission, diagnosis at admission, and surgical or nonsurgical follow-up plan. These forms are

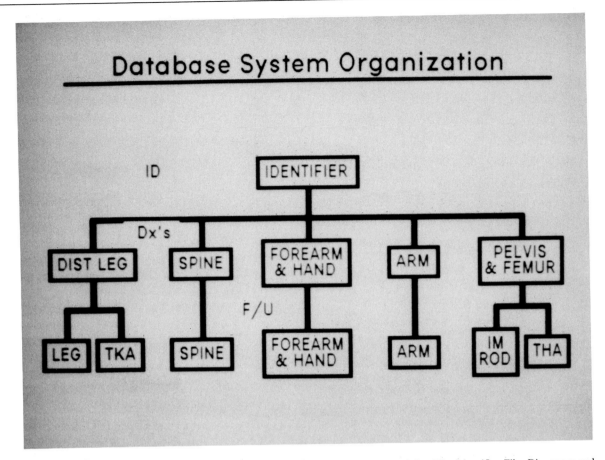

Fig. 40-5 Database system organization. The system is divided into three categories: The Identifier File, Diagnoses and Procedures, and Follow-Up.

returned on a daily basis to the department and the data are entered into the computer via a keyboard (Fig. 40–6).

Inpatient data sheets are returned to the department after discharge. Coding, editing, and data entry are done at this point. It is not necessary to enter the name and file number of the patient and other general data again, because we can transfer data from the identifier file to the surgical file with which we are currently working. An identical operation is performed on the data-collection forms obtained at the outpatient clinic. This process avoids typographic errors caused by entering data twice.

Data Quality Control

Data processing is the treatment given to the data after collection.[7] The control of data quality is the most important aspect of any research process.[7] Once the data have been collected and coded, the quality control generally proceeds in stages. The first stage relates to completeness and the second to internal consistency among the various items constituting the data set. The preliminary controls for completeness of the data are usually done after the coding of the diagnoses and pro-

cedures has been completed. When reviewing the forms, we check for (1) the appropriate selection of the items and their classification, (2) the correct usage of key words in the diagnosis and procedure (we use as key words the anatomic names of bones), and (3) placement of the correct dates for every surgical procedure and diagnosis.

When the preliminary procedures for quality control are applied after collection and coding, it is often possible to recover missing bits of data by reviewing the chart.

Data Bank

Once quality control is assured, we have clean files for each category of the data collected. The identifier file contains general information concerning the patient and the diagnosis and the other files contain information on diagnostic and surgical procedures and follow-up. This set of data files is called the data bank.

We cannot overemphasize the importance of complete and full documentation in the structure of the identifier file. If the history, physical examination, and diagnosis sections are completed accurately, the master file will contain the appropriate basic information.

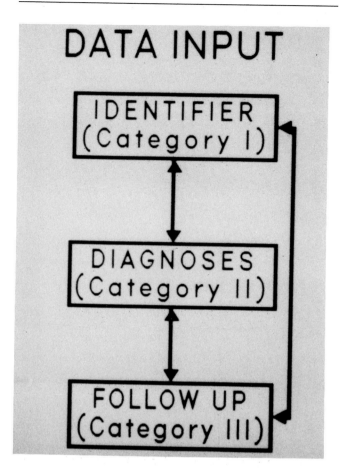

Fig. 40-6 Data entry system. Data can be entered in any of the three categories, thus giving flexibility to the system.

Data Analysis

The analysis of data is the interrelation of the type of data and the hypothesis posed by the investigator.[7] The first stage in the analysis of continuous variables consists of scanning the data set.[7] We retrieve information by searching the files from the fields we select for the particular conditions we want to study. This may be obtained from a single file or from a set of files, depending on the request posed by the researcher. Once the quality of data is documented, we can proceed with statistical testing of the specific hypothesis.

Reports

After all stages of data recording and processing have been accomplished, we report our conclusions, relating the results of the investigation and the statistical analysis performed.

Conclusion

We have used our database for 24 months and accumulated data from about 3,000 patients in the iden-

tifier file. We are now beginning to realize the fruits of the system. Our system is one in which clinical research papers can be prepared easily. At the same time, surveys to improve the quality of patient care are possible. It has been invaluable in analyzing outcomes in patients who have received the same diagnosis and undergone the same surgical procedure. This has ensured quality control without requiring a major search through hospital charts over a specified period.

The hospital chart should not, however, be discarded entirely. It remains valuable because all information about the patient is in the chart. The computer information may not reveal subtle trends that can only be found by a careful review of a record in the chart.

The word processing system can also be used by the faculty as an aid in the preparation of manuscripts. With the manuscript on a disk, editing can be done easily, making it unnecessary to retype the entire paper and thus avoiding new transcription errors.

The most used component is the capability for slide-making. Slides can be designed and produced in a quick and efficient manner. We can prepare and generate the slides for a presentation within hours.

Computer technology has advanced rapidly, especially in the areas of logic and memory. Such advances have made personal computers practical and affordable. During these past two years, our microcomputer system has been especially useful in monitoring and managing both inpatient and outpatient data. These data can be retrieved and statistically analyzed with ease. Such data can be also transformed into graphic displays.

We have identified information-handling problems and have designed a database system that can handle these problems in a cost-effective manner.

Acknowledgment

Portions of this chapter were adapted with permission from Guzman M, Sibriani R, Flores R: Methods for evaluating the impact of food and nutrition programmes: Data recording and processing. *Food Nutr Bull* 1984;6(suppl 8):233–251.

References

1. Aguilar EA, Swoop T, Dabezies EJ, et al: Clinical research database system for orthopaedic surgery. Presented at the 11th Annual Symposium on Computer Applications in Medical Care, Washington, DC, Nov 1–4, 1987.
2. Johnson AT: User friendliness in microcomputer programs. *Comput Programs Biomed* 1985;19:127–130.
3. Lustman F: SUMER: A database concept for clinical research and patient data-management. *Comput Programs Biomed* 1982;15:125–131.
4. Sadler CR: Orthopaedic computing: Bone and joint computer connection. *MD Computing* 1984;4:39–47.
5. Wiederhold G: Databases for health care, in Lindberg DAB,

Reichertz PL (eds): *Lecture Notes in Medical Informatics*. Berlin, Spring-Verlag, 1981, vol 12.

6. Walters RF: File structures for database management systems. *MD Computing* 1987;4:30–41.

7. Guzman M, Sibriani R, Flores R: Methods for evaluating the impact of food and nutrition programmes: Data recording and processing. *Food Nutr Bull* 1984;6(suppl 8):233–251.

8. D'Ambrosia RD: *Musculoskeletal Disorders*, ed 2. Philadelphia, JB Lippincott, 1986.

9. Hoppenfeld S: *Physical Examination of the Spine and Extremities*. Norwalk, Appleton-Century-Crofts, 1976.

10. AAOS Committee for the Study of Joint Motion: *Joint Motion: Method of Measuring and Recording*. Park Ridge, American Academy of Orthopaedic Surgeons, 1965.

11. Quattlebaum TG: An interactive data base system for assessing and managing outpatient experiences in residency training. *Comput Programs Biomed* 1983;17:157–165.

12. Quattlebaum TG: Microcomputer analysis and management of residency training experiences. *Comput Methods Programs Biomed* 1985;20:169–172.

13. Rockwood CA, Green DP: *Fractures in Adults*. Philadelphia, JB Lippincott, 1975.

Sports Medicine

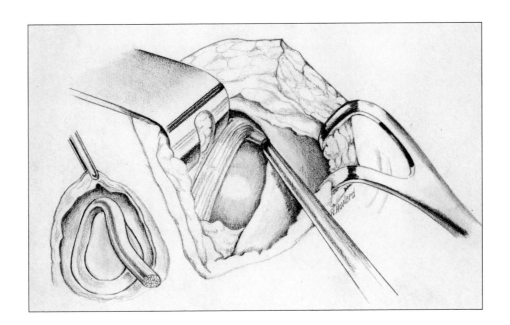

Rotator Cuff Tendinitis: Basic Concepts of Pathoetiology

Robert P. Nirschl, MD

Introduction

The pathologic changes and etiologic factors that clinicians have associated with rotator cuff tendinitis are being reassessed. Codman's[1,2] initial contributions have been augmented by the subsequent contributions of Moseley,[3] McLaughlin,[4,5] DePalma,[6] Rathbun and Mcnab,[7] Neer,[8] and Jobe and Jobe.[9] The increasing number of swimming, racket, and throwing-sport athletes who require examination and treatment for shoulder injuries has accelerated progress in diagnosing and treating this condition. In the athletically active patient, previous concepts concerning rotator cuff tendinitis were, at best, inconsistent in achieving the "true measure" of treatment success, namely, return to previous levels of athletic performance. Analysis of athletic techniques, the recent luxury of arthroscopic evaluation, and a careful review of the literature have resulted in a broader understanding of the etiology and pathology of rotator cuff tendinitis.

Etiology

The etiologic factors associated with rotator cuff tendinitis are multiple, varied, and often combined. The basic factors are categorized in the following outline:

I. Activity overuse
    A. Multiple repetitions
    B. Muscle-tendon imbalances
        1. Strength
        2. Flexibility
    C. Glenohumeral instability (secondary impingement)
        1. Upward humeral migration
        2. Anterior-superior subluxation
II. Age
    A. Physiologic
    B. Chronologic
III. Heredity
    A. Mesenchymal syndrome (predisposition to tendinitis)[10]
    B. Mechanical (primary impingement)
    C. Systemic factors (gout, estrogen deficiency)

The analysis of shoulder action in the racket and throwing sports demonstrates that many factors are occurring simultaneously. Jobe and associates[11] demonstrated the activity of the supraspinatus during the ac-celeration and follow-through phases of the throwing motion. Fowler[12] observed fatigue and weakness of the rotator cuff and scapular muscle groups in swimmers. In view of these and other reports,[13-16] it appears that a major etiologic factor in tendinitis (whether of the supraspinatus or other structures, such as the extensor carpi radialis brevis at the elbow) is multiple contractile overload (usually eccentric) of a tendon in a key, high-stress area.

Pathoetiology: Secondary Role of Impingement

The pathologic phases of rotator cuff tendinitis are not unlike those reported by this author for tennis elbow.[17-19] These changes occur primarily in the supraspinatus and are categorized as follows: (1) Inflammation only; (2) angiofibroblastic hyperplasia of tendon; (3) angiofibroblastic hyperplasia combined with fibrosis, iatrogenic cortisone change, soft calcification; and partial or total rupture.

Lindblom and Palmer,[20] Moseley and Goldie,[21] Rothman and Parke,[22] and Rathbun and Mcnab[7] all identified a critical zone of vascular supply in the rotator cuff. The consensus of these authors is that vascular compromise results in tissue devitalization. Nirschl and Pettrone[19] called this tendon devitalization "angiofibroblastic hyperplasia."

The etiologic factors outlined above have not been assigned relative responsibility for these changes. Since the report of Neer[8] in 1972, it has been common to equate rotator cuff tendinitis with primary anterior acromial impingement, predicated on the presence of a hereditary acromial excess (slope or exostosis) with resultant coracoacromial arch stenosis, abnormal rotator cuff compression (impingement), and subsequent pathologic change (tendinitis). This concept, although theoretically plausible, has some demonstrable practical deficiencies, especially in athletic patients, as outlined in the following:

Response of Symptomatic Shoulder Tendinitis to Exercise Neer[23]
reported major success in alleviating the symptoms of patients with stage I and stage II rotator cuff tendinitis by rehabilitative exercise programs. Many authors, including myself, have noted similar success. Since exercise does not alter the inherited bony architecture (for example, acromial slope or exostosis), reasons for this treatment success other than an effect on bony coracoacromial arch stenosis must be sought.

Absence of Pathologic Changes in the Coracoacromial Ligament
Direct surgical observation and histologic evaluation

have failed to identify the major pathologic changes that would be anticipated if impingement occurs in this area.

Lack of Consistent Objective Clinical Evidence of Acromial Distortion My observations of patients operated on for rotator cuff tendinitis with and without cuff tear indicate a directly observable acromial beak or exostosis in only 10% of cases, with another 18% having suggested coracoacromial arch stenosis without observable acromial changes. In the 1972 series involving older individuals (average age, 59 years) with full rotator cuff tears, Neer[8] noted only 25% with observable acromial variations or exostosis. Bigliani and associates'[24] series of cadaver dissections showed 41% with some acromial variance. From neither the Neer clinical surgical series nor the Bigliani cadaver series can it be concluded that the changes are primary, hereditary rather than secondary, reactionary changes. Indeed, it is quite likely that the conclusions concerning the Neer series were misinterpreted.

At present, there are no known clinical criteria or data to define or identify the presence of primary, hereditary coracoacromial arch stenosis.

Pathology

An understanding of the dense connective tissue that constitutes the fiber making up the tendon is necessary to understand the pathologic process in rotator cuff tendinitis. In tendons, collagen fibers or primary tendon bundles run in parallel courses. Each fiber or bundle is composed of a number of fibrils. Fibroblasts are the only type of cell present, and in longitudinal sections are lined in rows between collagen fibers. The cytoplasm is often indistinct and in cross sections the cells appear stellate, with cytoplasmic extension between the collagenous bundles. Surrounding the primary bundles, there is a small amount of loose connective tissue termed the endotendineum. Groups of primary bundles form secondary bundles or fascicles. These in turn are surrounded by a coarse type of connective tissue, the peritendineum. The tendon, thus, is composed of a variable number of fascicles and is sheathed by a thick connective tissue covering, called the epitendineum. In normal tendons, nerves and blood vessels extend through the major connective tissue septae but do not invade the fascicles. On gross examination, the tendon appears firm, taut, and shiny yellow-white.

In rotator cuff tendinitis, the tissue appears abnormal and is distinct from normal tendon. External examination usually reveals gray, dull, sometimes edematous and friable immature tissue, closely resembling early scar tissue, and similar to that seen in tennis elbow tendinitis. Superimposed superficial reddened hyperemia adherent to inflamed bursa may be present clinically. Microscopically, the normal, orderly tendon fibers are disrupted by a characteristic invasion of fibroblasts and vascular granulation-like tissue that can be described as an angiofibroblastic hyperplasia (Fig. 41–1). Adjacent to this early proliferating vascular reparative tissue, the tendon appears hypercellular, degenerative, and microfragmented. This angiofibroblastic tissue insinuates itself through these abnormal regions as well as focally, extending into adjacent, normal-appearing tendinous fibers. The degree of angiofibroblastic infiltration appears to correlate with the duration of clinical symptoms.

In advanced lesions, the characteristic reaction occurs in supporting tissues as well as in the tendon itself. The fibroadipose, connective, and even skeletal muscle tissue may reveal infiltration by the angiofibroblastic proliferation. Degeneration of skeletal muscle fibers, fibrosis and degeneration of fat, and vascular sclerosis may be seen in these supporting tissues. A mild sprinkling of chronic inflammatory cells may be scattered about in these supportive tissues, but it is highly unusual to detect inflammatory cells in the tendinous tissue itself, even in cases of long duration. Acute inflammatory cells are virtually absent in all cases. If chronic inflammatory cells are evident, the features are usually those of posttraumatic repair rather than tendinitis per se and include typical granulation tissue, either new or organizing, as well as early to late cicatricial fibrous tissue (scar).

Occasional lesions concomitant with rotator cuff tendinitis can also be identified in the supporting tissues. These include mild osteoarthritis and a nonspecific mild chronic synovitis. Again, however, inflammatory cells, even in these concomitant lesions, are relatively scanty. In cases treated by corticosteroid injection, a clear distinction can be made between the characteristic angiofibroblastic proliferation and the injection site. At the injection site, nonpolarized amorphous eosinophilic material can be identified, often without any foreign-body response and usually without evidence of calcification. Indeed, the proliferating vascular reparative tissue often insinuates itself between normal and abnormal tissue in regions very close to the injection site.

Functional Anatomy of the Rotator Cuff

The functional anatomy of the shoulder joint complex is quite sophisticated. This sophistication includes but is not restricted to the rotator cuff. Inman and associates[25] demonstrated a complex interrelationship of shoulder movement. Saha[26] stated that locking of the greater tuberosity against the acromion never takes place "in any position of abduction" if healthy relationships exist. He further noted that a rolling-down movement of the humeral head in the glenoid cavity inevitably takes place with active humeral flexion or abduction. Saha's greatest contribution to shoulder mechanics,

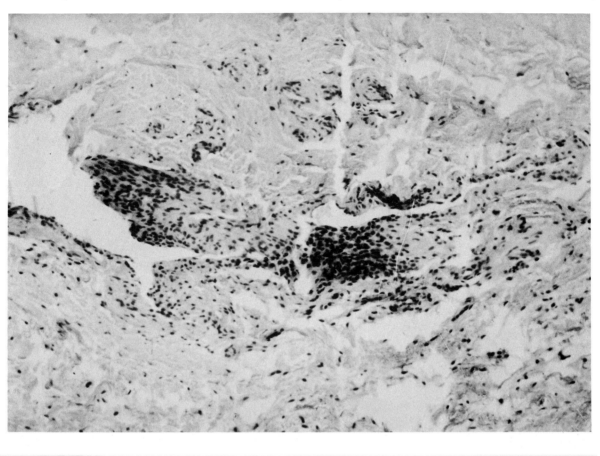

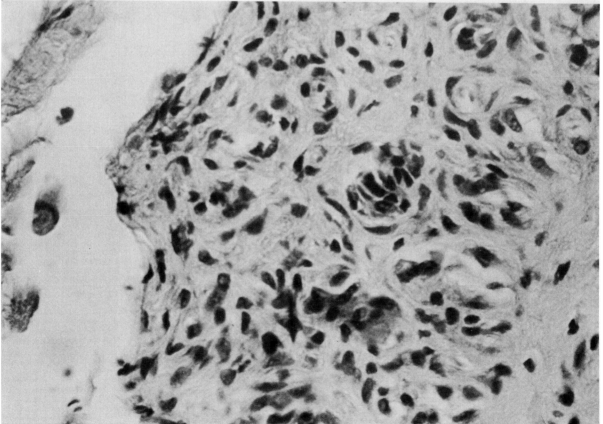

Fig. 41–1   Angiofibroblastic hyperplasia. **Top:** Low-power view (×100). **Bottom:** Higher-power view (×450).

however, was in recognizing the "zero position" of approximately 150 degrees of elevation and 45 degrees of forward flexion where the shear and compression forces generated by the deltoid and rotator cuff are equally balanced.

Sarrafan[27] noted that compression at the level of the glenohumeral joint is essential for stability. At 90 degrees of abduction and beyond, the pull of the deltoid passes through the glenohumeral joint, providing this stability. At less than 90 degrees, the forces generated by the deltoid pass outside the joint, thereby causing upward humeral displacement unless counteracted by the counterforcing joint compression forces of the transversely positioned rotator cuff muscles. Sarrafan confirmed Saha's report that compression and shear forces are maximum at 90 degrees of elevation and essentially nonexistent at 150 degrees. Clinical experience in reference to the rotator cuff in athletes using the upper extremity confirms that the most punishing position is 90 degrees of abduction in association with aggressive rotation (external to internal).

Sports Technique and Rotator Cuff Tendinitis

Clinical experience shows that aggressive internal rotation at 90 degrees of abduction is punishing to the rotator cuff (Fig. 41-2, *left*). Using sports techniques with abduction above 135 degrees is clinically less punishing (Fig. 41-2, *right*). This observation correlates well with Saha's report of "zero balance" at higher humeral elevations.

Hollingshead[28] stated that the supraspinatus is a shoulder abductor. J. Perry identified the role of the supraspinatus as a primary humeral head depressor, as well as a possible external rotator (personal communication, 1985). Andrews and associates[29] and D. Blatz (personal communication, 1985) suggested that the long head of the biceps may also act as a humeral head depressor. It is likely that the scapular and upper thoracic muscle groups also contribute to humeral head control. In addition, Andrews[30] pointed out the vulnerability of the superior anterior glenoid labrum in the acceleration phase of baseball throwing, with the potential of anterior superior subluxation when labral injury occurs in association with capsular laxity.

Present evidence indicates that the rotator cuff is important in the overall control of the glenohumeral joint. Instability of the joint (upward humeral migration) is likely to occur when the normal balance of strength and stability among the rotator cuff, deltoid, glenoid labrum, and scapular muscle groups is distorted.

Mechanisms of Rotator Cuff Injury

Basic Mechanical Forces

The basic mechanical forces to which a tendon is subjected are tension, compression, and shear. Analysis of sports activities, as well as activities of daily living, suggests that the most prevalent force is tension secondary to intrinsic muscular contraction. It is quite clear clinically that multiple repetitions can result in abusive overload. As pointed out by Curwin and Stanish,[13] eccentric tensile overloading is often more prevalent than concentric loading and is probably a common cause of tendon overuse. These patterns of mechanical force are, of course, present in the noncompartmentalized tendons (for example, in the lateral and medial elbow and the patellar, Achilles, and plantar fascia) as well as the compartmentalized rotator cuff (supraspinatus). Indeed, the supraspinatus is a small, relatively weak muscle in a key position and is highly stressed by eccentric tensile overloading in the swimming, racket, and throwing sports. Multiple occupational and living activities also take their toll. Since histologic changes of angiofibroblastic hyperplasia occur in the compartmentalized rotator cuff as well as in the noncompartmentalized tendons, the evidence is strong that the major mechanism of injury in the majority of patients with rotator cuff tendinitis is intrinsic muscular contractile tension overload. The clinical success of rehabilitative exercises designed to restore health and proper function to the rotator cuff supports this conclusion.

Impingement: Alternative Concepts

It is evident that mechanical compression forces (impingement) also occur in and about the rotator cuff. The question is not whether they occur, but how and why. Neer[8] in 1972 advanced the premise of primary impingement by acromial variance and subsequent coracoacromial arch stenosis. For the majority of patients, this premise has been noted to be theoretically and clinically suspect. My surgical experience indicates that acromial variance does occur, but only in 10% of patients. Other authors are now reaching this conclusion.[12] Unusual acromial variants such as os acromiale have also been reported by Mudge and associates[31] and Neer,[32] but these variants are extremely uncommon.

Review of the functional anatomy of the rotator cuff supports the concept that a major rotator cuff function is to stabilize the glenohumeral joint by counteracting the upward humeral migration forces of the deltoid (for example, when the shoulder is abducted below 90 degrees). Functional weakness of the rotator cuff probably results in upward humeral migration. Under these circumstances, compression via "secondary impingement" is likely to occur, further damaging the rotator cuff and causing secondary alterations in the subdeltoid bursa. Major progression of this process probably results in rotator cuff rupture and bony abutment of the humeral greater tuberosity under the acromion, with resultant bony changes (erosion and/or exostosis) in the areas of the subacromion and the greater tuber-

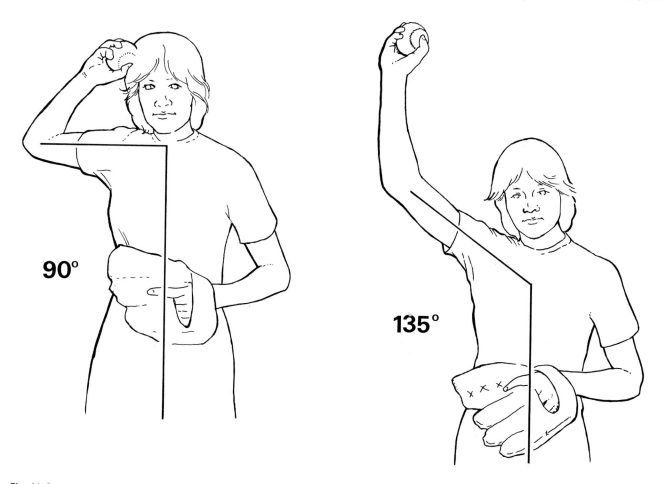

Fig. 41-2 Sports technique and rotator cuff tendinitis. **Left:** Clinical experience indicates that aggressive internal rotation at 90 degrees of abduction is punishing to the rotator cuff. **Right:** Sports techniques that use abduction of more than 135 degrees are less punishing. This observation correlates well with Saha's[26] report of "zero balance" at higher elevations. (Reproduced with permission from Nirschl RP: *Arm Care.* Arlington, Virginia, Medical Sports Publishing, 1981.)

osity. The data as presented by Neer[8] support these concepts.

The preliminary reports of Andrews and associates[29,30] posited a contributing factor to the loss of glenohumeral control, especially in throwing athletes: the forward humeral thrust at the interface of the cocking and acceleration phases of throwing probably places substantial stress on the biceps attachment to the supraglenoid rim and on the superior glenoid labrum. Injuries to these tissues can result in further anterior-superior subluxation, magnifying the "secondary impingement" phenomenon. It is well to keep this additional factor in mind, although I suspect it will not be statistically significant.

Role of the Coracoacromial Ligament

It is clear that control of the humeral head is essential for normal shoulder function. Rotator cuff muscle strength and tendon health are vital to this control.

This important function probably has passive, back-up support. The size, placement, and position of the coracoacromial ligament make it ideal for this function, and I speculate that this is the function of this ligament.

If this is the case, aggressive resection of the coracoacromial ligament may be detrimental to the long-term normal balance and function of the glenohumeral joint and may cause rotator cuff reinjury. The existence of "secondary impingement" and the absence of major pathologic changes in the coracoacromial ligament at the time of rotator cuff surgery lead to the conclusion that aggressive resection is unnecessary and possibly harmful. This concept is supported by the recent report of Watson.[33] In addition, I[16] reported that the coracoacromial ligament should not be incised without specific indication and noted, if anything, improved postoperative function with this approach. Conversely, there is no evidence to support the belief that failure to resect the coracoacromial ligament compromises the success of rotator cuff surgery.

Biologic-Pathologic Considerations

It has been generally accepted that tendon injury often results from multiple repetitions of overload. The concept has been advanced that this overload results in small mechanical microruptures and that the resultant response is an inflammatory reparative tissue. The concept is plausible, but not supported by microscopic evaluations of surgical specimens, which consistently fail to identify evidence of inflammatory reparative changes. Indeed, the microscopic evaluation of chronic tendinitis shows a characteristic pattern (angiofibroblastic hyperplasia) without inflammatory cells that is not characteristic of a true reparative pattern. This microscopic evidence of chronic tendinitis better supports the theory of those authors who have reported an avascular element in rotator cuff tendinitis.[7,20-22] It is likely that in the common situation, tensile overload of the supraspinatus results in fatigue, weakness, and ultimate avascular changes, progressing to angiofibroblastic hyperplasia. Mechanical dissociation may be associated, but is more likely a later phenomenon in the usual case.

Resultant loss of humeral control is anticipated to subsequently result in "secondary impingement" with the observed secondary changes of tendon rupture (partial or total), tendon fibrosis and inflammation, bursitis, and bony changes.

Concepts of Treatment

The etiologic-pathologic algorithm (described more fully in Chapter 42) has major implications for the treatment of rotator cuff tendinitis. The emphasis of treatment has shifted from enlarging the coracoacromial space to restoring health to the rotator cuff. If a clear indication exists that space compromise is a factor, certainly this should be included in the treatment scheme. Space problems are, however, in my experience, in the minority (28% overall) and are more likely to be caused by secondary factors. Treatment directed at enlarging the coracoacromial space, whether by open surgical techniques or by arthroscopy, should have specific indications now lacking in contemporary surgical reports. Conversely, Neer and Marberry[34] reported on the hazards of radical acromionectomy.

As noted by Neer,[23] Fowler,[12] and myself,[15] the majority of patients with rotator cuff tendinitis respond to a good rehabilitation program. An overview of the treatment protocol as practiced in our clinic is as follows: (1) relief of inflammation; (2) rehabilitative exercise for all weakened shoulder muscle groups (especially external rotators, abductors, and scapular muscle groups) and for flexibility (especially internal rotators and adductors); (3) general fitness conditioning; (4) review of activities to prevent overload, including evaluation of sports techniques (training), sports equipment, and counterforce bracing (biceps-deltoid)

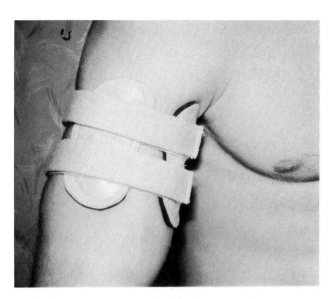

Fig. 41–3 Clinical observations indicate that symptomatic relief of activity-related rotator cuff pain can be obtained by counterforce support of the biceps and lower deltoid in some patients.

(Fig. 41–3); and (5) surgery. The primary indications for surgery are the failure of an appropriate rehabilitation effort and a significant alteration of the quality of the patient's life. Discussion of surgical technique is beyond the scope of this report, but traditional acromioplasty is not recommended, and present arthroscopic concepts and techniques appear limited for long-term consistent success.

Summary

A discussion of the etiologic and pathologic factors associated with rotator cuff tendinitis and rupture concludes that intrinsic muscle contractile tension overload rather than primary impingement is the major factor in the etiology of rotator cuff tendinitis. Treatment is predicated on restoring health to the rotator cuff rather than enlarging the coracoacromial space.

Acknowledgment

Ellsworth J. Stay, MD, Department of Pathology, Arlington Hospital, Arlington, Virginia, made a major contribution to the section on pathology and provided Figure 41–1.

References

1. Codman EA: Complete rupture of the supraspinatus tendon: Operative treatment with report of 2 successful cases. *Boston Med Surg J* 1911;164:708.
2. Codman EA: *The Shoulder: Rupture of the Supraspinatus Tendon*

and Other Lesions in or About the Subacromial Bursa. Boston, Thomas Todd, 1934.

3. Moseley HF: *Shoulder Lesions*, ed 2. New York, Paul B Hoeber, 1953.

4. McLaughlin HL: Muscular and tendinous defects at the shoulder and their repair, in Thomson JEM (ed): American Academy of Orthopaedic Surgeons *Instructional Course Lectures, II.* Ann Arbor, JW Edwards, 1944, p 343.

5. McLaughlin HL: Lesions of the musculotendinous cuff of the shoulder: The exposure and treatment of tears with retraction. *J Bone Joint Surg* 1944;26A:31.

6. DePalma AF: *Surgery of the Shoulder*, ed 2. Philadelphia, JB Lippincott, 1973.

7. Rathbun JB, Mcnab I: The microvascular pattern of the rotator cuff. *J Bone Joint Surg* 1970;52B:540–553.

8. Neer CS II: Anterior acromioplasty for the chronic impingement syndrome in the shoulder: A preliminary report. *J Bone Joint Surg* 1972;54A:41–50.

9. Jobe FW, Jobe CM: Painful athletic injuries of the shoulder. *Clin Orthop* 1983;173:117–124.

10. Nirschl RP: Mesenchymal syndrome. *Va Med Mon* 1969;96:659.

11. Jobe FW, Tibone JE, Perry J, et al: An EMG analysis of the shoulder in throwing and pitching: A preliminary report. *Am J Sports Med* 1983;11:3–5.

12. Fowler PJ: Swimming injuries to the rotator cuff. Presented at the 52nd Annual Meeting of the American Academy of Orthopaedic Surgeons, Las Vegas, Jan 24–29, 1985.

13. Curwin S, Stanish WD: *Tendinitis: Its Etiology and Treatment.* Lexington, Mass, Collamore Press, 1984.

14. Nirschl RP: Throwing or swinging the shoulder pays. *Phys Sports Med* 1984, No. 12.

15. Nirschl RP: *Arm Care.* Arlington, Virginia, Medical Sports Publishing, 1981.

16. Nirschl RP: Shoulder tendinitis, in Pettrone FP (ed): American Academy of Orthopaedic Surgeons *Symposium on Upper Extremity Injuries in Athletes.* St. Louis, CV Mosby, 1986, chap 28, pp 322–337.

17. Nirschl RP: Muscle and tendon trauma: Tennis elbow, in Morrey BF (ed): *The Elbow and Its Disorders.* Philadelphia, WB Saunders, 1985, pp 481–496.

18. Nirschl RP: Rehabilitation of the athletes elbow, in Morrey BF (ed): *The Elbow and Its Disorders.* Philadelphia, WB Saunders, 1985, pp 523–529.

19. Nirschl RP, Pettrone FA: Tennis elbow: The surgical treatment of lateral epicondylitis. *J Bone Joint Surg* 1979;61A:832–839.

20. Lindblom J, Palmer F: Rupture of the tendon aponeurosis of the shoulder joint: The so-called supraspinatus rupture. *Acta Chir Scand* 1939;82:133.

21. Moseley HF, Goldie I: The arterial pattern of the rotator cuff on the shoulder. *J Bone Joint Surg* 1963;45B:780–789.

22. Rothman RH, Parke WW: The vascular anatomy of the rotator cuff. *Clin Orthop* 1965;41:176.

23. Neer CS II: Impingement lesions. *Clin Orthop* 1983;173:70–77.

24. Bigliani LU, Morrison DS, April EW: The morphology of the acromion and its relationship to rotator cuff tears. *Orthop Trans* 1986;10:216.

25. Inman VT, Saunders JB, Abbot LC: Observations on the function of the shoulder joint. *J Bone Joint Surg* 1944;26A:1.

26. Saha AK: The classic: Mechanism of shoulder movements and a plea for the recognition of "zero position" of glenohumeral joint. *Clin Orthop* 1983;173:3–10.

27. Sarrafan SK: Gross and functional anatomy of the shoulder. *Clin Orthop* 1983;173:11–19.

28. Hollingshead WH: *Anatomy for Surgeons: Vol 3. The Back and Limbs.* New York, Hoever-Harper, 1958.

29. Andrews JR, Broussard TS, Carson WG: Arthroscopy of the shoulder in the management of partial tears of the rotator cuff: A preliminary report. *Arthros Rel Surg* 1985;162:117–122.

30. Andrews JR: Shoulder arthroscopy. Presented at the 52nd Annual Meeting of the American Academy of Orthopaedic Surgeons, Las Vegas, Jan 24–29, 1985.

31. Mudge MK, Wood VE, Frykman GK: Rotator cuff tears associated with os acromiale. *J Bone Joint Surg* 1984;66A:427–429.

32. Neer CS II: Rotator cuff tears associated with os acromiale, letter. *J Bone Joint Surg* 1984;66A:1320–1321.

33. Watson M: Major ruptures of the rotator cuff: The results of surgical repair in 89 patients. *J Bone Joint Surg* 1985;67B:618–624.

34. Neer CS II, Marberry TA: On the disadvantages of radical acromionectomy. *J Bone Joint Surg* 1981;63A:416–419.

Rotator Cuff Surgery

Robert P. Nirschl, MD

Introduction

In the past, surgical techniques for the rotator cuff have reflected a standardized approach. Indications for surgery have been primarily for repair of a full-thickness rupture. Neer[1] focused on rotator cuff tendinitis as a primary hereditary impingement from the anterior acromion. He therefore introduced the addition of acromioplasty to the repair procedure. Since his report, the impingement concept has been so widely accepted that the acromioplasty described by Neer has become a traditional and almost automatic aspect of rotator cuff surgery. The difficulties with this universal acceptance and implementation have received little recognition to date.

High-quality surgery requires identification of the pathologic or injured tissue, correction of the abnormality if possible, and avoidance of injury to normal structures. Accurate identification of the pathologic tissue presumes the presence of specific criteria for the indicated surgery and specific techniques to accomplish the desired goals most effectively. Unfortunately, no specific criteria have been developed for acromioplasty since it has been presumed that this technique is almost always indicated. Major reservations have now surfaced concerning the concept of primary impingement and its treatment implications, primarily because of growing experience with swimming, racket, and throwing-sport injuries and the availability of arthroscopic evaluation.

Etiology of Rotator Cuff Tendinitis

The contemporary view of the etiology of rotator cuff tendinitis is shown in Figure 42–1. The basic premise is that the etiologic and pathologic factors are multiple and varied. Overall, my view is that the primary etiologic factor in most symptomatic patients is multiple tendon tension overload of the rotator cuff (especially the supraspinatus). Subsequent fatigue, injury, and weakness of the cuff result in instability and imbalances that produce upward humeral migration and potential injury from secondary impingement. Primary impingement (for example, hereditary acromial variance or os acromiale) as described by Neer[2] and others[3,4] occurs but, in my experience, only in a minority of cases (10%). Subacromial exostosis was present in only 25% of Neer's cases and is better explained by secondary reactionary changes rather than primary acromial variance.

The pathologic change that occurs in the rotator cuff (usually in the supraspinatus), probably from tension overload, varies from minor to major angiofibroblastic hyperplasia with or without partial to complete rupture. Fibrosis may occur via tension overload or impingement (usually secondary) (Fig. 42–2).

Additional factors to consider concerning humeral head instability have been advanced by Andrews and associates.[5,6] These reports suggested an undetermined incidence of anterior shoulder subluxation in throwing athletes. This instability is also now noted in individuals participating in swimming, tennis, volleyball, and other aggressive upper-extremity sports. The cause of anterior subluxation is theorized to be associated with forward humeral thrust at the start of the acceleration phase of the throwing motion, thereby either injuring the anterior superior labrum, the anterior capsule, or both. This subluxation may contribute to upward humeral migration, with secondary impingement, or increase the eccentric tension load on the supraspinatus tendon, or both. Andrews[6] and D. Blatz (personal communication, 1985) also theorized a role for the long head of the biceps in this process, namely as a humeral head depressor. The biceps attachment to the supraglenoid rim has been arthroscopically identified as injured in association with superior labrum injuries.

It is also clear that muscular scapular support is also a factor in humeral head control.[7] Stretched and weakened scapular and midthoracic muscle groups in association with thoracic kyphosis are a common companion of symptomatic rotator cuff tendinitis.

Associated Findings

Subdeltoid bursitis is commonly found during surgery for rotator cuff tendinitis. A thickened, inflamed bursa would be anticipated in the impingement process (both primary and secondary).

Andrews[6] suggested that the biceps acts as a humeral head depressor and is also important in humeral head control. Tensile overload and tendinitis of the biceps tendon would, therefore, not be unexpected in athletes participating in sports involving the upper extremity. Secondary biceps impingement may also occur with upward humeral migration. Neviaser and associates[8] reported a 100% incidence of biceps involvement in a series of 63 rotator cuff surgical cases. My experience and that of others suggest an incidence in the 10% range.

Subacromial exostosis has been noted by many au-

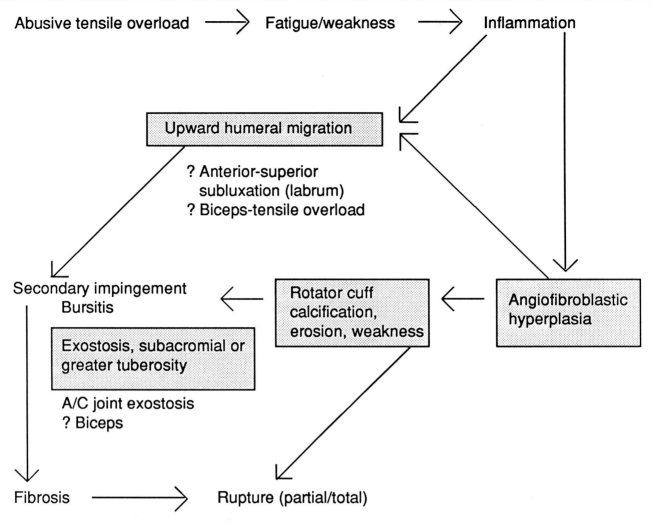

Abusive tensile overload $\longrightarrow$ Fatigue/weakness $\longrightarrow$ Inflammation

Upward humeral migration

? Anterior-superior
subluxation (labrum)
? Biceps-tensile overload

Secondary impingement
Bursitis

Rotator cuff
calcification,
erosion, weakness

Angiofibroblastic
hyperplasia

Exostosis, subacromial or
greater tuberosity

A/C joint exostosis
? Biceps

Fibrosis $\longrightarrow$ Rupture (partial/total)

Fig. 42-1 Etiologic-pathologic algorithm for rotator cuff tendinitis.

thors. Neer[1] reported an incidence of 25% in a rotator cuff surgical series. There are no published reports of incidences greater than 25%. My experience is in the 10% range. Although Neer initially concluded that the cause of the exostosis was a primary acromial variant, it can also be concluded that these findings are a bony reaction secondary to the impingement of upward humeral migration.

Greater tuberosity erosion or exostosis also occurs in about 20% of cases. Secondary reactionary changes are also the probable cause of these findings.

Acromioclavicular osteoarthritis is common in patients who overuse the upper extremity. Adolescent weight-lifters may have isolated acromioclavicular changes but the more common presentation is a combination of rotator cuff tendinitis and acromioclavicular osteoarthritis in patients 40 to 60 years old. In this age group, acromioclavicular osteoarthritis is present in most symptomatic rotator cuff cases that require surgery. Acromioclavicular osteoarthritis appears to be in-

dependent of rotator cuff tendinitis. However, with the exception of direct trauma, the cause (overload) is similar in both conditions. Osteophytic spur formation at the acromioclavicular joint may occur at the underside of the distal clavicle, the underside of the acromion, or both. Inferior osteophytic spur formation at the acromioclavicular joint can be a contributing factor to coracoacromial arch compromise.

The true incidence of anterior subluxation with or without anterior labral tear (partial flap or major tear) is not yet clear. When it is present, the response to nonsurgical and surgical treatments is unknown.

Scapular and midthoracic muscle weakness are common problems in association with rotator cuff tendinitis.[7] Indeed, these changes may be part of the causative process. Levator scapulae tendinitis is common in this situation. Rehabilitative restoration of the scapular and thoracic muscle groups is critical to long-term success.

Flexibility deficiencies are also commonly associated

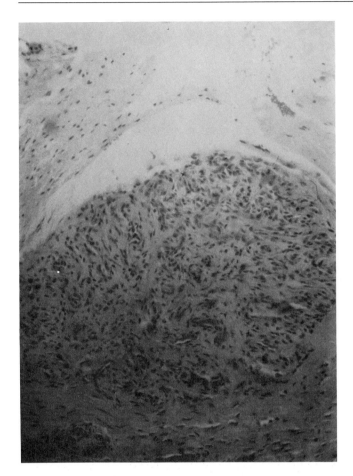 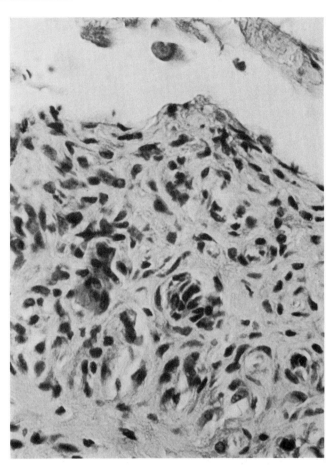

Fig. 42-2 Angiofibroblastic hyperplasia. Characteristic microscopic appearance of tendinitis. Vascular and fibroblastic elements of typical pathologic change. **Left:** Low-power view (×100). **Right:** Higher-power view (×450).

with symptomatic rotator cuff injuries. Flexibility abnormalities include a spectrum ranging from tight adductors and internal rotators to adhesive capsulitis.

This discussion of additional problems is not meant to be all-inclusive. Many other diagnoses are possible. Those discussed are, however, the more common problems encountered in recalcitrant shoulder tendinitis.

Surgical Indications

An accurate diagnosis, obtained by a comprehensive history and physical examination, is critical to surgical success. As noted, a wide variety of associated problems may be present and all must be addressed. An adequate trial of rehabilitation is indicated in most cases. It has been my observation, however, that many preoperative attempts at rehabilitation are inadequate and depend heavily on the use of pharmacologic agents for the relief of pain. Rehabilitation should encompass restoration of balanced strength and flexibility to all weakened structures, including the forearm, arm, shoulder, scapular, and trunk muscle groups. The primary surgical indications are as follows:

(1) Lack of response to a high-quality rehabilitation program.

(2) Objective evidence of rotator cuff abnormality. Ultrasonography, an arthrogram with or without computed tomographic scan, magnetic resonance imaging (utilizing improved shoulder coil and mature learning curve), and diagnostic arthroscopy can all be helpful. The history, the results of the physical examination, (including detailed strength testing), and routine radiographs can differentiate most problems. In addition to routine radiographs (anteroposterior, lateral, and axillary views), supraspinatus and West Point views can be used to assess the subacromial space and anterior glenoid. A positive arthrogram defines a full-thickness rotator cuff tear and a computed tomographic scan with arthrogram aids in diagnosing labral tears. A negative arthrogram does not imply, however, that major tendon damage (without rupture) has not occurred. Sonography can be of help in identifying tendon damage without rupture but a major learning curve is still present for many radiologists. Diagnostic arthroscopy can differentiate among injuries to the biceps, labrum, and

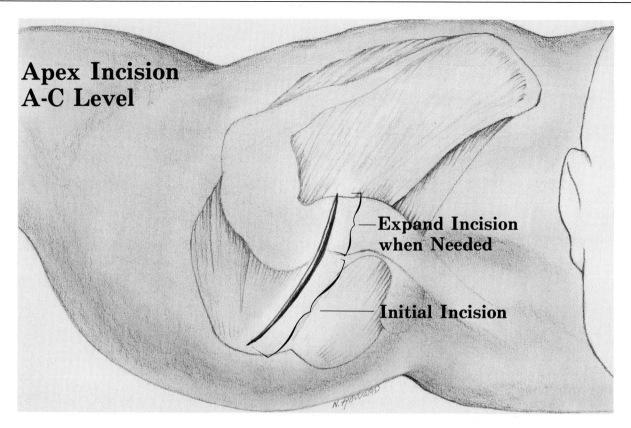

**Apex Incision
A-C Level**

—Expand Incision
when Needed

—Initial Incision

N. HOWARD

Fig. 42-3 Saber incision on the apex of the shoulder just anterior to the acromioclavicular joint. The primary incision parallels the deltoid fibers and extends approximately 6.5 cm to the level of the greater tuberosity. The incision is extended to the posterior border of the acromioclavicular joint when the distal clavicle is resected.

rotator cuff and may be a last resort in difficult diagnostic problems before definitive surgical procedures.

(3) Unacceptable quality of life for the individual patient in association with acceptable surgical risk.

Surgical Considerations

The surgical concepts and techniques employed are predicated on the findings. This point cannot be overemphasized as, in my opinion, a "cookbook mentality" has pervaded shoulder tendinitis surgery (whether by open or arthroscopic techniques).

The surgical goal is restoration of health to the rotator cuff on a permanent basis (if possible) without harm to normal or uninvolved tissue. If coracoacromial arch stenosis (either primary or secondary) is present (in my experience, this occurs in about 28% of cases), the arch should be enlarged to allow adequate humeral clearance. This may include removal of combinations of subacromial osteophytes, acromioclavicular osteoarthritis, greater tuberosity exostosis, thickened bursae, or thickened rotator cuff tendon. It is not necessary, however, to perform the traditional acromioplasty or to resect the coracoacromial ligament to accomplish these surgical goals.

Adhesive capsulitis is best worked out before surgery

if possible. At the very least, ensure full range of shoulder motion at the start of surgery by manipulation. Major adhesive capsulitis at the time of surgery may result in serious postoperative rehabilitation problems.

Identifiable subluxation may be treated by surgical means and is now responsive to the limited open technique. High-quality rehabilitation, under certain circumstances, may also be successful in controlling subluxation preoperatively. Full dislocation is not a significant factor in rotator cuff tendinitis.

Caution There are, at present, no control studies demonstrating the need for or effectiveness of acromioplasty (whether by open or arthroscopic techniques) in cases in which specific visual or palpable coracoacromial arch compromise are not identified. The same statement may be made for resection of the coracoacromial ligament. Indeed, in those surgical series in which other conclusions were reached, the diseased or injured rotator cuff was also surgically corrected, negating the conclusions. Neer and Marberry[9] reported on the harm caused by aggressive acromioplasty and Watson[10] reported that resection of the coracoacromial ligament in association with rotator cuff repair gave poorer results than ligament incision alone. It is my opinion that

Deltoid Split

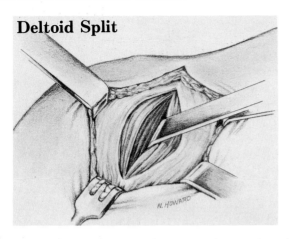

Fig. 42–4 The deltoid is split parallel to the direction of its fibers down to the level of the greater tuberosity.

Bursal Exposure

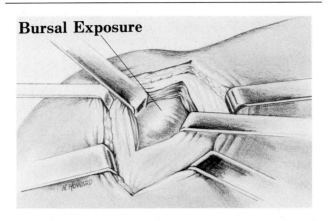

Fig. 42–5 The subdeltoid bursa is exposed. Resection of abnormal bursa is undertaken as indicated. Normal bursa may occasionally be resected to achieve exposure but should be spared as much as possible.

the coracoacromial ligament is an important passive constraint to upward humeral migration and should not be sacrificed without specific indication.[11] Indeed, in my present surgical series, using my preferred technique, there have been no identified failures on the basis of inadequate decompression of the coracoacromial arch. This technique spares most of the coracoacromial ligament and avoids the traditional acromioplasty.

Preferred Surgical Technique

The goal of surgery is to correct the pathologic alteration while protecting normal tissue. To protect the deltoid origin, the traditional anterior acromioplasty should be avoided. Adequate exposure in most rotator cuff operations can be achieved by a deltoid-splitting incision at the level of the acromioclavicular joint. In major rotator cuff tears, cuff retraction generally occurs laterally, and the incision allows access, if needed, to the retracted tissue. If supraspinatus retraction occurs proximally, the supraspinatus fossa is easily reached by resection of the distal clavicle and extension of the incision to the supraspinatus fossa.

Rotator cuff tendinitis may be accompanied by adhesive capsulitis. If this occurs, a full manipulation of the shoulder before the surgical incision is made is an important preliminary procedure.

The preferred incision extends from the anterior edge of the acromioclavicular joint in the direction of the deltoid fibers approximately 6.5 cm distally (Fig. 42–3). If acromioclavicular osteoarthritis is present or if it is necessary to expose the supraspinatus fossa, the incision is expanded posteriorly to the supraspinatus fossa. The decision to expand the incision is usually made

after exposure and inspection of the coracoacromial arch.

The deltoid is easily split longitudinally, since the muscle is relatively thin and flat at this level (Fig. 42–4). The subdeltoid bursa and coracoacromial ligament come into view promptly (Fig. 42–5). Normal bursa is protected and is incised only for exposure. Pathologic bursa is excised. Inflamed bursa adherent to the rotator cuff is indicative of significant rotator cuff pathologic change.

The rotator cuff and coracoacromial arch can now be inspected. Palpation is undertaken first as the palpating finger can also release any adhesions for enhancement of visualization. Clearance for the palpating finger is enhanced by the assistant applying downward traction on the arm. The palpating finger examines the underside of the coracoacromial ligament for tightness; the subacromial space for beaking, spurs, or excessive slope; the area below the acromioclavicular joint for spurs; the bicipital groove for location, subluxation, or tears; and the rotator cuff for tears, thinning, or adhesions.

Next, visual inspection is begun. The coracoacromial ligament is inspected for signs of inflammation and pathologic alteration. The assistant releases the arm traction to allow visual assessment of the functional relationship between the rotator cuff and the leading edge of the coracoacromial ligament through a passive full range of motion. Next, the rotator cuff is visually inspected (by rotating through a full range of motion) for thinning, hyperemia, roughened or eroded areas, flap tears, and partial-thickness and full-thickness tears. A normal rotator cuff is smooth, shiny, and white, with an even palpable density. Slight softness and laxity over the bicipital groove area and slight thinning at the area of attachment to the greater tuberosity are, however, normal.

Signs of abnormality usually occur in the supraspinatus tendon (just lateral to the bicipital groove, approximately 2.5 cm wide) extending from the greater tuberosity proximal for 6.5 cm. Bursal adhesion to the rotator cuff, hyperemia, and roughness are common signs of full-thickness tendinitis. Erosions, partial-thickness flap tears, and varying degrees of full-thickness tears are also common. Full-thickness tears characteristically occur at or in the region of the greater tuberosity. The common denominator of all these observed changes is underlying pathologic supraspinatus tendinitis (Fig. 42–6).

One final check for shoulder subluxation is now undertaken by passive manipulation, both in the sagittal plane and in forced abduction and external rotation.

The best surgical technique from this point forward is totally dependent on the findings.

Coracoacromial Ligament

The coracoacromial ligament rarely demonstrates obvious pathologic changes (either visually or microscopically). Palpable tightness, however, varies dramatically. In ligaments that are palpably tight, my usual approach is to incise the anterior third of the ligament obliquely, close to its acromial attachment (Fig. 42–7). If greater exposure is needed, further release is undertaken; the entire ligament only rarely needs to be released (even with resection of the distal clavicle and the expanded exposure needed to repair some major full-thickness cuff tears).

Acromioclavicular Joint

If acromioclavicular osteoarthritis is present (as it is about 30% of the time) or wide cuff exposure is needed, the skin incision is expanded to the posterior edge of the acromioclavicular joint. The acromioclavicular ligament is incised, and the metaphyseal flare of the distal end of the clavicle is removed with an oscillating saw. During the osteotomy, a large periosteal elevator is placed over the supraspinatus for its protection. It is unnecessary to remove more than the clavicular metaphyseal flare but be sure that any underside osteophytic spurs are resected. The distal clavicle is smoothed with a rasp at the completion of the resection (Fig. 42–8). It is unnecessary to incise the entire coracoacromial ligament when resecting the distal clavicle.

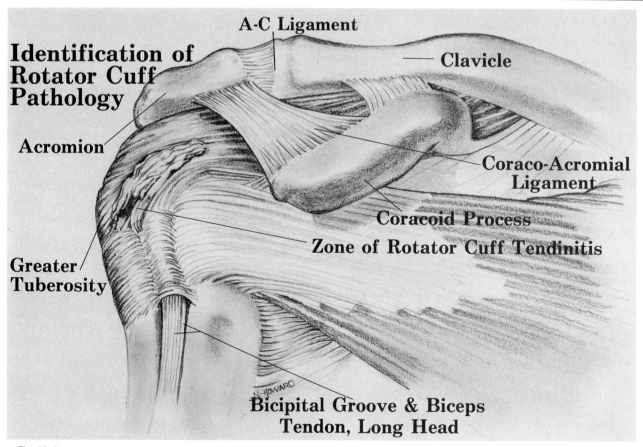

Fig. 42–6 There are wide variations in rotator cuff abnormality. Adherent, thickened bursa and hyperemia are clues to underlying angiofibroblastic degeneration. Erosions, partial tears, calcification, and full-thickness tears may be present. The abnormality is usually located in the supraspinatus tendon just lateral to the bicipital groove and just proximal to the greater tuberosity.

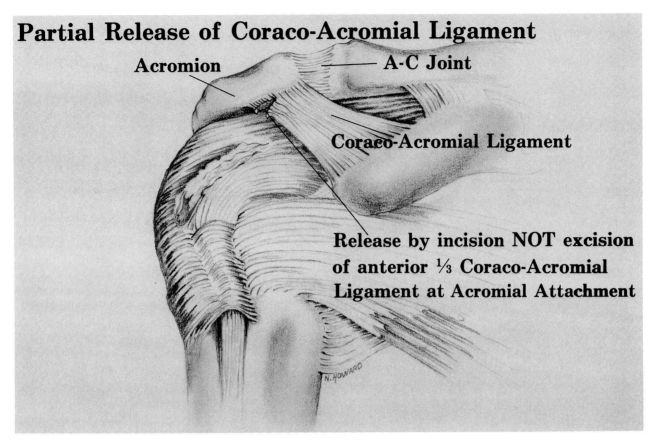

Partial Release of Coraco-Acromial Ligament

Acromion — **A-C Joint**

Coraco-Acromial Ligament

Release by incision NOT excision of anterior ⅓ Coraco-Acromial Ligament at Acromial Attachment

N. HOWARD

Fig. 42–7 In the typical situation, the anterior-third edge of the coracoacromial ligament is incised obliquely at the acromial attachment. Further release is unnecessary unless the circumstances are unusual.

Subacromial Space

The subacromial space is then inspected for possible compromise. It is conceivable, as Neer[1] and Bigliani and associates[4] suggested, that the downward slope of the anterior acromion may be hereditarily exaggerated, thus compromising the coracoacromial space, but there is no objective clinical or laboratory test to make this determination. Indiscriminate surgery on the acromion is, in my opinion, therefore unwarranted, since harm to the deltoid often results.

Subacromial pathologic change is most commonly associated with bony exostosis mirroring clavicular alteration in acromioclavicular osteoarthritis. The isolated anterior acromial lesion, as described by Neer,[1] is less common in my experience (10% of cases) but does occur in long-standing problems (most often noticed with full rotator cuff tear). If anterior subacromial exostoses are present (as found by palpation), they are easily removed with an instrument such as an oscillating saw (Fig. 42–9). It is unnecessary to remove any deltoid from the anterior acromion with this technique. The traditional full-thickness anterior acromioplasty is thus avoided unless some unusual circumstance is present.

In addition to the 10% incidence of subacromial (an-terior) exostosis, another 18% of surgical cases include a palpably tight coracoacromial arch. It has been my practice to expand the coracoacromial arch in this group of patients as well, despite the lack of a definite subacromial change.

Rotator Cuff

Visual inspection of the rotator cuff is easily obtained by humeral rotation and abduction.

Inspection of the cuff may reveal a wide variety of pathologic changes. These changes are usually located in the supraspinatus tendon.

In those tendons that display angiofibroblastic degeneration without rupture (for example, bursal adhesions, calcifications, erythema, erosions), the normal shiny surface is replaced by abnormal hyperemic and roughened areas that are often thin to palpation. These changes appear in the stress riser seam of the supraspinatus just lateral to the bicipital groove. An elliptical excision of the abnormal tendon is done (usually 6.5 cm long by 2.5 cm wide, extending proximally from the greater tuberosity) (Fig. 42–10). Excision of a width greater than 2.5 cm may compromise closure and it may be necessary to leave a small segment of abnormal

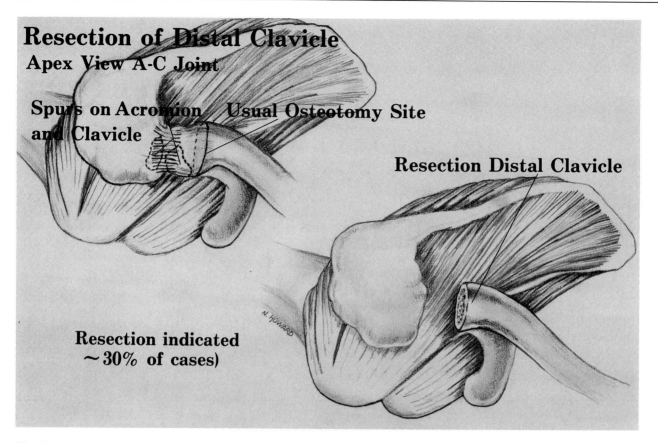

Fig. 42-8 Acromioclavicular osteoarthritis is commonly associated with rotator cuff tendinitis. Symptomatic acromioclavicular joints or exostosis compromising the coracoacromial arch can be resolved by resection of the metaphyseal flare (usually the outer 1.25 cm) of the distal clavicle. Exostoses on the acromial side are also removed if present.

tissue. It has been my experience, however, that this does not compromise the operation's success. In the typical case, angiofibroblastic degeneration pervades the entire thickness of the tendon. Full-thickness excision is indicated to eradicate most of the abnormal tendon.

In those cases in which there is a full-thickness tear, resection of the pathologic residual tissues at the rim of the tear is important for pain relief and to maintain the quality of the repair. These ruptures are usually vertical and are primarily in the area of the supraspinatus stress riser. Typically, the tear is shaped like an inverted V with the base of the V at the greater tuberosity. Tears larger than 2 cm are unusual in competitive athletes, but may occur in older, recreational athletes. Tears larger than 4 cm are unusual. Even in this situation, however, major tendon retraction, either lateral or proximal, is not common. Repair is undertaken (primarily with absorbable No. 1 sutures). Residual frail tissue or residual defects warrant augmentation with an autogenous tendon "patch graft."[12]

If proximal retraction into the supraspinatus fossa occurs, resection of the distal clavicle may be necessary for maximum supraspinatus mobilization and exposure. If the retracted cuff cannot be returned to its anatomic

position, repair into the humeral head is indicated. It is helpful to abduct the arm during this operative phase. In my view, however, the tension at the anastomatic site must not preclude the return of the arm to the patient's side at the time of surgery (that is, if it is necessary to maintain the arm in abduction at the time of surgery, it is unlikely that the repair can be protected during the postoperative rehabilitative process).

In those cases in which a major posterolateral cuff retraction occurs, a substantial amount of tendon may be present but hidden. Palpate thoroughly with the humeral head in full internal rotation before giving up any attempt at repair.

Biceps Tendon

The biceps tendon is involved in pathologic change by tension (in its role as humeral head depressor), compression (secondary to upward migration), and shear (via subluxation from the bicipital groove). Weaver[13] reported pathologic changes in the biceps in approximately 10% of surgical cases; this correlates well with my findings.[11] These changes include tendon sheath inflammation (the most common), partial angiofibroblastic changes, partial traumatic avulsion from the supra-

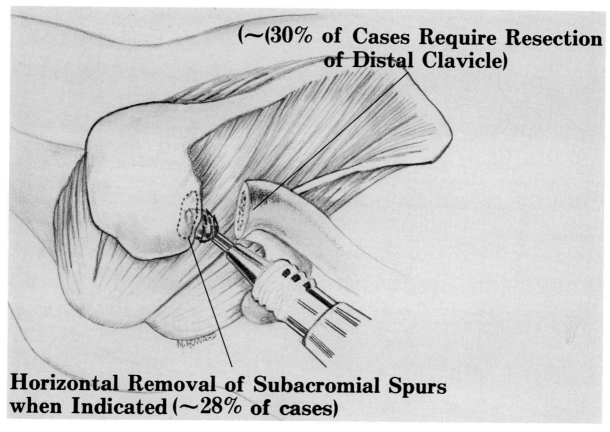

Fig. 42-9 Excision of subacromial exostosis. Subacromial exostosis or beaking occurs in approximately 10% of cases. Removal with an oscillating saw or motorized abrasion technique is recommended. Traditional acromioplasty is unnecessary and possibly harmful. A tight coracoacromial arch without evidence of subacromial exostosis or beaking occurs in an additional 18% of patients.

glenoid rim, and full tendon rupture at the level of the bicipital groove.

Since the biceps is probably a humeral head stabilizer, it is best to leave it undisturbed unless it is clearly symptomatic and major changes are present. In this instance, resection of pathologic tissue is recommended (Fig. 42-11). Total resection and distal bicipital groove attachment are rarely needed. My findings and those of Weaver[13] are in conflict with those of Neviaser and associates.[8]

Greater Tuberosity Exostosis

Reactive changes of exostosis are common with upward humeral migration and secondary impingement of the greater tuberosity. If exostoses are present, as happens in about 20% of cases, they are removed (usually by ronguer) (Fig. 42-12). Removal often enhances the ease of rotator cuff repair and ensures a new source of vascular supply in the repair area. Do not remove so much of the greater tuberosity as to compromise the stability of the bicipital groove.

Surgical Closure

With the limited exposure technique as described, deep closure is quite straightforward. Since the deltoid

acromial attachment is not altered, the deltoid muscle is merely approximated with absorbable suture. With this exposure technique, rehabilitation is faster and the danger of deltoid disruption is avoided.

In those cases in which resection of the distal clavicle has been done, a firm repair of the acromioclavicular ligament by several nonabsorbable sutures oversewn with a running absorbable suture enhances deltoid repair and postoperative rehabilitation (Fig. 42-13).

Special Techniques

Open Inspection of Labrum

General Considerations Exposure of the glenohumeral joint has been necessitated by the identification of shoulder subluxation in athletes. The analysis of baseball throwing and diagnostic arthroscopic investigation by Andrews and associates[5,6] advanced our understanding of this phenomenon. It is now clear that rotator cuff tendinitis may be aggravated and perhaps initiated by glenohumeral instability. This can be caused by rotator cuff functional and anatomic deficiency but also

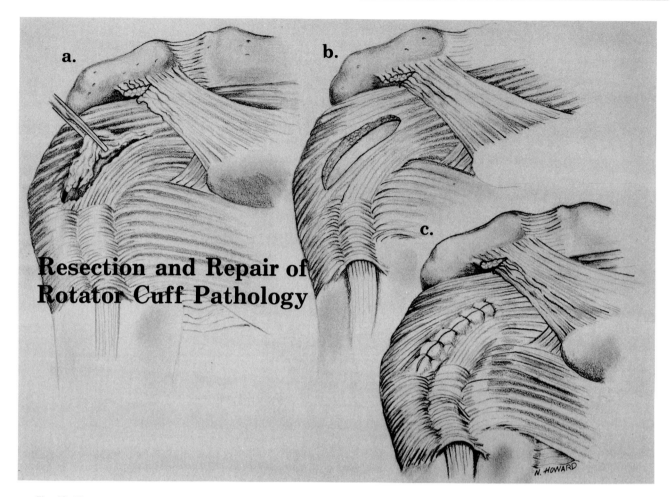

Fig. 42-10 Identified tendon changes are excised vertically in an elliptical fashion (**a** and **b**). The typical resection is a seam 1.9 to 2.5 cm wide and 6.5 cm long just lateral to the bicipital groove. The resection defect is repaired with absorbable sutures (**c**).

by anterior capsule, labrum, and biceps deficiencies. These deficiencies can result either in secondary impingement or tension overload of the rotator cuff.

Although the overall incidence of shoulder subluxation among all cases of shoulder tendinitis undergoing surgery is unknown (and probably small), this possibility must now be kept in mind.

The clinical criteria to support the diagnosis of shoulder subluxation are limited but include the historical account of slipping, sliding, or catching in the glenohumeral joint, a feeling of a "dead arm," and rotator cuff pain—often posterior in the region of the infraspinatus insertion to the cuff. The Virginia Sportsmedicine Institute subluxation test with passive forward humeral thrust may initiate anterior rotator cuff pain and duplicate the feeling of subluxation. A positive apprehension sign is not usual except in full dislocation. Congenitally lax shoulders present a diagnostic dilemma and both shoulders must always be examined. Helpful laboratory tests to outline the labrum include an arthrogram with computed tomographic scan. The West

Point radiographic view may show calcification at the anterior edge of the glenoid. The axillary view may reveal distortion of either the anterior or posterior glenoid edge.

To date, the most effective tool for diagnosing anterior labral defects (including labral flap tears), a capsular laxity, and tears to the biceps attachment of the supraglenoid rim has been arthroscopy.

By the open exposure, it is now possible to directly palpate and visually observe the upper hemisphere of the glenoid, the superior and posterior labrum, the capsule, and the biceps insertion into the supraglenoid tubercle. Synovitis and flap tears may be trimmed, debris removed, and, importantly, the capsule tightened at the time of rotator cuff repair (Fig. 42–14).

This is now my routine technique when the degenerated rotator cuff tendon is removed (the usual reason for surgery) or when a tear is present (either circumstance automatically allows convenient intra-articular access to the glenohumeral joint). Arthroscopy is used in other circumstances.

Technical Aspects In the typical surgical situation, the supraspinatus is significantly degenerated with or without rupture. The characteristic area of degeneration, as noted, extends from the greater humeral tuberosity proximally 6.5 cm just lateral (0.6 cm) to the bicipital groove. The width of the degenerated tissue is typically 1.9 to 2.5 cm. Thus, without rupture, a segment of degenerated tissue 6.5 cm long and 1.9 cm wide is removed. If rupture is present, the degenerated tendon margins are removed. In either circumstance, the biceps tendon is easily exposed and debrided if necessary. To expose the glenohumeral joint, a 0.25-inch Penrose drain is slid around the biceps tendon, an assistant applies downward traction on the humerus, and a palpating finger is easily introduced inside the rotator cuff and under the long head of the biceps. The biceps tendon is followed to its attachment on the supraglenoid tubercle; the palpating finger is then swept anteriorly and posteriorly over the glenoid labrum and capsule. The humeral head is maintained in distraction by the assistant applying traction at approximately 30 degrees of external rotation and 30 degrees of abduction.

Palpation is revealing and undue laxity or tears are detectable by palpation alone. Direct visual inspection can be undertaken by placing an Army-Navy retractor inside the rotator cuff either anterior or posterior to the humeral head and retracting in the direction desired. Retracting the long head of the biceps with the Penrose drain enhances the visual possibilities. Labral flap tears can be trimmed or debrided through this exposure with standard arthroscopic instruments. To date, I have found no major capsular or labral tears that required deep suturing, but I believe this could be accomplished if necessary by the newer arthroscopic suture placement techniques described by R. Caspari and J. Myers (unpublished data). If superior capsular laxity with subluxation does exist, my preliminary observation is that closure of the rotator cuff's surgical elliptical defect (that is, the defect left by excision of degenerated tissue) may suffice to resolve the subluxation.

This open technique resolves the dilemma of intraarticular inspection without the limitations inherent in arthroscopic techniques when definitive surgical resection and repair are indicated.

Augmentation Autogenous Tendon "Patch Graft"

In certain circumstances, the quality of the repaired tendon is severely compromised. This discussion is directed primarily at defects that have allowed full or almost full side-to-side repair but in which the residual repaired tissue remains compromised and of poor quality. In these circumstances, the reinforcement of this compromised tissue and repair by an autogenous tendon graft has proved to be extremely promising in preliminary follow-up of ten cases.[12] The speed of rehabilitation, return of strength, and relief of pain have

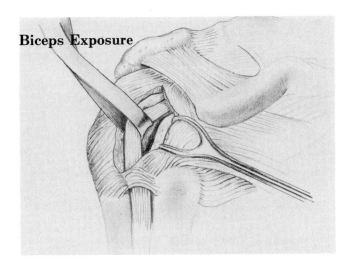

Fig. 42-11 Exposure of the long head of the biceps is achieved by retraction of the medial edge of the rotator cuff. Debridement of the paratenon or substance of the tendon is done as needed. In most cases, there is no abnormality and no treatment is needed.

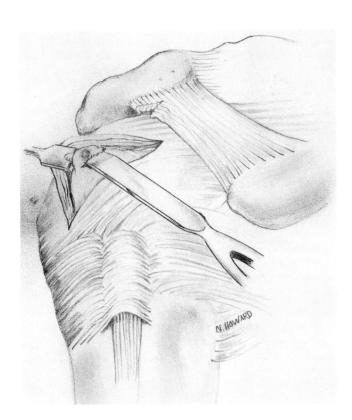

Fig. 42-12 Osteophytic spur. Bony exostoses are present in about 20% of cases. Removal with a rongeur or osteotome is recommended.

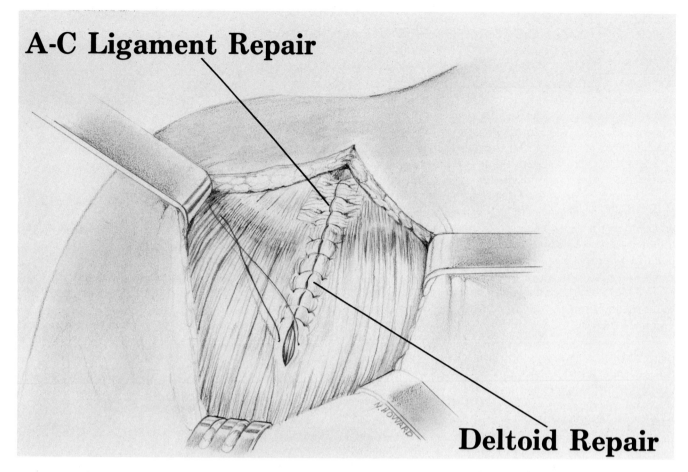

A-C Ligament Repair

Deltoid Repair

Fig. 42-13 Closure. If the distal clavicle has been resected, a firm repair of the acromioclavicular ligament enhances deltoid repair and postoperative rehabilitation. Avoiding the traditional acromioplasty simplifies deltoid repair. Because the deltoid's acromial attachment is not harmed, rehabilitation is faster and the danger of deltoid disruption is avoided.

exceeded those in similar cases when the autogenous tendon graft technique was not used.

It should be emphasized that this technique is used in circumstances when side-to-side closure has been essentially accomplished. This is a departure in concept from techniques to fill a major unrepairable gap when tissue is absent. I have used the proximal iliotibial band as the donor tendon in all my cases. I have noted no functional deficiency, residual pain, or cosmetic deformity at the donor site. A rectangular segment of the proximal iliotibial band is removed. This tendon donor is patched over the compromised rotator cuff by perimeter suturing with absorbable suture. The tendon is placed shiny side up and sutured under modest tension (Fig. 42–15).

Unrepairable Tendon Gaps

This situation is rare in younger competitive athletes (other than wheelchair athletes), but may occur in older (60 to 70 years) recreational athletes and is more commonplace in the nonathletic older patient (including those with rheumatoid arthritis). The major symptom is pain. Clinical preoperative function can be surprisingly good but is often poor. In this circumstance, major upward humeral migration is the rule and secondary subacromial osteophytes and acromioclavicular osteoarthritis are common. Modified acromioplasty with protection of the deltoid is critical to any functional success. Excision of the coracoacromial ligament merely allows further upward humeral migration and should be avoided. Oblique limited incision of the anterior third edge of the coracoacromial ligament in association with resection of an osteoarthritic distal clavicle may be indicated in certain circumstances, however (Fig. 42–16).

The goal of treatment in unrepairable tears is the relief of pain. It is best to resect all visible pathologic tissue to ensure maximum pain relief. An autogenous iliotibial patch graft may be tried, but in gaps larger than 2 cm (after attempted repair), the results are not likely to be better than those in debridement alone. Wide exposures, attempts at infraspinatus advance-

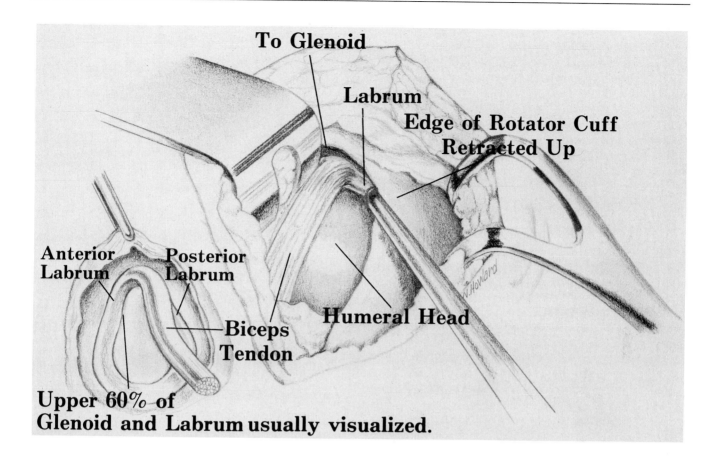

Fig. 42-14 Glenohumeral exposure. With the usual 6.5-cm elliptical resection of the abnormal segment of the rotator cuff, exposure of the upper hemisphere of the glenohumeral joint by palpation and direct visualization is possible. Labral and biceps tears, capsular laxity, synovial inflammation, and glenohumeral osteoarthritis can be diagnosed accurately. Arthroscopic debridement is possible and the capsule tightens when the rotator cuff is repaired.

ment, and large autografts may actually disturb the remaining normal tissues and compromise the potential for any function. These techniques, therefore, should be used only with extreme caution.

In my experience, if all pathologic tissue is resected, pain relief is generally excellent and functional performance can be surprisingly good if the deltoid function (origin) and the coracoacromial ligament are not significantly disturbed. C. Rockwood reported similar short-term experience but he is less protective of the coracoacromial ligament and acromion (personal communication, 1986). In my opinion, aggressive resection of the acromion and coracoacromial ligament is likely to compromise long-term results.

Principles of Postoperative Care

For the large majority of patients undergoing shoulder surgery, relaxed immobilization with a sling and swathe is customary. When healing is sufficient for the patient to tolerate comfortable activities of daily living without immobilization (usually two to three weeks), use of the sling is eliminated. Codman exercises are started a few days postoperatively. Control of edema and pain, as well as muscle reeducation, appear to be enhanced by the use of high-voltage electrical stimulation. This treatment is usually started two or three days postoperatively. Active exercise against gravity is begun when the patient can tolerate it (usually one week), with the exception of external rotation and direct abduction (these activities are usually started after two to four weeks, depending on the quality of repair). Resistance exercises in all motion arcs are usually underway by four weeks. The progression of rehabilitation exercise must be closely supervised by physical therapists. Easy sport activities, such as light swimming, gentle golf swings, and gentle tennis groundstrokes often can be started at six to eight weeks (again, depending on the quality of repair).

Those patients who have had only resection and repair progress more quickly. Overall, the rehabilitation

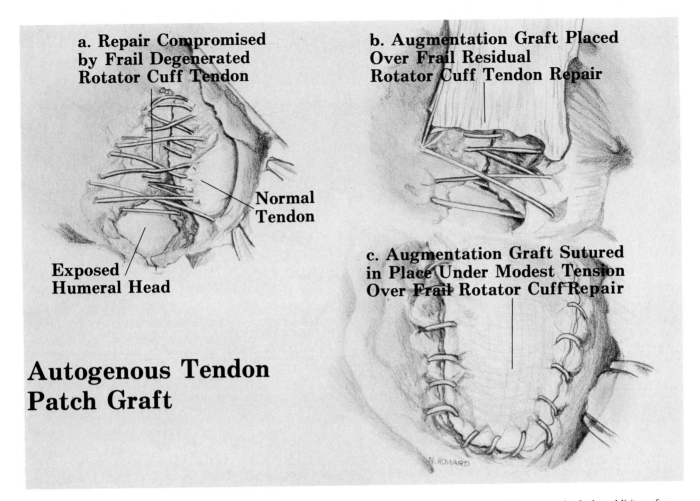

a. Repair Compromised by Frail Degenerated Rotator Cuff Tendon

Normal Tendon

Exposed Humeral Head

Autogenous Tendon Patch Graft

b. Augmentation Graft Placed Over Frail Residual Rotator Cuff Tendon Repair

c. Augmentation Graft Sutured in Place Under Modest Tension Over Frail Rotator Cuff Repair

N. HOWARD

Fig. 42–15 Augmentation graft for compromised tissue (**a**). When repair is possible but the tissue is compromised, the addition of an autogenous tendon patch graft enhances rehabilitation and the quality of the final result. Patch graft technique (**b**). A rectangular segment of tendon is harvested from the iliotibial band of the leg and sutured over the compromised tissue around the perimeter. Final placement (**c**). The patch graft is placed and sutured under modest tension with absorbable sutures.

of those patients who required an augmentation tendon graft progresses as quickly as that of patients who have a firmly repaired rotator cuff tear with remaining good-quality tissue. This is a marked improvement over frail repairs without the benefit of the graft.

Return to Sports

In the resection and repair group, a high level of function is usually evident by four months. The function of patients with full-thickness tears varies considerably with the size of the tear and the quality of the repaired tissue. The augmentation tendon patch graft technique,[12] however, appears to enhance both the quality and the predictability of the results. In those with full-thickness tears larger than 1 cm, good function is usually present by one year. In those patients with tears smaller than 1 cm, the speed of rehabilitation and

the quality of function are usually improved compared with those of patients who have larger tears. These findings relative to the size of the initial tear are consistent with the report of Tibone and associates.[14]

Overall, the success of surgery is measured by a full return to the pre-injury level of sports activity. Total success depends on a number of factors. These include the magnitude of the injury or tissue degeneration, the quality of the remaining tissues, the ultimate quality of the repair, maintaining the normal condition of the uninjured tissues, the intrinsic biologic healing capacity of the patient, the intensity and quality of the rehabilitation effort, psychological factors, and the ultimate demand of the sports activity.

Suffice it to say, when major injury occurs to competitive athletes in a very demanding sport (such as baseball pitching or swimming), the return to high-level competition is more challenging.[15] With favorable factors and the newer techniques described, the oppor-

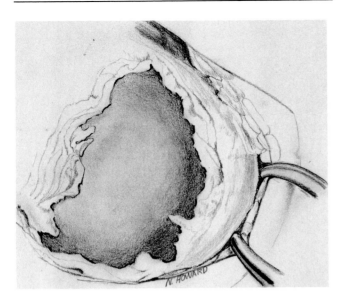

Fig. 42-16 Unrepairable gap with massive degeneration of the rotator cuff. In full-thickness tears with retraction, the displacement is more likely to be posterolateral (toward the infraspinatus fossa) than proximal (toward the supraspinatus fossa). When gaps cannot be repaired, full debridement of the remaining edges of the abnormal rotator cuff tissue usually results in satisfactory relief of pain. It is important to protect the deltoid and coracoacromial ligament because these structures are critical for remaining compensatory function. The traditional acromioplasty, therefore, is not recommended. Only one third or less of the coracoacromial ligament is incised.

tunity to return to high-level competition is enhanced but never certain. In contradistinction, the average recreational athlete (who has lower sports demands) can ordinarily expect to return to a reasonable level of sports performance if the repair is satisfactory and the rehabilitation adequate.

The rehabilitative techniques for return vary with the sport. When the patient achieves adequate rehabilitative progress (adequate flexibility, strength, and endurance as measured objectively by the usual physical therapy techniques), progression to conditioning and sports technique exercises commences. The intensity, duration, and technique of these exercises should be monitored by coach, trainer, and medical professionals for best long-term results.

Arthroscopy

Conceptual Deficiencies and Practical Limitations

There has been substantial progress in the application of arthroscopy to the shoulder[5,6,16,17] (and Caspari and Myers, unpublished data). As a diagnostic tool, it has been of immeasurable help in defining the problems of subluxation and reaffirming my belief in the high incidence of rotator cuff degenerative changes occurring without rupture.

At present, however, arthroscopic definitive treat-

ment remains investigational. The areas of potential treatment use are the following: (1) identification and debridement of labral flap tears; (2) possible stabilization of subluxation or dislocation; (3) synovectomy or removal of intra-articular debris; (4) debridement of rotator cuff degeneration with or without tears; and (5) expansion of the coracoacromial arch via acromioplasty and excision or incision of the coracoacromial ligament.

With respect to rotator cuff debridement, it has been my experience that palpation and visualization are necessary to identify the full extent of pathologic tendon changes because these changes usually encompass the entire thickness of the tendon. Arthroscopy is quite limited for accurately identifying the area and depth of tendon degeneration. Full-thickness resection is indicated in most surgical cases and arthroscopy offers no opportunity for repair of full-thickness resections.

Along with the primary proponents of arthroscopy,[5,16] I strongly support the concept of avoiding the traditional acromioplasty. I disagree, however, with those proponents who espouse acromioplasty (arthroscopic or otherwise) as a routine.[16] The diagnostic criteria for primary coracoacromial arch stenosis have not been defined. Since the usual arthroscopic techniques (such as coracoacromial arch expansion) are predicated on the concept of primary impingement (which, in my experience, occurs only in a minority of cases), the results of such surgery are likely to be inconsistent. As better criteria are developed concerning the diagnosis of primary vs secondary impingement, arthroscopic techniques may become more reliable. Until such time, these techniques are best described as developmental. My concepts are consistent with those of Ogilvie-Harris and Wiley.[17]

Summary

The surgical concepts and techniques presented here are superior to the traditional techniques that I used previously. The primary goal is to restore health to the rotator cuff. The new techniques of glenohumeral joint exposure and the augmentation tendon patch graft have expanded the possibilities of surgical shoulder care. The concept of primary impingement and traditional acromioplasty techniques warrant strong cautions.

Acknowledgment

Ellsworth J. Stay, MD, Department of Pathology, Arlington Hospital, Arlington, Virginia, provided Figure 42-2.

References

1. Neer CS II: Anterior acromioplasty for the chronic impingement syndrome in the shoulder: A preliminary report. *J Bone Joint Surg* 1972;54A:41–50.

2. Neer CS II: Rotator cuff tears associated with os acromiale, letter. *J Bone Joint Surg* 1984;66A:1320–1321.

3. Mudge MK, Wood VE, Frykman GK: Rotator cuff tears associated with os acromiale. *J Bone Joint Surg* 1984;66A:427–429.

4. Bigliani LU, Morrison DS, April EW: The morphology of the acromion and its relationship to rotator cuff tears. *Orthop Trans* 1986;10:216.

5. Andrews JR, Broussard TS, Carson WG: Arthroscopy of the shoulder in the management of partial tears of the rotator cuff: A preliminary report. *J Arthros Rel Surg* 1985;1:117–122.

6. Andrews JR: Shoulder arthroscopy. Presented at the 52nd Annual Meeting of the American Academy of Orthopaedic Surgeons, Las Vegas, Jan 24–29, 1985.

7. Fowler PJ: Swimming injuries to the rotator cuff. Presented at the 52nd Annual Meeting of the American Academy of Orthopaedic Surgeons, Las Vegas, Jan 24–29, 1985.

8. Neviaser TJ, Neviaser RS, Neviaser JS, et al: The four-in-one arthroplasty for the painful arc syndrome. *Clin Orthop* 1982;163:107.

9. Neer CS II, Marberry TA: On the disadvantages of radical acromionectomy. *J Bone Joint Surg* 1981;63A:416.

10. Watson M: Major ruptures of the rotator cuff: The results of surgical repair in 89 patients. *J Bone Joint Surg* 1985;67B:618–624.

11. Nirschl RP: Shoulder tendinitis, in Pettrone FP (ed): American Academy of Orthopaedic Surgeons *Symposium on Upper Extremity Injuries in Athletes*. St. Louis, CV Mosby, 1986, pp 322–337.

12. Nirschl RP: Autogenous patch graft as augmentation in rotator cuff surgery. *Video J Orthop*, 1988, vol 3, No. 1.

13. Weaver JK: A systematic approach to the surgical treatment of chronic shoulder pain. *Orthopedics* 1984;7:1697–1700.

14. Tibone JE, Elrod B, Jobe FW, et al: Surgical treatment of tears of the rotator cuff in athletes. *J Bone Joint Surg* 1986;68A:887–891.

15. Tibone JE, Jobe FW, Kerlan RK, et al: Shoulder impingement syndrome in athletes treated by an anterior acromioplasty. *Clin Orthop* 1985;198:134–140.

16. Ellman H: Arthroscopic subacromial decompression: Analysis of one to three year results. *Arthroscopy* 1987;3:173–181.

17. Ogilvie-Harris DJ, Wiley AM: Arthroscopic surgery of the shoulder: A general appraisal. *J Bone Joint Surg* 1987;68B:201–207.

CHAPTER 43

Compartment Syndromes

Pathophysiology of Compartment Syndromes

Frederick A. Matsen III, MD

A compartment syndrome is a condition in which increased tissue pressure within a limited space compromises the circulation and the function of the contents of that space.[1] Familiarity with the causes and effects of increased tissue pressure is central to the understanding of compartment syndromes. Unfortunately, the concept of "tissue pressure" is itself somewhat confusing: a nonhomogenous and nonisotropic material such as tissue cannot have a pressure in the same sense as a liquid or a gas. There are at least two definitions of "tissue pressure" that must be distinguished: the fluid tissue pressure and the net force per unit area applied to vessel walls.

The fluid tissue pressure ($P_T(H)$) is an important determinant of the fluid equilibrium across the walls of exchange vessels. This fluid tissue pressure, along with the capillary fluid pressure (P_C) and the effective osmotic pressures of tissue fluid (π_T) and plasma (π_C) determine the exchange of fluid across the vessel wall. These quantities are important in considerations of the fluid balance between intravascular and extravascular spaces of the compartment: the net fluid transfer out of the vessel is proportionate to

$$P_C - P_T(H) - \sigma(\pi_C - \pi_T)$$

where σ is the capillary membrane reflection coefficient.[2]

However, in discussing the effects of increased tissue pressure on local circulation in compartment syndromes, the tissue pressure to be considered is the net force per unit area exerted on the walls of intracompartmental vessels (P_O). In the remainder of this chapter, the term "tissue pressure" will be used to indicate this net pressure exerted on the outside of vessel walls.[1] Cells, fibers, fluids, gels, and matrices may all contribute to this tissue pressure. The law of Laplace determines the equilibrium about the vessel wall:

$$P_I - P_O = \frac{T}{R}$$

where P_I is the pressure inside the vessel, P_O is the pressure outside the vessel, T is the tension in the vessel wall, and R is the radius of the vessel.

When the vessel walls are flaccid (T = 0), the inside pressure (P_I) and the outside pressure (P_O) are equal. In a vessel with collapsible walls (such as a vein), the pressure of the blood inside the vessel cannot be less than the tissue pressure outside it. Increases in local tissue pressure, therefore, produce a corresponding increase in local venous pressure.[1]

Pathogenesis of Compartment Syndromes

A prerequisite for the development of increased tissue pressure is an envelope restricting the volume available to the enclosed tissue. Such envelopes include the epimysium, the fascia, the skin, and casts or other circumferential dressings. Examples of fascial envelopes include those surrounding the volar compartment of the forearm, the anterior compartment of the leg, and the deep posterior compartment of the leg. Pressure within an envelope may increase from a wide variety of causes, including bleeding and increased capillary permeability. Common clinical causes of compartment syndromes include fractures, diaphyseal osteotomies, crush injuries, prolonged limb compression (for example, in a patient with a drug overdose), unaccustomed exercise, and postischemic swelling, as can occur after prolonged femoral artery occlusion. Tissue pressure may also be increased iatrogenically by tight closure of fascial defects and the application of excessive traction to a fractured limb.[1] Furthermore, the external application of pressure to a limb further increases the pressure within it. It has been demonstrated, for example, that external application of 40 mm Hg of pressure to an intracompartmental muscle with a tissue pressure of 30 mm Hg produces a tissue pressure of 70 mm Hg.[1]

Increased tissue pressure also affects the local circulation. Hargens and associates[2] showed that in the normal canine anterolateral compartment the capillary pressure is approximately 25 mm Hg, the postcapillary venular pressure is 16 mm Hg, and the venular pressure is 6 mm Hg. Initially, one might suspect that a tissue pressure of 10 mm Hg would collapse the local venules, arresting local circulation, or that a pressure of 33 mm Hg would arrest local circulation by collapsing the local capillaries. Increased tissue pressure applied to the walls of collapsible vessels produces, however, a corresponding increase in the pressure within those vessels.[1] Thus, increased tissue pressure increases local venous pressure, lowering the local arteriovenous pressure gradient. No vascular occlusion occurs, as blood continues to flow down the pressure gradient from the arteries to the veins.[1]

Local blood flow is determined by the local arteriovenous gradient ($P_A - P_V$) and the local vascular resistance (R):

$$LBF = \frac{P_A - P_V}{R}$$

Thus, changes in local arteriovenous gradient have a direct effect on local blood flow. Ischemia is a potent stimulus for local vasodilatation, so that with the onset of ischemia, the local vascular resistance is reduced to a minimal value (R_{MIN}). Thus, the maximum local blood flow for a given arteriovenous gradient is:

$$LBF_{MAX} = \frac{P_A - P_V}{R_{MIN}}$$

This theory is consistent with the clinically observed ineffectiveness of sympathectomy and vasodilatory drugs in the treatment of compartment syndromes.[1]

Our model of the pathophysiology of a compartment syndrome may be summarized as follows (Fig. 43A–1): increased local tissue pressure increases the pressure within intracompartmental veins. The local arteriovenous gradient is thereby reduced, and with it the local blood flow. When local blood flow is no longer adequate to meet the metabolic demands of the tissue, the tissue loses function and eventually viability. Because the intracompartmental tissue pressure is usually less than the arterial blood pressure, the distal arterial blood flow and peripheral pulses often remain intact. Because the digital capillary bed drains into extracompartmental veins, the digital arteriovenous gradient and blood flow remain intact. Thus, peripheral pulses and digital circulation are poor indicators of the blood flow within the compartment.[1]

Experimental Studies

Having considered the theoretical aspects of compartment syndromes, let us turn to some experimental data concerning the effect of locally increased tissue pressure on local circulation. Reneman and associates[3] used intravital microscopy to evaluate the effect of increased tissue pressure on the microcirculation of the rabbit tenuissimus muscle. They observed that capillary blood flow ceased when the applied pressure was 25 to 30 mm Hg less than mean arterial pressure. No evidence of microvascular occlusion was found, even with applied pressures as high as 60 mm Hg.

Hargens and associates,[4] Akeson and associates,[5] and Mubarak and Hargens[6] conducted several studies demonstrating the greater compromise of neuromuscular viability and function by higher intracompartmental pressures.[5] For example, the severity of muscle damage as reflected by uptake ratios of technetium Tc 99m and pyrophosphate increased progressively with increased intracompartmental pressures. These same researchers quantitated the decrement in nerve conduction velocity as a function of intracompartmental pressure, again in the canine anterolateral compartment. Once more, the physiologic effect of tissue pressure became more severe as higher pressures were applied.[4] A pressure of

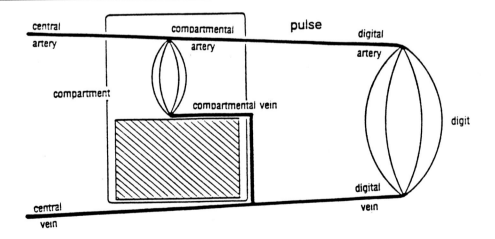

Fig. 43A–1 Comparison of local distal effects of increased tissue pressure. Within the affected compartment, locally increased tissue pressure (shaded block) increases local venous pressure and reduces the local arteriovenous gradient. The artery is not obstructed by its passage through the compartment; thus, the peripheral pulse remains intact. Because digital veins empty into veins that have a normal low pressure, the digital arteriovenous gradient is unaffected. Therefore, digital color, temperature, and capillary filling may be normal even in the presence of severely compromised intracompartmental circulation.

40 mm Hg applied for as long as 840 minutes did not arrest nerve conduction, whereas pressure of 50 mm Hg arrested nerve conduction in 330 minutes. Higher pressures required progressively less time to arrest nerve conduction.[4] Rorabeck and Clarke[7] demonstrated that the duration of pressure application was also a critical determinant of the recovery of nerve conduction in a dog model system. When pressures ranging from 40 to 80 mm Hg were applied for only four hours, full recovery of nerve conduction ensued. Complete recovery did not occur when these same pressures were applied for 12 hours.

The legs of human volunteers have also been used to investigate the effect of increased tissue pressure on local muscle oxygenation and nerve function. For example, when external pressure was applied to these normal limbs, higher applied pressures produced a greater reduction in anterior compartment muscle Po_2 (measured by mass spectrometry).[1] When external pressures were applied for a maximum of 80 minutes, pressures from 55 to 75 mm Hg were required to arrest peroneal nerve function in a group of three adult male subjects.[8]

Some clinical data are available on the tolerance of limbs for increased tissue pressure. Table 43A–1 shows tabulated results from three reports in which tissue pressure measurements were correlated with the results from surgical decompression. In the first group, function was normal at follow-up without surgical decompression despite pressures as high as 29 mm Hg. In the second group, a few patients had normal function at follow-up evaluation without surgical decompression despite pressures as high as 55 mm Hg. In the third group, consisting only of children, pressures as high as 45 mm Hg were consistent with normal follow-up function without surgical decompression. In the first group, 30 mm Hg was taken as the absolute indication for surgical decompression, so there are no data on patients with higher pressures who did not receive surgical decompression. In the second and third groups, clinical criteria were used as the prime indications for surgical decompression. The lowest intracompartmental pressure in the adult series requiring surgical decompression on clinical grounds was 45 mm Hg, and the corresponding value for the pediatric series was 33 mm Hg.

Variability in Pressure Tolerance

It is apparent that pressure tolerance varies among individual patients. One factor is the duration of the pressure increase. Lower tissue pressures can be tolerated for longer periods of time than can higher tissue pressures. Another factor appears to be the local arterial pressure. This effect can be predicted from our formula for local blood flow:

$$LBF = \frac{P_A - P_V}{R}$$

For a given local tissue and venous pressure (P_V), the resulting local blood flow depends largely on the local arterial pressure (P_A). A simple way to lower the local arterial pressure experimentally in a human volunteer is to raise the compartment above the level of the heart. This lowering of local arterial pressure can be measured directly or calculated by dividing the centimeters of elevation of the part by 1.3 cm of whole blood per mm Hg. Thus, raising the leg 55 cm above the level of the heart lowers the local arterial pressure by 43 mm Hg. This decrease in local arterial pressure is accompanied by a greater effect of increased tissue pressure in elevated limbs. For example, a pressure of 60 mm Hg applied to a limb level with the heart reduces the muscle oxygen tension to the same value as a pressure of 20 mm Hg applied to an elevated limb.[1] As another example, a pressure of 70 mm Hg was required to arrest nerve conduction when a subject's limb was level with the heart, whereas a pressure of only 35 mm Hg was required to arrest conduction in the peroneal nerve of the same subject when the limb was elevated 43 cm above the heart.[8] Thus, we predict that for a given increase in tissue pressure, any cause of lowered arterial pressure will further compromise the local arteriovenous gradient and blood flow. Clinically, decreased local arterial pressure may result from shock, peripheral vascular disease, or elevation of the limb.

While we are discussing the effects of limb elevation, it is essential to point out that elevation of the extremity above the level of the heart cannot reduce local venous

Table 43A-1
Clinical data on pressure tolerance

Study	No. of Patients	Pressure (mm Hg)	
		Maximum Without Decompression	Minimum With Decompression
Mubarak and Hargens[6]	135	29	30
Matsen et al[8]	31	55	45
Matsen and Veith[9]	11*	45	33

*This group consisted only of children.

pressure below the value of local tissue pressure.[1] Thus, it appears safe to state that local venous pressure can be greater than or equal to local tissue pressure but cannot be less than local tissue pressure.

We have seen that the tolerance for increased tissue pressure varies; that is, the physiologic effect of a given tissue pressure depends on the duration of pressure application and the local arterial pressure. Another factor that may alter local tissue pressure tolerance is the metabolic demands of the tissue. Rapidly metabolizing, traumatized tissue may require more blood flow to maintain its viability than does resting, uninjured muscle.

References

1. Matsen FA III: *Compartmental Syndromes*. New York, Grune & Stratton, 1980.
2. Hargens AR, Akeson WH, Mubarak SJ, et al: Fluid balance within the canine anterolateral compartment and its relationship to compartment syndromes. *J Bone Joint Surg* 1978;60A:499–505.
3. Reneman RS, Slaaf DW, Lindbom L, et al: Muscle blood-flow disturbances in compartment syndromes and the role of elevated total muscle-tissue pressure in these disturbances, in Hargens AR (ed): *Tissue Fluid Pressure and Composition*. Baltimore, Williams & Wilkins, 1981, pp 209–214.
4. Hargens AR, Romine JS, Sipe JC, et al: Peripheral nerve-conduction block by high muscle-compartment pressure. *J Bone Joint Surg* 1979;61A:192–200.
5. Akeson WH, Hargens AR, Garfin SR, et al: Muscle compartment syndromes and snake bites, in Hargens AR (ed): *Tissue Fluid Pressure and Composition*. Baltimore, Williams & Wilkins, 1981, pp 215–226.
6. Mubarak SJ, Hargens AR: Clinical use of the wick-catheter technique, in Hargens AR (ed): *Tissue Fluid Pressure and Composition*. Baltimore, Williams & Wilkins, 1981, pp 261–268.
7. Rorabeck CH, Clarke KM: The pathophysiology of the anterior tibial compartment syndrome: An experimental investigation. *J Trauma* 1978;18:299–304.
8. Matsen FA III, Mayo KA, Krugmire RB Jr, et al: A model compartmental syndrome in man with particular reference to the quantification of nerve function. *J Bone Joint Surg* 1977;59A:648–653.
9. Matsen FA, Veith RG: Compartmental syndromes in children. *J Pediatr Orthop* 1981;1:33–41.

P A R T B

The Diagnosis and Management of Chronic Compartment Syndrome

Cecil H. Rorabeck, MD, FRCS(C)

History

Chronic compartment syndrome is an exercise-related compartment syndrome characterized by local pain, swelling, and dysesthesia in the territory of the nerve crossing the compartment. The condition has usually been reported in the lower leg, but it has also been described in other anatomic locations. A number of terms have been used to describe chronic exercise-related compartment syndrome, including exertional compartment syndrome, medial tibial stress syndrome, shin splints, marked synovitis, and medial tibial syndrome.[1-5] All of these, however, should be looked upon as forms of chronic exercise-related compartment syndrome.

In 1881 Volkmann described the contracture that now bears his name. In his original monograph he believed that it was caused by prolonged blockage of arterial blood associated with the simultaneous occurrence of massive venous stasis. This original description of the acute compartment syndrome was later elaborated by others.[6-8] The existence of a chronic exercise-related compartment syndrome was not appreciated until Horn[9] and Hughes[10] noted the appearance of a compartment syndrome in army recruits after strenuous activity (route march) to which they were unaccustomed. They coined the term "march gangrene" to describe this condition. More recently, with the increasing emphasis on physical fitness and participatory sports among our population, the incidence of chronic compartment syndrome has undoubtedly increased. Mavor[11] pointed out that chronic exercise-related compartment syndrome could occur in the anterior tibial compartment of the leg. Others confirmed the presence of the condition and have recommended fasciotomy of the compartment involved as a method of treatment.[4,5,12,13] Although several investigators have pointed out that fasciotomy can relieve symptoms in most patients with chronic exertional compartment syndrome, the indications for this procedure have not, for the most part, been well defined.[4] Currently the clinical criteria for diagnosis remain uncertain, as is the role of tissue pressure measurements in the diagnosis.

Pathophysiology

The underlying cause of pain in the patient with chronic compartment syndrome is not entirely understood. Most investigators have suggested that the pain experienced by the athlete during exercise is probably related to muscle ischemia, because the symptoms rapidly subside after cessation of the activity. Others have suggested that the pain may be the result of metabolic breakdown products within the muscle itself.[4,14] When a muscle contracts during exercise, it increases its bulk by approximately 20%. There appears to be a group of patients who have relatively tight, unyielding fascia so that when the muscle expands during a normal contraction, tissue pressure is increased within that muscle. As the tissue pressure rises, muscle arteriolar blood flow is compromised. With repetitive muscle contractures, the tissue pressure increases between each contraction until ischemic muscle pain is felt. Blood flow studies have demonstrated diminished flow to muscles in experimental models of compartment syndrome.[1,14,15]

Clinical Studies

Patients with chronic compartment syndrome have clinical symptoms related to the anterior compartment, the anterior and posterior compartments, or the posterior compartments alone. Thus, there are three modes of clinical presentation. Those patients with chronic anterior compartment syndrome give histories of pain centered diffusely over the anterior compartment and occurring at variable periods following the initiation of the activity (usually running). The pain is frequently, although not always, bilateral. It usually radiates down toward the ankle and is associated with a feeling of swelling in the leg and/or dysesthesia on the dorsum of the foot. Physical findings in these patients are invariably normal. The patients are usually unable to "run through" the pain they are experiencing.

The second group of patients are those who have pain involving both the anterior and posterior compartment of the leg. The pain, again, is activity-related. The anterior pain is in the same location as described above and the posterior pain typically occurs along the posteromedial border of the tibia. It generally occurs in the middle or distal third and is spread out over an area several centimeters long. It begins at variable times after exercise, may or may not be bilateral, and is frequently associated with a sensation of swelling as well as dysesthesia on the medial or plantar aspect of the foot.

The third group of patients, those with posterior pain alone, have pain located along the posteromedial border of the tibia, usually radiating toward the ankle. The patients' posterior pain pattern is identical to that described above. Once again, the patients are usually unable to "run through" their pain and the posteromedial pain is sufficiently severe to prevent them from engaging in their activity.

Clinical findings in all three groups are almost always normal; the occasional exception is some discomfort deep along the posteromedial border of the tibia. The differential diagnosis includes stress fracture, deep venous thrombosis, and periostitis.

The Role of Tissue Pressure Measurements

Patients with histories compatible with a clinical diagnosis of chronic compartment syndrome should undergo tissue pressure studies. Most investigators agree that the diagnosis of chronic anterior compartment syndrome of the leg depends on the clinical history and physical findings. A history of exercise-induced pain with a subjective feeling of fullness or swelling of the extremity, with or without impairment of muscle function and dysesthesia in the area of the terminal branch of the deep peroneal nerve, may be diagnostic of chronic anterior compartment syndrome of the leg. Although these clinical symptoms and signs are clearly important, an unequivocal diagnosis of chronic exertional compartment syndrome cannot be made without dynamic studies, including pre-exercise and postexercise tissue pressure measurements.

A number of techniques are available to measure intramuscular pressure. These include the needle manometer, the constant-infusion technique, the wick catheter method, the slit catheter monitoring system, and microtip pressure transducers with or without continuous infusion.[15-18] Although all of these techniques were originally developed to measure compartment pressure at rest, a number of them have also been tried successfully and are currently recommended for monitoring dynamic intramuscular pressure during exercise.[17] Because of the various methods used to measure compartment pressure and the variation in measurement parameters, the interpretation of the pressure values elicited is sometimes confusing. For example, some investigators have suggested that resting pressures of more than 10 mm Hg are diagnostic of chronic exertional compartment syndrome. Others have suggested that postexercise pressure measurements are more important than resting or dynamic pressure studies. There is also confusion about the role of dynamic pressure studies. McDermott and associates,[3] as well as Puranen and Alavaikko,[19] pointed out that mean muscular pressure in excess of 50 mm Hg was a useful diagnostic measurement of chronic anterior compartment syndrome. Others, however, have questioned the validity of this.[4]

When choosing a system to measure compartment pressure in patients with suspected compartment syndrome, it is important to understand the strengths and limitations of each system. The technique used to measure compartment pressures should allow the investigator to measure pre-exercise pressure, dynamic pressure measurements (during exercise), and postexercise pressure measurements. All three measurements are important and techniques that do not allow all three to be made are substantially limited in usefulness. Thus, while the needle and needle-manometer techniques are useful for measuring pre-exercise and postexercise pressures, they nevertheless are not suitable for measuring dynamic pressure while the patient is running. The wick and slit catheter systems allow both static and dynamic pressure measurements. The Stryker system allows static pressure measurements but, because the unit is hand-held and has to be strapped to the leg, its accuracy may suffer during dynamic pressure studies.

Resting Pressure Studies

At University Hospital, we use the slit catheter system. The history indicates the compartment to be studied. We introduce 1 ml of lidocaine into the skin and subcutaneous tissue, so that it infiltrates the fascia overlying the affected compartment. A 16-gauge needle is then introduced at an acute angle to the long axis of the extremity. The needle can be felt to pierce the deep fascia and enter the muscle of the compartment. The slit catheter is hooked to the recording system and flushed so that there are no air bubbles in the system. It is imperative that the catheter be able to suspend a drop of saline so that an air bubble (and hence an artificially low reading) is not introduced into the compartment at the time of resting pressure measurements. The catheter is then passed along the barrel of the needle into the compartment and the needle is withdrawn. The catheter is taped firmly to the skin. Care must be taken to avoid circumferential taping that can artificially increase resting pressure values. With the patient in the supine position and with the machine at zero, resting pressures are now recorded.

Dynamic Pressure Measurements

The patient, who is in shorts and running shoes, walks to the treadmill and is asked to run on the treadmill until symptoms are reproduced (Fig. 43B–1). It is extremely important that the patients be able to reproduce their symptoms during the pressure studies for if they cannot, then the true meaning of normal or low pressure values cannot be evaluated. While the patient is running, pressure measurements are made continuously. These are recorded graphically as peak-to-peak pressure and mean muscular pressure.

Postexercise Pressure Measurements

Once the symptoms have been reproduced, the patient is asked to lie supine and postexercise pressure measurements are made immediately. Two important observations are the value immediately after exercise and the time taken for this value to return to the normal resting value. Normal values should be achieved within 15 minutes.

In a group of 75 asymptomatic university athletes, the normal pre-exercise resting value for anterior and deep posterior compartment pressure measurements was 10.9 ± 1.1 mm Hg. Similarly, the immediate postexercise pressure in this same group of normals was 18.1 ± 2 mm Hg. The postexercise value had returned to normal after 15 minutes (Fig. 43B–2). In contrast, patients with chronic compartment syndrome involving either the anterior or the deep posterior compartment often had resting pressures little different from those of controls (Fig. 43B–3). The sine qua non of an accurate tissue pressure diagnosis, therefore, is the immediate postexercise pressure and a sluggish return to pre-exercise values.

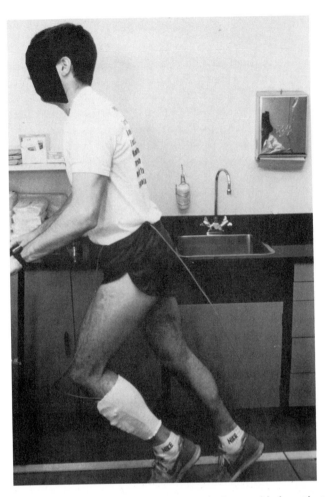

Fig. 43B–1 The dynamic phase of testing is shown, with the patient running on the treadmill.

Role of Magnetic Resonance Imaging

Newer, noninvasive techniques allow the assessment of changes in cross-sectional areas of muscle or in muscle density. Studies are underway to determine the role of magnetic resonance imaging as an adjunct to the diagnosis of chronic compartment syndrome. This may help the surgeon identify those patients who are likely to be helped by surgery.

Treatment

Nonsurgical Treatment

Not all patients with chronic anterior or posterior leg pain and increased tissue pressure during exercise require surgical treatment. Many patients will respond to a change in footwear, physiotherapy, anti-inflammatory drugs, and the like. The indication for surgery, therefore, is failure to respond to nonsurgical treatment in the presence of abnormal pressure values.

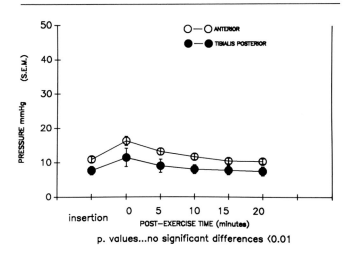

Fig. 43B-2 Insertional and postexercise pressures of normal volunteers are shown in mm Hg for both the anterior and tibialis posterior compartments.

Surgical Procedure

Fasciotomy of the anterior compartment is best done through two vertical incisions (Fig. 43B–4). The incision should be centered approximately 3 cm lateral to the crest of the tibia. The fascia is exposed proximally and distally and separated from the overlying fat. The terminal branch of the deep peroneal nerve must be identified at the point where it pierces the intermuscular septum in the distal third of the leg. If the nerve is cut, anesthesia on the dorsum of the foot may result. An incision is made in the fascia 1 cm in front of the anterior intramuscular septum both proximally and distally. The fasciotomy sites are connected by means of long Metzenbaum scissors. It is not ordinarily necessary to do a fasciotomy of the lateral compartment; if, however, one does need to be done, it can be completed easily through this incision by retracting posteriorly and incising the fascia 1 cm behind the intermuscular septum.

The technique of surgical fasciotomy of the deep posterior compartment is shown in Figure 43B–5. Again, two vertical incisions are made in the leg 1 cm behind the posteromedial border of the tibia. The saphenous vein is identified in the proximal incision and retracted anteriorly along with the nerve. The deep fascia is incised. To expose the deep compartment, it is necessary to detach the soleal bridge. This gives access to the deep posterior compartment, including the flexor digitorum and the tibialis posterior. The neurovascular bundle and the tibialis posterior tendon are identified and the fascia overlying the tendon is incised proximally and distally. The tibialis posterior, which is the key to posterior compartment decompression, is usually constricted proximally between the two origins of the flexor hallucis longus. It is important to enlarge that opening and to look for possible constriction during the surgical

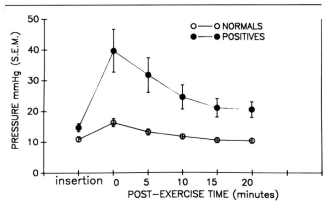

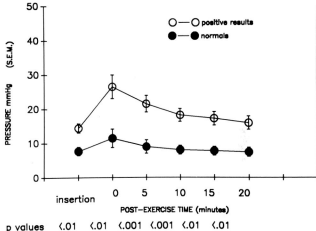

Fig. 43B-3 The postexercise pressures of patients with chronic compartment syndrome and normal volunteers are shown for the anterior (**top**) and the tibialis posterior compartments (**bottom**).

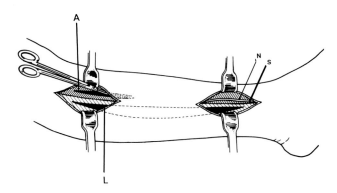

Fig. 43B-4 Anterior (A) and lateral (L) fasciotomies are shown with the terminal branch of the deep peroneal nerve (N) and intermuscular septum (S) identified.

procedure. The tourniquet is then released. Meticulous hemostasis is essential. The tissue and skin are closed over a ⅛-inch drain to minimize the risk of hematoma formation.

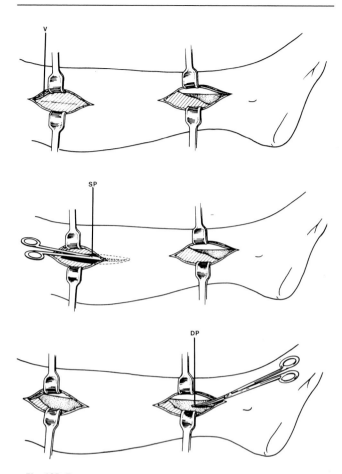

Fig. 43B–5 Deep posterior fasciotomy. **Top:** Two vertical incisions are made. The saphenous vein (V) is identified and retracted anteriorly. **Center:** The superficial posterior compartment (SP) is then entered and released. **Bottom:** Deep fascia is incised and the deep posterior compartment (DP) released.

Postoperative Management

The patients are examined postoperatively in the recovery room. They immediately begin active range-of-motion exercises for the ankle. They are advised to ice the leg. Fasciotomy is normally done as an outpatient procedure, but the patients are monitored very closely by the physiotherapist to ensure maintenance of the range of motion. If this is not instituted immediately, there is increased risk of scarring and recurrent compartment syndrome. The dressings are removed after 48 hours and a simple bandage is applied. The patients are advised to discontinue using their crutches as soon as they feel able to. Once soft-tissue healing has occurred, unrestricted walking is prescribed. Gentle straight-line jogging begins two weeks postoperatively and progresses over the next six weeks. Total rehabilitation time varies between six weeks and three months. Patients undergoing release of the deep posterior compartment generally need longer for rehabilitation than those undergoing simple anterior compartment fasciot-

omy. It is important to point this out to the patient in advance.

Results

To date, 25 patients have undergone fasciotomy at University Hospital for either anterior or deep posterior compartment syndrome. These patients have been followed up for a minimum of two years and the results of their surgery have been reported in detail elsewhere.[20,21] All patients had abnormal pressure values with an average resting pressure of 15 mm Hg. Dynamic or peak-to-peak studies were done in all patients, but these studies were found to be less useful. Although the amplitude of the peak was not thought to be particularly important, the shape of the peak and in particular the widening of the peak appeared to be more prominent as symptoms began to develop during running. The single most important study in this group of patients was the postexercise pressure measurement. The average postexercise pressure measurement was 37.3 mm Hg; this decreased to approximately 20 mm Hg after 20 minutes. It is important to note that none of the symptomatic patients in this study returned to the pre-exercise level within the time constraints of the study. Thus, a delayed return to pre-exercise values persisting beyond 15 minutes in patients with symptomatic leg pain is the single most important diagnostic pressure study.

A minimum of one year after surgery, the 25 patients were asked to evaluate the results of the fasciotomy and their level of physical activity. All 13 patients who had undergone fasciotomy for chronic anterior compartment syndrome had relief of their symptoms. In addition, ten of the 13 reported that they had been able to increase their physical activity as a result of the surgery. Three patients in this group reported that their level of physical activity had not changed as a result of the surgery but they were still satisfied with the procedure.

Three patients of the 25 were not satisfied with the procedure and were considered treatment failures. All three had recurrence of symptoms with physical activity; their level of physical activity was either unchanged or had decreased after the surgery. It is important to note that these three patients all underwent decompression of the deep posterior compartment. Repeat pressure studies showed prolonged elevation of the post-exercise pressure measurements in all three. Two patients underwent a second surgical procedure to decompress the deep posterior compartment. This procedure was successful in one.

Subsequent investigation of these patients and further experimental work demonstrated that failures of decompression of the deep posterior compression are probably related to failure to decompress the tibialis posterior muscle adequately at the time of fasciotomy.[1] Currently, as part of the decompression of the deep posterior compartment, we expose the tibialis posterior muscle and the musculotendinous junction and release the fascia covering the tibialis posterior. Also, the dissection is taken proximally and the bipennate origin of flexor hallucis longus is released to allow the tibialis posterior to glide freely through this hiatus. These patients now participate in a very early aggressive physiotherapy program that begins in the recovery room and consists of range-of-motion exercises to minimize the possibility of scarring and, thus, reformation of the fascia covering the compartment.

Discussion

The diagnosis of chronic compartment syndrome in patients with symptomatic leg pain is made on the basis of an accurate clinical history supplemented with intramuscular pressure studies. The medical history of a patient with chronic compartment syndrome includes exercise-related pain beginning at variable times after the initiation of the activity. Although it has been reported that patients with symptomatic chronic anterior compartment syndrome have increased intramuscular pressure at rest when compared to a group of normal controls, a resting pressure above 10 mm Hg is not by itself sufficient for the diagnosis of chronic anterior compartment syndrome. The standard deviations reported in the literature are too great and, thus, resting pressure values must be supplemented with a careful study of dynamic and postexercise pressure studies.

Although there is a tendency for patients with symptomatic chronic compartment syndrome to have higher peak-to-peak pressures during exercise than normal controls, careful analysis revealed no statistically significant difference when the height and the width of the peak were compared. Thus, dynamic pressure studies alone are unreliable for identifying a patient with chronic compartment syndrome who is likely to be helped by surgical fasciotomy. Part of the reason for the wide variation in values of dynamic peak-to-peak pressure measurements may be the depth of calf at which the catheter is placed, a variable that cannot be completely controlled and one that has been shown to produce variable dynamic pressure measurements.[22] Some investigators have suggested that dynamic pressure measurements are extremely helpful in identifying the patient with chronic compartment syndrome who is likely to be helped by fasciotomy, but our experience suggests the opposite.[3]

A prolonged increase in intramuscular pressure recorded immediately after a period of exercise remains the most helpful study. It has been demonstrated that the mean postexercise pressure taken at time zero in symptomatic patients with chronic compartment syndrome is significantly different from that in a comparable group of normal controls.[20,21] Thus, postexercise pressures in excess of the insertional pressure or pressures in excess of 15 mm Hg persisting for longer than 15 minutes are useful signs of chronic compartment syndrome likely to benefit from surgical fasciotomy.

Fasciotomy is an effective way of relieving chronic compartment syndrome. The success rate reported here is comparable to those in other series.[5,13] Nevertheless, the three reported failures of fasciotomy of the deep posterior compartment are of concern. A careful review of these patients, combined with a careful assessment of our surgical technique, leads us to believe that the failures resulted from failure to decompress the tibialis posterior adequately. The other possible cause of failure is the postoperative management. We recommend that these patients begin vigorous physiotherapy immediately postoperatively, with the knee, ankle, and foot put through a full range of motion. Weightbearing as tolerated is allowed immediately; the patients are encouraged to use crutches for the first few days but to discontinue them as quickly as possible. After wound healing, the patient is encouraged to begin swimming, cycling, and straight-line running. If these guidelines are followed, the success rate will be high.

References

1. Davey JR, Rorabeck CH, Fowler PJ: The tibialis posterior muscle compartment: An unrecognized cause of exertional compartment syndrome. *Am J Sports Med* 1984;12:391–397.
2. Leach RE, Hammond G, Stryker WS: Anterior tibial compartment syndrome: Acute and chronic. *J Bone Joint Surg* 1967;49A:451–462.
3. McDermott AG, Marble AE, Yabley RH, et al: Monitoring dynamic anterior compartment pressures during exercise: A new technique using the STIC catheter. *Am J Sports Med* 1982;10:83–89.
4. Rorabeck CH, Bourne RB, Fowler PJ: The surgical treatment of exertional compartment syndrome in athletes. *J Bone Joint Surg* 1983;65A:1245–1251.
5. Wallenstein R: Results of fasciotomy in patients with medial tibial syndrome or chronic anterior-compartment syndrome. *J Bone Joint Surg* 1983;65A:1252–1255.
6. Murphy JB: Myositis. *JAMA* 1914;63:1249–1255.
7. Petersen F: Über Ischämische Muskellähmung. *Arch Klin Chir* 1888;37:675–677.
8. Thomas JJ: Nerve involvement in the ischaemic paralysis and contracture of Volkmann. *Ann Surg* 1909;49:330–370.
9. Horn CE: Acute ischaemia of the anterior tibial muscle and the long extensor muscles of the toes. *J Bone Joint Surg* 1945;27:615–622.
10. Hughes JR: Ischaemic necrosis of the anterior tibial muscles due to fatigue. *J Bone Joint Surg* 1948;30B:581–594.
11. Mavor GE: The anterior tibial syndrome. *J Bone Joint Surg* 1956;38B:513–517.
12. Reneman RS: *The Anterior and Lateral Compartment Syndrome of the Leg.* The Hague, Mouton, 1968, p 176.
13. Styf FJ, Korner L: Chronic anterior compartment syndrome of the lower leg: Results of treatment by fasciotomy. *J Bone Joint Surg*, in press.

14. Baumann JU, Sutherland DH, Hänggi A: Intramuscular pressure during walking: An experimental study using the wick catheter technique. *Clin Orthop* 1979;145:292–299.

15. Mubarak SJ, Hargens AR, Owen CA, et al: The wick catheter technique for measurement of intramuscular pressure: A new research and clinical tool. *J Bone Joint Surg* 1976;58A:1016–1020.

16. Matsen FA III, Mayo KA, Sheridan GW, et al: Monitoring of intramuscular pressure. *Surgery* 1976;79:702–709.

17. Rorabeck CH, Castle GS, Hardie R, et al: Compartmental pressure measurements: An experimental investigation using the slit catheter. *J Trauma* 1981;21:446–449.

18. Whitesides TE, Haney TC, Morimoto K, et al: Tissue pressure measurements as a determinant for the need of fasciotomy. *Clin Orthop* 1975;113:43B–51.

19. Puranen J, Alavaikko A: Intracompartmental pressure increase on exertion in patients with chronic compartment syndrome in the leg. *J Bone Joint Surg* 1981;63A:1304–1309.

20. Rorabeck CH, Bourne RB, Fowler PJ, et al: The role of tissue pressure measurement in diagnosing chronic anterior compartment syndrome. *Am J Sports Med* 1988;16:143–146.

21. Rorabeck CH, Fowler PJ, Nott L: The results of fasciotomy in the management of chronic exertional compartment syndrome. *Am J Sports Med* 1988;16:224–227.

22. Kirkebo A, Wisnes A: Regional tissue fluid pressure in rat calf muscle during sustained contraction or stretch. *Acta Physiol Scand* 1982;114:551–556.

CHAPTER 44

Office Management of Athletic Injuries of the Hand and Wrist

James E. Culver, Jr., MD

Hand injuries occur frequently in sports activities. These injuries are often ignored or minimized because they are not totally disabling. Delay in treatment is unfortunate because prompt and proper care often shortens overall recovery time and prevents long-term sequelae. In addition, many of these injuries can be treated adequately with simple splinting or taping techniques.

While this discussion deals with those hand and wrist injuries that can be treated nonsurgically in an office setting, it is important for the physician to recognize when an injury is more serious and needs surgical care.

In acute injuries there is often a tendency to examine the radiograph and ignore the patient. However, careful history-taking and examination often point to the diagnosis. It is important to obtain a detailed history of how the injury occurred and to determine the consequences of the injury and what type of treatment, if any, was provided. Was there immediate deformity? Was there an open wound? What was the location of swelling? What was the extent of swelling? Where was the pain located and how intense was it? Did someone "pop" a joint back in place? Is there any numbness? Is there any loss of motion? Does it hurt when it moves? Was there a previous injury? The answers to these and other questions help to establish the diagnosis.

A careful physical examination is then carried out. Clinical findings such as pain, swelling, deformity, ecchymosis, and tenderness should be critically evaluated, for they are signs that there has been a significant injury. The severity of the injury is usually in proportion to these physical findings. The examination should be systematic and complete. Sensation must be checked and specific areas of tenderness sought. Joint range of motion and stability are tested, with special attention paid to pain during these manipulations.

Radiographic evaluation is important and multiple views may be needed. Special radiographic studies should focus on the specific area of injury discovered during the history-taking and physical examination. Special studies include various oblique views, carpal tunnel views, bone scan, tomograms, and arthrograms. Computed tomographic scans and magnetic resonance imaging are still being investigated, but these techniques are proving to be helpful in diagnosing hidden fractures.

The treatment of an acutely injured hand includes immobilization of the injured part, ice, and elevation. This treatment should be initiated immediately, even before the patient is referred for medical evaluation.

Swelling, ecchymosis, and pain, including pain on motion, should not be ignored even if a fracture or dislocation cannot be identified radiographically. Follow-up is important until the patient is completely asymptomatic and the hand is fully rehabilitated.

Types of Immobilization for Hand and Wrist Injuries

Immobilization of the injured part may be accomplished by a variety of taping, splinting, or casting techniques. For minor finger injuries, "buddy" taping may be adequate.

Molded dorsal aluminum splints lined with a layer of moleskin make good finger splints (Fig. 44–1). These splints can be molded to fit a particular finger and trimmed to treat just the part involved. Placing the splint on the dorsum of the digit allows the palmar side to be free so that the finger can be used in a limited way. These splints may also be made of a thermoplastic material and held on with Velcro straps. These plastic splints are particularly useful when healing has progressed enough for the splint to be removed for active exercises. Carefully molded plaster finger splints can provide good fixation, but they are more difficult to apply and remove and less durable than metal or plastic splints.

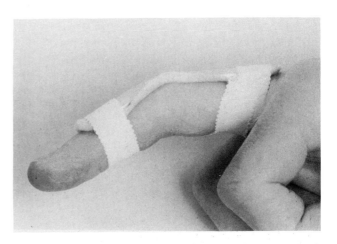

Fig. 44–1 A dorsal aluminum splint molded into a semicircle by pounding over a metal pipe, bent to accommodate the desired joint position, and lined with a layer of moleskin. Placing it on the dorsum of the finger leaves the palmar surface free to function.

More extensive splints for the hand and wrist made from plaster or the newer casting materials can provide good immobilization. Plaster makes an ideal splint because it can be molded to fit the injured part precisely. For longer-term treatment, the splint can be made from the newer casting materials or from a thermoplastic splinting material. Velcro straps can be used for easy removal. The various prefabricated orthoses—with or without thumb extensions—provide good fixation if the preset angle for the wrist is appropriate. These are useful once healing has progressed sufficiently for range-of-motion exercises to be initiated. They also provide good protection for activities, including sports, but may not be allowed in certain contact sports.

Custom-made splints are superior to prefabricated splints because they fit better. The extra time required to make them is worthwhile. In general, the splint or cast should immobilize only the injured part, leaving the rest of the hand free.

A rubberized cast[1] or orthosis, which can be made by an orthotist or a trainer, may be allowed in contact sports at the high school and college levels. These "playing casts" provide adequate fixation for most fractures, but are bulky and cumbersome and interfere with effective use of the hand. Enough of the hand must be immobilized to protect the injured part. A finger fracture generally requires a forearm cast that includes the involved and adjacent fingers. Whether or not these orthoses are allowed in an individual event is up to the officials.

Contusions

Contusions usually result from a direct blow to the dorsum of the hand or a fall onto the palm of the hand. Occasionally they appear on the palm because of the impact of a racket handle or bat. Treatment of a contusion is designed primarily to relieve symptoms and includes ice, elevation, rest, and protection. Usually, the hand is splinted in the correct position with the wrist in slight extension, the metacarpophalangeal joints flexed, and the proximal interphalangeal joints in near extension. In general, when there is contusion to the dorsum of the hand, the entire hand should be splinted from the proximal forearm to the fingertips. The patient must be examined frequently so that treatment can progress as swelling and pain subside. The injured part must be protected until the swelling has subsided completely and there is full range of motion without pain. The patient may participate in sports if the contused area can be protected adequately by a splint, brace, cast, or padding (depending on the nature of the injury and the sport involved).

Mallet Injuries

A mallet deformity consists of a flexed distal interphalangeal joint that cannot be extended actively to neutral because of an injury to the extensor tendon over the dorsum of the joint. The mechanism of injury is a blow to the extended fingertip that forces the distal interphalangeal joint into flexion against a tightly contracted extensor tendon, which gives way under the excessive flexion force. The patient experiences swelling, pain, and tenderness over the dorsum of the joint and is unable to extend the joint actively. Passive extension is usually possible unless hindered by pain. There is a spectrum of injury from stretching of the extensor tendon to avulsion of the tendon, to avulsion of a small bony fragment, to a large fracture fragment involving a significant portion of the articular surface of the proximal end of the distal phalanx.

A true lateral radiograph of the distal interphalangeal joint is important to rule out an avulsion fracture or a fracture involving the articular surface. It is even more important to recognize any volar subluxation of the joint indicating additional significant injury to the collateral ligaments. If joint subluxation is present, along with a fracture fragment involving more than 30% of the articular surface of the distal phalanx, surgery may be indicated.

Less severe injuries can be treated by simple splinting of the joint in full extension. Forced extension of a swollen distal interphalangeal joint can lead to necrosis of the skin over the dorsum of the joint. In this situation, it is better to splint the joint in near extension initially and then, as the swelling subsides, to increase the extension. My preference is a lightly padded dorsal metal splint (Fig. 44–2) that holds the joint in a neutral position. A variety of other available splints (Fig. 44–3) can provide adequate treatment. Only the distal interphalangeal joint should be splinted, leaving the proximal interphalangeal joint free to move.[2] Immobiliza-

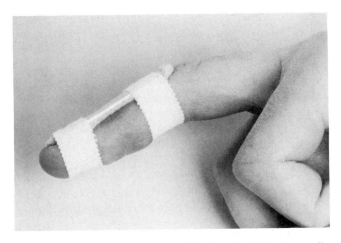

Fig. 44–2 A dorsal mallet finger splint. A molded aluminum splint lined with moleskin holds the distal interphalangeal joint in full extension. It is not necessary to immobilize the proximal interphalangeal joint; it can be left free for active exercise.

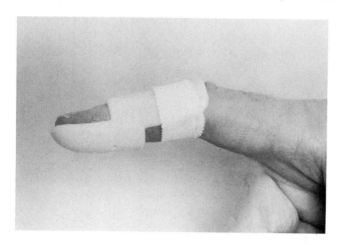

Fig. 44–3 A plastic prefabricated mallet finger splint that is commercially available in many sizes.

tion should be continuous for at least six weeks, followed by an additional two weeks of night-time splinting while active flexion exercises are begun. There may be some mild residual deformity. This type of splinting can produce a satisfactory result even in mallet injuries untreated for as long as four to six weeks.

Boutonnière Injury

A boutonnière injury is a flexion deformity of the proximal interphalangeal joint with a secondary extension contracture of the distal interphalangeal joint, secondary to an injury to the extensor mechanism overlying the proximal interphalangeal joint. The extensor mechanism injury involves disruption of the central slip from its attachment to the base of the middle phalanx and a volar subluxation of the lateral bands, secondary to a tear in the triangular ligament distal to the proximal interphalangeal joint. Active extension forces then pass through the volarly subluxated lateral bands, resulting in excessive extension at the distal interphalangeal joint with limited extensor force at the proximal interphalangeal joint. This injury is usually secondary to a blow to the end of a finger that forcefully flexes the proximal interphalangeal joint against a tight extensor mechanism. It may also occur from a direct blow to the dorsum of the finger distal to the proximal interphalangeal joint.

At the time of the injury there is swelling, pain, and tenderness localized over the dorsum of the proximal interphalangeal joint. The patient is unable to extend the joint actively but usually can do so passively. If the joint can be fully extended passively, the patient can often maintain that position. This is possible because the lateral bands relocate to the dorsum of the joint and, in that position, can hold the joint in full exten-

sion. However, with flexion, the lateral bands again subluxate volarly and active extension is impossible.

Treatment consists of splinting only the proximal interphalangeal joint in full extension (Fig. 44–4) continuously for eight weeks. It must be stressed that at no time should the joint be allowed out of the splint unless it is held in full extension. Joint motion should not be tested, and the splint should not be removed for showers. During this period, active flexion exercises for the distal interphalangeal joint are encouraged. After eight weeks, active flexion and extension exercises are initiated with the splint worn at night for an additional two to three weeks. If the athlete is to continue participating in sports, the proximal interphalangeal joint must be securely immobilized in full extension for at least 12 weeks.

If the proximal interphalangeal joint cannot be fully extended passively at the time of the initial injury, the lateral bands may be subluxated and trapped under the condyles of the proximal phalanx. Surgery is then indicated. If the patient is being treated with an extension splint, it is imperative that full extension has been obtained and maintained. If full extension cannot be obtained initially, a dynamic extension splint (Fig. 44–5) can be tried for one to two weeks, after which there is usually full extension. If full extension cannot be obtained after one to two weeks, surgery is indicated to reposition and repair the extensor mechanism.

Failure to treat the boutonnière injury will result in a permanently stiff and contracted proximal interphalangeal joint, significantly limiting the function of the finger. The ligaments, including the palmar plate, become secondarily contracted, making surgical correction very difficult and the outcome hard to predict.

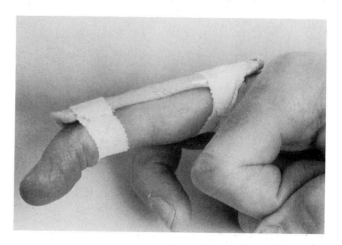

Fig. 44–4 A dorsal boutonnière splint holding the proximal interphalangeal joint in full extension. The distal interphalangeal joint is left free for active flexion.

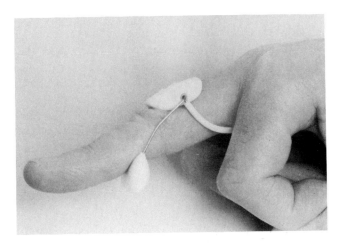

Fig. 44–5 A dynamic extension splint that is commercially available in various sizes. It is important that the extension force be confined to the proximal interphalangeal joint and that the distal pad be proximal to the distal interphalangeal joint so that this joint is not hyperextended. The splint must be adjusted so that there is minimal tension or the patient will not be able to wear it for more than a few minutes. The patient is instructed not to flex the proximal interphalangeal joint actively.

Ligament Injuries

Ligament injuries are frequently referred to as sprains. A first-degree sprain is a mild injury of the ligament. A second-degree sprain signifies a partial tear of the ligament. A third-degree sprain is a complete tear of the ligament. Ligament injuries are common in the hand and wrist. Treatment depends on the severity of the injury. A first-degree sprain needs little treatment, whereas second- and third-degree sprains should be treated carefully. The swelling that accompanies a severe ligament injury may last for 12 to 18 months and even then the joint may never return to its original size. This prolonged swelling is often disturbing to the patient who expects the swelling to resolve in a couple of weeks.

Proximal Interphalangeal Joint

The proximal interphalangeal joint is especially susceptible to ligament injury. Partial tears of the collateral ligaments are common in sports because of forces applied to the side of the finger. The swelling is localized to the side of the injury and may be extensive. Mild sprains can be treated with buddy taping to the adjacent finger, generally the finger adjacent to the side of the injury. Taping should continue until the swelling and tenderness have subsided. Most partial tears and even some complete collateral ligament tears are stable because of the joint configuration. However, if a portion of the palmar plate is also torn, instability may be present. It is, therefore, important to test for joint stability by stressing the injured collateral ligament. If the joint

is stable, it should be splinted for approximately three weeks, usually in 20 to 30 degrees of flexion. Only the proximal interphalangeal joint itself need be splinted. A molded aluminum splint can be applied either dorsally or palmarly. After three weeks, guarded range of motion exercises are begun. As the discomfort and swelling subside, the rehabilitation program is advanced.

The joint should be protected during any sports activities until there is full range of painless motion. Radiographs often show small avulsion fractures adjacent to one side of the joint. These avulsion fragments represent partial tears of the collateral ligaments. They are treated as ligament injuries.

When a proximal interphalangeal joint dislocates, one or more ligaments are torn. The palmar plate is avulsed from the base of the middle phalanx and portions of one or both collateral ligaments are torn. These dislocations can usually be easily reduced by manipulation with the patient under local anesthesia. Following reduction, the joint is usually stable. They must be immobilized in about 20 degrees of flexion for three weeks to allow ligament healing adequate to prevent joint hyperextension. If the joint is stable, active flexion exercises are encouraged after the first week, but the joint is prevented from extending beyond 20 degrees of flexion by means of a dorsal extension-block splint. If one of the collateral ligaments is unstable under stress but the joint is functionally stable, motion may hinder healing and should not be started for three to four weeks. As healing progresses, the splinting may be changed to buddy taping. The joint must be protected from hyperextension forces for at least eight weeks or until it is asymptomatic. If the joint is functionally unstable, surgical repair is needed.[3]

Small chip fractures, which are often seen at the base of the middle phalanx, are avulsion fractures representing a small tear in the palmar plate. These injuries are treated with a metal splint until swelling and discomfort subside and then by buddy taping and flexion exercises.

For most sports the proximal interphalangeal joint can be protected sufficiently for the athlete to participate. Whether or not to participate is an individual decision based on the severity of the injury and the sport involved.

Metacarpophalangeal Joints

Ligament injuries of the metacarpophalangeal joints are not nearly as common as those of the proximal interphalangeal joint. When the joint is in full extension, the collateral ligaments are lax. Therefore, a deviating force applied to the extended finger does not place much stress on the collateral ligament. However, when the joint is fully flexed, the ligaments are tight and any deforming force may injure a collateral ligament. The collateral ligaments, therefore, are tested for stability by fully flexing the metacarpophalangeal joint and then applying stress in the lateral direction. If there is pain on stress of one of the collateral ligaments in the metacarpophalangeal joint, the joint should be splinted to avoid stress to that ligament. After three weeks, guarded flexion exercises should be encouraged. Splinting is often needed for six to eight weeks until there is painless flexion. As discomfort subsides, the finger can be treated by taping it to the finger adjacent to the side of the injury.

Metacarpophalangeal Joint of the Thumb

Injury to the ulnar collateral ligament of the metacarpophalangeal joint of the thumb is common in athletics. This injury is particularly common in skiers, who often get their thumbs caught in the straps of the ski poles when they fall. It is important to distinguish between a partial and a complete tear of the ligament, because a complete tear requires surgical treatment. Before ligament stability is tested, a radiograph should be obtained to rule out an avulsion fracture. If an avulsion fracture is present, stressing the ligament is unnecessary and might even displace the fracture. If there is more than minimal displacement of the fracture, or there is rotation of the fracture, surgery is recommended. If no fracture is seen radiographically, the ligament should be stressed with the metacarpophalangeal joint in maximal flexion.[4] The fully flexed position places the stress entirely on the collateral ligament itself. Because of the pain that occurs with testing, using local anesthesia on the joint makes the examination more reliable. Stress on the injured thumb should be compared with stress on the uninjured thumb. Stress radiographs of both thumbs can be made for documentation. Angulation of 30 degrees, or more than 20 degrees over that of the contralateral thumb, indicates a high probability of complete rupture of the ligament. Surgical repair is then indicated because the ligament may be flipped back on itself and have become trapped in that position by the adductor aponeurosis. This would prevent healing.[5]

A partial tear is treated by means of a short arm thumb spica cast with the thumb in a neutral to slightly overcorrected (ulnar deviation) position for a total of five weeks. The patient may then start exercising, but should avoid stressing the unprotected collateral ligament until it is completely asymptomatic. The ligament can be protected by various taping techniques (Fig. 44–6) designed to hold the thumb adjacent to the index metacarpal or to absorb the stress of pinching activities. An alternative to the plaster cast is taping the thumb to the index metacarpal and keeping it there continuously for the first four to five weeks. Participation in sports is allowed at any time if the thumb is in a cast or is taped snugly to the index metacarpal. Protection during sports can be discontinued after three months if the symptoms have resolved. First-degree sprains of

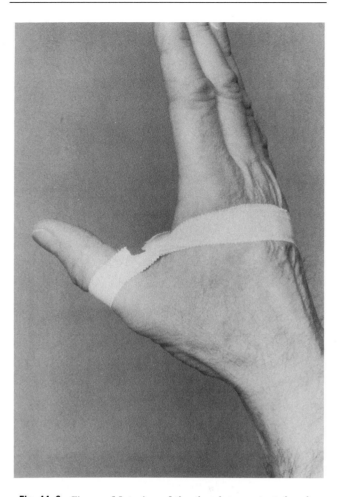

Fig. 44–6 Figure-of-8 taping of the thumb to protect the ulnar collateral ligament of the metacarpophalangeal joint while it is healing. The portion of the tape around the thumb should be just proximal to the interphalangeal joint. The thumb should not be allowed too much abduction with this technique.

the ulnar collateral ligament can be treated by a dorsal metal splint (Fig. 44–7) or by taping.

Hyperextension injuries to the metacarpophalangeal joint of the thumb produce pain and tenderness on the palmar aspect of that joint. These injuries should be treated with a dorsal splint that holds the joint in approximately 30 degrees of flexion (Fig. 44–7). Dorsal dislocations of the joint of the thumb, unlike those of the metacarpophalangeal joints of the fingers, can usually be reduced in a closed fashion. The best way to reduce the dislocation is not by traction, but by actually compressing the joint surfaces and attempting to slide the dislocated proximal phalanx over the end of the first metacarpal. The joint is then immobilized at 30 degrees of flexion for three weeks. This is followed by an exercise program. The joint must be protected from hyperextension forces during sports participation for at least eight weeks or until completely asymptomatic.

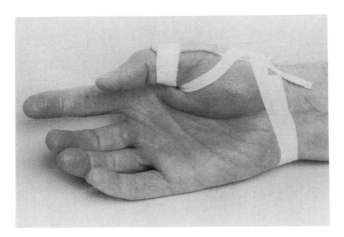

Fig. 44-7   A dorsal metal splint for the metacarpophalangeal joint can be used to protect minor injuries of the ulnar collateral ligament, or after a more severe injury has been treated initially with a plaster cast. The proximal end of the splint is difficult to keep in place and usually requires circumferential tape around the wrist. An elastic wrap over the proximal end of the splint also helps.

Wrist

Injuries of the wrist require very careful evaluation. The amount of swelling, pain, and tenderness is a good indicator of the severity of the injury. The initial radiographs, which may appear to be normal, should be evaluated not only for fracture but for abnormal position of the various carpal bones. If any malalignment or separation of the carpals is seen on either anteroposterior or lateral views, then a significant ligament injury has probably occurred. Comparison views of the other wrist are helpful. Any significant ligament injury is best treated surgically.[6] Beware of an avulsion or "chip" fracture about the wrist, which may indicate a significant ligament injury.

Wrist injuries should be treated with a wrist splint, brace, or short arm cast for two to four weeks and then reevaluated. Longer immobilization may be needed. As pain and swelling subside, range-of-motion exercises are started. These progress to strengthening exercises. The patient should not participate in sports unprotected until full range of painless motion has been obtained and strength has been restored.

Some athletes, especially females, have generalized laxity of the wrist ligaments and appear to be predisposed to overuse stress and recurrent wrist sprains. This generalized laxity leads to an increase in flexibility, which in turn leads to increased performance in such sports as gymnastics. However, the same increased flexibility that aids their performance also increases their risk of injury. It is extremely important for these individuals to learn proper techniques and to protect the wrist from injury. These athletes must learn to set the wrist, or position it in neutral, and to maintain this position as much as possible. Taping and wearing elastic

supports about the wrist are helpful. A brace to prevent extremes of range of motion is also very helpful if it is feasible in that particular sport. Conditioning of the forearm muscles is also important so that the athlete can maintain the wrist in a neutral position; this takes stress off the lax ligaments. In some situations, modification of activity or even a change of sport may be necessary.

Fractures

Stable displaced and adequately reduced fractures should be immobilized for three to four weeks. This is followed by a rehabilitation program. These fractures should be protected during athletic participation for at least two additional months. Articular fractures can be managed in the same way if they are nondisplaced. Displaced or unstable fractures may need surgical fixation. Any disruption of the articular surface must be corrected surgically.

Immobilization should involve only the affected parts. In general, the joint proximal and distal to the fracture is immobilized. Other joints should be left free to prevent unnecessary stiffness. However, for athletic participation more extensive protection and immobilization may be needed to prevent additional injury.

Phalangeal Fractures

Fractures of the distal phalanx generally result from a crushing injury to the fingertip. They result in subungual hematoma. If the hematoma is painful, it can be drained under sterile conditions by a variety of techniques, including a paper clip heated by an alcohol flame, an electric cautery unit, a scalpel blade, or a hypodermic needle. Crush fractures of the tuft of the distal phalanx require only symptomatic treatment—usually a short period of immobilization for protection and comfort. Stable nondisplaced fractures of the shaft of the distal phalanx can be treated with a simple splint immobilizing the digit distal to the proximal interphalangeal joint.

Nondisplaced or reduced and stable fractures of the middle and proximal phalanges are treated as described above. Reduction can usually be accomplished with the patient under local digital block anesthesia. Rotational as well as longitudinal alignment must be restored. The entire digit is usually immobilized for three weeks. Early guarded motion is then started, but the fracture must be carefully protected during sports participation until it is solidly healed. This may take two to three months. Epiphyseal fractures, especially of the proximal phalanx, are common in the young athlete and are often angulated. Reduction is easily accomplished by manipulation. If these phalangeal fractures are unstable, they need surgical fixation. It is especially important that articular fractures be anatomically reduced and internally fixed.

Proximal Interphalangeal Joint Fractures

Subluxation of a proximal interphalangeal joint fracture is a complex injury, the significance of which is frequently overlooked. A lateral radiograph shows a fracture at the palmar base of the middle phalanx with dorsal subluxation of the middle phalanx (Fig. 44–8). The fracture fragment represents the avulsion of the palmar plate. In addition, a portion of the collateral ligament is also avulsed from the middle phalanx with this fragment. This combination renders the joint unstable and subject to recurrent subluxation. The subluxation must be reduced and the reduction maintained. If the articular fracture involves one third or less of the articular surface, closed treatment is usually successful.

A metacarpal block with a local anesthetic agent is usually needed for the reduction of the subluxation. After reduction, the subluxation will recur if the joint is allowed to extend beyond a certain point. For this reason, the joint must be immobilized in flexion just short of the point at which resubluxation occurs. This is generally 30 to 50 degrees. Immobilization is accomplished by a dorsal splint that blocks extension[7] but allows flexion (Figs. 44–9 and 44–10). Flexion exercises are encouraged, but the patient is warned not to try to overcome the effect of the splint and extend the joint beyond the intended stop. During weekly examinations the splint is adjusted so that the joint can extend an additional 10 degrees. Lateral radiographs must verify that the joint has not subluxated. It takes four to six weeks to obtain full joint extension, but by that time flexion should be complete.

The joint must be protected during athletic participation for ten to 12 weeks after the injury. For sports, the joint should be immobilized in 30 to 40 degrees of flexion. If the articular fracture involves 30% to 50% of the articular surface, the above treatment may be adequate. A fracture involving more than 50% of the articular surface should be treated surgically.

Metacarpal Fractures

Fractures of the metacarpal necks, particularly of the ring and small fingers, are common. Reduction can usually be accomplished with the patient under local anesthesia, but maintaining reduction is often difficult. Angulation of no more than 20 degrees is certainly acceptable for the fourth and fifth metacarpals. No more than minimal angulation of the second and third metacarpal necks is acceptable. Immobilization after reduction is best accomplished by anterior and posterior plaster splints. These should be carefully molded so that pressure is applied from the palmar side of the metacarpal head and dorsally on the metacarpal shaft. The splint should be adequately padded so that there are no pressure points. The adjacent digits are included in the splints. In my experience, separate anterior and posterior splints are easier to mold than an ulnar gutter splint. The proximal interphalangeal joints can be left free, but the splints must continue to the proximal forearm. These fractures should be immobilized for four weeks before active metacarpophalangeal motion is begun. Some type of short arm cast is needed for athletic participation for two to three months. If angulation cannot be controlled, internal fixation is required.

Nondisplaced or reduced and stable fractures of the metacarpal shafts and bases can be treated by splint or cast immobilization that includes the metacarpophalangeal joints, wrist, and forearm. Displaced fractures of the bases of the metacarpals are often unstable and require internal fixation. An example is Bennett's fracture, which occurs at the base of the metacarpal of the thumb.

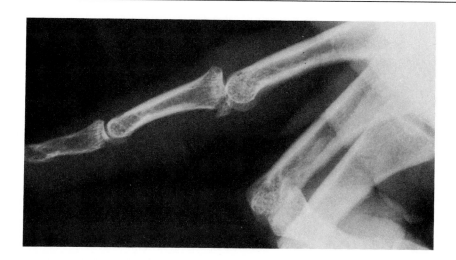

Fig. 44–8 Lateral radiograph of a finger demonstrating a fracture subluxation of the proximal interphalangeal joint. There is a small avulsion fracture at the palmar base of the middle phalanx and the joint is subluxated dorsally.

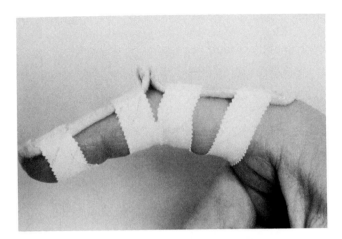
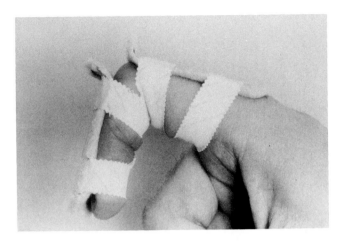

Fig. 44-9 A dorsal extension-block splint made from two pieces of molded aluminum. One end of each of the splints is bent at right angles. **Left:** The two splints are taped to the segments of the finger on each side of the proximal interphalangeal joint in such a way that the bent portions of the splint make contact when the joint is in the desired position. Moving the two splints closer together while the finger is flexed allows extension to be blocked with the joint in more flexion. The patient is instructed not to extend the joint forcefully beyond the point where the splints make contact.[9] **Right:** The dorsal extension-block splint demonstrating flexion of the proximal interphalangeal joint.

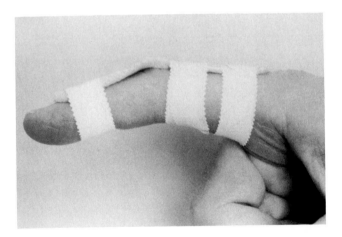
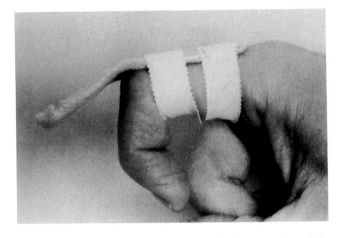

Fig. 44-10 An alternative dorsal extension-block splint showing static positioning of the joint. **Left:** For active flexion exercises of the proximal interphalangeal joint, the tape distal to the joint is removed, allowing the joint to flex. During the exercises, the joint is actively extended to the splint. **Right:** The alternative dorsal extension-block splint demonstrating flexion of the proximal interphalangeal joint. The tape distal to the joint can also be left on and the tape proximal to the joint removed. When the joint flexes, the proximal end of the splint is then lifted off the proximal phalanx. The advantage of this splint is that the joint is more securely immobilized when at rest with the entire splint taped in place.

Scaphoid Fractures

Scaphoid fractures are common in sports. Inadequate initial treatment often results in symptomatic nonunion. For this reason, nondisplaced fractures must be treated vigorously with complete immobilization in a cast. My preference is a long arm thumb spica cast for six weeks, followed by a short arm thumb spica cast until the fracture is healed, usually an additional two to three months. After the first two weeks the athlete can participate in sports while wearing a rubberized wrist-thumb playing cast. If there is any doubt about

fracture displacement, open reduction and internal fixation is indicated.

After a wrist injury, initial radiographs are frequently normal (Fig. 44-11, *left*). The wrist, however, must be treated. If there is tenderness over the scaphoid, a short arm thumb spica cast is advised although other types of splints and orthoses are usually adequate. The wrist must be reevaluated and radiographed again at two, four, and six weeks, until either the patient is asymptomatic or a fracture becomes apparent (Fig. 44-11, *right*). A nondisplaced fracture of the scaphoid may not

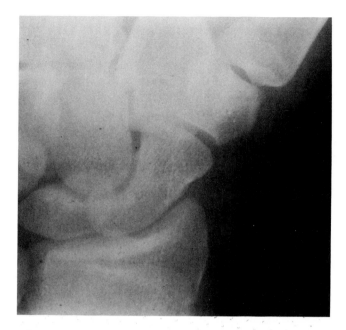 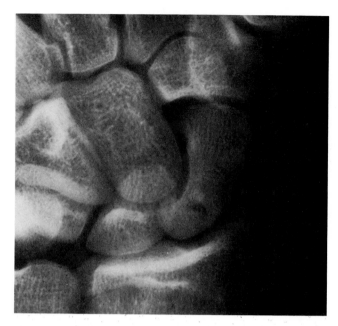

Fig. 44-11 A hyperextension injury produced pain and tenderness over the scaphoid. **Left:** A wrist radiograph taken two days later. No fracture can be identified. **Right:** Radiograph of the same wrist taken three weeks after the injury. A fracture of the scaphoid is now evident. This demonstrates the importance of follow-up radiographs when a scaphoid fracture is suspected but cannot be identified on the initial radiograph.

be radiographically apparent until four to six weeks after the initial injury. Therefore, if the patient with a wrist injury is not monitored for this length of time, the fracture will be missed and a scaphoid nonunion may result.

Fractures of the other carpals may also occur. These fractures are sometimes difficult to diagnose on routine radiographs. If the wrist continues to be painful despite apparently normal radiographs, a bone scan will almost always rule out the presence of a fracture or localize the area of the injury. Tomograms or a computed tomographic scan can then demonstrate the fracture. If the fracture is nondisplaced and stable, it usually heals in two to three months. Rigid immobilization should be carried out for the first four to six weeks, followed by guarded mobilization and protective splinting or casting. Fractures of the hook of the hamate may best be treated by excision of the fracture fragment.[8]

Rehabilitation

A rehabilitation program is important for returning the athlete to full participation. A therapist who is knowledgeable and skilled in upper extremity rehabilitation is invaluable. Range-of-motion exercises for nonimmobilized joints should be initiated immediately. Early motion for joints involved or adjacent to the injury should be started as soon as feasible. Active range-of-motion exercises are the most effective, and passive manipulation is to be discouraged. Various treatments, such as ice massage, ice packs, heat, and diathermy are useful. Ice massage is useful over muscles but should be avoided over tendons, for which ice packs are more useful. Strengthening exercises are started once the joints have been mobilized and healing has progressed to the point at which the extra stress will not be harmful. The injured hand should continue to be protected during athletic participation until pain and tenderness have resolved and full motion and strength have been restored.

Summary

Most common hand injuries occurring in athletics can be simply treated and the athlete returned to participation at an early date. Delayed or inadequate treatment may result in an unacceptable outcome, including permanent deformity. The injured athlete must be carefully examined, treated, and monitored until fully rehabilitated.

References

1. Bergfeld JA, Weiker GG, Andrish JT, et al: Soft playing splint for protection of significant hand and wrist injuries in sports. *Am J Sports Med* 1982;10:293–296.

2. McCue FC III, Baugher WH, Kulund DN, et al: Hand and wrist injuries in the athlete. *Am J Sports Med* 1979;7:275–286.

3. Burton RI, Eaton RG: Common hand injuries in the athlete. *Orthop Clin North Am* 1973;4:809–838.

4. Palmer AK, Louis DS: Assessing ulnar instability of the metacarpophalangeal joint of the thumb. *J Hand Surg* 1978;3:542–546.

5. Stener B: Displacement of the ruptured ulnar collateral ligament of the metacarpophalangeal joint of the thumb: A clinical and anatomical study. *J Bone Joint Surg* 1962;44B:869–879.

6. Culver JE: Instabilities of the wrist. *Clin Sports Med* 1986;5:725–740.

7. McElfresh EC, Dobyns JH, O'Brien ET: Management of fracture-dislocation of the proximal interphalangeal joints by extension-block splinting. *J Bone Joint Surg* 1972;54A:1705–1711.

8. Stark HH, Jobe FW, Boyes JH, et al: Fracture of the hook of the hamate in athletes. *J Bone Joint Surg* 1977;59A:575–582.

9. Strong ML: A new method of extension block splinting for the proximal interphalangeal joint: Preliminary report. *J Hand Surg* 1980;5:606–607.

Specific Rehabilitation for the Injured Recreational Runner

William G. Clancy, Jr., MD

Lower-extremity injuries in the runner are perplexing and often difficult diagnostic problems. Also, it is difficult to predict when symptoms will resolve and allow a return to asymptomatic running. Nonsurgical treatment programs are often based on little scientific data. Indeed, nonsteroidal anti-inflammatory medication is widely used in the treatment of acute and subacute injuries to inhibit an inflammatory reaction. Yet, the inflammatory reaction in these injuries should be considered a necessary part of the healing response—a desirable effect, it is logical to assume. Almekinders and Gilbert[1] recently reported that the use of piroxicam in experimentally created partial muscle strain in rats appeared to inhibit the healing reaction and muscle regeneration. Krejci and Kock[2] showed that steroid use can significantly delay the normal healing response in animals.

Little is really known about the etiology of these various injuries. It appears that the injury is essentially one of muscle, tendon, or bone overload. This means that the body was not able to respond sufficiently to the accumulated stress concentration, and breakdown was sufficient to produce an inflammatory reaction.

The involved area may have decreased genetic strength and may fail because of inferior biomechanical properties. Failure may occur if loads are greater than normal because of an anatomic variation that concentrates stress at a particular site. Failure may also result from inadequate muscular protection because of inadequate muscular strength, endurance, or flexibility.

Errors in training may lead to the overload causing the injury. The use of inappropriate training techniques (such as too frequent training with a high-intensity interval training program) is but one example. Other factors, such as prolonged use of poor or worn-out shoes or running on the side of a road that has a significant incline (such as a drainage ditch), may also contribute to stress concentration or overload.

The treatment and rehabilitation program for each type of injury must be based on (1) accurate diagnosis of the injury (not always easy); (2) classification of the injury as acute (symptoms present for less than two weeks), subacute (symptoms present for two to six weeks), or chronic (symptoms present for more than six weeks); (3) evaluation of the possible cause or causes of the injury; (4) treatment and rehabilitation of the injured part; and (5) a running prescription as part of the rehabilitation program.

History-taking should include investigations of the following:

(1) Is there a history of other overuse injuries to the same leg or foot?

(2) The athlete's training program. Was the weekly mileage program reasonable? Was an interval training program used and, if so, was the intensity level appropriate? Was there a sudden change in the training program (an increase in mileage or workout pace per minute, or a switch to interval or hill training)?

(3) Any change in running environment. Did the runner change from grass to roads or from soft surfaces to hard surfaces? Evaluation of the athlete's running shoes is important. Are the shoes new or old and worn down?

The physical examination should include an evaluation of lower-extremity muscle flexibility and significant anatomic variations such as leg-length discrepancy, femoral anteversion, valgus or varus alignment of the knee, patellofemoral tracking, excessive tibial internal or external rotation, and excessive supination or pronation of the foot and the presence of any other foot deformity.

General Guidelines for a Running Prescription

The most difficult aspect of the rehabilitation program is the development of a running prescription for the various lower-extremity problems. The running prescription is one of the most important aspects in the rehabilitation program of running injuries. The running prescription requires a thorough history of the running schedule that the athlete was trying to maintain before the injury. Next, it is necessary to determine whether the athlete is a runner or a jogger. A brief history of the athlete's background and goals as a runner or jogger is needed.

A jogger, in my opinion, is one whose pace is slower than eight minutes a mile and whose workout distance is seldom over 4 miles and is usually 2 to 3 miles. He or she usually runs three to five days a week. The goal is one of fitness, however, and the workout is usually sufficient to produce the so-called endorphin high.

A runner is one whose pace per mile is generally eight minutes or faster and who usually runs at least five days a week. The runner usually varies the training intensity and distance to improve performance. Most, but not all, such runners compete in "fun runs" or competitive

5K or 10K races, or even longer races. Participation in competitive races is not, however, the real criterion of whether the person is a jogger or runner, as many joggers participate in half or full marathons. The athlete's attitude is more important. The jogger trains for fitness, whereas the runner competes either against the clock or against other runners. The runner has a very strong inner drive that must be recognized and appreciated by the treating physician. This at times overwhelming drive must be taken into consideration when making decisions about treatment and rehabilitation options.

The next facts to be ascertained are the athlete's normal training routine before the injury and whether there was a change in the training program that might have contributed to the injury. The goal of the treatment and rehabilitation program is to return the athlete to the preinjury training schedule. One must also determine whether the athlete's goals and training program are realistic.

To develop a running prescription, one must have a general understanding of the various training programs.

Most joggers use the LSD (long slow distance) system. This program was originally developed by competitive distance runners who rebelled against the high-injury interval training programs used during the 1950s and 1960s in the United States. LSD is basically an offshoot of the preseason conditioning program used by Arthur Lydiard in developing the great New Zealand runners of the 1960s and 1970s.

Interval training consists of repetitions of shorter-than-race distances run at a pace much faster than race pace with a minimal recovery period between each repetition (interval). This is still the main training regimen of middle-distance runners and is used to some extent by distance runners. It is the sine qua non of a successful training program. However, it probably has the highest correlation with injury production. Unfortunately, interval training is a necessary evil if improved performance is desired. Excessive hill training in the early cross-country season has a similarly high correlation with injury, as does running stadium steps.

In cross-training, one sport is substituted for another. The second sport does not duplicate the original sport but exercises some of the muscle groups involved in the original sport. It can produce the same cardiovascular effort but not necessarily the same musculoskeletal effect. The substitution of bicycling or roller-skiing for running is an example of cross-training. The substitution of cross-country skiing for running is a more closely related cross-training activity. Cross-training does not provide the same benefits as the original sport but does appear to produce a reasonably high sport-specificity benefit.

For example, a bike racer who can average 23 mph for 30 minutes is unlikely to go out and run 6 miles at a pace of six minutes per mile without significant training, even though the athlete's maximum rate of oxygen consumption (VO_2 max) may show that he or she is more than capable of doing so. This is called sports specificity. Cross-training means that while the injured area is rested, the athlete can use another sport to maintain a reasonable lower-extremity and cardiovascular training level that carries over to the desired sport. Someone with a significant case of acute Achilles tendinitis may not be able to run but could perform bike training (without toe clips) at a very high intensity level without adversely affecting the resolution of the Achilles tendinitis. Thus, cross-training becomes an integral part of the rehabilitation program used before the athlete is allowed to resume a graduated running program (the running prescription).

It is impossible to present a specific rehabilitation program for each injury because the running prescription depends on whether the athlete is a jogger or runner and on the previous training program as well as on the specific injury. The following rehabilitation programs are generalizations that should be modified for individual cases.

Trochanter Bursitis and Iliotibial Band Syndromes

Both of these entities are theoretically caused by a relative tightness of the iliotibial band or its contributing muscles, the tensor fascia and the gluteus maximus, producing a friction effect on either the greater trochanter or the lateral femoral epicondyle.[3] There may, indeed, be a contracture of these muscles, the iliotibial band, or both, or an environment-induced relative tightness of the iliotibial band. Ober's test is positive in many of these patients. Running on the side of a road where there is a small but definite drainage contour produces a compensatory varus load at the knee, bowstringing the iliotibial band over the bony prominences of the hip and knee, producing a friction syndrome and a secondary bursitis. It usually takes a minimum of six weeks of rest before running can be resumed.

The patient is switched to a cross-training program and is placed on a flexibility program for the tensor fascia and gluteus maximus muscles. Local injection of a soluble steroid into the bursa is occasionally effective for trochanteric bursitis, but is rarely effective for the bursa over the lateral femoral epicondyle. In either case, we routinely give the patient a two-week course of nonsteroidal anti-inflammatory medication.

Cross-Training Activities that do not produce pain are allowed during the six-week rest period. If the patient has trochanter bursitis, any activity that produces hip extension is eliminated. Cycling appears to be the best tolerated sport. If the patient has iliotibial band syndrome located at the lateral femoral epicondyle, then activities that produce knee flexion with varus loading are eliminated. Cycling while wearing an orthosis with a ⅛-inch lateral wedge is allowed if this activity does not produce symptoms.

Running Prescription When there is no pain on palpation of either the greater trochanter or the lateral femoral epicondyle, resumption of running is allowed. The patient is shown how to reproduce the pain by palpation. When the patient can no longer produce pain by palpation, a graduated running program can be resumed. This usually takes six weeks. Resumption of running is begun with the patient wearing a ⅛-inch lateral heel wedge. The athlete is instructed to run only on level surfaces. For the first three weeks, running is allowed every other day for one-half the usual distance and at three-quarters the normal pace. At four weeks the patient may resume running without the orthosis and on a daily basis, but the distance run should be only two thirds to three quarters of the normal daily mileage. The intensity level should be alternated every other day for at least two more weeks.

Stress Fractures of the Lower Extremity

Cross-Training Cross-training is initiated once the injury has been diagnosed and is used while the athlete cannot tolerate the pain of impact loading. The aerobic training devices to be substituted are either an exercise bicycle or a rowing machine. If tolerated, cross-country skis, rollerblades, or rollerskis can be used if no pain is present. Running in a pool may also be utilized.

Running Prescription Once there is minimal pain to palpation of the area of the stress fracture, we allow the athlete to resume a graduated running program. For the first week we allow running every other day and recommend that the distance be approximately one-half the preinjury distance and that the pace be one minute per mile slower than the normal training pace. If there is no pain at the stress fracture site during or after the first week, the athlete is allowed to increase the distance to three fourths of the preinjury distance and to run as frequently as before the injury. By the third week, we expect the athlete to increase this intensity or training pace to within 30 seconds per mile of the normal training pace. If the athlete is asymptomatic after these three weeks, a full return should be well tolerated. For most stress fractures, the average time before running can be tolerated without pain is six to eight weeks from the onset of the first symptoms. This appears to be reasonably consistent for stress fractures of the tibia, fibula, and metatarsals, as well as femoral shaft stress fractures.

Stress fractures of the navicular, femoral neck, and pubic rami vary considerably as to when asymptomatic running can and should be allowed.

Compartment Syndromes

Symptomatic compartment syndromes, when documented by vascular studies, are probably best treated surgically.[4] A graduated running program is usually be-

gun about three to four weeks after surgery. Cross-training, as well as flexibility work, is begun the second week after surgery and consists of either cycling or swimming or the use of rollerblades. For the first two weeks after resumption of running, training consists of running approximately one-third the usual daily training distance every third day. In the third week, training consists of running one-half the usual daily distance every other day. During the fourth week, the athlete runs on the normal number of days of training but decreases the distance and intensity on alternate days. No interval training is performed during the first four weeks after running is resumed.

Tendinitis About the Foot and Ankle (Achilles, Peroneal, and Posterior Tibial Tendinitis)

True tendinitis about the foot and ankle, when seen within the first two weeks of symptoms, usually resolves with approximately two to three weeks of rest from running. Subacute tendinitis (symptoms present for more than two weeks but less than six weeks) usually takes at least six weeks of rest from running to resolution. Chronic tendinitis (symptoms present for more than six weeks) takes a minimum of six weeks and frequently several months of rest for symptoms to resolve.[5,6] A flexibility and eccentric weight training program is initiated.

Cross-Training During the rest period from running, the most effective cross-training program is cycling. Toe clips may not be desirable for those with Achilles tendinitis but appear to be well tolerated in those with other forms of tendinitis. Swimming is also well tolerated but may not be quite as effective a cross-training sport.

Running Prescription Once the tendon is no longer tender to palpation, resumption of running is allowed. The first two weeks consist of running only every other day for one-half the normal daily mileage and at only one-half to two-thirds the intensity level. If this program is tolerated and the patient is symptom-free, then the patient is allowed to resume running on a daily basis. The intensity level, however, should markedly decrease on alternate days.

Plantar Fasciitis

This entity, probably a fatigue microscopic failure of the plantar fascia, is usually well tolerated for several months until the athlete eventually develops chronic symptoms.[6,7] Whether the injury is acute or chronic, the athlete is placed on a cross-training program. A flexible leather orthosis with a ⅛-inch medial heel wedge is placed in the street shoe. The patient is placed on a regimen of nonsteroidal anti-inflammatory medication. Local steroid injections are not used as they appear to provide only temporary symptomatic relief and a false sense of success. A flexibility program for the toe flexors is begun.

Cross-Training Substitution of outdoor cycling, weather permitting, or utilization of an exercise bike or a rowing device appears to be the most effective cross-training program.

Running Prescription Once the proximal plantar fascia is no longer tender to palpation (usually after a minimum of six weeks of rest from impact loading), the athlete is allowed to begin running. The flexible leather orthosis with the 1/8-inch medial heel wedge is worn in street and running shoes for approximately six to 12 weeks.

Running every third day for the first two weeks is initiated with cross-training performed the other two days. The distance is kept at one-third to one-half the usual daily program. After two weeks of painless running, the athlete may run every other day for two more weeks; if the runner remains asymptomatic, a normal training program may be resumed. Hill training is not recommended during the first six to eight weeks.

References

1. Almekinders LC, Gilbert JA: Healing of experimental muscle strains and the effects of nonsteroidal antiinflammatory medication. *Am J Sports Med* 1986;14:303–308.
2. Krejci V, Kock P: *Muscle and Tendon Injuries in Athletes.* Chicago, Year Book Medical Publishers, 1979, pp 24–29.
3. Zoltan DJ, Clancy WG Jr, Keene JS: A new operative approach to snapping hip and refractory trochanteric bursitis in athletes. *Am J Sports Med* 1986;14:201–204.
4. Detmer DE, Sharpe K, Sufit RL, et al: Chronic compartment syndrome: Diagnosis, management, and outcomes. *Am J Sports Med* 1985;13:162–170.
5. Clancy WG Jr, Neidhart D, Brand RL: Achilles tendonitis in runners: A report of five cases. *Am J Sports Med* 1976;4:46–57.
6. Clancy WG Jr: Tendinitis and plantar fasciitis in runners, in D'Ambrosia R, Drez D Jr (eds): *Prevention and Treatment of Running Injuries.* Thorofare, New Jersey, CB Slack, 1982, pp 77–87.
7. Snider MP, Clancy WG, McBeath AA: Plantar fascia release for chronic plantar fasciitis in runners. *Am J Sports Med* 1983;11:215–219.

Specific Rehabilitation Programs for the Throwing Athlete

Thomas E. Anderson, MD

Jeffrey Ciolek, PT, ATC

The rehabilitation of the injured athlete in throwing sports begins after the initial diagnosis or surgical intervention. Rehabilitation or reconditioning of the athlete for the coordinated motion of throwing can be as important as the surgical procedure. Inappropriate rehabilitation can often negate an exquisitely performed surgical procedure or allow a relatively minor problem to end a throwing career.

The throwing motion is a complex, coordinated movement involving energy transfer through the legs, pelvis, trunk, and upper extremity to the ball or racket.[1-3] Any interruption of these integrated movements produces additional stress to the shoulder and elbow and their surrounding soft-tissue structures that results in decreased performance. The risk of injury and altered performance is decreased by normal articular biomechanics, muscular balance, and flexibility of the upper extremity.

Shoulder

There are four components of shoulder rehabilitation: (1) restoring normal passive and active range of motion, (2) reestablishing synchrony of motion, (3) increasing muscle strength and endurance, and (4) progressively resuming throwing activities.

Range of Motion

Normal glenohumeral and scapulothoracic motion is required for normal motion and flexibility of the throwing arm. Restoring adequate range of motion should be the first priority of the rehabilitation program, and strengthening exercises should be slowly phased into the program. Less than full range of motion contributes to abnormal movement patterns, thereby continuing to compromise the individual's performance.

Initially, simple pendulum exercises can be used as a warm-up and relaxation technique. These exercises provide a generalized warm-up for the athlete and decrease pre-exercise anxiety. Pendulum exercises can help the athlete regain the initial part of the range of motion, and they provide gentle distraction and mobilization for the joint. Treatment modalities, such as heat, transcutaneous electrical nerve stimulation, or electrical stimulation may be used in conjunction with the range-of-motion program. Heat should not be applied immediately postoperatively or during periods of acute inflammation because it may aggravate the injury. Cold applied at the end of the workout will help control swelling and inflammation and modulate pain. Active and active-assisted range-of-motion exercises can be added to the program until full range of motion is accomplished. This can be accomplished by working initially in isolated planes, then in combined planes, and finally in diagonal patterns.

External rotation is the type of motion that should be given the most attention in the range-of-motion and stretching exercise programs.[4,5] The shoulder must go into the extremes of external rotation during the cocking phase of the pitching act; therefore, the internal rotators should be stretched in various angles (90 degrees of abduction, 135 degrees of abduction, and full abduction). With the patient in the supine position, keep the elbow bent 90 degrees and at the side. Then, with a stick or assistive device, rotate the arm outward. In an additional position with the patient supine, the arm is abducted to 90 degrees; slow external rotation of the arm is performed and the stretch is sustained for 30 to 60 seconds. This will help the patient gain additional motion in external rotation.

Horizontal adduction can be regained by the patient performing the initial exercises in a supine position. In this position, the scapula is stabilized while the patient tries to improve motion of the glenohumeral joint. The arm is brought across the chest in a slow, sustained stretch. The importance of slow, sustained stretching should be emphasized to the patient. As the arm is brought across the body, the elbow of the involved arm can be grasped and pulled further and more tightly across the body to help the patient regain this motion. This horizontal adduction stretch is important for regaining the flexibility of the posterior shoulder. As the patient's mobility improves, these exercises can also be performed in the standing position.

Initially, forward flexion or elevation of the shoulder is done in the supine position. The patient uses the opposite arm to grasp the forearm of the injured arm to help elevate the arm. When the 90-degree position is reached, which should be easily accomplished with the range of motion gained by gentle pendulum exercises, gravity assists the patient to reach full forward flexion of the shoulder. Again, these stretches are slow, sustained stretches held for 20- to 30-second intervals. Rapid or jerking motions may cause microhemorrhages within the stretched tissues. These microhemorrhages increase inflammation in this area and may result in decreasing rather than increasing the range of motion.

A towel can be used to assist the patient in combined abduction and external rotation. In the standing position, the patient holds the involved arm overhead while pulling the opposite arm behind the back with a towel, taking the involved arm into positions of combined abduction, extension, and external rotation. In the throwing athlete, the throwing shoulder has increased external rotation and decreased internal rotation in the abducted position. These differences should be considered when defining full range of motion for that particular individual.

Contract-relax, or hold-relax, stretching can also be used to increase shoulder motion. This stretching has been called proprioceptive neuromuscular facilitation stretching. This technique takes advantage of reflex inhibition of the muscle, and should be done under the supervision of a therapist or athletic trainer. Proprioceptive neuromuscular facilitation can also help the patient exercise using diagonal motions.

Synchrony of Motion

When range of motion has been regained and no significant weakness is noted, synchrony of motion is the next goal. Emphasis here is on the motions of the cocking phase, because the thrower must accomplish smoothly the sequence of shoulder abduction, horizontal extension, and external rotation.[1] In the standing position, the individual practices the throwing motion. This can be done in front of a mirror and may be performed twice each day with 25 repetitions each time. The scapula must be stabilized at the end of the cocking motion, at which time the shoulder is abducted in full horizontal extension and externally rotated. Performing this exercise in a fluid fashion helps the individual regain proprioceptive feedback about the shoulder position.

Progressive-Resistance Exercises

In attempts to increase the strength and endurance of the shoulder, both the glenohumeral and scapulothoracic areas need to be involved. Usually, light weights are used in a high-repetition regimen. Resistance is increased to a maximum of 5 to 10 lb depending on the size of the individual. Often, light weights of 3 to 5 lb are used. These exercises are best performed using both concentric and eccentric motion in a slow, controlled fashion. The eccentric mode should be emphasized. This is primarily the mode of contraction used by the external rotators of the shoulder when attempting to decelerate the arm during the follow-through phase. With this exercise program, the tissues about the shoulder act according to Wolff's law and, by resisting the acting forces, gradually become stronger. Therefore, the activities need to be performed with very light weights to avoid further injury to the tissues. The use of high repetitions is incorporated to increase both the strength and endurance of the tissues. Approximately three sets of these exercises should be performed. As heavier weights are attempted, the coordination of motion between the deltoid and rotator cuff musculature is lost as the deltoid begins to dominate the motion. Once the deltoid dominates, there is a loss of the synchrony of motion about the shoulder, and there is an increased risk for developing or redeveloping an injury.

Recent electromyographic studies[4] show that the supraspinatus can be isolated in the prone position. The major emphasis of the strength program should be on the external rotators. This is where the greatest imbalance in strength is usually noted. In the prone position, the patient can gain external rotation strength with the arm dependent at 90 degrees of forward flexion. Abduction, performed in the prone position with the thumb pointed toward the ceiling, strengthens the rotator cuff. Sidelying rotation is usually the first and easiest of the external-rotation positions. Once this is accomplished easily and without pain, the patient can move to the standing position to perform shoulder flexion and abduction and concentrate on full range-of-motion exercises. Abduction is performed with the arm in the externally and internally rotated positions. The internally rotated position, with the arm horizontally forward-flexed approximately 30 degrees, best isolates supraspinatus muscle and tendon activity.[5,6] When these standing exercises are performed using weights, the arm should be brought to 80 degrees of abduction only, so that impingement is not created.

Specific areas can be addressed while the patient is in the prone position. The motion of the scapula can be controlled to strengthen the rhomboids and lower trapezius. Wall push-ups aid scapulothoracic stabilization because the serratus anterior is strengthened for scapular stabilization, and this stimulates contraction of the latissimus dorsi.[4]

When strength and endurance exercises can be accomplished without pain, the next step is a more integrated muscle action to increase strength and endurance. This can be accomplished by early throwing and isokinetic training as a conditioning tool. Isokinetic training can provide a valuable adjunct to conventional weight-lifting exercises. This mode of training can be integrated at various phases of the rehabilitation and conditioning program. The main advantage of the isokinetic program is that the muscle can be strengthened at various velocities and at higher functional speeds. The most common program is called a velocity spectrum of isokinetic training. Most isokinetic exercise equipment can isolate and exercise effectively the important rotational muscle and can work in diagonal patterns. Recommended speeds are 180 to 300 degrees per second. Fifteen repetitions per set are accomplished approximately three times per week. Maximal activities are not recommended at speeds slower than 180 degrees per second. Slower speeds may increase the likelihood of muscular imbalance or may stress the tissues too vigorously, causing problems with muscle soreness and subsequent loss of range of motion. Submaximal work, however, is beneficial. The isokinetic conditioning program is an adjunct to the previously mentioned progressive-resistance exercise program. Although it strengthens the muscles, the isokinetic program does not address the use of eccentric contractions, an important form of contraction incorporated during the throwing mechanism.

Return to Throwing

Initially, the athlete may return to throwing by practicing the throwing motions without weights in front of a mirror. Subsequently, the patient may practice throwing using an object of the same weight as a baseball in the hand. When practicing in front of the mirror, the athlete should concentrate on each phase of throwing. Initially, the posterior excursion of the throwing arm and the fixation in the shoulder girdle should be observed for a smooth follow-through so that the stress of the deceleration is distributed throughout the soft tissues and not concentrated in one area. If this does not cause pain, short-distance throwing can begin. The purpose of this phase is to gain a more coordinated motion, and fluidity of motion with accuracy is emphasized. Velocity is not important during this early phase of return to throwing. The use of proper throwing mechanics is much more important; however, mechanics can be more difficult to observe in short-distance throwing. Long-distance arc throwing (long toss) is accomplished next. Level throwing should be attempted before throwing from the mound. Long toss should be used as a warm-up to the other phases. Again, the patient should concentrate on fluid motion and accuracy, and distance may be increased gradually to 150 ft. Again, the main emphasis is on proper mechanics and transfer of energy through the legs, pelvis, trunk, and upper extremity. The individual can begin actual pitching from the mound when the short toss can be done without any discomfort. Second in importance to proper mechanics is accuracy of the throw, and then velocity. A sample of a throwing program is given in the Addendum.

Individuals need two- to three-day rests between workouts during the initial phase of throwing from the mound. At any particular velocity of throwing, the number of throws is gradually increased until approximately 40 to 45 throws at that particular velocity can be accomplished without difficulty. These 40 to 45 throws can be divided initially into sets of ten to 15 pitches each with a subsequent period of rest, thus simulating innings. The velocity is gradually increased from a 60% initial velocity up to 100%. This is often divided into stages of 60%, 75%, 90%, and 100% velocity. After warm-up, the number of pitches is counted. We increase the number of pitches at a particular velocity and then decrease the number when proceeding to the next higher velocity. It is very helpful to write out this program for the individual athlete to follow, including the specific number of pitches and velocities (Addendum). An adequate number of days between throwing workouts must also be included in this program, particularly if the athlete is throwing from the pitcher's mound. The athlete should use the normal mix of pitches, that is, the individual's own style and combination of fastballs and breaking pitches. However, it is extremely difficult to throw a breaking pitch at a lower velocity; therefore, this pitch may not be possible for the athlete to perform at the lower velocity. The initial rehabilitation program at the lower velocity is composed primarily of fastball pitching. Again, of primary importance is proper mechanics, then accuracy, and finally velocity. If possible, the individual's coach should observe the athlete's throwing exercises to help avoid the introduction of abnormal mechanics, or to correct any preexisting abnormal mechanics. These are often easily corrected while the athlete is working through the lower-velocity phase of the program.

Elbow

Rehabilitation of the elbow is often accomplished by avoiding the activities that either initially or subsequently caused discomfort for the individual during throwing. As with the shoulder, restoring full active and passive range of motion is the first goal. After range of motion is achieved, progressive-resistance exercises are performed to allow conditioning and strengthening of the musculature and the tendinous structures about the elbow. After the athlete achieves a baseline strength for these tissues, gradual return to throwing can be accomplished.

Range of Motion

Full range of motion about the elbow is best gained by using active range of motion. If the rehabilitation and injury permit, continuous passive motion machines can be helpful in the postoperative period to regain motion and prevent tightening of the anterior and posterior capsular structures. Passive and active-assisted range-of-motion exercises are also beneficial. These exercises should be performed with a slow, steady stretching motion and not with a jerky or rapid motion. Gentle mobilization techniques applying longitudinal traction are also beneficial.

Full extension is the range of elbow motion that is often the most difficult to obtain. Frequently, nighttime splinting is used to maintain full extension, because the anterior capsule is more susceptible to contracture than the posterior capsule.

When range of motion is regained, progressive-resistance exercises can then be emphasized. The exercises most commonly used for progressive resistance are wrist curls and extensions, as well as pronation and supination with a fixed weight. Various spring-loaded grip-strengthening devices or putty can be used to strengthen the flexor musculature to increase grip strength. Biceps curls and triceps extensions strengthen the tissues acting at the elbow. These are performed with light weights and a high number of repetitions. The maximum weight is 5 to 10 lb. When adequate baseline strength and endurance have been obtained, the patient can progress to throwing.

Return to Throwing

The athlete's return to throwing for most elbow problems is very similar to that described for shoulder problems. Once again, recurrence or exacerbation of any pain must be avoided. The period of rest between throwing intervals may be extended or the velocity of throwing may be decreased if recurrence of discomfort or any significant tenderness or soreness develops. It is often beneficial to decrease swelling after workouts with ice therapy. For elbow problems, ice therapy needs to be limited somewhat, because the ulnar nerve, in its subcutaneous position, may be susceptible to an ice injury. Therefore, ice should be applied to the elbow for a maximum of ten to 15 minutes.

Conditioning

A program for the athlete to regain total strength is a necessary part of an effective conditioning program for the thrower. This program should include a spectrum of lower-extremity exercises and trunk strengthening for the abdominal and back muscles, because much of the power during the throwing motion comes from the legs and trunk. Endurance training should be included in the total program. This training should consist of one to two hours of continuous exercise per week (three to five sessions per week). Endurance exercises include running and biking.

General flexibility programs should be emphasized, particularly during the regimen of progressive-resistance exercises, because gradual loss of flexibility may occur. Loss of flexibility may also occur throughout the season if the athlete does not concentrate on stretching. Strength loss during the season of up to 5% has been documented,[1] even in individuals who have no shoulder and elbow problems throughout the season. More significant strength loss occurs if there have been such problems.

Psychological Aspects

In training and rehabilitation, the athlete often does more exercises and is more active than before the injury. Throughout the rehabilitation phase, the athlete may work harder and throw less than ever before. It should be emphasized to the athlete that this program of increasing strength and endurance decreases the likelihood of re-injury in the future. The rehabilitation program may be very frustrating for the individual who has had few problems prior to the injury. In addition, periodically the athlete will have a number of questions for the physician, therapist, and trainer. Therefore, the goals of therapy and the rationale behind the program must be communicated to the patient on a continuing basis.

References

1. Pappas AM, Zawachi RM, McCarthy CF: Rehabilitation of the pitching shoulder. *Am J Sports Med* 1985;13:223–235.
2. Zarins B, Andrews JR, Carson WG: *Injuries To the Throwing Arm.* Philadelphia, WB Saunders, 1985.
3. Moynes DR: Prevention of injury to the shoulder through exercises and therapy. *Clin Sports Med* 1983;2:413–422.
4. Blackburn TA: Throwing injuries to the shoulder, in Donatelli R (ed): *Clinics in Physical Therapy: Physical Therapy of the Shoulder.* New York, Churchill Livingstone, 1987, vol 2, pp 209–239.
5. Jobe FR, Tibone JE, Perry J, et al: An EMG analysis of the shoulder in throwing and pitching. *Am J Sports Med* 1983;2:3–5.
6. Moynes DR, Perry J, Antonelli DJ, et al: Electromyography and motion analysis of the upper extremity in sports. *Phys Ther* 1986;66:1905–1911.

Addendum

The goal of this program to return to throwing is safe and efficient reconditioning of your arm to normal functional ability. The program gradually increases the intensity and volume of throwing each week. Intervals of brief throwing combined with short rest periods will help you adjust to a normal game situation. Be sure to discuss the details of this program with your physical therapist or physician before beginning. Parts of the program may need to be revised based on your injury, progress, or playing position. Remember: a well-designed strength and flexibility program should be done in conjunction with the throwing program.

Begin each session with light jogging or a stationary bike ride, and then a thorough stretching program. Your stretching exercises should consist of specific shoulder and arm exercises and trunk and leg stretches assigned by your physician or physical therapist. Proper warm-up is critical to a safe throwing sequence. Do not perform your weight-lifting exercises immediately before throwing.

Begin Program

Start throwing approximately ten to 15 light warm-up throws a distance of about 30 ft. It may be helpful to mimic the throwing motion before throwing the ball.

Long Toss Long-toss exercises are very gentle, high lobs thrown a distance of 90 to 180 ft. The throw should be done in a rainbow fashion with minimal cocking effort. It is important to follow through smoothly.

Short Toss This is the most important phase of the program. Short-toss throwing progresses from a distance of 30 to 60 ft. Level throwing should be attempted before throwing from the mound.

Phase 1

Long Toss: 90 ft, ten to 12 throws, 50% intensity. Stretch ten minutes.
Short Toss: 30 ft, 15 to 20 throws, 50% intensity.

Phase 2

Long Toss: 90 to 120 ft, ten to 12 throws, 50% intensity. Stretch ten minutes.
Short Toss: 60 ft, 15 to 20 throws, 50% intensity.

Long Toss: 90 to 120 ft, ten to 12 throws, 50% intensity. Stretch ten minutes.
Short Toss: 60 ft, 25 to 30 throws, 50% intensity.

Long Toss: 90 to 120 ft, ten to 12 throws, 50% intensity. Stretch ten minutes.
Short Toss: 60 ft, 30 to 40 throws, 50% intensity.

Phase 3

Long Toss: 120 to 150 ft, ten to 12 throws, 50% intensity. Stretch ten minutes.
Short Toss: 60 ft, 15 to 20 throws, work to 75% intensity.

Long Toss: 120 to 150 ft, ten to 12 throws, 50% intensity. Stretch ten minutes.
Short Toss: 60 ft, 25 to 30 throws, work to 75% intensity.

Long Toss: 120 to 150 ft, ten to 12 throws, 50% intensity. Stretch ten minutes.
Short Toss: 60 ft, 30 to 40 throws, work to 75% intensity.

Phase 4: Interval Sequence
(Begin on the mound)

Short Toss: 60 ft, ten to 20 throws, work to 75% intensity. Stretch ten minutes. Ten to 20 throws.

Phase 5: Interval Sequence
(Begin on the mound, include breaking balls)

Short Toss: 60 ft, 15 throws, work to 75% intensity. Rest. Ten throws. Rest. Five throws.

Short Toss: 60 ft, 15 throws. Rest. Fifteen throws. Rest. Ten throws.

Short Toss: 60 ft, 15 throws. Rest. Fifteen throws. Rest. Fifteen throws.

Phase 6
(On the mound)

Short Toss: 60 ft, 20 to 30 throws, 75% to full intensity.

Short Toss: 60 ft, 30 to 40 throws, 75% to full intensity.

Short Toss: 60 ft, 75% to full intensity.

Simulate game situation with work and rest intervals.

Approximately 15 throws per inning; ten-minute rest.

Progress innings as tolerated, checking endurance and throwing speed.

Index